Neurological Disorders in Pregnancy

Gaurav Gupta · Todd Rosen
Fawaz Al-Mufti · Anil Nanda
Priyank Khandelwal
Sudipta Roychowdhury
Editors

Michael S. Rallo · Sanjeev Sreenivasan
Associate Editors

Neurological Disorders in Pregnancy

A Comprehensive Clinical Guide

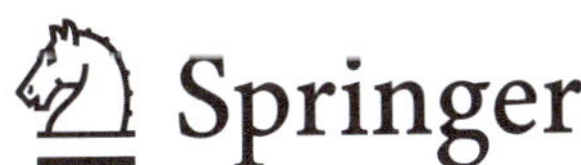

Editors
Gaurav Gupta
Department of Neurosurgery
Rutgers Robert Wood Johnson Medical
School
New Brunswick, NJ, USA

Fawaz Al-Mufti
Department of Neurology, Neurosurgery
and Radiology
New York Medical College -
Westchester Medical Center
Valhalla, NY, USA

Priyank Khandelwal
Department of Neurology
Robert Wood Johnson University
Hospital
New Brunswick, NJ, USA

Todd Rosen
Department of Obstetrics, Gynecology
and Reproductive Sciences
Rutgers Robert Wood Johnson Medical
School
New Brunswick, NJ, USA

Anil Nanda
Department of Neurosurgery
Robert Wood Johnson University
Hospital
New Brunswick, NJ, USA

Sudipta Roychowdhury
Department of Neuroradiology
University Radiology
New Brunswick, NJ, USA

Associate Editors
Michael S. Rallo
Department of Neurosurgery
Robert Wood Johnson University
Hospital
New Brunswick, NJ, USA

Sanjeev Sreenivasan
Department of Cerebrovascular &
Endovascular Neurosurgery
Rutgers - Robert Wood Johnson
Medical Sc
New Brunswick, NJ, USA

ISBN 978-3-031-36492-1   ISBN 978-3-031-36490-7   (eBook)
https://doi.org/10.1007/978-3-031-36490-7

Editorial Contact: Gregory Sutorius

This Springer imprint is published by the registered company Springer Nature Switzerland AG
The registered company address is: Gewerbestrasse 11, 6330 Cham, Switzerland

Foreword

The journey into the complex world of neurological disorders in pregnancy is an exploration that bridges neurosurgery, neurology, and obstetrics. This textbook, meticulously crafted by experts in these fields, serves as a guidepost to navigate the intricate landscape where maternal health and neurological well-being intersect.

Pregnancy is a transformative period in a woman's life where profound physiological changes and adaptations occur in support of the developing fetus. In some instances, the emergence or exacerbation of neurological disorders complicates the care of the obstetric patient. To provide the best possible care, it is necessary to understand the delicate balance between maternal health and fetal development.

In this comprehensive textbook, the authors explore both common and uncommon neurologic conditions affecting pregnancy. The interdisciplinary approach taken by our contributors brings together the latest insights from neurology, neurosurgery, neuroradiology, and obstetrics, ensuring a holistic understanding of these conditions and their management. The insights shared are valuable not only for healthcare professionals but also for researchers, educators, and students seeking to expand their knowledge in this specialized field.

Our hope is that this textbook will serve as an indispensable resource, fostering interdisciplinary collaboration, and ultimately improving the care and outcomes for women facing neurological challenges during pregnancy.

Amy P. Murtha
Dean, Rutgers Robert Wood Johnson Medical School
Professor of Obstetrics and Gynecology
New Brunswick, NJ, USA

Preface

This book is a product of an extraordinary team effort. The multidisciplinary management of any pregnant patient with neurological disorders includes experts in this field from neurosurgery, neurology, high-risk obstetrics—maternal fetal medicine, and neuroradiology.

The knowledge about the pathophysiology of neurological conditions in pregnancy can be complex. As we encounter a significant number of pregnant patients with varied spectrum of neurological disorders, we realized that the management of such conditions is loosely based on old and outdated evidence and not supported by well-defined or systematic literature reviews or meta-analysis. For instance, pregnant patients with certain neurological conditions, e.g., diagnosis of brain aneurysm in pregnancy, are being managed with elective cesarean section even though there is data suggesting that in most uncomplicated cases, the patient should be allowed to deliver vaginally without an associated increase in fetal or maternal morbidity/mortality. Taking motivation from our successful management of pregnant cases with neurological disorders at Rutgers Robert Wood Johnson Medical School and Hospital, we decided to pen this book to help guide our medical community in better management of these perplexing issues. It is an attempt to encourage "evidence-based practices" in treating such patients.

New Brunswick, NJ, USA   Gaurav Gupta

Acknowledgments

'Neurological Disorders in Pregnancy- a comprehensive clinical guide' is the work of a multi-disciplinary team a at Rutgers-Robert Wood Johnson Medical School in New Brunswick, New Jersey, USA. The team consists of dedicated physicians and experts in this field who have contribute from their knowledge, experience, and evidence mased medicine to guide us towards better management of pregnant patients with neurological disorders. I would like to thank my colleagues Dr Todd Rosen (High risk Maternal Fetal Medicine) Anil Nanda (Neurosurgery), Drs Priyank Khandelwal and Dr Fawaz Al-Mufti from Neurology, and Dr Sudipta Roychowdhury from Neuro-radiology. I would like to thank my Associate Editors- Michael Rallo, who is an MD, PhD candidate in training at Rutgers Robert Wood Johnson Medical School, and Dr Sanjeev Sreenivasan, our clinical research fellow at Rutgers Neurosurgery. I would also like to thank all the authors who have contributed to this text.

Thank you,
Gaurav Gupta

Contents

Part I

Obstetric, Anesthetic, and Radiologic Considerations

Pre-conception Planning for Patients with Neurological Disorders

1

Jessica C. Fields and Todd Rosen

Introduction

Pre-conception Planning for All Patients

In general, pre-conception planning is imperative to maximize successful and healthy pregnancy outcomes for both mothers and babies. A discussion of patient health care before conception provides the opportunity to review lifestyle, medical conditions and medications, immunizations, and nutrition and weight to make changes to improve pregnancy.

While it is important to screen reproductive-aged patients for interest in pursuing pregnancy [1], pre-conception planning should be a priority for all care because health status and risk factors continually change, and pregnancies are often unintentional. Furthermore, the American College of Obstetricians and Gynecologists (ACOG) and American Society for Reproductive Medicine (ASRM) are both proponents of coverage for and access to pre-conception counseling and services [2]. In addition to individualized care, all patients should be offered genetic counseling if desired and be recommended initiation of folic acid every day starting at least 1 month prior to conception with continuation for the entire pregnancy to prevent fetal malformations [3, 4]. Counseling should be provided on the importance of a healthy diet, regular exercise, attainment of a normal body mass index, and smoking cessation to enhance pregnancy outcomes.

Pre-conception Planning for Patients with Specific Neurological Disorders

For those with neurological disorders, pre-conception planning provides an opportunity for discussion of pregnancy impact on disease, the effect that disease impairment may have on pregnancy, and use of treatment for disease control during pregnancy. Pre-conception counseling plays an integral role because neurologic disease holds potential for significant contribution to morbidity and mortality in pregnancy. It is crucial to identify possible risks and reduce harm for the patient, fetus, and neonate [5]. Planning not only allows for optimization of neurologic health but also fosters patient education about pregnancy risks and provides time and integrated care to intervene for ultimate pregnancy success [6].

J. C. Fields · T. Rosen (✉)
Division of Maternal-Fetal Medicine, Department of Obstetrics, Gynecology and Reproductive Sciences, Rutgers Robert Wood Johnson Medical School, New Brunswick, NJ, USA
e-mail: rosentj@rwjms.rutgers.edu

The key integral components of pre-conception assessment for patients with neurological disorders include understanding patient history, performing a physical exam, and reviewing neuroimaging and medications. Additional considerations may be important for the postpartum period or breastfeeding. Moreover, it is critical that all women with pre-existing neurological disorders have excellent communication between all involved physicians. Counseling and risk assessment should involve a multidisciplinary care team such as obstetricians, neurologists, neurosurgeons, anesthesiologists, geneticists, and neonatologists.

Given that various neurological disorders have intricacies to their impact on pregnancy, specific neurological disorders will each be discussed separately to address all unique planning tools and concerns.

Spinal Cord Injury

Women with spinal cord injury (SCI) who are considering pregnancy should have pre-conception counseling and planning [7–9]. It is important to start with an understanding of a patient's history given that there are concomitant chronic medical problems and adaptations associated with SCI. The approach to patients with neurotrauma, including SCI, is discussed in detail in Chap. 25.

There is increased risk of complications with SCI in pregnancy including anemia (i.e., from iron deficiency, anemia of chronic disease, and chronic renal insufficiency), asymptomatic bacteriuria, lower urinary tract infections (up to 35% incidence), pyelonephritis, decubitus ulcers, and respiratory problems. Risk of pre-term birth ranges from 8 to 13%, which is similar to the general population [10–14]. Given the association with urinary tract infections, serial or frequent urine cultures or antibiotic suppression is recommended, although there is no definitive evidence to suggest this management [14–16]. Additionally, due to risk for pulmonary compromise, baseline pulmonary function studies, specifically vital capacity, should be performed pre-pregnancy and serially re-assessed during pregnancy to determine which patients may need ventilatory support in labor; this is especially important for those with high thoracic or cervical spinal lesions, typically above T5 [7, 14, 16]. Frequent skin exams and position changes to prevent decubitus ulcers as well as stool softeners and a high fiber diet to aid with worsening constipation in pregnancy are recommended [16].

Additionally, venous thromboembolism (VTE) incidence is higher in this population at about 8%, yet there is insufficient data to recommend universal thromboprophylaxis during pregnancy or postpartum [7, 17]. Each case must have an individualized risk assessment with stronger consideration of mechanical or pharmacologic prophylaxis if a patient has additional risk factors [18]. Range of motion exercises in the lower extremities, leg elevation, and leg stockings can be utilized for VTE prevention as well as upper body exercises to improve strength for those who are not quadriplegic [15, 18, 19].

A multidisciplinary team should involve specialists including but not limited to maternal-fetal medicine subspecialists, anesthesiologists, spinal rehabilitation physicians, physiotherapists, occupational therapists, lactation consultants, and neonatologists [15, 20]. Specifically, a discussion about risk for autonomic dysreflexia should occur pre-conception since this is the most serious of pregnancy complications, is potentially fatal, and affects about 90% of those with SCI lesions at or above level T6 [11, 21]. The most common sign is often severe systemic hypertension and this must be monitored for closely.

Patients should understand that they are not at higher risk than the general obstetric population for congenital malformations or fetal death [22]. Pregnancies may be at increased risk for small for gestational age infants and serial fetal growth ultrasounds may be performed [23]. Some SCIs may be congenital or hereditary in origin, and genetic counseling may be helpful to patients who desire understanding of inheritance in offspring in addition to other risk factors for pregnancy. For example, specific syndromes like

Kippel-Trenaunay or von Hippel-Lindau are associated with augmented risk for epidural or subdural hemangiomas and should receive a pre-conception MRI to determine if neuraxial anesthesia is a safe option [24]. Congenital spinal cord lesions such as meningomyeloceles have a higher risk in offspring and these patients should be on a higher dose of about 4 mg/day of folic acid for prevention [25].

Anesthesia consultation is advised so that a plan for epidural can be made with onset of labor. Early epidural is important in prevention of autonomic dysreflexia [14, 21]. Vaginal delivery is feasible for women with SCI. Moreover, postpartum issues should be anticipated such as difficulty with breastfeeding and need for additional support as well as an increased risk of mental health problems and need for rehospitalization for postpartum depression [26–28].

History of Hydrocephalus with Ventriculoperitoneal (VP) Shunt

Patients with VP shunts placed in the brain secondary to hydrocephalus may consider pregnancy. For these patients, pre-conception planning should include a description of risks with VP shunts during pregnancy and an MRI to establish baseline ventricular size and to verify appropriate shunt function. Considerations for management of pregnant patients with hydrocephalus are discussed at length in Chap. 16.

Risks of VP shunts in pregnancy include shunt malfunction, found in studies to occur in up to 25–50% of pregnancies [29, 30]. In the third trimester of pregnancy, functional occlusion of the shunt can be seen secondary to the increase in intra-abdominal pressure from a large uterus and in turn, obstructed cerebrospinal fluid drainage and elevation in intracranial pressure [31]. Symptoms of shunt malfunction—confusion, nausea/vomiting, tiredness, headache, or nystagmus, for example—should be explained to patients so that they can seek urgent neurosurgical care.

Vascular Disorders of the Brain

Stroke

Women with a history of stroke, ischemic or hemorrhagic, who are planning pregnancy should have full evaluation to prevent recurrence of stroke in pregnancy. It is well known that the pregnancy and postpartum periods are associated with an increased stroke risk [32–36]. Despite this higher risk, overall recurrence rate is low. It is important that women considering conception reduce modifiable risk factors such as smoking or substance use and be aware of risk factors inherent to pregnancy such as gestational hypertension, infection, and cesarean delivery [34, 37–39]. Review of imaging studies such as CT or MRI as well as echocardiography or carotid Doppler studies are useful in discussing prognosis. A review of medications should occur as many patients with a history of stroke may not only have underlying disorders but be on aspirin, clopidogrel, venous thromboembolism prophylaxis, blood pressure medication, or lipid lowering statin therapy. Of these agents, statins must be discontinued due to risk of spontaneous abortion and teratogenicity. There are safe antihypertensive drugs that may be used in pregnancy including labetalol, methyldopa, nifedipine, and hydralazine. However, angiotensin converting enzyme (ACE) inhibitors and angiotensin II receptor blockers (ARBs) are contraindicated in pregnancy due to risk of fetal renal damage. Diuretics are not the preferred antihypertensive medication in pregnancy, but may be continued if the patient conceives on hydrochlorothiazide or other medications of this class. Long-acting beta-blockers such as atenolol may cause prolonged beta-blockade of the newborn and may be associated with intrauterine growth restriction (IUGR); a move to an antihypertensive with less risk may be appropriate [40–46]. Additional consideration of prophylactic enoxaparin during pregnancy with plan to switch to heparin around 36 weeks gestation should be discussed for women with a prior history of ischemic/thrombotic stroke [47, 48]. The relative risk of gestational and peripartal stroke and nuances of treatment are discussed at length in Chaps. 3 (Ischemic) and 4 (Hemorrhagic).

Arteriovenous Malformation (AVM)

It is inconclusive whether there is increased risk for arteriovenous malformation (AVM) rupture in pregnancy. The physiologic hemodynamic changes of pregnancy including larger plasma volume, increased cardiac output, and higher cerebral blood flow may theoretically increase the risk of hemorrhage but the magnitude of this risk is unknown [49]. There is a paucity of data given the low AVM prevalence in the pregnant population. Some evidence suggests increased rupture risk. Very early studies of AVMs in pregnancy showed as high as 21–48% risk for spontaneous hemorrhage [50–53]. Robinson et al. studied 24 women with AVMs who had high rates of adverse fetal outcomes including a 49% fetal complication rate and 26% fetal mortality rate [53]. However, the high risk for adverse outcomes in these early studies may be a result of publication bias.

More recently, Porras et al. provided evidence of a 5.7% hemorrhage risk in pregnant women compared to 1.3% in nonpregnant counterparts [54]. Additional studies have shown approximate AVM hemorrhage rates of 3–9% in pregnancy versus 3–4% when not pregnant [55, 56]. Another study involving 54 women with AVM highlighted an annual hemorrhage rate of 11% during pregnancy compared to 1% outside of gestation [57]. When AVM rupture in pregnancy does occur, it is usually in the third trimester at a mean of 30 weeks gestation, and high maternal mortality rates have been suggested [58].

Yet, other studies must be recognized that suggest no significantly higher risk of AVM hemorrhage in pregnancy [55, 58, 59]. Given the limited and inconclusive evidence [60–62] but continued concern for rupture, some experts recommend treatment of AVMs pre-conception [63]. However, intervention is not without risk, suggesting that curative treatment should be guided by general neurosurgical considerations. This counseling may be impacted by other risk factors for AVM hemorrhage in addition to pregnancy such as prior rupture [64–68], AVM location [67–69], deep venous drainage [70], and associated aneurysms [71]. Moreover, the approach to treatment might also influence rupture risk: a 2014 retrospective review of 253 women with AVMs showed an annual hemorrhage rate of 11.1% for those who became pregnant in the 3-year latency interval between stereotactic radiosurgery and complete AVM obliteration compared to an annual hemorrhage rate of 2.5% for those not pregnant [72]. There are no randomized trials to confirm which treatment is better; one randomized trial comparing medical to interventional treatment of unruptured AVMs was stopped early because of the superiority of medical management [73]. Thus, pre-conception history and imaging are necessary investigations to provide optimal counseling to patients. The evidence relating to risk of AVM hemorrhage and approach to management is discussed in detail in Chap. 19.

Intracranial Aneurysm

Similar to AVMs, intracranial aneurysms may have increased risk of rupture in pregnancy, but the literature is controversial. Studies have shown an increased risk of subarachnoid hemorrhage as a consequence of hemodynamic changes induced by pregnancy [53, 58, 74, 75].

More recently, studies have refuted this increased association [74, 76, 77]. Specifically, a Dutch analysis of 244 women showed no increase in rupture risk [76]. Kim et al. analyzed the Nationwide Inpatient Sample (NIS) from 1988 to 2009 showing aneurysm rupture risk of 1.4% during pregnancy and 0.05% during delivery, which is similar to the annual aneurysm rupture risk in the general population [77]. Since these more current population-based analyses do not suggest worsened risk of bleeding during pregnancy and while an individualized risk assessment must still be performed, the evidence suggests no need to prophylactically intervene pre-conception for asymptomatic and unruptured aneurysms [76, 77].

Nevertheless, an aneurysm has the potential to rupture in pregnancy and if this were to occur, maternal and fetal morbidity and mortality are increased [58]. During pre-conception counseling, the patient should be informed that pre-pregnancy treatment is far preferable to having to treat an unruptured aneurysm during the pregnancy. If the patient conceives before appropriate treatment, or if she refuses advice to undergo treatment prior to conception, it is important to discuss a possible plan for management of a ruptured aneurysm in pregnancy. Immediate neurosurgical intervention with possible clipping or coiling of the aneurysm would be needed during pregnancy to better both maternal and fetal outcomes [78]. From the NIS study, maternal mortality from untreated aneurysmal rupture was significantly higher than in treated ruptured aneurysms [79]. This decision for an emergency operation during pregnancy would be based on neurosurgical need, not obstetrical considerations. In general, the decision to treat an unruptured aneurysm should be based on neurosurgical assessment of risk relating to aneurysm size, enlargement, morphology, and/or associated symptoms. A more detailed discussion of cerebral aneurysm risk assessment and treatment in pregnancy is provided in Chap. 2.

Cavernous Malformations (CM)

Cavernous malformations are not a contraindication to pregnancy. Previous studies, mostly case series and reports, have shown an association between pregnancy and increased risk of growth or hemorrhage of CMs [79–81]. One such study by Porter et al. demonstrated that in 100 patients with brain stem CM, 7 (11%) of 62 women had a hemorrhage in pregnancy [82]. Suggestions for biologic plausibility at that time involved hypotheses around greater expression of vascular endothelial growth factor and basic fibroblast growth factor triggered by the hormones of pregnancy [82].

However, follow-up investigations have not demonstrated this association, and suggest that pregnancy causing enlargement or higher bleeding rates of CMs is likely not true [83–87]. Two more recent large clinical cohorts showed a similar risk of bleeding from CM in pregnant women compared to women not pregnant during childbearing years [88, 89]. Specifically, Kalani et al. [88] showed in a retrospective study of 168 pregnancies that pregnancy or delivery was associated with a 3% risk of CM rupture or 3.4% per patient-year which is not significantly different from the overall annual hemorrhage rate of CM in the general population at 2.4%. Furthermore, a prospective study assessing hemorrhage risk of CM in pregnant women confirmed these findings of no conferred risk and that vaginal delivery is a safe option for appropriate candidates [90]. This literature and the management of CMs in pregnancy is further described in Chap. 19.

Moyamoya

Pregnancy outcomes are generally good in those patients with moyamoya if the disease is known in advance and involves multidisciplinary care. One study involving 70 cases of known moyamoya in pregnancy resulted in only one patient with a poor outcome [91] and another study highlighted reassuring fetal outcomes [92].

The key principles to moyamoya management in pregnancy stem from prevention of ischemic and/or hemorrhagic events. While moyamoya is an uncommon disease, it has potentially fatal consequences due to the progressive nature of the disease with continued stenosis of the internal carotid, anterior, and middle cerebral arteries ultimately resulting in hypoxia and subsequent formation of collaterals and dilation of these perforating arteries, which can possibly rupture causing brain hemorrhage [68, 92–100]. Thus, as long as disease status is known, imaging can be performed pre-pregnancy to determine disease severity. Per Lu et al., the annual hemorrhage rate was 3.9% among 96 female patients regardless of pregnancy [95]. There are limited high-quality studies examining the risk of stroke in patients with moyamoya during pregnancy; case series have suggested a high risk for ischemic or hemorrhagic stroke, yet there is no data to support a protective benefit of surgical revascularization prior to pregnancy [101, 102]. These concepts are discussed in detail in Chap. 20.

Cerebral Venous Thrombosis (CVT)

In general, a worse prognosis is associated with CVT if associated with hemorrhagic venous infarction, regardless of pregnancy status. It is recommended that patients with history of CVT considering pregnancy be placed on anticoagulation, usually a heparin derivative, for both treatment and secondary prophylaxis. If deemed refractory to medical management, case series and anecdotal reports suggest that invasive endovascular procedures such as mechanical thrombectomy or direct chemical thrombolysis are acceptable [103]. Ideally, any procedure would be performed prior to pregnancy to limit fetal risk. The occurrence of CVT in pregnancy is discussed in Chap. 5, while considerations for gestational anticoagulation are described in Chap. 28.

Headaches (Migraines)

Headaches can be difficult to manage during pregnancy, and it is crucial for pre-conception planning to include review of individualized headache history and discussion of migraine course over pregnancy and options for prevention and treatment as well as awareness of warning signs for ominous headaches. Headaches are a common problem for women during childbearing years, and migraine peak prevalence reaches approximately 40% in those aged between 30 and 50 [104].

There are numerous studies focused on migraine course in pregnancy [105]. The majority of women (about 60–70%) have improvement in migraines during pregnancy [106], especially by the second and third trimesters, and only about 5% have worsened migraines, while the rest have no change [106]. Women who typically have migraines with menstruation or without auras have improvement in the first trimester and often resolution of their headaches [106, 107]. Moreover, the MIGRA study followed 2000 women with headaches over the course of pregnancy and found a significant reduction in migraine frequency, especially in the second and third trimesters [108].

While migraines have not been associated with increased fetal risks such as miscarriage, stillbirth, or teratogenicity [109], studies have linked migraines with a greater prevalence of hypertensive disorders of pregnancy. A 2019 national population-based cohort study compared 22,841 pregnant women with migraines with 228,324 matched controls and found that those with migraines had a 50% increase in adjusted prevalence ratio for hypertensive disorders [110].

Most of pre-conception planning for migraines surrounds treatment strategy. Prior to pregnancy, women employ numerous pharmacologic agents for symptom control and prevention from acetaminophen to nonsteroidal anti-inflammatory drugs (NSAIDs) to triptans, caffeine-barbiturate combinations, and opioids. Medication adjustments should occur prior to pregnancy for the best pregnancy outcomes. In pregnancy, patients should be counseled that acetaminophen is the recommended first-line acute therapy and 1000 mg can be an effective treatment [111] without evidence of fetal risk. Aspirin and NSAIDs are potential next options in early pregnancy, however, are not safe beyond 20 weeks due to risk for premature ductus arteriosus closure in the fetus and neonatal pulmonary hypertension [112]. In general, the use of NSAIDS for more than a few days even in early pregnancy is uncommon. Opioids can potentially be used in pregnancy as well but these are not advised for chronic use due to risk for addiction, medication overuse, and development of chronic daily headaches [113, 114]. Furthermore, chronic opioid use specifically in the third trimester, such as meperidine, codeine, or morphine, can lead to neonatal withdrawal syndrome [107]. If migraines are refractory to these treatments, triptans (5-HT IB/ID receptor agonists) may be considered [115]. A large study including prospective pregnancy data has been unable to fully delineate risks associated with sumatriptan or naratriptan but has not shown a large increase in risk of major birth defects [116]; thus, lack of data for these medications in pregnancy has prevented creation of clear guidelines.

Steroids such as prednisone can also be used, however there are potential complications with prolonged steroid use [107]. After 14 weeks of pregnancy, the fetus is largely protected from nonfluorinated steroids because these are oxidized by placental 11-β hydroxysteroid dehydrogenase [117, 118].

The use of ergotamine is contraindicated in pregnancy due to potential adverse fetal outcomes from hypertonic uterine contractions or vasospasm/vasoconstriction [119, 120].

Other drugs have proven to be helpful for control of headaches in pregnancy. Caffeine can be utilized alone or in combination with other medications. During pregnancy, intake of up to about 200 mg of caffeine per day is considered low risk [121, 122], keeping in mind that a cup of drip coffee has approximately 100 mg of caffeine [123]. Adjuncts such as metoclopramide, promethazine, and prochlorperazine are safe and have proven to be efficacious with concomitant symptoms such as nausea/vomiting and pain [116].

Education is paramount for prevention and includes nutritional counseling to avoid specific headache triggers as well as recommendations for sleep and exercise. Additionally, randomized clinical trials provide evidence for benefit of non-pharmacologic treatment such as relaxation training, thermal biofeedback, and cognitive behavior therapy [124]. Since there are no prospective randomized clinical trials focused on migraine prophylaxis in pregnancy, prophylaxis for migraines is generally only recommended if migraines persistently get worse over the course of pregnancy. Propranolol or verapamil are drug options for prophylaxis in pregnancy [107, 125]. A detailed discussion to evaluation and management of migraine and other headache syndromes in pregnancy is provided in Chap. 8.

Epilepsy and Seizure Disorders

Pre-conception planning is crucial to confirm the diagnosis of epilepsy or specific seizure disorder after review of patient history, imaging, and electroencephalogram (EEG) results. The latter may be required if a diagnosis of epilepsy is not well established, especially given the presence of mimics for epilepsy or seizures. Furthermore, one study underscored that women with epilepsy have limited knowledge about pregnancy and childbirth [126] and potential complications can be reduced via pre-conception intervention [127]. Providers should discuss pregnancy with all childbearing aged women at each visit [128] to address need for good seizure control if desiring pregnancy or otherwise learning about birth control options and interaction between birth control and certain antiepileptic drugs (AEDs).

Prior to pregnancy, review of a patient's seizure medication by a neurologist is important in order to optimize AED regimen and to potentially switch medications for safety in pregnancy. Patients should be well-informed of the risks and benefits of AED use [129] and specifically the risk of seizure must be weighed against AED risk, such as propensity for congenital malformation, poor neonatal outcome, or adverse neurodevelopment. If a patient has been seizure-free for over 2 years with normal electroencephalogram (EEG), then one may consider tapering off or stopping the AED. Stopping use of an AED is recommended at least 6 months prior to attempting conception to ensure disease-free status, especially because these women are at risk for seizure recurrence after withdrawal during this time period [130]. Women continuing on AEDs should conceive once a minimum dose of medication is being used with the goal of monotherapy when possible. In a recent retrospective cohort study, planned pregnancies were significantly more associated with AED monotherapy and less need for change in AED regimen during pregnancy [131].

There is no one trial delineating the safest AED for pregnancy but an abundance of evidence from epilepsy pregnancy registries shows that many AEDs should be avoided if possible, especially in the first trimester, including carbamazepine, phenobarbital, primidone, phenytoin, topiramate, and valproate given their association with congenital malformations [132], specifically neural tube defects (NTDs), congenital heart anomalies, cleft lip/palate, and/or urogenital defects. Overall, levetiracetam or lamotrigine are generally the first-line seizure control medications due to data supporting low risk of these complications. There is compiled evidence from the North American Antiepileptic Drug (NAAED) Pregnancy Registry supporting increased rate of major fetal malformations with AED use, including a 9% malformation rate with valproate, for example [133]. Since valproate has been shown to be significantly more teratogenic than other medications, it should be avoided and all other AED options should be considered first. After the first trimester, most medications can be utilized, and specifically, valproate and phenobarbital can be employed especially if seizures cannot be adequately controlled with other agents [134, 135]. If valproate or phenobarbital must be used, the recommendation is for prevention of high plasma levels and administration in a three or four time daily dosing regimen. IQ in children exposed to in utero low dose valproate was about the same as IQ of children exposed to other AEDs in one prospective study [136]. However, in other studies, valproate and phenobarbital have shown potential to cause decreased intelligence in offspring when given after the first trimester and can be stopped if there is an effective alternative for the patient [137, 138].

Moreover, it is key to provide patient education about the need for medication compliance with good seizure control prior to conception. Having no seizures for at least 9 months prior to pregnancy is associated with remaining seizure-free during pregnancy. Patients should also be aware of the possible need to make AED adjustment in pregnancy based on changing AED levels. This may occur because of pregnancy-related physiologic changes like increased hepatic metabolism, alteration in volume distribution, and rise in glomerular filtration rate which in turn may decrease AED levels by increasing renal clearance and decreasing protein binding. Thus, some studies suggest active monitoring of AED levels in pregnancy, especially lamotrigine which has been tied to increased seizure frequency during pregnancy [130]. Optimal target concentration of AED should be established prior to pregnancy so that this can be the goal in pregnancy [128]. After reviewing published evidence in 2009, the American Academy of Neurology (AAN) did not find that epileptic pregnant women on AEDs were at higher risk of cesarean delivery, pre-term labor, or late pregnancy bleeding [129, 139, 140].

With multidisciplinary care and good understanding and treatment of disease, patients should understand that about 90% of women with epilepsy have excellent outcomes with healthy neonates [141]. Yet, patients should be counseled that seizures can be harmful to mother and/or baby in pregnancy [142], and that there is some evidence supporting increased morbidity and mortality in women with epilepsy including complications like pre-eclampsia, pre-term labor, bleeding, placental abruption, fetal growth restriction, or maternal or fetal death [143–147]. None of these risks should be considered a contraindication to pregnancy. AED exposure has been associated with risk of pre-term birth and delivery of a small for gestational age (SGA) infant [128]. The magnitude of increased risk is small for most of these problems, i.e., ranging from 1 to 1.7 times expected rates, except for maternal mortality, which has been shown to be as much as ten-fold higher among women with epilepsy in delivery hospitalization [128]. Studies have not been consistent regarding an increase in fetal death or stillbirth in women with epilepsy. Small increases in risk for miscarriage or stillbirth were shown in a 2015 systematic review and meta-analysis [143] and a population-based retrospective cohort study [144]. Data shows that tonic-clonic seizures can cause hypoxia and lactic acidosis and in turn, harm the fetus [128].

Pre-conception folic acid supplementation is particularly important in this population to reduce risk for congenital malformations like neural tube defects [148], and is shown to be beneficial in cognitive and behavioral studies of children born to women on AEDs. Guidelines differ regarding suggested dose of folic acid; the ACOG recommends taking 4 mg daily for women at high risk of having a child with a neural tube defect [149] but does not recommend dose above 0.4 mg daily for women on AEDs [150] nor do the 2009 guidelines from the AAN [140]. In the Neurodevelopmental Effects of Antiepileptic Drugs (NEAD) study by Meador et al., mean IQ was higher in 6-year-old children of mothers who adhered to periconceptional folic acid when compared to children of mothers who did not take periconceptional folic acid and started folic acid later [136, 147]. Genetic counseling can also provide insight into risk of offspring development of epilepsy. Studies suggest a modestly higher risk of having epilepsy in children who have a parent with epilepsy, but the degree of this risk is dependent upon specific epilepsy syndrome [151–153]. Furthermore, in discussion regarding neonatal risk, there is some suggestion that specific antiepileptics like carbamazepine can be associated with a bleeding problem in the neonate and that Vitamin K can be utilized in both mother and neonate for prevention [129, 154]. Considerations for management of acute seizures, epilepsy, and fetal protection are discussed in detail in Chap. 6.

Myasthenia Gravis

Pre-conception planning is important to first confirm a diagnosis of myasthenia gravis with neurology if it has not been confirmed. Methods for diagnosis range from detection of antibodies against nicotinic acetylcholine receptors or other postsynaptic antigens to detection of neuromuscular junction dysfunction through repetitive nerve stimulation testing or single-fiber electromyography [155]. If a diagnosis has been established, treatment goals and options should be discussed with the patient before becoming pregnant. The disease severity may vary over time and patients must know how to monitor for changes in symptoms and adjust to treatments with plan for optimization of treatment prior to pregnancy. It is important to be aware that MG most commonly affects the periocular, oropha-

ryngeal, and proximal limb muscles with muscles involved in respiration being impacted in severe cases [156]. Furthermore, triggers for worsening of MG can occur in pregnancy and include surgery, infection, select medications, and emotional stress or fatigue [156].

If a patient is considering pregnancy but has yet to have a thymectomy, this should be considered prior to conception to help improve clinical outcomes [157]. Thymectomy has proven effective in disease control with less need for immunosuppressive agents and is generally recommended for all patients under age 65 as standard of care [158, 159]. Clinical benefit over a 3-year time period was found in a randomized single-blinded clinical trial of thymectomy in patients with non-thymomatous, seropositive MG [160]. Moreover, thymectomy appears to confer protection against neonatal MG [161, 162]. The Medical Birth Registry of Norway performed a retrospective analysis showing that neonates born to MG mothers with a prior thymectomy had a lower incidence of neonatal MG when compared to those born to MG mothers without thymectomy [162]. Most experts recommend young women with MG have a thymectomy as soon as possible, as long as they are not pregnant, although thymectomy in the year before conception may not lead to remission of MG symptoms prior to pregnancy given delayed therapeutic benefit [157, 161, 163].

Medications must be discussed and modified if necessary prior to conception to reduce teratogenicity. Two common MG drugs that must be stopped are methotrexate (MTX) and mycophenolate mofetil (MMF); they are contraindicated in pregnancy and recommendation is for stopping MTX at least 3 months and MMF at least 6 weeks prior to conception [164]. Data clearly shows teratogenicity of these medications with MTX being associated with increased miscarriages [165] and MMF with miscarriage and congenital malformations of the lip and palate, distal limbs, esophagus, kidney, and central nervous system of the fetus [166, 167].

Many medications can safely be continued in pregnancy, and necessity for MG treatment should be tailored to disease severity. The recommended treatment for MG in pregnancy is the acetylcholinesterase inhibitor pyridostigmine and corticosteroids like prednisone at the lowest effective dose, if needed [157, 159]. Rituximab (RTX) can also be employed with no increase in adverse outcomes [165, 168]. Other medications such as azathioprine and cyclosporine may be added to help with MG exacerbations [159]. High-dose intravenous immune globulin (IVIG) and plasmapheresis may be used for acute exacerbations of disease or myasthenic crisis [159, 163, 169–171] and have generally been well tolerated in pregnancy for numerous autoimmune conditions [160, 172].

Understanding the variable impact of pregnancy on MG is important [155, 169]. MG has not been associated with increased risk of spontaneous abortion [162]. Similar to other neurologic disease, optimal control prior to pregnancy usually predicts a stability of disease during pregnancy, although highest risk for exacerbation is during the first trimester and postpartum period [157, 159, 163, 173–175]. Postpartum exacerbation may be triggered by fatigue in caring for a newborn or hormonal plus immunologic changes. Even with well-controlled MG, anxiety remains and discussions between MG patients and care providers must be thoughtful and respectful when discussing pregnancy [176]. All pregnancies may be different for MG patients as well [177] since the disease course is unpredictable. It is suspected that improvement in MG occurs in the second or third trimester due to immunosuppression caused by high AFP [175, 178, 179]. Baseline forced vital capacity should be assessed because respiratory function can become compromised over the course of pregnancy due to the enlarged uterus [175]. Of note, long-term outcomes of MG are not impacted by pregnancy [174].

It should be understood that there is increased risk for complications (about 30% of MG patients) during delivery thus stressing the importance of a multidisciplinary care team involving obstetrics, neurology, and anesthesiology [157, 159]. The disease itself does not affect smooth muscle but given that labor and delivery is impacted by striated muscle, especially in the second phase of delivery, fatigue can occur and it

can be prolonged and involve fetal distress [155, 162, 180]. Forceps or vacuum extraction are beneficial, however, MG itself is not an indication for cesarean delivery [161]. Therefore, spontaneous vaginal delivery should be encouraged with cesarean delivery performed for indicated obstetrical reasons [159]. Stress dose steroids should also be considered during labor and delivery if patients have been on long-term oral steroids [157].

Additionally, medications delivered during labor must be monitored closely. Parenteral anticholinesterase medications can potentially strengthen the muscle since oral absorption may be limited. More importantly, it is important to identify and mitigate effects of medications that make MG symptoms worse [155]. Specifically, nondepolarizing muscle relaxants and magnesium should be avoided since they can significantly worsen MG [159]. Magnesium which is commonly employed for management of pre-eclampsia, eclampsia, or pre-term labor is contraindicated due to precipitation of severe MG crisis [181, 182]. Anesthesiology consultation prior to labor is recommended; MG patients who need general anesthesia may have a higher risk for needing mechanical ventilation [183] and general anesthesia should be avoided if possible. Epidural or combined spinal-epidural anesthesia is recommended by expert opinion to reduce respiratory issues as well as to help with overexertion and fatigue [184]. Spinal anesthesia can also be safely used for MG patients needing cesarean delivery [178].

Neonatologists play an important role in assessing and supporting the needs for an infant born to a patient with MG given the risk for transient neonatal MG or arthrogryposis. Incidence of transient neonatal MG is about 10–30% [174], can be seronegative or involve different antibodies [185–187], and has symptoms ranging from generalized hypotonia to poor suck or respiratory problems. Monitoring for symptoms in the several days after birth is needed because symptom onset can be delayed but this usually all resolves within 1–7 weeks [188]. The issues surrounding pre-conception counseling, gestational and peripartal management, and neonatal monitoring are discussed in detail in Chap. 17.

Brain Tumors

While rare, there are a myriad of brain tumors that occur in childbearing aged women such as gliomas, meningiomas, or metastatic brain tumors. It is important to discuss risks and benefits of pregnancy with a brain tumor because symptoms and treatment can be difficult in pregnancy. Management of brain tumors is vast and if surgical resection, radiation and/or chemotherapy are needed, pregnancy should be deferred until these therapies have been delivered. Radiation can have poor outcomes such as spontaneous abortion, malformations, growth, and mental retardation, and possible higher childhood cancer risk [189, 190]. Chemotherapy for malignant brain tumors is also not ideal during pregnancy because most cross the placenta and are teratogenic [191]. Moreover, there may be subtle changes in cardiac and neurocognitive outcomes in these fetuses, which requires more data to be conclusive [192].

There are pregnancy risks for women with brain tumors that should be known since pregnancy can impact tumor symptoms and growth [193, 194]. For example, there is evidence to suggest that some brain tumors such as meningiomas may be negatively impacted by pregnancy hormones [195]. Changes in sex hormones, such as progesterone, during pregnancy can promote growth in meningiomas and vestibular schwannomas due to expression of hormonal receptors [196, 197]. Additionally, 1 study of 11 pregnant women with grade II gliomas showed significant radiologic enlargement of the brain mass during pregnancy when compared to times outside of pregnancy [198]; in this study, there was concomitant increase in seizure frequency suggesting the need for close monitoring for changing neurologic findings and awareness to differentiate adverse events from brain tumors versus eclampsia [198].

Generally, benign or asymptomatic tumors may be observed whereas malignant or symptomatic tumors should be treated regardless of pregnancy with neurosurgical recommendation superseding obstetrical consideration. Management may require use of steroids or mannitol due to potential for pregnancy to promote a higher intracranial pressure or cerebral edema [199–201]. In some cases, this is due to the ability of pregnancy to promote fluid retention and thus contribute to enlargement of vascular tumors [194]. Here, excessive hydration is not recommended given potential for cerebral edema [202]. Clinically, it is important to be able to recognize seizures as a potential complication of tumor enlargement and differentiate these from eclampsia; in a case series by Pallud et al., increased seizure frequency was found in pregnant women with grade II gliomas [198].

Prenatal genetic counseling is important prior to conception because many hereditary tumor syndromes are associated with brain tumors and autosomal dominant diseases such as neurofibromatosis types I and II, tuberous sclerosis, Turcot syndrome, von Hippel-Lindau syndrome, Li-Fraumeni, and Gorlin syndrome [203, 204]. If a genetic syndrome is identified, pre-implantation genetic testing with in vitro fertilization can potentially be an option to mitigate risk. Use of a gestational carrier may also be indicated when patients have neurologic tumors that may be hormonally responsive with an increased potential for accelerated growth in pregnancy. For more details on considerations for counseling, diagnosis, and management of brain tumors in pregnancy, please refer to Chap. 11.

Pituitary Adenomas (Prolactinomas)

Pituitary adenomas comprise about 15% of intracranial neoplasms and are often undiagnosed [205]. Prolactinoma is the most common type of pituitary adenoma and presents particular issues for pregnant patients. One of the biggest concerns for women with lactotroph adenomas, or prolactinomas, is growth of the tumor. Adenoma growth is likely caused by increased serum estradiol in pregnancy, which promotes lactotroph hyperplasia. Studies have shown evidence of more than doubling in pituitary size using magnetic resonance imaging (MRI) in pregnant versus nonpregnant women [206]. Risk of growth for those with microadenomas (<10 mm in diameter) is low [207, 208]. A review of 14 studies by Molitch et al. showed that only 2.4% of patients with microadenomas showed a symptomatic increase in size during pregnancy whereas 22.9% of women who had macroadenomas without prior treatment with surgery or radiation had significant enlargement [209]. Women should be counseled about neurologic symptoms that could develop, more often in those with macroadenomas (about 13–36%), such as new headaches or visual changes. Additionally, if there is concern during pregnancy about adenoma growth or pituitary apoplexy secondary to ischemia or hemorrhage, MRI can be utilized due to lower fetal risk compared to CT [210]. There may be a small risk for developing pituitary apoplexy during pregnancy in women who have pre-existing pituitary adenomas, which is caused by the pituitary gland enlarging by about 3 mm at the end of pregnancy [211].

Treatment of prolactinomas is usually with dopamine agonists such as bromocriptine or cabergoline, and often these medications are needed to correct prolactin levels and allow for normal ovulation and restoration of fertility. These medications are usually stopped with pregnancy, although there are no known adverse fetal outcomes after exposure to these medications. For example, a study involving over 6000 pregnancies with exposure to bromocriptine during the first month of pregnancy did not harm the fetus and incidence of spontaneous abortion, multiple births, and fetal malformations were comparable to those not on the medication [208]. The same has been found in a large study of cabergoline use at time of conception [209]. Another study followed children up to age 9 who were exposed to bromocriptine in utero and no negative outcomes were found [212]. Interestingly, there is some data that bromocriptine may reduce the risk of miscarriage in women with a history of recurrent pregnancy loss [213, 214].

Women with a macroadenoma should be advised to delay pregnancy until they have a reduction in adenoma size with either a dopamine agonist or surgery, if necessary, due to an adenoma refractory to medication or elevating the optic chiasm, especially given their increased risk for clinically significant enlargement in pregnancy [208]. Surgery lowers the risk for symptomatic enlargement in pregnancy [209].

In regard to planning pregnancy with microadenomas, routine visual field testing is not needed and the Endocrine Society guidelines recommend against measuring prolactin because prolactin can be elevated from pregnancy alone [215]. If a pregnant woman were to develop visual symptoms, then visual testing should be performed. If a pregnant woman has a macroadenoma that extends above the sella, visual testing should be serially checked in pregnancy and subsequent MRI without contrast can be performed if needed. The approach to workup and management of pituitary and sellar tumors is discussed in detail in Chap. 12.

Multiple Sclerosis (MS)

Pre-conception planning for women with MS generally involves understanding disease course in pregnancy and optimizing medications that are safe during pregnancy. MS is a disease that largely impacts childbearing aged women [216], but it significantly improves in pregnancy [217] with fewer relapses. A 2011 meta-analysis of 13 studies that included 1221 pregnancies provided evidence that the period of pregnancy was associated with less MS disease activity whereas the postpartum state was associated with a rise in disease activity [218].

Important data is derived from the Pregnancy in Multiple Sclerosis Study (PRIMS) in which 254 women were followed throughout 269 pregnancies and 12 months postpartum. PRIMS reported mean rates of relapse prior to pregnancy, in the first trimester, in the second trimester, in the third trimester, and in the first 3 months postpartum of 0.7, 0.5, 0.6, 0.2, and 1.2 per woman per year, respectively [217]. Multiple other studies have suggested the same with decreased MS disease in pregnancy and an increase postpartum

[219, 220]. Reasons for postpartum relapses are not fully understood but postpartum triggers may include stress, fatigue, infection, or loss of antenatal immunosuppression impacted by estrogen [221]. Long-term sequelae from MS secondary to pregnancy is less clear [222–224].

While there is some controversy about the impact of MS on obstetrical outcomes, most data suggest that MS usually does not adversely affect pregnancy [225]. For example, spontaneous abortion and congenital malformations have not been higher in women with MS [218, 226, 227]. Also, studies are controversial as to whether birth weight is less [226, 228]; one study analyzing 4730 women with MS showed a small but significant increase in risk for intrauterine growth restriction [227]. Some patients with MS may have increased need for a vacuum-assisted vaginal delivery or cesarean section [227, 228]. Delivery is usually not more difficult in MS however there can be issues with fatigue or spasticity of the pelvic floor. Delivery mode should be determined by obstetrical considerations; the largest prospective study looking at risk of postpartum relapses did not show increased risk of postpartum relapses by delivery mode or epidural anesthesia [229]. Epidural anesthesia is safe for patients with MS and anesthesia should be based on obstetric needs [230].

Women with MS should plan for pregnancy once MS activity has been minimal for at least 1 year and in good control for optimal pregnancy outcome [231]. Women with MS may be on numerous medications such as disease-modifying antirheumatic drugs (DMARDs), antimuscarinics such as oxybutynin for bladder disorders, antispasmodics such as baclofen or diazepam, and anti-depressants. There are conflicting expert opinions regarding medication use and pregnancy, and it ultimately must involve weighing benefits and risk of specific drugs in pregnancy. There is limited evidence on use of DMARDs in pregnancy, and some drugs can be considered in pregnancy whereas others should be stopped [231–234]. Data from review of 761 pregnancies with exposure to interferon-beta showed a lower mean birth weight, shorter mean birth length, and pre-term birth but no increase in spontaneous abortions, congenital malformations, birth weight under 2500 g, or increased cesarean sections [235]. In this same study, data did not show adverse outcomes with either glatiramer acetate or natalizumab. While data on pregnancies exposed to such drugs is limited [235–238], patients should not abort pregnancy for these exposures [235, 239].

Patients with MS should not avoid pregnancy due to fear of passing the disease to their offspring. While there are some MS associated genetic variants [240] that have been studied in large cohorts, MS is not a Mendelian trait and risk of passing on MS is low. Evidence suggests that about 2% of those with MS will have affected children [241, 242]. Chapter 9 provides a detailed response to some of the most commonly encountered questions related to the evaluation and management of MS during pregnancy.

Conclusion

It is clear that pre-conception planning is ideal for all pregnancies and particularly important for women affected by neurologic disorders in which multiple issues may be at play. The key tenants to care include proper diagnosis of neurologic disease and optimal pre-pregnancy management of disease with history and physical, neuroimaging, or medications if necessary. Continued discussion of the risks and benefits to pregnancy as well as multidisciplinary collaboration for those with neurologic disease is paramount to providing education to patients and power for shared decision-making to make the best pre-conception plan.

References

1. Bellanca HK, Hunter MS. ONE KEY QUESTION®: preventive reproductive health is part of high quality primary care. Contraception. 2013;88(1):3–6.
2. ACOG Committee Opinion No. 762: prepregnancy counseling. Obstet Gynecol. 2019;133(1):e78–89.
3. Crider KS, Bailey LB, Berry RJ. Folic acid food fortification its history, effect, concerns, and future directions. Nutrients. 2011;3(3):370–84.

4. Centers for Disease Control. Use of folic acid for prevention of spina bifida and other neural tube defects--1983-1991. MMWR Morb Mortal Wkly Rep. 1991;40(30):513–6.

5. ACOG Committee Opinion No. 755: Well-Woman Visit. Obstet Gynecol. 2018;132(4):e181–6.

6. Johnson K, et al. Recommendations to improve preconception health and health care--United States: a report of the CDC/ATSDR Preconception Care Work Group and the Select Panel on Preconception Care: (506902006-001). Washington, DC: American Psychological Association; 2006.

7. Pereira L. Obstetric management of the patient with spinal cord injury. Obstet Gynecol Surv. 2003;58(10):678–86.

8. Thierry JM. The importance of preconception care for women with disabilities. Matern Child Health J. 2006;10(5 Suppl):S175–6.

9. McLain AB, Massengill T, Klebine P. Pregnancy and women with spinal cord injury. Arch Phys Med Rehabil. 2016;97(3):497–8.

10. Wanner MB, Rageth CJ, Zäch GA. Pregnancy and autonomic hyperreflexia in patients with spinal cord lesions. Spinal Cord. 1987;25(6):482–90.

11. Verduyn WH. Spinal cord injured women, pregnancy and delivery. Paraplegia. 1986;24(4):231–40.

12. Westgren N, et al. Pregnancy and delivery in women with a traumatic spinal cord injury in Sweden, 1980-1991. Obstet Gynecol. 1993;81(6):926–30.

13. Hughes SJ, et al. Management of the pregnant woman with spinal cord injuries. Br J Obstet Gynaecol. 1991;98(6):513–8.

14. American College of Obstetricians and Gynecologists. ACOG Committee Opinion: Number 275, September 2002. Obstetric management of patients with spinal cord injuries. Obstet Gynecol. 2002;100(3):625–7.

15. Skowronski E, Hartman K. Obstetric management following traumatic tetraplegia: case series and literature review: obstetric management following traumatic tetraplegia. Aust N Z J Obstet Gynaecol. 2008;48(5):485–91.

16. Greenspoon JS, Paul RH. Paraplegia and quadriplegia: special considerations during pregnancy and labor and delivery. Am J Obstet Gynecol. 1986;155(4):738–41.

17. Ghidini A, et al. Pregnancy and women with spinal cord injuries. Acta Obstet Gynecol Scand. 2008;87(10):1006–10.

18. Baschat AA, Weiner C. Chronic neurologic diseases and disabling conditions in pregnancy. In: Welner SL, Haseltine F, editors. Welner's guide to the care of women with disabilities. Philadelphia: Lippincott, Wiliams & Wilkins; 2004. p. 145–58.

19. Ditunno JF, Formal CS. Chronic spinal cord injury. N Engl J Med. 1994;330(8):550–6.

20. Le Liepvre H, et al. Pregnancy in spinal cord-injured women, a cohort study of 37 pregnancies in 25 women. Spinal Cord. 2017;55(2):167–71.

21. Krassioukov A, et al. A systematic review of the management of autonomic dysreflexia after spinal cord injury. Arch Phys Med Rehabil. 2009;90(4):682–95.

22. Goller H. Pregnancy damage and birth-complications in the children of paraplegic women. Spinal Cord. 1972;10(3):213–7.

23. Signore C, et al. Pregnancy in women with physical disabilities. Obstet Gynecol. 2011;117(4):935–47.

24. Vercauteren M, et al. Neuraxial techniques in patients with pre-existing back impairment or prior spine interventions: a topical review with special reference to obstetrics. Acta Anaesthesiol Scand. 2011;55(8):910–7.

25. Wilson RD, et al. Pre-conceptional vitamin/folic acid supplementation 2007: the use of folic acid in combination with a multivitamin supplement for the prevention of neural tube defects and other congenital anomalies. J Obstet Gynaecol Can. 2007;29(12):1003–13.

26. Cesario SK. Spinal cord injuries: nurses can help affected women & their families achieve pregnancy birth. AWHONN Lifelines. 2002;6(3):224–32.

27. Holmgren T, et al. The influence of spinal cord injury on breastfeeding ability and behavior. J Hum Lact. 2018;34(3):556–65.

28. Crane DA, et al. Pregnancy outcomes in women with spinal cord injuries: a population-based study. PM&R. 2019;11(8):795–806.

29. Yu JN. Pregnancy and extracranial shunts: case report and review of the literature. J Fam Pract. 1994;38(6):622–6.

30. Maheut-Lourmiere J, Chu Tan S. [Hydrocephalus during pregnancy with or without neurosurgical history in childhood. Practical advice for management]. Neurochirurgie. 2000;46(2):117–21.

31. Ng J, Kitchen N. Neurosurgery and pregnancy. J Neurol Neurosurg Psychiatry. 2008;79(7):745–52.

32. Petitti DB, et al. Incidence of stroke and myocardial infarction in women of reproductive age. Stroke. 1997;28(2):280–3.

33. James AH, et al. Incidence and risk factors for stroke in pregnancy and the puerperium. Obstet Gynecol. 2005;106(3):509–16.

34. Bateman BT, et al. Intracerebral hemorrhage in pregnancy: frequency, risk factors, and outcome. Neurology. 2006;67(3):424–9.

35. Lanska DJ, Kryscio RJ. Risk factors for peripartum and postpartum stroke and intracranial venous thrombosis. Stroke. 2000;31(6):1274–82.

36. Kamel H, et al. Risk of a thrombotic event after the 6-week postpartum period. N Engl J Med. 2014;370(14):1307–15.

37. Miller EC, et al. Infections and risk of peripartum stroke during delivery admissions. Stroke. 2018;49(5):1129–34.

38. Miller EC, et al. Infection during delivery hospitalization and risk of readmission for postpartum stroke. Stroke. 2019;50(10):2685–91.

39. Ros HS, et al. Pulmonary embolism and stroke in relation to pregnancy: how can high-risk women be identified? Am J Obstet Gynecol. 2002;186(2):198–203.

40. Bellos I, et al. Safety of non-steroidal anti-inflammatory drugs in postpartum period in women with hypertensive disorders of pregnancy: systematic review and meta-analysis. Ultrasound Obstet Gynecol. 2020;56(3):329–39.

41. Lydakis C, et al. Atenolol and fetal growth in pregnancies complicated by hypertension. Am J Hypertens. 1999;12(6):541–7.

42. ACOG Practice Bulletin No. 203: chronic hypertension in pregnancy. Obstet Gynecol. 2019;133(1):e26–50.

43. Collins R, Yusuf S, Peto R. Overview of randomised trials of diuretics in pregnancy. Br Med J (Clin Res Ed). 1985;290(6461):17–23.

44. Cooper WO, et al. Major congenital malformations after first-trimester exposure to ACE inhibitors. N Engl J Med. 2006;354(23):2443–51.

45. Hosokawa A, Bar-Oz B, Ito S. Use of lipid-lowering agents (statins) during pregnancy. Can Fam Physician. 2003;49:747–9.

46. Karalis DG, et al. The risks of statin use in pregnancy: a systematic review. J Clin Lipidol. 2016;10(5):1081–90.

47. Sibai BM, Coppage KH. Diagnosis and management of women with stroke during pregnancy/postpartum. Clin Perinatol. 2004;31(4):853–68.

48. Kearon C, et al. Antithrombotic therapy for VTE disease: antithrombotic therapy and prevention of thrombosis, 9th ed: American College of Chest Physicians Evidence-Based Clinical Practice Guidelines. Chest. 2012;141(2 Suppl):e419S–96S.

49. Trivedi R, Kirkpatrick P. Arteriovenous malformations of the cerebral circulation that rupture in pregnancy. J Obstet Gynaecol. 2003;23(5):484–9.

50. Amias AG. Cerebral vascular disease in pregnancy. I. Haemorrhage. J Obstet Gynaecol Br Commonw. 1970;77(2):100–20.

51. Fliegner JR, Hooper RS, Kloss M. Subarachnoid haemorrhage and pregnancy. J Obstet Gynaecol Br Commonw. 1969;76(10):912–7.

52. Robinson JL, Hall CJ, Sedzimir CB. Subarachnoid hemorrhage in pregnancy. J Neurosurg. 1972;36(1):27–33.

53. Robinson JL, Hall CS, Sedzimir CB. Arteriovenous malformations, aneurysms, and pregnancy. J Neurosurg. 1974;41(1):63–70.

54. Porras JL, et al. Hemorrhage risk of brain arteriovenous malformations during pregnancy and puerperium in a North American Cohort. Stroke. 2017;48(6):1507–13.

55. Horton JC, et al. Pregnancy and the risk of hemorrhage from cerebral arteriovenous malformations. Neurosurgery. 1990;27(6):867–72.

56. Forster DMC, Kunkler IH, Hartland P. Risk of cerebral bleeding from arteriovenous malformations in pregnancy: the Sheffield experience. Stereotact Funct Neurosurg. 1993;61(1):20–2.

57. Gross BA, Du R. Hemorrhage from arteriovenous malformations during pregnancy. Neurosurgery. 2012;71(2):349–56.

58. Dias MS, Sekhar LN. Intracranial hemorrhage from aneurysms and arteriovenous malformations during pregnancy and the puerperium. Neurosurgery. 1990;27(6):855–66.

59. Liu X-J, et al. Risk of cerebral arteriovenous malformation rupture during pregnancy and puerperium. Neurology. 2014;82(20):1798–803.

60. Skidmore FM, et al. Presentation, etiology, and outcome of stroke in pregnancy and puerperium. J Stroke Cerebrovasc Dis. 2001;10(1):1–10.

61. Lanzino G, et al. Arteriovenous malformations that rupture during pregnancy: a management dilemma. Acta Neurochir (Wien). 1994;126(2–4):102–6.

62. Crawford PM, et al. Arteriovenous malformations of the brain: natural history in unoperated patients. J Neurol Neurosurg Psychiatry. 1986;49(1):1–10.

63. Can A, Du R. Neurosurgical issues in pregnancy. Semin Neurol. 2017;37(6):689–93.

64. da Costa L, et al. The natural history and predictive features of hemorrhage from brain arteriovenous malformations. Stroke. 2009;40(1):100–5.

65. Hernesniemi JA, et al. Natural history of brain arteriovenous malformations. Neurosurgery. 2008;63(5):823–31.

66. Forster DMC, Steiner L, Håkanson S. Arteriovenous malformations of the brain: a long-term clinical study. J Neurosurg. 1972;37(5):562–70.

67. Yamada S, et al. Risk factors for subsequent hemorrhage in patients with cerebral arteriovenous malformations. J Neurosurg. 2007;107(5):965–72.

68. Gross BA, Du R. The natural history of moyamoya in a North American adult cohort. J Clin Neurosci. 2013;20(1):44–8.

69. Stapf C, et al. Predictors of hemorrhage in patients with untreated brain arteriovenous malformation. Neurology. 2006;66(9):1350–5.

70. Kader A, et al. The influence of hemodynamic and anatomic factors on hemorrhage from cerebral arteriovenous malformations. Neurosurgery. 1994;34(5):801–7; discussion 807–8.

71. Meyers PM, et al. Endovascular treatment of cerebral artery aneurysms during pregnancy: report of three cases. AJNR Am J Neuroradiol. 2000;21(7):1306–11.

72. Tonetti D, et al. Hemorrhage during pregnancy in the latency interval after stereotactic radiosurgery for arteriovenous malformations: clinical article. J Neurosurg. 2014;121(Suppl_2):226–31.

73. Mohr JP, et al. Medical management with or without interventional therapy for unruptured brain arteriovenous malformations (ARUBA): a multicentre, non-blinded, randomised trial. Lancet. 2014;383(9917):614–21.

74. Jaigobin C, Silver FL. Stroke and pregnancy. Stroke. 2000;31(12):2948–51.

75. Salonen Ros H, et al. Increased risks of circulatory diseases in late pregnancy and puerperium. Epidemiology. 2001;12(4):456–60.
76. Tiel Groenestege AT, et al. The risk of aneurysmal subarachnoid hemorrhage during pregnancy, delivery, and the puerperium in the Utrecht population: case-crossover study and standardized incidence ratio estimation. Stroke. 2009;40(4):1148–51.
77. Kim YW, Neal D, Hoh BL. Cerebral aneurysms in pregnancy and delivery: pregnancy and delivery do not increase the risk of aneurysm rupture. Neurosurgery. 2013;72(2):143–50.
78. Robba C, et al. Aneurysmal subarachnoid hemorrhage in pregnancy-case series, review, and pooled data analysis. World Neurosurg. 2016;88:383–98.
79. Katayama Y, et al. Surgical management of cavernous malformations of the third ventricle. J Neurosurg. 1994;80(1):64–72.
80. Yamasaki T, et al. Intracranial and orbital cavernous angiomas: a review of 30 cases. J Neurosurg. 1986;64(2):197–208.
81. Zauberman H, Feinsod M. Orbital hemangioma growth during pregnancy. Acta Ophthalmol (Copenh). 1970;48(5):929–33.
82. Porter RW, et al. Cavernous malformations of the brainstem: experience with 100 patients. J Neurosurg. 1999;90(1):50–8.
83. Simonazzi G, et al. Symptomatic cerebral cavernomas in pregnancy: a series of 6 cases and review of the literature. J Matern Fetal Neonatal Med. 2014;27(3):261–4.
84. Kaya AH, et al. There are no estrogen and progesterone receptors in cerebral cavernomas. Surg Neurol. 2009;72(3):263–5.
85. Pozzati E, Musiani M. Cavernous hemangioma. J Neurosurg. 1998;89(3):498–9.
86. Flemming KD, Goodman BP, Meyer FB. Successful brainstem cavernous malformation resection after repeated hemorrhages during pregnancy. Surg Neurol. 2003;60(6):545–7.
87. Robinson JR, Awad IA, Little JR. Natural history of the cavernous angioma. J Neurosurg. 1991;75(5):709–14.
88. Kalani MYS, Zabramski JM. Risk for symptomatic hemorrhage of cerebral cavernous malformations during pregnancy: clinical article. J Neurosurg. 2013;118(1):50–5.
89. Witiw CD, et al. Cerebral cavernous malformations and pregnancy. Neurosurgery. 2012;71(3):626–31.
90. Joseph NK, et al. Influence of pregnancy on hemorrhage risk in women with cerebral and spinal cavernous malformations. Stroke. 2021;52(2):434–41.
91. Fukushima K, et al. A retrospective chart review of the perinatal period in 22 pregnancies of 16 women with moyamoya disease. J Clin Neurosci. 2012;19(10):1358–62.
92. Komiyama M, et al. Moyamoya disease and pregnancy: case report and review of the literature. Neurosurgery. 1998;43(2):360–8.
93. Scott RM, Smith ER. Moyamoya disease and moyamoya syndrome. N Engl J Med. 2009;360(12):1226–37.
94. Ikezaki K, et al. A clinical comparison of definite moyamoya disease between South Korea and Japan. Stroke. 1997;28(12):2513–7.
95. Liu X-J, et al. Intracranial hemorrhage from moyamoya disease during pregnancy and puerperium. Int J Gynecol Obstet. 2014;125(2):150–3.
96. Sato K, et al. Vaginal delivery under epidural analgesia in pregnant women with a diagnosis of moyamoya disease. J Stroke Cerebrovasc Dis. 2015;24(5):921–4.
97. Takahashi JC, et al. Pregnancy and delivery in moyamoya disease: results of a nationwide survey in Japan. Neurol Med Chir. 2012;52(5):304–10.
98. Tanaka H, et al. Vaginal delivery in pregnancy with moyamoya disease: experience at a single institute: pregnancy with moyamoya disease. J Obstet Gynaecol Res. 2015;41(4):517–22.
99. Sei K, Sasa H, Furuya K. Moyamoya disease and pregnancy: case reports and criteria for successful vaginal delivery. Clin Case Rep. 2015;3(4):251–4.
100. Miller EC, Leffert L. Stroke in pregnancy: a focused update. Anesth Analg. 2020;130(4):1085–96.
101. Maragkos GA, et al. Moyamoya disease in pregnancy: a systematic review. Acta Neurochir (Wien). 2018;160(9):1711–9.
102. Inayama Y, et al. Moyamoya disease in pregnancy: a 20-year single-center experience and literature review. World Neurosurg. 2019;122:684–691.e2.
103. Kernan WN, et al. Guidelines for the prevention of stroke in patients with stroke and transient ischemic attack: a guideline for healthcare professionals from the American Heart Association/American Stroke Association. Stroke. 2014;45(7):2160–236.
104. Stewart WF, et al. Prevalence of migraine headache in the United States. Relation to age, income, race, and other sociodemographic factors. JAMA. 1992;267(1):64–9.
105. Loder E, Silberstein SD. Headaches in women. In: Silberstein SD, Lipton RB, Dodick D, editors. Wolff's headache and other head pain. New York: Oxford University Press; 2008. p. 691–710.
106. MacGregor EA. Headache in pregnancy. Neurol Clin. 2012;30(3):835–66.
107. Macgregor EA. Headache in pregnancy. Continuum (Minneap Minn). 2014;20:128–47.
108. Kvisvik EV, et al. Headache and migraine during pregnancy and puerperium: the MIGRA-study. J Headache Pain. 2011;12(4):443–51.
109. Wainscott G, et al. The outcome of pregnancy in women suffering from migraine. Postgrad Med J. 1978;54(628):98–102.
110. Skajaa N, et al. Pregnancy, birth, neonatal, and postnatal neurological outcomes after pregnancy with migraine. Headache. 2019;59(6):869–79.
111. Lipton RB, et al. Efficacy and safety of acetaminophen in the treatment of migraine: results of a

randomized, double-blind, placebo-controlled, population-based study. Arch Intern Med. 2000;160(22):3486–92.

112. Morris JL, Rosen DA, Rosen KR. Nonsteroidal anti-inflammatory agents in neonates. Paediatr Drugs. 2003;5(6):385–405.

113. Mathew NT. Transformed migraine, analgesic rebound, and other chronic daily headaches. Neurol Clin. 1997;15(1):167–86.

114. Rapoport A, et al. Analgesic rebound headache in clinical practice: data from a physician survey. Headache. 1996;36(1):14–9.

115. Evans EW, Lorber KC. Use of 5-HT1 agonists in pregnancy. Ann Pharmacother. 2008;42(4):543–9.

116. Cunnington M, Ephross S, Churchill P. The safety of sumatriptan and naratriptan in pregnancy: what have we learned? Headache. 2009;49(10):1414–22.

117. Yang K. Placental 11 beta-hydroxysteroid dehydrogenase: barrier to maternal glucocorticoids. Rev Reprod. 1997;2(3):129–32.

118. Edwards CR, et al. Dysfunction of placental glucocorticoid barrier: link between fetal environment and adult hypertension? Lancet. 1993;341(8841):355–7.

119. Banhidy F, et al. Ergotamine treatment during pregnancy and a higher rate of low birthweight and preterm birth. Br J Clin Pharmacol. 2007;64(4):510–6.

120. Hughes HE, Goldstein DA. Birth defects following maternal exposure to ergotamine, beta blockers, and caffeine. J Med Genet. 1988;25(6):396–9.

121. Jahanfar S, Jaafar SH. Effects of restricted caffeine intake by mother on fetal, neonatal and pregnancy outcomes. Cochrane Database Syst Rev. 2015;(6):CD006965.

122. Maslova E, et al. Caffeine consumption during pregnancy and risk of preterm birth: a meta-analysis. Am J Clin Nutr. 2010;92(5):1120–32.

123. Service, U.S.D.o.A.A.R., National Nutrient Database for Standard Reference Release. USDA.gov.

124. Campbell JK, Penzien DB, Wall EM, the US Headache Consortium. In: Evidence-based guidelines for migrane headache: behavioral and physical treatments. AOA.net.

125. Silberstein SD, Dodick DW, Bigal ME. Migraine treatment. In: Silberstein SD, Lipton RB, Dodick DW, editors. Wolff's headache and other head pain. New York: Oxford University Press; 2008. p. 177–292.

126. McGrath A, et al. Pregnancy-related knowledge and information needs of women with epilepsy: a systematic review. Epilepsy Behav. 2014;31:246–55.

127. Sabers A. Influences on seizure activity in pregnant women with epilepsy. Epilepsy Behav. 2009;15(2):230–4.

128. Tomson T, et al. Management of epilepsy in pregnancy: a report from the International League Against Epilepsy Task Force on Women and Pregnancy. Epileptic Disord. 2019;21(6):497–517.

129. Harden CL, et al. Practice parameter update: management issues for women with epilepsy--focus on pregnancy (an evidence-based review): teratogenesis and perinatal outcomes: report of the Quality Standards Subcommittee and Therapeutics and Technology Assessment Subcommittee of the American Academy of Neurology and American Epilepsy Society. Neurology. 2009;73(2):133–41.

130. Pennell PB, et al. Lamotrigine in pregnancy: clearance, therapeutic drug monitoring, and seizure frequency. Neurology. 2008;70(22 Pt 2):2130–6.

131. Abe K, et al. Impact of planning of pregnancy in women with epilepsy on seizure control during pregnancy and on maternal and neonatal outcomes. Seizure. 2014;23(2):112–6.

132. Tomson T, et al. Pregnancy registries: differences, similarities, and possible harmonization. Epilepsia. 2010;51(5):909–15.

133. Wyszynski DF, et al. Increased rate of major malformations in offspring exposed to valproate during pregnancy. Neurology. 2005;64(6):961–5.

134. Tomson T, et al. Valproate in the treatment of epilepsy in girls and women of childbearing potential. Epilepsia. 2015;56(7):1006–19.

135. Sen A, Nashef L. New regulations to cut valproate-exposed pregnancies. Lancet. 2018;392(10146):458–60.

136. Meador KJ, et al. Fetal antiepileptic drug exposure and cognitive outcomes at age 6 years (NEAD study): a prospective observational study. Lancet Neurol. 2013;12(3):244–52.

137. Reinisch JM, et al. In utero exposure to phenobarbital and intelligence deficits in adult men. JAMA. 1995;274(19):1518–25.

138. Meador KJ, et al. Cognitive function at 3 years of age after fetal exposure to antiepileptic drugs. N Engl J Med. 2009;360(16):1597–605.

139. Harden CL, et al. Practice parameter update: management issues for women with epilepsy--focus on pregnancy (an evidence-based review): obstetrical complications and change in seizure frequency: Report of the Quality Standards Subcommittee and Therapeutics and Technology Assessment Subcommittee of the American Academy of Neurology and American Epilepsy Society. Neurology. 2009;73(2):126–32.

140. Harden CL, et al. Practice parameter update: management issues for women with epilepsy--focus on pregnancy (an evidence-based review): vitamin K, folic acid, blood levels, and breastfeeding: report of the Quality Standards Subcommittee and Therapeutics and Technology Assessment Subcommittee of the American Academy of Neurology and American Epilepsy Society. Neurology. 2009;73(2):142–9.

141. McAuley JW, Anderson GD. Treatment of epilepsy in women of reproductive age: pharmacokinetic considerations. Clin Pharmacokinet. 2002;41(8):559–79.

142. Fountain NB, et al. Quality improvement in neurology: Epilepsy Update Quality Measurement Set. Neurology. 2015;84(14):1483–7.

143. Viale L, et al. Epilepsy in pregnancy and reproductive outcomes: a systematic review and meta-analysis. Lancet. 2015;386(10006):1845–52.
144. MacDonald SC, et al. Mortality and morbidity during delivery hospitalization among pregnant women with epilepsy in the United States. JAMA Neurol. 2015;72(9):981–8.
145. Richmond JR, et al. Epilepsy and pregnancy: an obstetric perspective. Am J Obstet Gynecol. 2004;190(2):371–9.
146. Borthen I, et al. Complications during pregnancy in women with epilepsy: population-based cohort study: complications during pregnancy in women with epilepsy. BJOG. 2009;116(13):1736–42.
147. Meador KJ, et al. Fetal loss and malformations in the MONEAD study of pregnant women with epilepsy. Neurology. 2020;94(14):e1502–11.
148. Pennell PB, Davis A. Selecting contraception in women treated with antiepileptic drugs. In: Klein A, Angela O'Neal M, Scrifres C, et al., editors. Neurological illness in pregnancy: principles and practice. New York: Wiley Publishing; 2016. p. 110.
149. Practice Bulletin No. 187: neural tube defects. Obstet Gynecol. 2017;130(6):e279–90.
150. Gynecologists., A.C.o.O.a. Preconception and interconception care. In: ACOG, editor. Guidelines for women's health care; 2014.
151. Ottman R, et al. Higher risk of seizures in offspring of mothers than of fathers with epilepsy. Am J Hum Genet. 1988;43(3):257–64.
152. Schupf N, Ottman R. Risk of epilepsy in offspring of affected women: association with maternal spontaneous abortion. Neurology. 2001;57(9):1642–9.
153. Peljto AL, et al. Familial risk of epilepsy: a population-based study. Brain. 2014;137(Pt 3):795–805.
154. Bruno MK, Harden CL. Epilepsy in pregnant women. Curr Treat Options Neurol. 2002;4(1):31–40.
155. Hamel J, Ciafaloni E. An update. Neurol Clin. 2018;36(2):355–65.
156. Amato AA, Russell J. Neuromuscular disorders. Boston: Mc-Graw-Hill Educational Medical; 2016.
157. Norwood F, et al. Myasthenia in pregnancy: best practice guidelines from a U.K. multispecialty working group. J Neurol Neurosurg Psychiatry. 2014;85(5):538–43.
158. Wolfe GI, et al. Randomized trial of thymectomy in myasthenia gravis. J Thorac Dis. 2016;8(12):E1782–3.
159. Sanders DB, et al. International consensus guidance for management of myasthenia gravis: executive summary. Neurology. 2016;87(4):419–25.
160. Wolfe GI, et al. Randomized trial of thymectomy in myasthenia gravis. N Engl J Med. 2016;375(6):511–22.
161. Djelmis J, et al. Myasthenia gravis in pregnancy: report on 69 cases. Eur J Obstet Gynecol Reprod Biol. 2002;104(1):21–5.
162. Hoff JM, Daltveit AK, Gilhus NE. Myasthenia gravis in pregnancy and birth: identifying risk factors, optimising care. Eur J Neurol. 2007;14(1):38–43.
163. Massey JM, De Jesus-Acosta C. Pregnancy and myasthenia gravis. Continuum. 2014;20(1):115–27.
164. Durst JK, Rampersad RM. Pregnancy in women with solid-organ transplants: a review. Obstet Gynecol Surv. 2015;70(6):408–18.
165. Gotestam Skorpen C, et al. The EULAR points to consider for use of antirheumatic drugs before pregnancy, and during pregnancy and lactation. Ann Rheum Dis. 2016;75(5):795–810.
166. Perez-Aytes A, et al. In utero exposure to mycophenolate mofetil: a characteristic phenotype? Am J Med Genet A. 2008;146A(1):1–7.
167. Kylat R. What is the teratogenic risk of mycophenolate? J Pediatr Genet. 2017;6(2):111–4.
168. Chakravarty EF, et al. Pregnancy outcomes after maternal exposure to rituximab. Blood. 2011;117(5):1499–506.
169. Varner M. Myasthenia gravis and pregnancy. Clin Obstet Gynecol. 2013;56(2):372–81.
170. Watson WJ, Katz VL, Bowes WA Jr. Plasmapheresis during pregnancy. Obstet Gynecol. 1990;76(3 Pt 1):451–7.
171. Guidon AC, Massey EW. Neuromuscular disorders in pregnancy. Neurol Clin. 2012;30(3):889–911.
172. Clark AL. Clinical uses of intravenous immunoglobulin in pregnancy. Clin Obstet Gynecol. 1999;42(2):368–80.
173. Braga AC, et al. Myasthenia gravis in pregnancy: experience of a portuguese center. Muscle Nerve. 2016;54(4):715–20.
174. Batocchi AP, et al. Course and treatment of myasthenia gravis during pregnancy. Neurology. 1999;52(3):447–52.
175. Ciafaloni E, Massey JM. The management of myasthenia gravis in pregnancy. Semin Neurol. 2004;24(1):95–100.
176. Ohlraun S, et al. Impact of myasthenia gravis on family planning: how do women with myasthenia gravis decide and why? Muscle Nerve. 2015;52(3):371–9.
177. Edmundson C, Guidon AC. Neuromuscular disorders in pregnancy. Semin Neurol. 2017;37(6):643–52.
178. Ducci RD, et al. Clinical follow-up of pregnancy in myasthenia gravis patients. Neuromuscul Disord. 2017;27(4):352–7.
179. Ferrero S, et al. Myasthenia gravis: management issues during pregnancy. Eur J Obstet Gynecol Reprod Biol. 2005;121(2):129–38.
180. Hoff JM, Daltveit AK, Gilhus NE. Myasthenia gravis: consequences for pregnancy, delivery, and the newborn. Neurology. 2003;61(10):1362–6.
181. Benshushan A, Rojansky N, Weinstein D. Myasthenia gravis and preeclampsia. Isr J Med Sci. 1994;30(3):229–33.
182. Piura B. The association of preeclampsia and myasthenia gravis: double trouble. Isr J Med Sci. 1994;30(3):243–4.

183. Naguib M, et al. Multivariate determinants of the need for postoperative ventilation in myasthenia gravis. Can J Anaesth. 1996;43(10):1006–13.

184. Almeida C, et al. Myasthenia gravis and pregnancy: anaesthetic management--a series of cases. Eur J Anaesthesiol. 2010;27(11):985–90.

185. O'Carroll P, et al. Transient neonatal myasthenia gravis in a baby born to a mother with new-onset anti-musk-mediated myasthenia gravis. J Clin Neuromuscul Dis. 2009;11(2):69–71.

186. Niks EH, et al. A transient neonatal myasthenic syndrome with anti-musk antibodies. Neurology. 2008;70(14):1215–6.

187. Townsel C, et al. Seronegative maternal ocular myasthenia gravis and delayed transient neonatal myasthenia gravis. Am J Perinatol Rep. 2016;6(1):e133–6.

188. Ahlsten G, et al. Follow-up study of muscle function in children of mothers with myasthenia gravis during pregnancy. J Child Neurol. 1992;7(3):264–9.

189. Glick RP, Penny D, Hart A. The pre-operative and post-operative management of the brain tumor patient. In: Walsh J, Morantz RA, editors. Brain tumors. New York: Marcel Dekker; 1994. p. 345–66.

190. Doll DC. Management of cancer during pregnancy. Arch Intern Med. 1988;148(9):2058.

191. Sklar CA, et al. Premature menopause in survivors of childhood cancer: a report from the childhood cancer survivor study. JNCI. 2006;98(13):890–6.

192. Amant F, et al. Long-term cognitive and cardiac outcomes after prenatal exposure to chemotherapy in children aged 18 months or older: an observational study. Lancet Oncol. 2012;13(3):256–64.

193. Simon R. Brain tumors in pregnancy. Semin Neurol. 1988;8(3):214–21.

194. Michelsen JJ, New PF. Brain tumour and pregnancy. J Neurol Neurosurg Psychiatry. 1969;32(4):305–7.

195. Cohen-Gadol AA, et al. Neurosurgical management of intracranial lesions in the pregnant patient: a 36-year institutional experience and review of the literature: clinical article. J Neurosurg. 2009;111(6):1150–7.

196. Carroll RS, et al. Androgen receptor expression in meningiomas. J Neurosurg. 1995;82(3):453–60.

197. Carroll RS, Zhang J, Black PM. Expression of estrogen receptors alpha and beta in human meningiomas. J Neurooncol. 1999;42(2):109–16.

198. Pallud J, et al. Pregnancy increases the growth rates of World Health Organization grade II gliomas. Ann Neurol. 2010;67(3):398–404.

199. Effects of antenatal dexamethasone administration in the infant: long-term follow-up. J Pediatr. 1984;104(2):259–67.

200. Evans MI. Pharmacologic suppression of the fetal adrenal gland in utero: attempted prevention of abnormal external genital masculinization in suspected congenital adrenal hyperplasia. JAMA. 1985;253(7):1015.

201. Bain MD, et al. In vivo permeability of the human placenta to inulin and mannitol. J Physiol. 1988;399(1):313–9.

202. Stevenson CB, Thompson RC. The clinical management of intracranial neoplasms in pregnancy. Clin Obstet Gynecol. 2005;48(1):24–37.

203. Ostrom QT, et al. Risk factors for childhood and adult primary brain tumors. Neuro Oncol. 2019;21(11):1357–75.

204. Bondy ML, et al. Genetic epidemiology of childhood brain tumors: genetic epidemiology of CBT. Genet Epidemiol. 1991;8(4):253–67.

205. Ezzat S, et al. The prevalence of pituitary adenomas: a systematic review. Cancer. 2004;101(3):613–9.

206. Gonzalez JG, et al. Pituitary gland growth during normal pregnancy: an in vivo study using magnetic resonance imaging. Am J Med. 1988;85(2):217–20.

207. Casanueva FF, et al. Guidelines of the Pituitary Society for the diagnosis and management of prolactinomas. Clin Endocrinol. 2006;65(2):265–73.

208. Molitch ME. Prolactinoma in pregnancy. Best Pract Res Clin Endocrinol Metab. 2011;25(6):885–96.

209. Molitch ME. Endocrinology in pregnancy: management of the pregnant patient with a prolactinoma. Eur J Endocrinol. 2015;172(5):R205–13.

210. American College of Obstetricians and Gynecologists' Committee on Obstetric Practice. Committee Opinion No. 656 summary: guidelines for diagnostic imaging during pregnancy and lactation. Obstet Gynecol. 2016;127(2):418.

211. de Heide LJ, van Tol KM, Doorenbos B. Pituitary apoplexy presenting during pregnancy. Neth J Med. 2004;62(10):393–6.

212. Raymond JP, et al. Follow-up of children born of bromocriptine-treated mothers. Horm Res. 1985;22(3):239–46.

213. Hirahara F, et al. Hyperprolactinemic recurrent miscarriage and results of randomized bromocriptine treatment trials. Fertil Steril. 1998;70(2):246–52.

214. Chen H, Fu J, Huang W. Dopamine agonists for preventing future miscarriage in women with idiopathic hyperprolactinemia and recurrent miscarriage history. Cochrane Database Syst Rev. 2016.

215. Melmed S, et al. Diagnosis and treatment of hyperprolactinemia: an endocrine society clinical practice guideline. J Clin Endocrinol Metab. 2011;96(2):273–88.

216. Koch-Henriksen N, Sørensen PS. The changing demographic pattern of multiple sclerosis epidemiology. Lancet Neurol. 2010;9(5):520–32.

217. Confavreux C, et al. Rate of pregnancy-related relapse in multiple sclerosis. N Engl J Med. 1998;339(5):285–91.

218. Finkelsztejn A, et al. What can we really tell women with multiple sclerosis regarding pregnancy? A systematic review and meta-analysis of the literature: pregnancy in multiple sclerosis. BJOG. 2011;118(7):790–7.

219. Bove R, et al. Management of multiple sclerosis during pregnancy and the reproductive years: a systematic review. Obstet Gynecol. 2014;124(6):1157–68.
220. Hughes SE, et al. Predictors and dynamics of postpartum relapses in women with multiple sclerosis. Mult Scler J. 2014;20(6):739–46.
221. Devonshire V, et al. The immune system and hormones: review and relevance to pregnancy and contraception in women with MS. Int MS J. 2003;10(2):44–50.
222. Verdru P, et al. Pregnancy and multiple sclerosis: the influence on long term disability. Clin Neurol Neurosurg. 1994;96(1):38–41.
223. Ramagopalan S, et al. Term pregnancies and the clinical characteristics of multiple sclerosis: a population based study. J Neurol Neurosurg Psychiatry. 2012;83(8):793–5.
224. D'hooghe MB, Nagels G, Uitdehaag BMJ. Long-term effects of childbirth in MS. J Neurol Neurosurg Psychiatry. 2010;81(1):38–41.
225. Cavalla P, Gilmore W. Pregnancy in multiple sclerosis: data from an administrative claims database. Neurology. 2018;91(17):771–3.
226. Dahl J, et al. Pregnancy, delivery and birth outcome in different stages of maternal multiple sclerosis. J Neurol. 2008;255(5):623–7.
227. Kelly VM, Nelson LM, Chakravarty EF. Obstetric outcomes in women with multiple sclerosis and epilepsy. Neurology. 2009;73(22):1831–6.
228. van der Kop ML, et al. Neonatal and delivery outcomes in women with multiple sclerosis. Ann Neurol. 2011;70(1):41–50.
229. Vukusic S, et al. Pregnancy and multiple sclerosis (the PRIMS study): clinical predictors of postpartum relapse. Brain. 2004;127(6):1353–60.
230. Ferrero S, Pretta S, Ragni N. Multiple sclerosis: management issues during pregnancy. Eur J Obstet Gynecol Reprod Biol. 2004;115(1):3–9.
231. Freedman MS, et al. Treatment optimization in multiple sclerosis: Canadian MS Working Group Recommendations. Can J Neurol Sci. 2020;47(4):437–55.
232. Ghezzi A, et al. Current recommendations for multiple sclerosis treatment in pregnancy and puerperium. Expert Rev Clin Immunol. 2013;9(7):683–92.
233. Coyle PK, et al. Management strategies for female patients of reproductive potential with multiple sclerosis: an evidence-based review. Mult Scler Relat Disord. 2019;32:54–63.
234. Alroughani R, et al. Pregnancy and the use of disease-modifying therapies in patients with multiple sclerosis: benefits versus risks. Mult Scler Int. 2016;2016:1–8.
235. Lu E, et al. Disease-modifying drugs for multiple sclerosis in pregnancy: a systematic review. Neurology. 2012;79(11):1130–5.
236. Fragoso YD, et al. Long-term use of glatiramer acetate by 11 pregnant women with multiple sclerosis: a retrospective, multicentre case series. CNS Drugs. 2010;24:969–76.
237. Finkelsztejn A, et al. The Brazilian database on pregnancy in multiple sclerosis. Clin Neurol Neurosurg. 2011;113(4):277–80.
238. Salminen HJ, Leggett H, Boggild M. Glatiramer acetate exposure in pregnancy: preliminary safety and birth outcomes. J Neurol. 2010;257(12):2020–3.
239. Coyle PK, et al. Final results from the Betaseron (interferon β-1b) Pregnancy Registry: a prospective observational study of birth defects and pregnancy-related adverse events. BMJ Open. 2014;4(5):e004536.
240. International Multiple Sclerosis Genetics Consortium, et al. Genetic risk and a primary role for cell-mediated immune mechanisms in multiple sclerosis. Nature. 2011;476(7359):214–9.
241. Compston A, Coles A. Multiple sclerosis. Lancet. 2008;372(9648):1502–17.
242. Carton H, et al. Risks of multiple sclerosis in relatives of patients in Flanders, Belgium. J Neurol Neurosurg Psychiatry. 1997;62(4):329–33.

Mode of Delivery in Pregnant Women with Neurological Disorders

2

Jessica C. Fields and Todd Rosen

Introduction

Mode of Delivery in Pregnancy

Delivery options in pregnancy include a vaginal delivery, assisted vaginal delivery with utilization of a vacuum or forceps, or a cesarean delivery. In general, for pregnancies that are low risk, the safest mode of delivery is vaginally, as it is known that cesarean delivery is associated with increased risk of maternal morbidity and mortality [1], especially because of augmented risk from repeat cesarean deliveries in future pregnancies [2]. Over time, countries such as the USA have become witness to a rising cesarean delivery rate, which is in part due to modifiable factors [3, 4]. Therefore, an effort has been set forth to prevent the first cesarean for each patient because it may lead to problems in subsequent pregnancies [5]. Ultimately, optimal mode of delivery should be determined after in-depth multidisciplinary evaluation of potential medical or obstetrical indications and analysis of benefits and risks to each option.

J. C. Fields · T. Rosen (✉)
Division of Maternal-Fetal Medicine, Department of Obstetrics, Gynecology and Reproductive Sciences, Rutgers Robert Wood Johnson Medical School, New Brunswick, NJ, USA
e-mail: rosentj@rwjms.rutgers.edu

Mode of Delivery in Pregnancy Complicated by Neurosurgical Disorders

Management of pregnant women with neurosurgical disorders is difficult, with two lives at stake, and determining optimal mode of delivery can be quite challenging. As in the general population, a vaginal delivery is recommended if minimal risks are at stake. The general consensus is that cesarean delivery should be recommended in cases of obstetric indication or neurologically unstable patients. Otherwise, there is an overall paucity of definitive guidance for neurosurgical patients undergoing labor and delivery.

It is important to understand how pregnancy and labor may contribute to clinically significant changes in the brain to understand the special considerations one must address in the neurosurgical patient. Large hemodynamic changes occur in pregnancy due to high metabolic demand that begin in the first trimester and increase even more during labor and delivery. Such changes includ increased cardiac output and plasma volume with a rise of about 40–50% [6–8] which predispose pregnant women to circulatory issues. Yet, unlike other organs which can accommodate these changes more easily, the brain and cerebral circulation must adapt to maintain homeostasis in ways such as preventing constriction of cerebrovascular circulation and maintaining adequate cerebrovascular resistance and flow in addition to protecting from increases in blood–brain barrier permeability [9]. At the same time, there may be brain changes secondary to hormones such as estrogen, progesterone, and vascular endothelial growth factor [10]. Furthermore, pregnancy may impact blood vessel integrity with an initial higher vascular distensibility that is later replaced by more vulnerable vessel walls that can be damaged by hemodynamic stress [6, 11].

In addition to these vascular changes, studies have focused on characterizing changes in cerebrospinal fluid (CSF) pressure during pregnancy. Marx et al. in the 1960s studied lumbar CSF pressure in pregnancy at rest and in labor and found that increased CSF pressure occurred with contractions and simultaneous panting, bearing down, or changing respiratory function of the patient [12]. Hopkins et al. followed up this study to determine that CSF pressure increased with contractions and pushing as well [13]. These studies suggest that painful contractions and Valsalva can increase intracranial pressure (ICP), potentially worsening an already elevated ICP in a neurosurgical patient [14]. Moreover, mean cerebral blood flow velocity decreases with hyperventilation and increases with blood pressure secondary to pain from uterine contractions [15, 16]. Thus, during labor, the impact of uterine contractions, pain, and pushing with Valsalva on cerebrovascular and pressure dynamics raises concern about the potential for neurological complication.

Anesthesiology in Pregnancy Complicated by Neurosurgical Disorders

In all cases, anesthesiology consultation should be performed pre-delivery to allow for a comprehensive review of prior records including imaging studies. An anesthesia consult is a crucial adjunct to the mode of delivery conversation for patients. General anesthesia concerns include increased ICP, intracranial mass effect, risk for brain herniation, reactions to medications such as succinylcholine, difficulty in performing neuraxial procedures from changes in anatomy, and difficulty in managing the airway [17–20].

Neuraxial anesthesia is usually preferred as long as it is deemed safe and feasible because it provides the best labor pain management and anesthesia for a cesarean delivery. One goal of anesthesia is to minimize pain to mitigate acute changes in CSF pressure. In general, pregnancy may cause a slow rise in baseline lumbar epidural pressure likely from the space-occupying effect of increased blood volume in epidural veins. Evidence shows that those with baseline elevated ICP will have a transient rise in ICP after epidural [20–23] and this may be a source of concern in anesthesia selection. When considering safe placement of neuraxial anesthesia, there should be maintenance of continued CSF flow without large pressure differences between the intracranial and intraspinal compartments to prevent loss of CSF volume through the dural puncture and brain herniation [20].

Cases in which general anesthesia is preferred must be determined; for the most part, pregnant women with altered mental status or inability to cooperate cannot receive neuraxial anesthesia [24]. Furthermore, when considering postpartum or post-operative analgesia, use of acetaminophen and nonsteroidal anti-inflammatory agents can reduce opioid use [25, 26] and other methods such as transverse abdominis plane blocks or catheters can be very effective in these patients if there is no contraindication [27, 28]. Considerations regarding selection of anesthesia and analgesia for pregnant patients is discussed in detail in Chaps. 19 and 20.

While we delineate general recommendations for mode of delivery below, it is important to recognize the need to individualize care with thorough assessment of one's neurosurgical condition before selecting the optimal delivery route. Given variability in neurosurgical disorders and specific clinical scenarios, pregnant women should be evaluated on a case-by-case basis with multidisciplinary collaboration among neurologists, neurosurgeons, obstetricians, and anesthesiologists to determine optimal mode of delivery.

Chiari Malformations (CM)

Delivery Considerations

Chiari malformation (CM) Type I has been the most well studied in pregnant women and will likely be more increasingly common during pregnancy due to the increasing rate of CM diagnosis [29, 30]. Due to limited evidence, there is no established universally accepted protocol guiding mode of delivery or anesthesia type in this population [31, 32]. Careful consideration of delivery route for each patient with CMI should be performed, however, review of the current literature leads us to a recommendation of vaginal delivery for most of these patients.

With CM, there is displacement of the cerebellar tonsils through the foramen magnum with risk for hydrocephalus, syringomyelia, and brainstem compression. Specifically, about 40–50% of those with CM-I will have syringomyelia [33]. Increased ICP and changes in CSF flow augment the risk of herniation or decreased cerebral perfusion pressure [34, 35], which have made selection of optimal delivery mode a challenge. Historically, cesarean delivery was recommended for women with CM-I or syringomyelia due to the perceived exacerbated neurological risks including worsened symptoms during maternal pushing and Valsalva maneuvers with the theoretical risk for a transient increase in ICP to result in a progressive hindbrain herniation over time [33, 36–39]. Symptoms vary but may include weakness, burning pain in the neck or back, parathesias in extremities, and referred chest pain [40, 41] as well as a "tussive headache" [42, 43], and it is important that a symptomatic patient undergo full formal neurological evaluation prior to delivery [39].

Despite historical recommendation for cesarean delivery, many recent case reports and studies provide evidence for uneventful vaginal deliveries in this population [44–46]. For example, Roper et al. performed a 14-year retrospective case series of women with CM and found vaginal delivery to be safe [46]. A recent retrospective cohort study by Knafo et al. showed no increased clinical or radiological neurological compromise in women with CM-I and/or syringomyelia who had a vaginal delivery with neuraxial anesthesia versus those who had a cesarean delivery under general anesthesia [47]. Two additional large case series involving 148 and 63 patients, respectively, found no neurologic deterioration in women undergoing vaginal deliveries [48, 49]. In the latter study, many women experienced symptomatic CM-I such as headaches yet vaginal delivery was not associated with worsening of these symptoms [49]. Moreover, for those undergoing a vaginal delivery, it is reasonable to offer a passive second stage with a vacuum or forceps assisted delivery to avoid risk for increased intracranial pressure with Valsalva [33]. Thus, this emerging body of evidence supporting vaginal delivery challenges the classic recommendation.

It is difficult to determine optimal delivery mode in the other types of CM given the dearth of research and rarity of these types. Due to worsened severity of Types II, III, and IV and concomitant symptoms with possible life-threatening complications, it may be reasonable to consider cesarean section for these patients.

Anesthesia Considerations

Optimal anesthesia for patients with CM continues to be debated. Previously, neuraxial anesthesia was not recommended due to concern for a dural puncture to exacerbate symptoms or cause worsening of tonsillar herniation [47, 50–52]. Traditionally, general anesthesia was the anesthetic of choice for patients with CM in order to prevent changes in CSF pressure and ICP elevation [53, 54]. Some studies have recommended cesarean delivery under general anesthesia to avoid the consequence of dural puncture [39] but other risks with general anesthesia remain, such as difficulties in securing an airway or hyperextension of the neck during intubation which can compress the foramen magnum [33, 52, 55].

Some recent studies suggest no harm with neuraxial anesthesia but given the low rates of dural tears in the general population of about 1–2% [44, 56, 57], more studies with larger case numbers are needed to fully understand risks. Spinal anesthesia has been administered without complication in women with surgically corrected CM I [33, 58, 59]. It is reasonable to provide neuraxial anesthesia to those with asymptomatic type 1 CM [20]. At the same time, there is theoretical concern for neuraxial anesthesia especially in those with uncorrected or symptomatic CMI due to possibility of compression of structures at the level of the foramen magnum or increased ICP [60] and two older case reports have highlighted poor neurological outcomes [51, 52]. Additionally, Choi et al. recommended a combined spinal-epidural as the safest anesthetic procedure [34] but superiority of technique has been difficult to establish [31]. Thus, when taken in sum, it is reasonable to offer neuraxial pain management to this population but anesthesia consultation prior to delivery should be performed due to need for an optimized individualized plan [44]. In general, early pain management has been suggested to promote a successful uncomplicated delivery [33, 34].

Details regarding the evaluation and management of CM in pregnant patients are discussed in Chap. 33.

Spinal Cord Injury (SCI)

Delivery Considerations

We recommend vaginal delivery for pregnancy in women with SCI. Spontaneous vaginal delivery rates vary and an assisted vaginal delivery with forceps or a vacuum may be needed. Approximately 30% of women with SCI need cesarean sections according to some studies [61–64]. Additionally, pre-term labor is controversial in those with SCI with some series reporting comparable numbers to the general population and others seeing increased pre-term delivery, up

to about 20% in one study for example [65]. Episiotomy is not usually advised given possible risk for dehiscence given the sedentary nature of SCI patients [66].

One issue with labor for women with SCI is the inability to detect labor pain which is dependent on the level of the spinal injury; specifically, transection above T10 is associated with unrecognized contractions whereas those with injury below T11 will detect labor pain. Despite the inability for some to feel pain, neuraxial anesthesia is still recommended; providing an early epidural extending to the T10 level may help prevent autonomic dysreflexia (ADR) even if not for pain [67–69]. Pre-hydration is also important before epidurals given the risk for hypotension. Furthermore, women with spinal cord transection above T10 require additional monitoring to prevent an unattended delivery including learning how to palpate the uterus for contractions, obtaining weekly cervical checks, and potentially being hospitalized near term. Additionally, symptoms that are driven by the sympathetic nervous system such as leg spasms, shortness of breath, or increased spasticity should be assessed for as surrogate signs of labor. While in labor, patients should have their position changed frequently along with skin examinations to prevent decubitus ulcer formation. Furthermore, use of an indwelling Foley catheter is helpful to avoid bladder distension and initiation of a bowel regimen is important to prevent constipation [70].

Another issue is risk for autonomic dysreflexia, which most often occurs in labor. Women with SCI should deliver in a unit that can perform invasive hemodynamic monitoring if needed. For patients with baseline pulmonary insufficiency, continuous hemodynamic monitoring with pulse oximetry, arterial line, and electrocardiogram should be performed [71]. For all patients, blood pressure and body temperature monitoring should be performed and monitored closely.

Precautions are particularly important for those with SCI above T5-T6 as they are more likely to deliver earlier (i.e., 36–40 weeks rather than 38–42 weeks) and about 85% develop autonomic dysreflexia in labor [65]. Other than severe hypertension, symptoms such as headache, facial erythema, swealing, arrhythmias, or fetal hypoxia should be monitored for closely. Contractions will exacerbate symptoms.

Anesthesia Considerations

As described above, neuraxial anesthesia is recommended for patients with SCI and is crucial to provide with vaginal delivery to prevent potentially devastating outcomes.

Considerations for the initial evaluation and management of pregnant patients with traumatic brain and spinal cord injury are discussed in Chap. 17.

Guillain-Barre Syndrome

Delivery Considerations

Women with Guillain-Barre Syndrome (GBS) may develop similar problems to those with SCI [72]. There is no reason to perform routine cesarean delivery in cases of GBS, even in women with severe disease. Assisted second stage may be needed for those with significant muscle weakness or lower extremity paralysis. Cesarean delivery should be reserved for obstetrical indications [72, 73].

Anesthesia Considerations

Regional anesthesia is recommended in patients with Guillain-Barre Syndrome [74]. While literature is scant, the limited evidence suggests no worsening or relapse of symptoms with use of neuraxial anesthesia [72]. Additionally, patients may have an amplified hemodynamic response to pain emphasizing the need for optimal pain control [75]. Epidural anesthesia helps to prevent autonomic instability from pain and it has been reported that these patients may

only need a small dose of anesthetic drug [76, 77]. General anesthesia may be considered in cases of respiratory compromise [78]; however, it poses risks such as difficult extubation and autonomic instability. If general anesthesia is necessary, succinylcholine should not be used due to the risk for serious hyperkalemia [72, 79]. Also, nondepolarizing muscle relaxants can cause a prolonged neuromuscular block so they must be used cautiously to prevent need for ventilation [76].

The impact of pregnancy on the clinical course, evaluation, and management of GBS is described in detail in Chap. 22.

Brain Tumors

Delivery Considerations

Literature is limited regarding optimal mode of delivery for pregnant women with brain tumors. Due to concern for raising intracranial pressure with vaginal pushing, cesarean delivery has historically been the preferred mode of delivery [80, 81]. Increased CSF pressure during painful uterine contractions could also lead to neurologic compromise in women who have baseline increased intracranial pressure secondary to a mass [12, 14, 82]. However, there is not enough evidence to make a general recommendation to support the benefit of cesarean section [83–85]. Rather than all women getting a cesarean section, consideration should be individualized based on the location, size of the mass, or need for general anesthesia [86]. One recent study by Girault et al. studied 23 pregnancies in women with brain tumors and while pregnancy outcomes varied, successful vaginal deliveries with epidural anesthesia were described [87]. Some evidence has suggested performing cesarean delivery at the same time as tumor resection to limit the risk of cerebral herniation and anesthesia for select patients [88, 89]. Vaginal delivery is the route of choice for women with microadenomas.

Anesthesia Considerations

Neuraxial anesthesia is not contraindicated in those with space-occupying lesions and both spinal and epidural anesthesia have been successfully performed for women with tumors [87, 90]. An individualized neurology consult should be performed to determine if dural puncture could result in brain herniation. Furthermore, neuroimaging should be reviewed to determine evidence of vasogenic edema, hydrocephalus, effaced cisterns or obstruction of CSF flow that could pose problems for neuraxial anesthesia. If these abnormalities are found and/or there is high risk of brain herniation, neuraxial anesthesia might not be appropriate. The decision for anesthesia in these patients should involve a multidisciplinary approach [20].

Pregnancy-related considerations pertaining to the evaluation and management of brain tumors, generally, and sellar neoplasms, more specifically, are discussed in detail in Chaps. 36 and 37.

Seizure Disorder/Epilepsy

Delivery Considerations

Patients with seizure disorder can labor with cesarean section reserved for the usual obstetric complications [91–93]. There is a higher seizure risk peripartum underscoring the necessity for anti-epileptic (AED) medications to be continued during labor and in the postpartum period. Studies such as the Kerala Registry of Epilepsy and Pregnancy showed that seizure relapse reached peaks the day before delivery, day of delivery, and day following delivery [94]. Studies suggest an approximate incidence of 2% for seizures during labor and this has been attributed to low serum AED concentrations [95, 96]. This further highlights the need for pregnant women to maintain target concentration of AEDs in the third trimester. It would be reasonable for women to bring their own medication for delivery to ensure they are taken at the correctly schedule

times [94]. Furthermore, intravenous medication can be given if oral formulation is not possible.

Anesthesia Considerations

Consultation with anesthesia prior to delivery is imperative to have an optimal pain management plan. Neuraxial anesthesia is recommended if desired by patients. Neuraxial anesthesia with a well-dosed epidural can allow women to rest during the first stage of labor and reduce potential seizure risk from lack of sleep and/or stress [97]. Minimizing external stimulation with appropriate delivery room environment such as dimmed lighting can additionally aid in reduction of sleep deprivation. All involved in the care of these patients should be alert for any signs of seizures to minimize harm to both the patient and fetus.

The approach to management of epilepsy and seizures during pregnancy, including safety guidance pertaining to fetal AED exposure, is presented in Chap. 28.

Cerebrovascular Disease and Malformations of the Brain

Ischemic and Hemorrhagic Stroke

Delivery Considerations

In general, for women who have suffered a stroke during pregnancy, vaginal delivery is preferred with cesarean avoided if possible [98, 99]. Special consideration regarding the optimal timing for delivery may be needed and if both mother and fetus are deemed stable, ideal delivery would involve a controlled induction close to or at term.

Anesthesia Considerations

Determination if neuraxial anesthesia is feasible includes a work-up involving assessment of coagulation status and knowledge of the effect the stroke had on body anatomy and physiology. Pregnant women with a prior or recent stroke may be on anticoagulation or antiplatelet therapy; thus, the Society for Obstetric Anesthesia and

Perinatology (SOAP) and American Society for Regional Anesthesia and Pain Medicine (ASRA) guidelines should be referred to for the selection of safe anesthesia [100, 101]. For women that have been on low-molecular weight heparin during pregnancy, they may switch to the shorter half-life unfractionated heparin in anticipation of delivery [101–103]. It is advised that heparin or other antithrombotic agents be stopped 24 h before induction or labor with the plan to start within 24 h after delivery [104]. Guidelines for the selection of an anticoagulant regimen during pregnancy are provided in Chap. 15.

The approach to evaluation and management of ischemic and hemorrhagic stroke during pregnancy is discussed in Chaps. 6 and 7, respectively.

Intracranial Aneurysm

Delivery Considerations

There is no established evidence-based optimal delivery management for a pregnant woman with an unruptured intracranial aneurysm, however, it is reasonable to offer a vaginal delivery to most of these patients with cesarean delivery reserved for obstetric indication if coordinated between neurosurgery, anesthesiology, and obstetrics. While many studies of pregnant women with aneurysms have shown an increased rate of cesarean deliveries, a large 2013 study by Kim et al. called this higher rate of cesarean deliveries into question. No increased association was reported between pregnancy or delivery and risk of aneurysm rupture [105]. This is controversial with studies suggesting increased hemorrhage risk in pregnancy [106–108] versus other studies showing that aneurysm rupture is not more prevalent in pregnancy [109, 110].

Studies that do support increased hemorrhage risk show increased rupture during pregnancy in the third trimester [107, 111], which may be plausible secondary to hemodynamic changes of pregnancy such as increased plasma volume, increased cardiac output, increased vascular stress on weakened vessel walls, and pregnancy-induced hypertension [112–115]. Some experts suggest that vaginal delivery be reserved for those with previously treated aneurysms due to no increased risk for complications in these patients [113, 116, 117]. Yet, on the contrary, there is limited evidence of maternal or fetal benefit in those who have a cesarean or vaginal delivery in this population [105, 118]. Specific situations may warrant cesarean delivery such as severe neurologic impairment of the mother, diagnosis of the aneurysm at term, aneurysm rupture requiring emergent delivery and surgery, or neurosurgical intervention within the week before delivery [116, 119, 120]. In addition, a patient's future childbearing plans should be considered. Family size should be limited in women who require delivery only by cesarean section because of increasing risk for placenta accreta and other complications with each surgery. The "cure" of cesarean section may be worse than the risk of aneurysm rupture in patients who intend to have large families.

While the evidence in pregnancy is not fully clear, there are studies assessing aneurysm rupture risk in the general population with two notable studies being the International Study of Unruptured Intracranial Aneurysms and the Unruptured Cerebral Aneurysms Study [121, 122]. Both of these studies emphasized the association between larger size (>7 mm) and location in posterior circulation with increased rupture risk [121–123]. Other factors may additionally interact to promote risk of rupture such as prior aneurysmal subarachnoid hemorrhage or familial history of cerebral aneurysms [122, 124]. Neurosurgeons and Maternal-Fetal Medicine Specialists should take these factors into account when making recommendations about mode of delivery.

Anesthesia Considerations

Epidural can be given to patients with brain aneurysms. This technique would allow for control over blood pressure to mitigate acute hemodynamic stress and allow for extended duration of anesthesia [125]. There is theoretical risk of persistent CSF leak and intracranial hypotension after spinal anesthetic or dural puncture with an epidural that could cause a resultant rise in cerebral blood volume and increased pressure across a weak aneurysmal wall, but this has not been reported [20].

The pathway for diagnosis and management of cerebral aneurysms during pregnancy, including a detailed discussion of the rupture risk, is provided in Chap. 8.

Arteriovenous Malformation (AVM)

Delivery Considerations

Pregnant women with AVMs should undergo multidisciplinary counseling to devise an optimal delivery plan. While cesarean delivery has long been utilized for these women [98], vaginal delivery may be the best option. Pregnancy involves increased blood volume and venous blood pressure and while one would think that AVMs would be more likely rupture in this environment, studies have shown similar rates of hemorrhage for AVMs in pregnant versus nonpregnant women. For example, Horton et al. [126] showed in a cohort of 451 women that risk of AVM rupture was similar for pregnant and nonpregnant women. In another retrospective analysis, risk of hemorrhage during pregnancy was not higher compared with the control period [127]. Furthermore, there is no clear evidence that vaginal delivery promotes AVM bleeding and cesarean delivery prevents it. Dias and Sekhar described ruptured AVMs in pregnancy in their study, however only two cases of rupture were during childbirth [111].

The risk of vaginal versus cesarean delivery must be weighed based on hemorrhage risk of AVM. Cerebral imaging may be helpful to determine the exact location and size of the AVM and assess flow rate, venous drainage, arteriovenous fistula, or coexisting aneurysm. Factors associated with increased risk of AVM rupture include deep location, deep venous drainage, arteriovenous fistula, and concomitant aneurysm [128, 129]. Cesarean delivery may seem reasonable in

high-risk AVMs due to enhanced control over maternal blood pressure and intracranial vascular pressure. Additionally, no statistically significant difference in fetal outcome has been shown with either mode of delivery in the setting of AVMs [111].

Pregnant women who have surgically repaired AVMs should not require any special considerations for mode of delivery or anesthetic management. Default should be to offer vaginal delivery to women who have had successful repair of their lesions.

Anesthesia Considerations

Neuraxial anesthesia has been used successfully in patients with AVMs [130–132]. The main goal is to prevent hypertension to reduce risk of increased pressure gradient across the wall of the AVM which might promote rupture [133]. It is additionally suspected that risk of AVM rupture with dural puncture is low likely due to many unknown intracranial lesions and spinal anesthesia being common, despite case reports in the literature of rupture secondary to spinal anesthesia or lumbar puncture [134, 135].

Considerations regarding the evaluation and management of cerebral arteriovenous malformations in pregnancy are discussed in Chap. 9.

Cavernous Malformations

Delivery Considerations

There is no consensus on optimal mode of delivery for those with cavernous malformations (CMs) [136]. In general, given the lack of benefit in cesarean delivery, vaginal delivery should be considered, and the mode of delivery should be made based upon obstetric indications for pregnant women with cavernous malformations.

There are conflicting theories regarding cavernous malformations. Some suggest increased bleeding risk due to hyperdynamic circulation and increased turbulent blood flow and pulse pressure in sinusoids as well as impact from hormonal stimulation such as estrogen and increased growth due to angiogenic processes from growth factors [137–143]. Similarly, there are studies reporting growth of these malformations in pregnancy [144, 145] which might imply increased rupture risk. Yet, many of these mechanisms are unclear [146–148]. There are few cases reports and studies to suggest an association between CMs and bleeding in pregnancy [149, 150]. Case reports of CMs have more frequently suggested cesarean delivery as the optimal method to reduce intracranial hemorrhage from increased intracranial pressure and Valsalva [150, 151].

Despite these ideas, there is lack of data to support increased bleeding in pregnancy [152]. A recent retrospective study involving 214 deliveries of women with known CMs showed no association with additional risk for adverse obstetric outcomes [153]. Another study from 2012 involving 186 patients demonstrated no increased risk of hemorrhage from CMs with pregnancy or delivery [154]. Kalani et al. [155] studied 149 vaginal deliveries in pregnant women with CM and there were no documented hemorrhages. In a more recent study this year, Joseph et al. showed no evidence of hemorrhage during vaginal deliveries in patients with CM [156].

Anesthesia Considerations

Neuraxial anesthesia should be offered to patients with CMs. Reports are limited specifically in addressing risks of anesthesia with CMs, and instead the focus of recent studies has been on risks with mode of delivery. Given that those with CM should be offered a vaginal delivery, epidural is a reasonable option for these patients. Similar to anesthesia for other cerebrovascular diseases, anesthesia for CMs should involve maintenance of hemodynamic stability. Additionally, successful general anesthesia for cesarean delivery in a case of a brainstem CM has been described [151]. There has been suggestion that those with CMs have imaging such as magnetic resonance imaging prior to delivery because patients can have CMs with multiple lesions in the supraspinal area or coexistence in the spinal cord which might complicate neuraxial approaches [157, 158].

Thus, the decision to perform neuraxial anesthesia should involve a multidisciplinary approach.

CMs in pregnancy are discussed in more detail in Chap. 9.

Moyamoya

Delivery Considerations

There is no definitive evidence to recommend route of delivery for pregnant women with Moyamoya. The incidence of stroke during delivery in this population has not been fully delineated [159]. Historically, given concern for cerebral infarction or intracranial hemorrhage and association with high morbidity and mortality, cesarean delivery has been more commonly the method of delivery for those with Moyamoya [15, 16, 160, 161]. The changes in cerebral blood flow including decreased blood flow velocity with hyperventilation and increased velocity with elevated blood pressure from painful, uterine contractions could result in cerebral ischemia [15, 16]. However, because there is no data to support pregnancy increasing the risk for perinatal stroke during delivery in patients with Moyamoya, vaginal delivery under epidural anesthesia may be recommended in those with asymptomatic disease [162]. Small studies and case reports have provided evidence for vaginal delivery with epidural in which no adverse outcomes were seen [159, 163, 164]. Vacuum or forceps have been recommended to shorten the second stage of labor in patients with Moyamoya [165], but these interventions carry risk and data that support this recommendation are limited.

Anesthesia Considerations

As discussed above, vaginal delivery with the use of neuraxial anesthesia has been described. Anesthesia should involve maintenance of normotension and normocapnia to provide optimal delivery outcomes. In general, epidural anesthesia can be offered to these patients if blood pressure is simultaneously maintained in a controlled range: hypotension risks ischemic brain infarction or lower placental perfusion while hypertension can result in hemorrhage [20, 111, 166].

Considerations pertaining to the evaluation and management of Moyamoya disease during pregnancy are described in Chap. 10.

Ventriculoperitoneal Shunt

Delivery Considerations

Vaginal delivery is the mode of delivery of choice despite no controlled studies of the optimal delivery method for pregnant women with ventriculoperitoneal (VP) shunts [167–169]. If the shunt is working properly, there should not be concern for increased ICP during the second stage of labor and thus a shortened second stage is not needed.

If a cesarean delivery is performed for obstetric indications or because a patient is unstable, it is important to prevent movement of the abdominal tip of the shunt when the peritoneal cavity is opened [170]. Infection risk is low in these cases and while there has been debate about use of prophylactic antibiotics for labor and delivery [167], they are generally recommended to prevent shunt infection [168].

Anesthesia Considerations

As for anesthesia considerations, the exact location of the VP shunt must be clear prior to neuraxial attempt. Often, the surgical scar from the shunt procedure provides the location, however, imaging may be needed if records or the physical exam are unclear [171]. For most VP shunts, neuraxial anesthesia is attempted. Reasons for general anesthesia would be due to higher ICP from a poorly functioning shunt or if there is thought that the shunt could be disrupted from a spinal or epidural catheter. An epidural is usually preferred over spinal due to unpredictable shortened duration of action for the spinal secondary to local anesthetic leak through the shunt into the peritoneal cavity. There is always risk that neur-

axial anesthesia will fail or be inadequate in such cases [172].

The approach to the evaluation and management of hydrocephalus in pregnancy, including patients with VP shunts, is provided in Chap. 32.

Idiopathic Intracranial Hypertension (IIH)

Delivery Considerations

Patients with idiopathic intracranial hypertension (IIH) may undergo vaginal delivery, and cesarean delivery should be again reserved for obstetric indications. Labor contractions and Valsalva may contribute to increased CSF pressure, however, evidence has not suggested cesarean delivery reduces the risk of this potential adverse outcome [173–175] and a vaginal-assisted delivery can be performed to reduce risk [176, 177]. Data shows vaginal delivery can occur in patients with papilledema without significant consequence [178].

Anesthesia Considerations

Neuraxial risk is minimal in patients with IIH and such patients are not usually at risk for brain herniation with dural puncture [179–181]. CSF drainage with serial lumbar punctures has been used as treatment for patients with IIH [182, 183]. Pregnant women with IIH may have transient rises in ICP, vision loss, or headache due to many events during labor and delivery such as contractions and pain, Valsalva, or epidural bolus. Evidence shows that continuous spinal, epidural, or combined spinal-epidural anesthesia can be used in those with IIH and help minimize ICP caused by pain and delivery [184, 185] as well as prevent the need for general anesthesia, which often involves a difficult intubation in these patients secondary to comorbid obesity.

Evaluation and management of the pregnant patient with IIH is discussed in detail in Chap. 35.

Conclusion

In summary, each of the above neurosurgical diseases has specific physiologic implications for the route of pregnancy delivery and anesthesia modality. A multidisciplinary approach with individualized assessment is crucial in determining the optimal mode of delivery and anesthesia choice for these pregnant women. Specific scenarios may necessitate prioritizing the neurosurgical state whereas often the decision should rely solely on obstetric indications. Analysis of risks and benefits in each case is needed to guide decision-making.

References

1. Clark SL, Belfort MA, Dildy GA, Herbst MA, Meyers JA, Hankins GD. Maternal death in the 21st century: causes, prevention, and relationship to cesarean delivery. Am J Obstet Gynecol. 2008;199:36.e31–5.
2. Solheim KN, Esakoff TF, Little SE, Cheng YW, Sparks TN, Caughey AB. The effect of cesarean delivery rates on the future incidence of placenta previa, placenta accreta, and maternal mortality. J Matern Fetal Neonatal Med. 2011;24:1341–6.
3. Declercq E, Menacker F, MacDorman M. Rise in "no indicated risk" primary caesareans in the United States, 1991-2001: cross sectional analysis. BMJ. 2005;330:71–2.
4. Declercq E, Menacker F, MacDorman M. Maternal risk profiles and the primary cesarean rate in the United States, 1991–2002. Am J Public Health. 2006;96:867–72.
5. Obstetric Care Consensus No. 1: safe prevention of the primary cesarean delivery. Obstet Gynecol. 2014;123:693–711.
6. Feske SK, Singhal AB. Cerebrovascular disorders complicating pregnancy. Continuum. 2014;20:80–99.
7. San-Frutos L, Engels V, Zapardiel I, et al. Hemodynamic changes during pregnancy and postpartum: a prospective study using thoracic electrical bioimpedance. J Matern Fetal Neonatal Med. 2011;24:1333–40.
8. Sanghavi M, Rutherford JD. Cardiovascular physiology of pregnancy. Circulation. 2014;130:1003–8.
9. Johnson AC, Cipolla MJ. The cerebral circulation during pregnancy: adapting to preserve normalcy. Physiology. 2015;30:139–47.
10. Nevo O, Soustiel JF, Thaler I. Cerebral blood flow is increased during controlled ovarian stimulation. Am J Physiol Heart Circ Physiol. 2007;293:H3265–9.
11. Poppas A, Shroff SG, Korcarz CE, et al. Serial assessment of the cardiovascular system in normal pregnancy: role of arterial compliance and pulsatile arterial load. Circulation. 1997;95:2407–15.
12. Marx GF, Zemaitis MT, Orkin LR. Cerebrospinal fluid pressures during labor and obstetrical anesthesia. Anesthesiology. 1961;22:348–54.
13. Hopkins EL, Hendricks CH, Cibils LA. Cerebrospinal fluid pressure in labor. Am J Obstet Gynecol. 1965;93:907–16.
14. Stevenson CB, Thompson RC. The clinical management of intracranial neoplasms in pregnancy. Clin Obstet Gynecol. 2005;48:24–37.
15. Miyakawa I, Lee HC, Haruyama Y, Mori N, Mikura T, Kinoshita K. Occlusive disease of the internal carotid arteries with vascular collaterals (moyamoya disease) in pregnancy. Arch Gynecol. 1986;237:175–80.
16. Saruki N, Ohtake T, Kawano M, et al. Anesthetic management of the cesarean section in a patient with moyamoya disease. Rinsho Masui. 1990;14:51–3.
17. Anson JA, Vaida S, Giampetro DM, McQuillan PM. Anesthetic management of labor and delivery in patients with elevated intracranial pressure. Int J Obstet Anesth. 2015;24:147–60.
18. Cottrell JE, Hartung J, Giffin JP, Shwiry B. Intracranial and hemodynamic changes after succinylcholine administration in cats. Anesth Analg. 1983;62:1006–9.
19. Kovarik WD, Mayberg TS, Lam AM, Mathisen TL, Winn HR. Succinylcholine does not change intracranial pressure, cerebral blood flow velocity, or the electroencephalogram in patients with neurologic injury. Anesth Analg. 1994;78:469–73.
20. Leffert LR, Schwamm LH. Neuraxial anesthesia in parturients with intracranial pathology. Anesthesiology. 2013;119:703–18.
21. Bromage PR. Continuous lumbar epidural analgesia for obstetrics. Can Med Assoc J. 1961;85:1136–40.
22. Grocott HP, Mutch WA. Epidural anesthesia and acutely increased intracranial pressure. Lumbar epidural space hydrodynamics in a porcine model. Anesthesiology. 1996;85:1086–91.
23. Hilt H, Gramm H-J, Link J. Changes in intracranial pressure associated with extradural anaesthesia. Br J Anaesth. 1986;58:676–80.
24. Miller EC, Leffert L. Stroke in pregnancy: a focused update. Anesth Analg. 2020;130:1085–96.
25. Mkontwana N, Novikova N. Oral analgesia for relieving post-caesarean pain. Cochrane Database Syst Rev. 2015;2015:CD010450.
26. Valentine AR, Carvalho B, Lazo TA, Riley ET. Scheduled acetaminophen with as-needed opioids compared to as-needed acetaminophen plus opioids for post-cesarean pain management. Int J Obstet Anesth. 2015;24:210–6.
27. Abdallah FW, Halpern SH, Margarido CB. Transversus abdominis plane block for postoperative analgesia after caesarean delivery performed

under spinal anaesthesia? A systematic review and meta-analysis. Br J Anaesth. 2012;109:679–87.

28. Krohg A, Ullensvang K, Rosseland LA, Langesæter E, Sauter AR. The analgesic effect of ultrasound-guided quadratus lumborum block after cesarean delivery: a randomized clinical trial. Anesth Analg. 2018;126:559–65.

29. Smith-Bindman R, Miglioretti DL, Johnson E, et al. Use of diagnostic imaging studies and associated radiation exposure for patients enrolled in large integrated health care systems, 1996-2010. JAMA. 2012;307:2400.

30. Wilkinson DA, Johnson K, Garton HJL, Muraszko KM, Maher CO. Trends in surgical treatment of Chiari malformation type I in the United States. J Neurosurg Pediatr. 2017;19:208–16.

31. Janjua MB, Haynie AE, Bansal V, et al. Determinants of Chiari I progression in pregnancy. J Clin Neurosci. 2020;77:1–7.

32. Parfitt SE, Roth CK. Chiari malformation in pregnancy. Nurs Womens Health. 2015;19:177–81.

33. Parker JD, Broberg JC, Napolitano PG. Maternal Arnold-Chiari type I malformation and syringomyelia: a labor management dilemma. Am J Perinatol. 2002;19:445–50.

34. Choi CK, Tyagaraj K. Combined spinal-epidural analgesia for laboring parturient with Arnold-Chiari type I malformation: a case report and a review of the literature. Case Rep Anesthesiol. 2013;2013:1–5.

35. Schijman E. History, anatomic forms, and pathogenesis of Chiari I malformations. Childs Nerv Syst. 2004;20:323–8.

36. Murayama K, Mamiya K, Nozaki K, et al. Cesarean section in a patient with syringomyelia. Can J Anaesth. 2001;48:474–7.

37. Nielsen JL, Bejjani GK, Vallejo MC. Cesarean delivery in a parturient with syringomyelia and worsening neurological symptoms. J Clin Anesth. 2011;23:653–6.

38. Penney DJ, Smallman JMB. Arnold-Chiari malformation and pregnancy. Int J Obstet Anesth. 2001;10:139–41.

39. Sicuranza GB, Steinberg P, Figueroa R. Arnold-Chiari malformation in a pregnant woman. Obstet Gynecol. 2003;102:1191–4.

40. Guyotat J, Bret P, Jouanneau E, Ricci A-C, Lapras C. Syringomyelia associated with type I Chiari malformation a 21-year retrospective study on 75 cases treated by foramen magnum decompression with a special emphasis on the value of tonsils resection. Acta Neurochir. 1998;140:745–54.

41. Heiss JD, Patronas N, DeVroom HL, et al. Elucidating the pathophysiology of syringomyelia. J Neurosurg. 1999;91:553–62.

42. McGirt MJ, Attenello FJ, Atiba A, et al. Symptom recurrence after suboccipital decompression for pediatric Chiari I malformation: analysis of 256 consecutive cases. Childs Nerv Syst. 2008;24:1333–9.

43. Rosen DS, Wollman R, Frim DM. Recurrence of symptoms after Chiari decompression and duraplasty with nonautologous graft material. Pediatr Neurosurg. 2003;38:186–90.

44. Chantigian RC, Koehn MA, Ramin KD, Warner MA. Chiari I malformation in parturients. J Clin Anesth. 2002;14:201–5.

45. Garvey GP, Wasade VS, Murphy KE, Balki M. Anesthetic and obstetric management of syringomyelia during labor and delivery: a case series and systematic review. Anesth Analg. 2017;125:913–24.

46. Roper JC, Al Wattar BH, Silva AHD, Samarasekera S, Flint G, Pirie AM. Management and birth outcomes of pregnant women with Chiari malformations: a 14 years retrospective case series. Eur J Obstet Gynecol Reprod Biol. 2018;230:1–5.

47. Knafo S, Picard B, Morar S, et al. Management of Chiari malformation type I and syringomyelia during pregnancy and delivery. J Gynecol Obstet Hum Reprod. 2021;50:101970.

48. Gruffi TR, Peralta FM, Thakkar MS, et al. Anesthetic management of parturients with Arnold Chiari malformation-I: a multicenter retrospective study. Int J Obstet Anesth. 2019;37:52–6.

49. Waters JFR, O'Neal MA, Pilato M, Waters S, Larkin JC, Waters JH. Management of anesthesia and delivery in women with Chiari I malformations. Obstet Gynecol. 2018;132:1180–4.

50. Barton JJS, Sharpe JA. Oscillopsia and horizontal nystagmus with accelerating slow phases following lumbar puncture in the Arnold-Chiari malformation. Ann Neurol. 1993;33:418–21.

51. Hullander RM, Bogard TD, Leivers D, Moran D, Dewan DM. Chiari I malformation presenting as recurrent spinal headache. Anesth Analg. 1992;75:1025–6.

52. Semple DA, McClure JH, Wallace EM. Arnold-Chiari malformation in pregnancy. Anaesthesia. 1996;51:580–2.

53. Agustí M, Adàlia R, Fernández C, Gomar C. Anaesthesia for caesarean section in a patient with syringomyelia and Arnold-Chiari type I malformation. Int J Obstet Anesth. 2004;13:114–6.

54. Ghaly R, Sauer R, Candido K, Knezevic N. Anesthetic management during cesarean section in a woman with residual Arnold-Chiari malformation type I, cervical kyphosis, and syringomyelia. Surg Neurol Int. 2012;3:26.

55. Mueller D. Pregnancy and Chiari malformation: review of the literature and current recommendations. Chiari Medicine; 2013.

56. Nath S, Koziarz A, Badhiwala JH, et al. Atraumatic versus conventional lumbar puncture needles: a systematic review and meta-analysis. Lancet. 2018;391:1197–204.

57. Pan PH, Bogard TD, Owen MD. Incidence and characteristics of failures in obstetric neuraxial analgesia

and anesthesia: a retrospective analysis of 19,259 deliveries. Int J Obstet Anesth. 2004;13:227–33.

58. Landau R, Giraud R, Delrue V, Kern C. Spinal anesthesia for cesarean delivery in a woman with a surgically corrected type I Arnold Chiari malformation. Anesth Analg. 2003;97:253.

59. Mueller DM, Oro' J. Chiari I malformation with or without syringomyelia and pregnancy: case studies and review of the literature. Am J Perinatol. 2005;22:67–70.

60. Teo MM. Spinal neuraxial anaesthesia for caesarean section in a parturient with type I Arnold Chiari malformation and syringomyelia. SAGE Open Med Case Rep. 2018;6:2050313X1878611.

61. Hughes SJ, Short DJ, Usherwood M, Tebbutt H. Management of the pregnant woman with spinal cord injuries. BJOG. 1991;98:513–8.

62. Slimani O, Jayi S, Fdili Alaoui F, et al. An aggressive vertebral hemangioma in pregnancy: a case report. J Med Case Rep. 2014;8:207.

63. Verduyn WH. Spinal cord injured women, pregnancy and delivery. Spinal Cord. 1986;24:231–40.

64. Wanner MB, Rageth CJ, Zäch GA. Pregnancy and autonomic hyperreflexia in patients with spinal cord lesions. Spinal Cord. 1987;25:482–90.

65. Westgren N, Hultling C, Levi R, Westgren M. Pregnancy and delivery in women with a traumatic spinal cord injury in Sweden, 1980-1991. Obstet Gynecol. 1993;81:926–30.

66. Verduyn WH. Pregnancy and delivery in tetraplegic women. J Spinal Cord Med. 1997;20:371–4.

67. ACOG Committee Opinion Number 275, September 2002: obstetric management of patients with spinal cord injuries, Obstet Gynecol. 2002;100:625–7.

68. Baker ER, Cardenas DD. Pregnancy in spinal cord injured women. Arch Phys Med Rehabil. 1996;77:501–7.

69. Krassioukov A, Warburton DE, Teasell R, Eng JJ. A systematic review of the management of autonomic dysreflexia after spinal cord injury. Arch Phys Med Rehabil. 2009;90:682–95.

70. Pereira L. Obstetric management of the patient with spinal cord injury. Obstet Gynecol Surv. 2003;58:678–86.

71. Greenspoon JS, Paul RH. Paraplegia and quadriplegia: special considerations during pregnancy and labor and delivery. Am J Obstet Gynecol. 1986;155:738–41.

72. Chan LY-S, Tsui MH-Y, Leung TN. Guillain-Barré syndrome in pregnancy. Acta Obstet Gynecol Scand. 2004;83:319–25.

73. Rockel A, Wissel J, Rolfs A. Guillain-Barre syndrome in pregnancy--an indication for caesarian section? J Perinat Med. 1994;22:393–8.

74. Pacheco LD, Saad AF, Hankins GDV, Chiosi G, Saade G. Guillain-Barré syndrome in pregnancy. Obstet Gynecol. 2016;128:1105–10.

75. Wiertlewski S, Magot A, Drapier S, Malinovsky J-M, Péréon Y. Worsening of neurologic symptoms after epidural anesthesia for labor in a Guillain-Barré patient. Anesth Analg. 2004;98:825–7.

76. Brooks H, Christian AS, May AE. Pregnancy, anaesthesia and Guillain Barré syndrome: case report. Anaesthesia. 2000;55:894–8.

77. McGrady EM. Management of labour and delivery in a patient with Guillain-Barré syndrome. Anaesthesia. 1987;42:899.

78. Wexner SD, Martz GM, Matjusko MJ. Neurologic diseases. In: Benumoff JL, editor. Anestheisia and uncommon diseases. Philadelphia: W.B. Saunders; 1998. p. 10–11.

79. Jeffrey M. Feldman, cardiac arrest after succinylcholine administration in a pregnant patient recovered from Guillain-Barré syndrome. Anesthesiology. 1990;72:942–4.

80. Cohen-Gadol AA, Friedman JA, Friedman JD, Tubbs RS, Munis JR, Meyer FB. Neurosurgical management of intracranial lesions in the pregnant patient: a 36-year institutional experience and review of the literature: clinical article. J Neurosurg. 2009;111:1150–7.

81. Glick RP, Penny D, Hart A. The pre-operative and post-operative management of the brain tumor patient. In: Morantz RA, Walsh JW, editors. Brain tumors. New York, NY: Marcel Dekker; 1994. p. 345–66.

82. Ravindra V, Braca J, Jensen R, Duckworth EM. Management of intracranial pathology during pregnancy: case example and review of management strategies. Surg Neurol Int. 2015;6:43.

83. Abd-Elsayed AA, Díaz-Gómez J, Barnett GH, et al. A case series discussing the anaesthetic management of pregnant patients with brain tumours. F1000Res. 2013;2:92.

84. Pallud J, Mandonnet E, Deroulers C, et al. Pregnancy increases the growth rates of World Health Organization grade II gliomas. Ann Neurol. 2010;67:398–404.

85. Peeters S, Pagès M, Gauchotte G, et al. Interactions between glioma and pregnancy: insight from a 52-case multicenter series. J Neurosurg. 2018;128:3–13.

86. Finfer SR. Management of labour and delivery in patients with intracranical neoplasms. Br J Anaesth. 1991;67:784–7.

87. Girault A, Dommergues M, Nizard J. Impact of maternal brain tumours on perinatal and maternal management and outcome: a single referral centre retrospective study. Eur J Obstet Gynecol Reprod Biol. 2014;183:132–6.

88. Tewari KS, Cappuccini F, Asrat T, et al. Obstetric emergencies precipitated by malignant brain tumors. Am J Obstet Gynecol. 2000;182:1215–21.

89. Wu J, Ma Y-H, Wang T-L. Glioma in the third trimester of pregnancy: two cases and a review of the literature. Oncol Lett. 2013;5:943–6.

90. Kasper E, Hess P, Silasi M, et al. A pregnant female with a large intracranial mass: reviewing the evi-

dence to obtain management guidelines for intracranial meningiomas during pregnancy. Surg Neurol Int. 2010;1:95.

91. Hiilesmaa VK. Pregnancy and birth in women with epilepsy. Neurology. 1992;42:8–11.

92. Källén B. A register study of maternal epilepsy and delivery outcome with special reference to drug use. Acta Neurol Scand. 2009;73:253–9.

93. Tomson T, Battino D, Bromley R, et al. Executive summary: management of epilepsy in pregnancy: a report from the international league against epilepsy task force on women and pregnancy. Epilepsia. 2019;60:2343–5.

94. Thomas SV, Syam U, Devi JS. Predictors of seizures during pregnancy in women with epilepsy: epileptic seizures during pregnancy. Epilepsia. 2012;53:e85–8.

95. Katz JM, Devinsky O. Primary generalized epilepsy: a risk factor for seizures in labor and delivery? Seizure. 2003;12:217–9.

96. Sveberg L, Svalheim S, Tauboll E. The impact of seizures on pregnancy and delivery. Seizure. 2015;28:35–8.

97. Huang C-Y, Dai Y-M, Feng L-M, Gao W-L. Clinical characteristics and outcomes in pregnant women with epilepsy. Epilepsy Behav. 2020;112:107433.

98. Camargo EC, Singhal AB. Stroke in pregnancy. Obstet Gynecol Clin N Am. 2021;48:75–96.

99. Shainker SA, Edlow JA, O'Brien K. Cerebrovascular emergencies in pregnancy. Best Pract Res Clin Obstet Gynaecol. 2015;29:721–31.

100. Horlocker TT, Vandermeulen E, Kopp SL, Gogarten W, Leffert LR, Benzon HT. Regional anesthesia in the patient receiving antithrombotic or thrombolytic therapy: American Society of Regional Anesthesia and Pain Medicine evidence-based guidelines (fourth edition). Reg Anesth Pain Med. 2018;43:263–309.

101. Leffert L, Butwick A, Carvalho B, et al. The Society for Obstetric Anesthesia and Perinatology consensus statement on the anesthetic management of pregnant and postpartum women receiving thromboprophylaxis or higher dose anticoagulants. Anesth Analg. 2018;126:928–44.

102. ACOG Practice Bulletin No. 196: thromboembolism in pregnancy. Obstet Gynecol. 2008;132:e1–17.

103. Bates SM, Rajasekhar A, Middeldorp S, et al. American Society of Hematology 2018 guidelines for management of venous thromboembolism: venous thromboembolism in the context of pregnancy. Blood Adv. 2018;2:3317–59.

104. Barghouthi T, Bushnell C. Prevention and management of stroke in obstetrics and gynecology. Clin Obstet Gynecol. 2018;61:235–42.

105. Kim YW, Neal D, Hoh BL. Cerebral aneurysms in pregnancy and delivery: pregnancy and delivery do not increase the risk of aneurysm rupture. Neurosurgery. 2013;72:143–50.

106. Mas J-L, Lamy C. Stroke in pregnancy and the puerperium. J Neurol. 1998;245:305–13.

107. Salonen Ros H, Lichtenstein P, Bellocco R, Petersson G, Cnattingius S. Increased risks of circulatory diseases in late pregnancy and puerperium. Epidemiology. 2001;12:456–60.

108. Simolke GA, Cox SM, Cunningham FG. Cerebrovascular accidents complicating pregnancy and the puerperium. Obstet Gynecol. 1991;78:37–42.

109. Hunt HB, Schifrin BS, Suzuki K. Ruptured berry aneurysms and pregnancy. Obstet Gynecol. 1974;43:827–37.

110. Tiel Groenestege AT, Rinkel GJE, van der Bom JG, Algra A, Klijn CJM. The risk of aneurysmal subarachnoid hemorrhage during pregnancy, delivery, and the puerperium in the utrecht population: case-crossover study and standardized incidence ratio estimation. Stroke. 2009;40:1148–51.

111. Dias MS, Sekhar LN. Intracranial hemorrhage from aneurysms and arteriovenous malformations during pregnancy and the puerperium. Neurosurgery. 1990;27:855–66.

112. Kittner SJ, Stern BJ, Feeser BR, et al. Pregnancy and the risk of stroke. N Engl J Med. 1996;335:768–74.

113. Nelson LA. Ruptured cerebral aneurysm in the pregnant patient. Int Anesthesiol Clin. 2005;43:81–97.

114. Selo-Ojeme DO, Marshman LAG, Ikomi A, et al. Aneurysmal subarachnoid haemorrhage in pregnancy. Eur J Obstet Gynecol Reprod Biol. 2004;116:131–43.

115. Stoodley MA, Macdonald RL, Weir BKA. Pregnancy and intracranial aneurysms. Neurosurg Clin N Am. 1998;9:549–56.

116. Meyers PM, Halbach VV, Malek AM, et al. Endovascular treatment of cerebral artery aneurysms during pregnancy: report of three cases. AJNR Am J Neuroradiol. 2000;21:1306–11.

117. Piotin M, de Souza Filho CB, Kothimbakam R, Moret J. Endovascular treatment of acutely ruptured intracranial aneurysms in pregnancy. Am J Obstet Gynecol. 2001;185:1261–2.

118. Davie CA, O'Brien P. Stroke and pregnancy. J Neurol Neurosurg Psychiatry. 2008;79:240–5.

119. Kopitnik TA, Samson DS. Management of subarachnoid haemorrhage. J Neurol Neurosurg Psychiatry. 1993;56:947–59.

120. Treadwell SD, Thanvi B, Robinson TG. Stroke in pregnancy and the puerperium. Postgrad Med J. 2008;84:238–45.

121. Investigators TUJ. The natural course of unruptured cerebral aneurysms in a Japanese cohort. N Engl J Med. 2012;366:2474–82.

122. Wiebers DO. Unruptured intracranial aneurysms: natural history, clinical outcome, and risks of surgical and endovascular treatment. Lancet. 2003;362:103–10.

123. Chien A, Liang F, Sayre J, Salamon N, Villablanca P, Viñuela F. Enlargement of small, asymptomatic, unruptured intracranial aneurysms in patients with no history of subarachnoid hemorrhage: the dif-

ferent factors related to the growth of single and multiple aneurysms: clinical article. J Neurosurg. 2013;119:190–7.

124. Broderick JP, Brown RD, Sauerbeck L, et al. Greater rupture risk for familial as compared to sporadic unruptured intracranial aneurysms. Stroke. 2009;40:1952–7.

125. Parikh N, Parikh N. Management of anesthesia for cesarean delivery in a patient with an unruptured intracranial aneurysm. Int J Obstet Anesth. 2018;36:118–21.

126. Horton JC, Chambers WA, Lyons SL, Adams RD, Kjellberg RN. Pregnancy and the risk of hemorrhage from cerebral arteriovenous malformations. Neurosurgery. 1990;27:867.

127. Liu X-J, Wang S, Zhao Y-L, et al. Risk of cerebral arteriovenous malformation rupture during pregnancy and puerperium. Neurology. 2014;82:1798–803.

128. Lv X, Wu Z, Jiang C, et al. Angioarchitectural characteristics of brain arteriovenous malformations with and without hemorrhage. World Neurosurg. 2011;76:95–9.

129. Stapf C, Mast H, Sciacca RR, et al. Predictors of hemorrhage in patients with untreated brain arteriovenous malformation. Neurology. 2006;66:1350–5.

130. Elias M, Abouleish E, Bhandari A. Arteriovenous malformation during pregnancy and labor--case review and management. Middle East J Anaesthesiol. 2001;16:231–7.

131. Sharma SK, Herrera ER, Sidawi JE, Leveno KJ. The pregnant patient with an intracranial arteriovenous malformation. Cesarean or vaginal delivery using regional or general anesthesia? Reg Anesth. 1995;20:455–8.

132. Viscomi C, Wilson J, Bernstein I. Anesthetic management of a parturient with an incompletely resected cerebral arteriovenous malformation. Reg Anesth Pain Med. 1997;22:192–7.

133. Carvalho CS, Resende F, Centeno MJ, Ribeiro I, Moreira J. Abordagem anestésica de grávida com malformação arteriovenosa cerebral e hemorragia subaracnoidea durante a gravidez: relato de caso. Rev Bras Anestesiol. 2013;63:223–6.

134. Eggert SM, Eggers KA. Subarachnoid haemorrhage following spinal anaesthesia in an obstetric patient. Br J Anaesth. 2001;86:442–4.

135. von Knobelsdorff G, Paris A. Intrazerebrale Blutung nach Sectio ceasarea in Spinalanästhesie: Koinzidenz oder Kausalität? Anaesthesist. 2004;53:41–4.

136. Xu Y-L, Liu J-T, Song Y-J, et al. Pregnancy combined with epilepsy and cerebral cavernous malformation. Chin Med J. 2017;130:619–20.

137. Aiba T, Tanaka R, Koike T, Kameyama S, Takeda N, Komata T. Natural history of intracranial cavernous malformations. J Neurosurg. 1995;83:56–9.

138. Deutsch H, Jallo GI, Faktorovich A, Epstein F. Spinal intramedullary cavernoma: clinical presentation and surgical outcome. J Neurosurg Spine. 2000;93:65–70.

139. Katayama Y, Tsubokawa T, Maeda T, Yamamoto T. Surgical management of cavernous malformations of the third ventricle. J Neurosurg. 1994;80:64–72.

140. Kiliç T, Pamir MN, Küllü S, Eren F, Ozek MM, Black PM. Expression of structural proteins and angiogenic factors in cerebrovascular anomalies. Neurosurgery. 2000;46:1179–92.

141. Pozzati E, Acciarri N, Tognetti F, Marliani F, Giangaspero F. Growth, subsequent bleeding, and de novo appearance of cerebral cavernous angiomas. Neurosurgery. 1996;38:662–70.

142. Shimizu Y, Nagamine Y, Fujiwara S, Suzuki J, Yamamoto T, Iwasaki Y. An experimental study of vascular damage in estrogen-induced embolization. Surg Neurol. 1987;28:23–30.

143. Zygmunt M, Herr F, Münstedt K, Lang U, Liang OD. Angiogenesis and vasculogenesis in pregnancy. Eur J Obstet Gynecol Reprod Biol. 2003;110:S10–8.

144. Yamasaki T, Handa H, Yamashita J, et al. Intracranial and orbital cavernous angiomas: a review of 30 cases. J Neurosurg. 1986;64:197–208.

145. Zauberman H, Feinsod M. Orbital hemangioma growth during pregnancy. Acta Ophthalmol. 2009;48:929–33.

146. Detwiler PW, Porter RW, Zabramski JM, Spetzler RF. De novo formation of a central nervous system cavernous malformation: implications for predicting risk of hemorrhage: case report and review of the literature. J Neurosurg. 1997;87:629–32.

147. Moriarity JL, Wetzel M, Clatterbuck RE, et al. The natural history of cavernous malformations: a prospective study of 68 patients. Neurosurgery. 1999;44:1166–71.

148. Zabramski JM, Wascher TM, Spetzler RF, et al. The natural history of familial cavernous malformations: results of an ongoing study. J Neurosurg. 1994;80:422–32.

149. Porter RW, Detwiler PW, Spetzler RF, et al. Cavernous malformations of the brainstem: experience with 100 patients. J Neurosurg. 1999;90:50–8.

150. Yamada S, Nakase H, Nakagawa I, Nishimura F, Motoyama Y, Park Y-S. Cavernous malformations in pregnancy. Neurol Med Chir. 2013;53:555–60.

151. Hayashi M, Kakinohana M. Obstetric anesthesia for a pregnant woman with brainstem cavernous malformations: a case report. A A Case Rep. 2017;9:54–6.

152. Merlino L, Del Prete F, Titi L, Piccioni MG. Cerebral cavernous malformation: management and outcome during pregnancy and puerperium. A systematic review of literature. J Gynecol Obstet Hum Reprod. 2021;50:101927.

153. Maor GS, Faden MS, Brown R. Prevalence, risk factors and pregnancy outcomes of women with vascular brain lesions in pregnancy. Arch Gynecol Obstet. 2020;301:665–70.

154. Witiw CD, Abou-Hamden A, Kulkarni AV, Silvaggio JA, Schneider C, Wallace MC. Cerebral cavernous malformations and pregnancy. Neurosurgery. 2012;71:626–31.

155. Kalani MYS, Zabramski JM. Risk for symptomatic hemorrhage of cerebral cavernous malformations during pregnancy: clinical article. J Neurosurg. 2013;118:50–5.
156. Joseph NK, Kumar S, Brown RD, Lanzino G, Flemming KD. Influence of pregnancy on hemorrhage risk in women with cerebral and spinal cavernous malformations. Stroke. 2021;52:434–41.
157. De Jong A, Benayoun L, Bekrar Y, Forget S, Wernet A. Anesthésie obstétricale chez des patientes porteuses de cavernomes cérébraux : à propos de deux cas. Annales Françaises d'Anesthésie et de Réanimation. 2012;31:635–7.
158. Gross BA, Du R, Popp AJ, Day AL. Intramedullary spinal cord cavernous malformations. Neurosurg Focus. 2010;29:E14.
159. Sato K, Yamada M, Okutomi T, et al. Vaginal delivery under epidural analgesia in pregnant women with a diagnosis of moyamoya disease. J Stroke Cerebrovasc Dis. 2015;24:921–4.
160. Hashimoto K, Fujii K, Nishimura K, Kibe M, Kishikawa T. Occlusive cerebrovascular disease with moyamoya vessels and intracranial hemorrhage during pregnancy. Neurol Med Chir. 1988;28:588–93.
161. Kato R, Terui K, Yokota K, Nakagawa C, Uchida J, Miyao H. Anesthetic management for cesarean section in moyamoya disease: a report of five consecutive cases and a mini-review. Int J Obstet Anesth. 2006;15:152–8.
162. Amias AG. Cerebral vascular disease in pregnancy I. Haemorrhage. BJOG. 1970;77:100–20.
163. Sei K, Sasa H, Furuya K. Moyamoya disease and pregnancy: case reports and criteria for successful vaginal delivery. Clin Case Rep. 2015;3:251–4.
164. Tanaka H, Katsuragi S, Tanaka K, et al. Vaginal delivery in pregnancy with moyamoya disease: experience at a single institute: pregnancy with moyamoya disease. J Obstet Gynaecol Res. 2015;41:517–22.
165. Sasaki J, Mesaki N. Pregnancy and delivery in a patient with moyamoya disease (in Japanese). Sanka To Fujinka. 1984;1:109–16.
166. Komiyama M, Yasui T, Kitano S, Sakamoto H, Fujitani K, Matsuo S. Moyamoya disease and pregnancy: case report and review of the literature. Neurosurgery. 1998;43:360–8.
167. Landwehr JB Jr, Isada NB, Pryde PG, Johnson MP, Evans MI, Canady AI. Maternal neurosurgical shunts and pregnancy outcome. Obstet Gynecol. 1994;83:134–7.
168. Maheut-Lourmière J, Chu Tan S. [Hydrocephalus during pregnancy with or without neurosurgical history in childhood. Practical advice for management]. Neurochirurgie. 2000;46:117–21.
169. Yu JN. Pregnancy and extracranial shunts: case report and review of the literature. J Fam Pract. 1994;38:622–6.
170. Littleford JA, Brockhurst NJ, Bernstein EP, Georgoussis SE. Obstetrical anesthesia for a parturient with a ventriculoperitoneal shunt and third ventriculostomy. Can J Anesth. 1999;46:1057–63.
171. Bedard JM, Richardson MG, Wissler RN. Epidural anesthesia in a parturient with a lumboperitoneal shunt. Anesthesiology. 1999;90:621–3.
172. Kaul B, Vallejo MC, Ramanathan S, Mandell GL, Krohner RG. Accidental spinal analgesia in the presence of a lumboperitoneal shunt in an obese parturient receiving enoxaparin therapy. Anesth Analg. 2002;95:441–3.
173. Bagga R, Jain V, Das CP, Gupta KR, Gopalan S, Malhotra S. Choice of therapy and mode of delivery in idiopathic intracranial hypertension during pregnancy. MedGenMed. 2005;7:42.
174. Digre KB, Varner MW, Corbett JJ. Pseudoturnor cerebri and pregnancy. Neurology. 1984;34:721.
175. Koontz WL, Herbert WNP, Cefalo RC. Pseudotumor cerebri in pregnancy. Obstet Gynecol. 1983;62:324–7.
176. Gumma AD. Recurrent benign intracranial hypertension in pregnancy. Eur J Obstet Gynecol Reprod Biol. 2004;115:244.
177. Peterson CM, Kelly JV. Pseudotumor cerebri in pregnancy. Case reports and review of literature. Obstet Gynecol Surv. 1985;40:323–9.
178. Huna-Baron R, Kupersmith MJ. Idiopathic intracranial hypertension in pregnancy. J Neurol. 2002;249:1078–81.
179. Bedson CR, Plaat F. Benign intracranial hypertension and anaesthesia for caesarean section. Int J Obstet Anesth. 1999;8:288–90.
180. Karmaniolou I, Petropoulos G, Theodoraki K. Management of idiopathic intracranial hypertension in parturients: anesthetic considerations. Can J Anesth. 2011;58:650.
181. Kim K-M, Orbegozo M. Epidural anesthesia for cesarean section in a parturient with pseudotumor cerebri and lumboperitoneal shunt. J Clin Anesth. 2000;12:213–5.
182. Fields JD, Javedani PP, Falardeau J, et al. Dural venous sinus angioplasty and stenting for the treatment of idiopathic intracranial hypertension. J Neurointerven Surg. 2013;5:62–8.
183. Wall M. Idiopathic intracranial hypertension. Neurol Clin. 2010;28:593–617.
184. Kassam SH, Hadi HA, Fadel HE, Sims W, Jay WM. Benign intracranial hypertension in pregnancy: current diagnostic and therapeutic approach. Obstet Gynecol Surv. 1983;38:314–21.
185. Palop R, Choed-Amphai E, Miller R. Epidural anesthesia for delivery complicated by benign intracranial hypertension. Anesthesiology. 1979;50:159–60.

Neuroimaging in the Pregnant Patient

3

Sri Hari Sundararajan, Srirajkumar Ranganathan,
Sanjeev Sreenivasan, Gaurav Gupta,
and Sudipta Roychowdhury

Neuroimaging in the pregnant patient is tailored to evaluating the neuraxis of either the patients themselves or their underlying gestation(s). Imaging indications can range from outpatient follow-up and pre-scheduled gestational anatomic surveys to emergent indications affecting either the expectant patient or fetus.

This chapter will review basic principles of neuroimaging relevant to this unique population, highlight theoretical concepts of image acquisition unique to each imaging modality potentially unfamiliar to physicians without a radiologic training background, summarize guidelines regarding imaging indications, and showcase select commonly identified conditions pertaining to their neuroimaging manifestations encountered in clinical practice. These points will be covered in sections reviewing available imaging modalities and commonly seen neuroimaging indications in the pregnant patient and the underlying gestation.

Section 1: Cross-Sectional Imaging Modalities and Principles of Use

Ultrasound

Ultrasound has been utilized in obstetric evaluation for more than 60 years [1, 2]. Its ubiquitous implementation widely permeates across all fields of Medicine, provides tomographic images that can be acquired and interpreted in real time, and is relatively inexpensive compared to the total costs required for CT and MRI maintenance and use. Additionally, relative to other cross-sectional imaging modalities, ultrasound is portable and is without radiation risk to the pregnant patient or the underlying gestation(s). The technology involves utilization of mechanical sound waves that are used travel through mediums of varying elasticity. These emitted waves are subsequently detected for alterations on their return to ascertain structural properties of the imaged target object. Sound waves are generated following passage of oscillating electric currents

S. H. Sundararajan (✉)
Department of Radiology, Rutgers Robert Wood Johnson Medical School, New Brunswick, NJ, USA

S. Ranganathan
Department of Radiology, Northwestern University Feinberg School of Medicine, Chicago, IL, USA

S. Sreenivasan
Cerebrovascular & Endovascular Neurosurgery, Robert Wood Johnson Medical School, Rutgers University, New Brunswick, NJ, USA
e-mail: sa2034@rwjms.rutgers.edu

G. Gupta
Neurosurgery, Rutgers Robert Wood Johnson Medical School, New Brunswick, NJ, USA
e-mail: guptaga@rutgers.edu

S. Roychowdhury
Neuroradiology, University Radiology, New Brunswick, NJ, USA
e-mail: sroychowdhury@univrad.com

© The Author(s), under exclusive license to Springer Nature Switzerland AG 2023
G. Gupta et al. (eds.), *Neurological Disorders in Pregnancy*,
https://doi.org/10.1007/978-3-031-36490-7_3

through piezoelectric crystals—the most common of which is lead zirconate titatanate (PZT). These crystals are embedded within ultrasound probes and result in the creation of sound waves of varying frequency type depending on crystal arrangement and electric current oscillation. Frequency is defined as the number of times the wave oscillates above and below its baseline axis per second (Hertz of Hz). Ultrasound frequencies are three orders of magnitude higher than the audible range to humans (ultrasound frequency between 1 and 20 MHz versus audible frequency between 20 Hz and 20 kHz) [3, 4].

The emitted waves are compressed or elongated (also known as rarefaction) during their delivery to and arrival from an imaged object, with these changes referred to as a sound wave's wavelength. Wavelength (lambda or λ) is inversely proportional to ultrasound frequency (f) and directly proportional to speed of propagation in a given medium (c). In short, $f = c/\lambda$, with c equaling 1540 m/s in standard soft tissues. These principles of ultrasound also allow for quantification of absolute blood flow velocities via Doppler [3, 4].

Sound wave height (i.e., amplitude) determines the strength and intensity of the resultant image. Certain mediums result in either significant disruption (i.e., attenuation) or propagation of sound waves and are dictated by fixed attenuation coefficients (alpha or α). Aerated lung (α >34) and corticated bone (α ~20) have high attenuation coefficients and therefore prevent passage of ultrasound waves. Water and blood (α ~0.18) possess low attenuation coefficients, and therefore allow passage of ultrasound waves without significant alteration in amplitude. These properties are of vital importance, as the soft-tissue properties of the abdominal compartment and pelvic viscera respectively allow for excellent visualization of the neuraxis of a growing fetus via either transabdominal or transvaginal approaches respectively (noting that air in overlying bowel gas may limit transabdominal sonography due to its high attenuation coefficient) [3, 4].

Thermal effects of ultrasound pertain to tissues or water absorbing ultrasound energy with increases in temperature. Mechanical effects pertain to the formation, growth, and dynamic behavior of gas bubbles formed when dissolved gases come out of solution due to local heat caused by sound energy. The manifestations of these effects are reflected in the Mechanical Index (MI) and Thermal Index (TI), respectively. These indices represent ratios of total acoustic power that needed to raise the maximum temperature by 1 °C (TI) or cause cavitation-related bioeffects (MI). Different tissues have different thermal and mechanical indices and indicate the potential for heating and cavitary microbubble creation within objects beyond the transducer [5].

In the USA, the FDA mandates the MI be less than 1.9 for all ultrasound exams [6]. For all prenatal imaging performed in the pregnant patient, MI values lower than 0.4 are recommended in the setting of pre-existing gas bodies to prevent further microbubble formation. TIs less than 0.5 are recommended, especially in the first trimester. TI values between 0.5 and 1 should be limited to scanning times less than 30 min. TI values greater than 2.5 should be limited to scanning times less than 1 min [7]. These indices are of importance in regard to fetal imaging, as non-human experiments have found that increases of greater than 4 °C for longer than 5 min can result in developmental abnormalities in fetal tissues [8]. High frequency ultrasound (HIFU) makes use of these mechanical-thermal properties of concentrated ultrasound waves and has been employed in therapeutic soft tissue ablations [9].

Fetal anatomy is typically evaluated by ultrasound during the end of first trimester/beginning of second trimester, typically starting at the 18 weeks of gestational age. The examination serves many purposes, providing information regarding gestational age, number of fetuses, orientation of placenta, and ability to initially screen for fetal malformations. When performing obstetric sonographic examinations, picking a fixed point for standardization of transducer alignment is important. The sonographer from this reference point then achieves multiplanar imaging in the axial, coronal, and sagittal planes accordingly. In the case of cranially directed neurosonography, the transducer is typically aligned with the sutures and fontanelle prior to examination of the intracranial contents [10].

With regard to the neurological portion of the ultrasound evaluation, the following structures are consistently evaluated for on ultrasound examination: lateral cerebral ventricles, choroid plexus, midline falx, cavum septum pellucidum, cerebellum, cisterna magna, and upper lip. Measurement of the nuchal fold is also useful when recorded between 16 and 20 weeks gestational in the assessment of aneuploidy risk. Examples of specific conditions that can be diagnosed with sonography in the fetus will be discussed in the following subsections [10].

Computed Tomography (CT)

Ionizing radiation dose exposures from diagnostic imaging during pregnancy can be a cause of concern to both referrers and patients. Following plain radiography or CT during early pregnancy, one study showed 6 of 208 family medicine physicians recommended termination of pregnancy after a first trimester radiograph or CT while 25 of the same 208 physicians were unsure regarding after-effects following a CT exam. Similarly, in this same study, 5 of 65 obstetricians recommended pregnancy termination following a first trimester CT scan [11]. Another study stated that 3/4th of surveyed emergency room physicians underestimated radiation dose from a CT scan and a scan's potential for increased cancer risk [12]. These public and medical community fears of ionizing radiation exposure to an intrauterine gestation after imaging should not be underestimated. As such, guidelines based on a combination of environmental exposures and clinical data dictate minimum levels of radiation exposure allowable in the general population, healthcare providers, and special populations (including pregnant patients).

Risks following ionizing radiation exposure are related to stage of fetal development, dose of exposure, and targeted location with the period of greatest sensitivity being first trimester fetal organogenesis. Dose from scatter radiation to areas outside the field of view are clinically insignificant to a fetus given the combination of scatter low penetration and abdominal lead or bismuth shielding employed during CT acquisition [13]. Based on such data, radiation exposures less than 5 rad have not been associated with increases in fetal anomalies or loss of pregnancy. Head CT examination results in a fetal exposure of less than 1 rad, noting that this is further reduced with the use of abdominal lead shielding. Childhood cancer development in utero from ionizing radiation is of equal concern. One in 2000 children exposed to ionizing radiation will develop leukemia, compared to the natural background rate of 1 in 3000. Although carcinogenesis risk is slightly higher, this was estimated to be no more than 1 in 1000 children for every 1 rad (i.e., 10 mSv) of exposure [14–16].

Iodinated contrast crosses the placental barrier and may depress fetal and neonatal thyroid activity. As such, contrast-enhanced imaging is seldom performed in the pregnant patient. One single high-dose of in utero exposure to iodinated IV contrast is unlikely to show any clinically apparent effect on the child's thyroidal function at birth [16, 17]. Nevertheless, neonatal thyroid function testing is recommended during the first week following delivery if iodinated contrast had been given during pregnancy, as studies have shown hospitalized post-natal and premature infants exposed to iodinated contrast are at risk of hypothyroidism [16, 18].

Neuroimaging of the pregnant patient typically does not include the abdominal compartment given this is outside the field of view needed for evaluation of the brain, head and neck, and cervical spine. However, thoracic, lumbar, or sacral region CT imaging potentially includes exposure to the abdominal compartment. As such, a brief discussion of radiation dose basics and relevant information pertaining to stochastic and deterministic radiation risks is warranted for a better understanding and allowance of informed consent in the event a provider needs to have such discussions with a pregnant patient.

In the early 1980s, the yearly per individual radiation dose was 3.6 mSv averaged over the

U.S. population. Medical radiation contributed only 0.54 mSv to this annual dose, with the remainder coming from radon, soil, construction materials, and cosmic rays. In 2006, medical radiation contributed 3 mSv to the annual dose. This raised the per individual dose to 6.2 mSv averaged over the U.S. population.

The national contributors to annual radiation exposure in descending order: Radon > CT > Nuclear Medicine > Occupational/Environmental. Brenner and Hall in 2007 reported in the New England Journal of Medicine on the relationship between CT scans, corresponding increase in radiation exposure, and increased cancer risk in adults and children. The paper cites an estimate of 1.5%–2% of all cancers from radiation maybe attributable to radiation from CT studies [19].

Awareness of dose specific terms is useful in differentiating the meaning behind reported numbers in any given diagnostic test. Absorbed Dose is the energy deposited in tissue per unit mass of tissue. In CT, absorbed dose is measured using an ionization chamber and phantoms. The unit is the Gray (Gy), with 1 Gy being equal to 1 J/kg. Doses for diagnostic studies are measured in milliGray (mGy). Equivalent dose is a measure of the absorbed dose to a specific tissue, allowing for relative biological effects. Equivalent dose (HT) = Absorbed Dose to Tissue (DT) × Radiation Weighting Factor (WR), noting that the WR for photons utilized in CT examinations is equal to 1. The unit is the Sievert (Sv). Effective dose is a single number accounting for the stochastic effects of non-uniform exposure to ionizing radiation. Effective dose = Equivalent dose (HT) × Tissue Weighting Factor (WT), noting that the WT for most organs is 0.12. Its unit is also the Sievert (Sv) [20].

CTDIvol is an estimate of a patient's absorbed dose in CT. It is reported as mGy. Dose-Length Product (DLP) is the product of CTDIvol and Scan Length (cm). It is reported as mGy cm. DLP values (mGy cm) are converted into Effective Dose (mSv) by multiplying the DLP to conversion factors published by the American Association of Physicists in Medicine: Chest: 0.014 mSv/mGy cm, Abdomen: 0.015 mSv/mGy cm, Pelvis: 0.015 mSv/mGy cm. Conversion of DLP values from mGy cm to Effective Dose is how an approximate whole-body dose from partial body exposure is extrapolated in various research studies. The Effective Dose (mSv) is a number approximating whole-body dose from non-uniform partial-body exposure. It is extrapolated in various research studies. A non-contrast head CT effective dose is average 2 mSV (range 0.9–4 mSV), compared to a chest CT angiogram for pulmonary embolism evaluation average of 15 mSV (range 13–40 mSV), noting that these mSV values continue to be lowered and optimized with advancing technologies [21].

The seventh iteration of United States' National Academies report published in 2005 extrapolated biological effects of ionizing radiation from exposure to ≤100 mSv and is referred to as the BEIR VII report. These estimations of solid cancers and leukemia stem mainly from the Hiroshima-Nagasaki Atomic Bomb survivors of 1945, though other sources include survivors of the Chernobyl Nuclear Accident of 1986, similar accidental radioactive release incident, and patients of medical imaging. The Linear-No-Threshold Model (LNTM) is a linear response model correlating radiation exposure and cancer development used in BEIR VII to develop future risks of developing cancer [14].

In a lifetime, approximately 42 in 100 patients (42%) will be diagnosed with cancer from causes unrelated to radiation. Approximately 1 in 100 patients (1%) are expected to develop solid cancer or leukemia from a single exposure of 100 mSv. Lower doses produce proportionally lower risks, noting that it is predicted that 1 individual in 1000 could develop cancer from a single exposure to 10 mSv [14]. The accuracy of these conclusions and linearly extrapolating biological effects from exposure from ≤100 mSv remains controversial however and continues to be scrutinized [22].

Children are more sensitive to radiation effects than adults. Children have a longer life expectancy than adults, resulting in a longer time-period for expressing radiation damage. Children may receive a higher radiation dose than necessary if CT settings are not adjusted for body size or gravid uterus. As such, the risk for developing radiation-related cancer and growth deficits from in-utero exposure can be several times higher for a fetus or young child compared with a non-pregnant adult exposed to a similar CT scan [23].

The risks and benefits of any imaging study must be considered. CT can be a life-saving tool, with high diagnostic accuracy and ability to arrive at rapid diagnoses. However, anywhere from 5% to 30% of CT exams have been reported medically unnecessary. Substitution of ionizing radiation based imaging with MRI, Ultrasound, or no medical imaging should be practiced when clinically possible and appropriate. The concept of "As Low As Reasonably Achievable" (ALARA) involves minimizing imaging-related radiation and release of radioactive materials and is often invoked when imaging pregnant patients or similar special populations. Therefore, when the benefits of CT imaging outweigh associated individual risks for medically indicated studies, the lowest possible dose while maintaining diagnostic accuracy should be pursued [24, 25].

CT is not indicated for evaluation of the fetal neuraxis. Risk of fetal outcomes such as prenatal death, growth retardation, organ malformation, head size, and cancer induction are associated with certain dose thresholds throughout fetal development, but specific periods of development pose even higher risk and lower dose thresholds [15]. However, in times of emergency or trauma afflicting the carrying host, fetal inclusion in the field of view may be unavoidable. CT utility is more applicable in initial evaluation of potential neurological pathologies in the pregnant patient. Examples of specific conditions will be discussed in following subsections.

Magnetic Resonance Imaging (MRI)

MRI utilizes a combination of induced magnetic fields and radiofrequency (RF) waves for the purpose of manipulating hydrogen nuclei orientations in order to generate composite images matching their emitted source's macroscopic appearance. As the human body is primarily made up of water, MRI works well in imaging viscera and soft tissues, particularly elements of the neuraxis. Intra-uterine gestations are especially well imaged given the high water content of fetuses and their respective pathologies [26]. In this discussion, the technique for acquiring traditional spin-echo MRI images will first be reviewed.

The unit Tesla (T) denotes the magnetic field strength, with commercially available magnets most frequently either 1.5 or 3 T. Lower-field strength magnets referred to as open-bore MRIs are available and are advantageous for patients unable to undergo image acquisition due to claustrophobic reactions or in larger or obese patients who cannot fit on standard MRI tables [27]. However, their image quality is significantly less compared to standard 1.5 or 3 T [28]. As such all fetal MRI should be performed on a minimum of 1.5 T, though the standard use of 3 T magnets continues to gain traction given their wider availability, improving strategies to resolve artifacts associated with higher field strengths, and generation of images with greater signal-to-noise ratios while maintaining comparable acquisition speeds relative to 1.5 T magnets [29–31].

Following hydrogen nuclei realignment by an external magnetic field (denoted as beta or β), RF waves are delivered to excite nuclei into opposite planes of orientation, typically into the transverse plane with a 90-degree RF pulse. These excited nuclei spin (or precess) around their new axis similar to a spinning top, eventually returning to their natural state. This Larmor precession (denoted as gamma or γ) is influenced by external magnetic fields and is measured as a function of nuclear rotation rate (measured as angular frequency and denoted as omega or ω). The Larmor equation dictates this relationship: $\omega = \gamma\beta$. The energy released during precession of the hydrogen nuclei is recorded and fill designated spaces encoded in either 2D or 3D arrays known as k-spaces. Data in these k-spaces are then processed and converted into stripe patterns via inverse Fourier transformations, a mathematical transformation named after French mathematician Jean Baptise Joseph Fourier (1786–1830). The resultant stripes possess unique densities, phasicities, angles, and amplitudes that are then summated into recognizable anatomic images [32–34].

Certain time variables are present in this imaging process that dictate the type of MRI sequence performed, two of which are inherent properties of the imaged body part and two of which are properties controlled at the time of image acquisition. T2 refers to the time taken for an excited hydrogen nucleus to lose 37% of its energy from the transverse plane after the 90-degree RF pulse delivery noted above. T1 refers to the flipped vantage point of this transverse magnetization loss and measures the time taken for the precessed hydrogen nucleus to return to 63% of its baseline longitudinal magnetization. Different tissues have different T1 properties, noting that larger magnetic field strengths lengthen individual tissues' T1 properties [32–34].

The echo time (TE) describes the time between hydrogen nucleus resting state and induction into its excited state following RF pulse delivery. The repetition time (TR) describes the time between the excited hydrogen nucleus having achieved its new excitatory precession state to the time taken to complete release of its energy and return to its initial resting state. The TR can be lengthened by delivery of 180-degree RF pulses before complete relaxation of the hydrogen nuclei is achieved, as this re-orients the nuclei into their opposite longitudinal axis. This provides more time for the nucleus to precess, release energy, and fill more arrays in a given k-space accordingly [32–34].

The two basic MRI images types are T1-weighted images and T2-weighted images, with differences in TEs and TRs implemented during scan acquisition dictating the type of image generated. T1-weighted images possess short TR (between 250 and 700 milliseconds or ms) and short TE (10–25 ms), while T2-weighted images possess long TR (greater than 2000 ms) and long TE (greater than 60 ms). The eventual loss of a nucleus's excitatory state is due to inhomogeneities in the external field and local magnetic fields of imaged tissues that predispose all excited nuclei to return to their resting longitudinal plane. Therefore, tissues with less inhomogeneity—such as cerebrospinal fluid (CSF) and fluids of water consistency—take longer to decay their transverse magnetization and are therefore bright on T2-weighted images [32–34].

The primary sequence of fetal MRI is the single shot sequence of the fetal brain, spine, and whole body performed in sagittal, coronal and axial planes. This is an ultra-fast spin echo sequence utilized for the purpose of obtaining anatomic details in structures with unavoidable or unpredictable motion degradation, as often exhibited by intrauterine gestation(s). In our institution, this is performed with both low (62 ms) and high (95 ms) Time-to-Echo (TE) values. These are images with T2-weighted properties that are rapidly acquired by maximizing k-space data through successive delivery of shortly spaced 180-degree RF pulses to obtain as much signal as possible in a single TR period. Body coils are placed on patients to further improve signal-to-noise (SNR) and reduce local field inhomogeneities [32–34].

In contrast to traditional spin-echo images described above, gradient echo images are generated following delivery of smaller flip-angles (ranging between 10° and 80° depending on the sequence) rather than traditional 90-degree RF pulses. Although this results in smaller energy spikes relative to spin-echo images, the TE and TR times used in these sequences are magnitudes smaller than spin echo images, with short TEs ranging between 1 and 5 ms, long TEs considered >10 ms, short TRs <50 ms, and long TRs considered >100 ms. The rapidity of acquisition makes these sequences of equal importance in the performance of fetal MRI. Gradient T1-weighted images are used to detect areas of fat, hemorrhage, calcium, and proteinaceous fluid in fetal MRIs, as these materials are usually bright on T1 weighted images. This property is used to replace dedicated susceptibility-weighted imaging that is difficult to perform during fetal MRI acquisition, noting that this technique will be discussed again shortly [32–34].

Fetal MRI gradient sequences are performed in our institution in the axial, coronal, and sagittal planes and include balanced gradient echo images with T2-weighted properties (referred to as

FIESTA by GE or True FISP by SIEMENS) and ultrafast gradient echo images with T1-weighted properties (referred to as SPGR by GE or VIBE by SIEMENS) with and without fat-saturation. Fat saturation is performed by delivery of a selective RF pulses tailored to flip only protons in fat pulse, thereby preventing fat-containing structures from achieving an excited state and subsequently precessing with delivery of the dedicated RF pulse at the TE interval. This differs from fat saturation via Short-Tau Inversion Recovery (STIR) in which a 180-degree inversion pulse is delivered at the T2 time of fat during MRI acquisition [32–34].

Three other sequences used in our institutional fetal MRI protocol will be briefly mentioned. The Time-of-Flight technique images the flow of blood in a specific direction, therefore allowing for its specificity to looking at either the venous or arterial system depending on which direction of flow the signal is saturated out [35]. Diffusion-weighted imaging (DWI) is a rapidly performed sequence acquired either via a fast gradient or echo-planar acquisition performed for assessing diffusivity of free water molecules within a given imaged structure. Live (often normal) tissues with maintained cell membranes and functioning Sodium-Potassium ATPase mediated pumps allow for free diffusivity of water between given tissues. In contrast, tissues with ongoing infarction, infection, or inflammation and tumors with densely packed cellular contents demonstrate restricted diffusion of water [36, 37]. Normal tightly packed structures—such as white-matter tracts—demonstrate a similar type of restricted diffusivity evaluated with an offset of DWI known as diffusion-tensor imaging (DTI). DTI evaluates the integrity and continuity of white matter tracts as a measure of either isotropic (movement in all spatial directions) or anisotropic (restricted movement in all spatial directions) water movement. Normal white matter tracts possess unique fractional anisotropic appearances in a three-dimensional axis that are conventionally color-coded for ease of interpretation—blue for craniocaudal, green for anteroposterior, and red for transverse [36, 37].

As opposed to fetal MRI sequences whose primary focus is speed of acquisition, conventional MRI examinations of the pregnant patient's neuraxis balances speed of acquisition with high signal-to-noise (SNR) acquisition in order to generate images with high contrast and spatial resolution and fewer artifacts. MRI tailored to imaging the pregnant patient's neuraxis is performed on either 1.5 or 3 T magnets with routine T1 and T2 weighted images (both gradient and spine-echo acquired) along with DWI images. Fluid-Attenuation Inverse Recovery (FLAIR) is similar to STIR and involves saturation of CSF by delivery of a 180-degree inversion pulse at the T2 time of CSF during MRI acquisition, thereby generating a T2-weighted image without fluid in order to highlight edema or other fluid-retentive pathologic states. Gradient Echo (GRE) imaging and associated susceptibility weighted imaging (SWI) are imaging techniques sensitive to hemorrhage and mineral (notably iron) localization, with continued advances in this technique allowing for better separation of overlapping susceptibility-inducing constituents such as superior iron distinction apart from other minerals with Quantitative Susceptibility Mapping (QSM) [38].

An important consideration regarding 1.5 and 3 T is the degree of energy deposition that occurs in each magnetic field, defined as the specific absorption rate (SAR) and measured in watts per kilogram (W/kg). Specifically, deposition of energy created by the excitatory RF pulses is dissipated as heat in surrounding tissues. The resultant released energy can result in unfavorable increases in body temperature or burns, with such adverse effects potentially translating to the pregnant patient and/or fetus. The FDA put regulations in place in 2014 that define maximum targeted and whole-body SAR values per unit time in various parts of the human body. Whole-body SAR averaged over 15 min should be less than 4 W/kg. Targeted head exposure SAR averaged over 10 min should be less than 3.2 W/kg. Exams that surpass these values trigger fail-safe mechanisms to halt acquisition in all modern MR units [39]. SAR is more closely monitored during 3 T fetal MRI examinations for these reasons [40]. Although no evidence is present to definitively prove harm to the fetus from these effects, given the unknown risks of RF energy depositions in this special population, ultrasound is preferred in initially evaluating the first trimester gestation and early second trimester while fetal MRI is reserved for evaluation of the late second and third trimester fetus.

The main possible posited risks and adverse outcomes from SAR include tissue heating, acoustic damage, and teratogenesis in both early and later pregnancy. Although mechanistically possible, these risks are largely theoretical, as research has failed to show any reproducible harmful effects of exposure of either the developing gestation(s) or pregnant patient to magnetic fields 3 T or less employed during clinical practice. It should be noted, however, that the majority of this data stems from magnetic fields of 1.5 T or less. Also, less is known regarding potential effects of varying gradient and radiofrequency magnetic fields employed during scan acquisition image generation. Therefore, theoretical risks need to be carefully balanced against potential benefits to patient undergoing any MRI examination. Proceeding with any MRI examination in the pregnant patient must therefore be performed following a thorough addressing of the potential benefits to the patient/fetus and risks associated with declining such examination [41].

Gadolinium based contrast agents are not routinely used during pregnancy. Once water-soluble gadolinium-chelated agents enter fetal circulation, subsequent excretion from the fetal bladder into amniotic fluid results in swallowing and redistribution through the fetal alimentary tract. While animal models have demonstrated stunted growth following administration, no human controlled studies exist to corroborate such. As such, its use is considered an FDA pregnancy category C substance (evidence exists supporting adverse effects from animal models) [16, 42]. No uniform agreement on its safety during pregnancy exists however, as the European Society of Urogenital Radiology guidelines state that because only a miniscule amount of contrast passes the maternal-fetal placental barrier, its use in pregnancy is safe [16, 43].

Section 2: Maternal Neuroimaging in Pregnancy

Headache

Headache is the most frequent indication for neurological evaluation in the pregnant patient. They may be divided into primary (pain is the disease) and secondary (pain is a symptom of an alternate underlying pathology) subtypes. Primary headaches that occur during pregnancy include migraines without aura, migraine with aura, tension-type, and cluster [44]. Aside from migraine headaches that may show a reduction in frequency and intensity during pregnancy, remaining primary headaches are common or exacerbated during the pregnant state, with tension-type being the most common with 26% prevalence in pregnant patients. Given a characteristic lack of neuroimaging features, neuroimaging is typically not indicated in classic primary-type headaches [45]. Secondary headaches are manifestations of an underlying intracranial or parenchymal pathology warranting urgent neuromedical or neurosurgical intervention. Recent research suggests that these secondary causes can account for up to 25%–42% of women who seek medical attention during pregnancy. As such, the threshold for neuroimaging as a whole is much lower in these patients. Specific "red flag" features of headaches indicating a secondary etiology include acute alterations in baseline neurological examination (aside from effects of auras in migraine headache), worst headache of life with 'thunderclap' sudden onset, headache in the setting of systemic illness, headache associated with visual disturbance (papilledema), post-traumatic headache, or headache worsened with Valsalva and upright position. Thunderclap headache is defined as any severe headache peaking within 1 min. Non-thunderclap headache is any headache with mild to severe intensity, peaking in more than 1 min. Several of these resultant entities are reviewed in the subsequent sections [46]. Headache in pregnancy is discussed in further detail in Chap. 27.

Idiopathic Intracranial Hypertension (IIH)

Idiopathic intracranial hypertension (IIH) refers to a disease entity involving the elevation of intracranial pressures unrelated to an intracranial space-occupying process (such as brain tumor) or infectious/inflammatory process (such as meningitis). Patient symptomology includes positional headaches, decreases in visual acuity (most severely as papilledema), and pulsatile tinnitus unrelated to direct inner ear pathology. Commonly, patients with classic IIH are female, obese, and relatively young/pre-menopausal. Increased frequency in the obese and pregnant state is mediated by a combination of elevations in adipokines and steroid hormones, noting dysregulation of 11 beta hydroxysteroid dehydrogenase activity in the liver and adipose tissue with resultant elevations in CSF resorption is a recently proposed biochemical pathway of development [47]. The elevation in intracranial pressure can be detected by a combination of clinical examination findings, lumbar puncture with elevation of opening pressure (greater than 20 cm H_2O in non-obese patients and greater than 25 cm H_2O in obese patients), and imaging [48, 49].

The leading hypothesis regarding its increased detection in pregnant patients is related to a combination of hormonally and hemodynamically induced effects. Notably, increased levels of estrogen lead to an associated increase in procoagulants, blood pressure, hyperlipidemia, and glucose intolerance. Similarly, increases in progesterone result in vasodilation with increases of plasma volume. Beginning in week 5 of gestation with subsequent elevations throughout pregnancy until delivery, changes in the coagulation system during pregnancy include increases in plasminogen activator inhibitor, rise in activated protein C resistance, increases in Facto VII, increases in fibrinogen levels, increasing Factor V activity, and drops in Protein S [16].

Classic MRI brain features of IIH include the detection of intraorbital optic nerves tortuosity, stretching/thinning of the posterior globes, empty sella, low-lying cerebellar tonsils, or a combination of these findings [50]. Dural venous sinus stenosis is often identified at the transverse—sigmoid junction of the dominant or codominant dural venous sinus system. The debate of venous sinus stenosis being a cause or consequence of IIH continues, noting that articles as recent as 2019 state the entity results in the incidental presence of an "empty sella" (i.e., flattened appearance of pituitary gland on imaging) rather than IIH itself [51]. Regardless of one's stance on the role of venous sinus stenosis in IIH symptomology, dural venous sinus stenting has become a progressively more performed procedure in the field of Interventional Neuroradiology, as its resultant effects of significant improvements of patient symptomology have been favorable (Fig. 3.1) [52–54]. IIH in pregnancy is discussed in further detail in Chap. 35.

Cerebral Venous Sinus Thrombosis (CVST)

Venous thromboembolism in the intracranial setting often poses a diagnostic dilemma in particularly the pregnant patient, as its clinical presentation may broadly range from acute neurological deficit, altered mental status, seizure, obtundation, or even coma. Its incidence is rare, estimated at 5 per million cases and accounts for 0.5%–1% of all strokes, though this incidence increases with pregnancy, puerperium, hormone replacement therapy, and oral contraceptive use. Its pathophysiology stems from achieving Virchow's triad of biophysical and chemical criteria, notably endothelial injury, coagulation cascade activation, and alterations in laminar blood flow with superimposed direct drug and hormonally induced thrombosis [55]. Approximately 0.004%–0.01% of all pregnancies are complicated by CVST, and up to 2% of pregnancy strokes can be attributed to CVST [56, 57]. Initial noncontract head CT may demonstrate increased density throughout the various superficial and/or deep venous drainage pathways. Depending on extent of thrombotic burden, increased density may be peripherally detected in the superior sagittal, transverse, and sigmoid dural venous sinuses and centrally detected in the straight

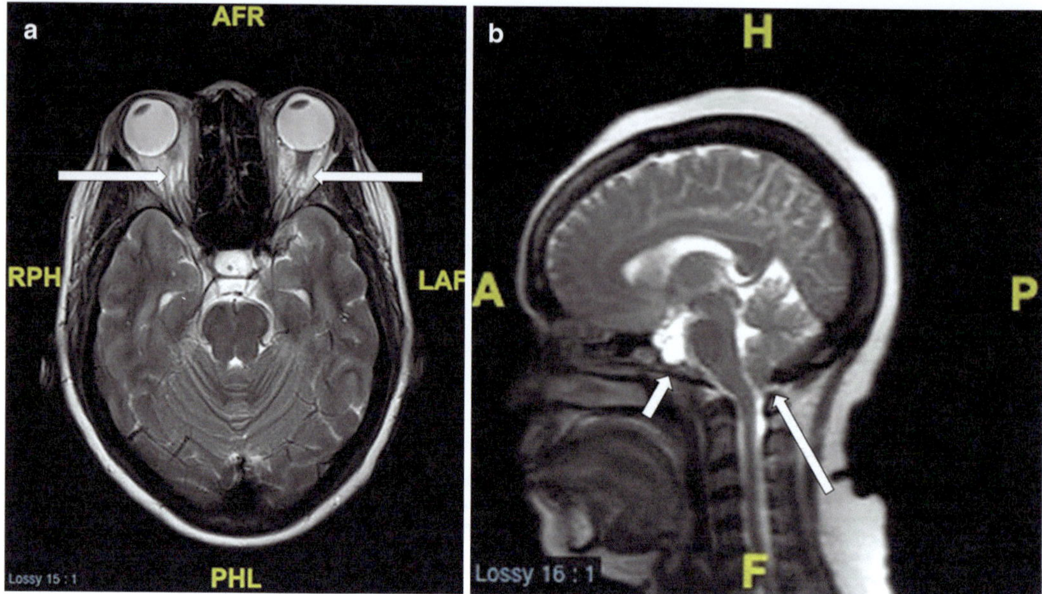

Fig. 3.1 Patient presenting with headaches and blurry vision, noting papilledema on ophthalmologic evaluation. Axial T2 (**a**) and Sagittal T2 (**b**) brain MRI images in a patient with IIH. Left image shows markedly tortuous optic nerves with prominent CSF around optic nerves (long arrows). Right image shows empty sella (short arrow) and ectopic cerebellar tonsils (long arrow). All these findings suggest diagnosis of IIH in this pregnant patient

sinus and internal cerebral veins on the noncontrast CT modality. MRI is more sensitive in its evaluation given its ability to detect thrombus in the involved superficial and deep cerebral veins and venous sinuses. Aside from increased susceptibility and intrinsically T1 bright signal related to the effects of thrombotic burden, secondary effects of thrombosis can be seen, including the evolution of infarcts with restricted diffusion and associated T2 abnormality typically affecting symmetric deep and superficial structures, noting that zones of venous infarction are not of the typical arterial stroke distributions [58]. Unfractionated heparin and low-molecular weight heparin do not cross the placental barrier and are the anticoagulants of choice in pregnancy. However, pregnancy may alter the metabolism of LMWH, requiring high doses than typical. Coumadin is contraindicated in the first trimester given its teratogenicity and ability to readily cross the placenta, though its uses after first trimester is within standards of clinical practice (Fig. 3.2) [16, 59]. CVST in pregnancy is discussed in further detail in Chap. 11.

Reversible Posterior Leukoencephalopathy (PRES)

Reversible posterior leukoencephalopathy (PRES) is seen in a wide age range from pediatric to geriatric, though it most commonly affects young to middle aged female adults even when excluding pregnant patients with eclampsia. PRES pathophysiology stems from a combination of systemic hypertension and impaired cerebral autoregulation resulting in increased blood flow. Simultaneous aberrant immunological activation with endothelial dysfunction is contributory in the pre-eclamptic pregnant state. Prognosis is usually good [60].

PRES is initially detected on noncontrast CT as vasogenic edema in a holohemispheric watershed, superior frontal sulcus, and/or dominant

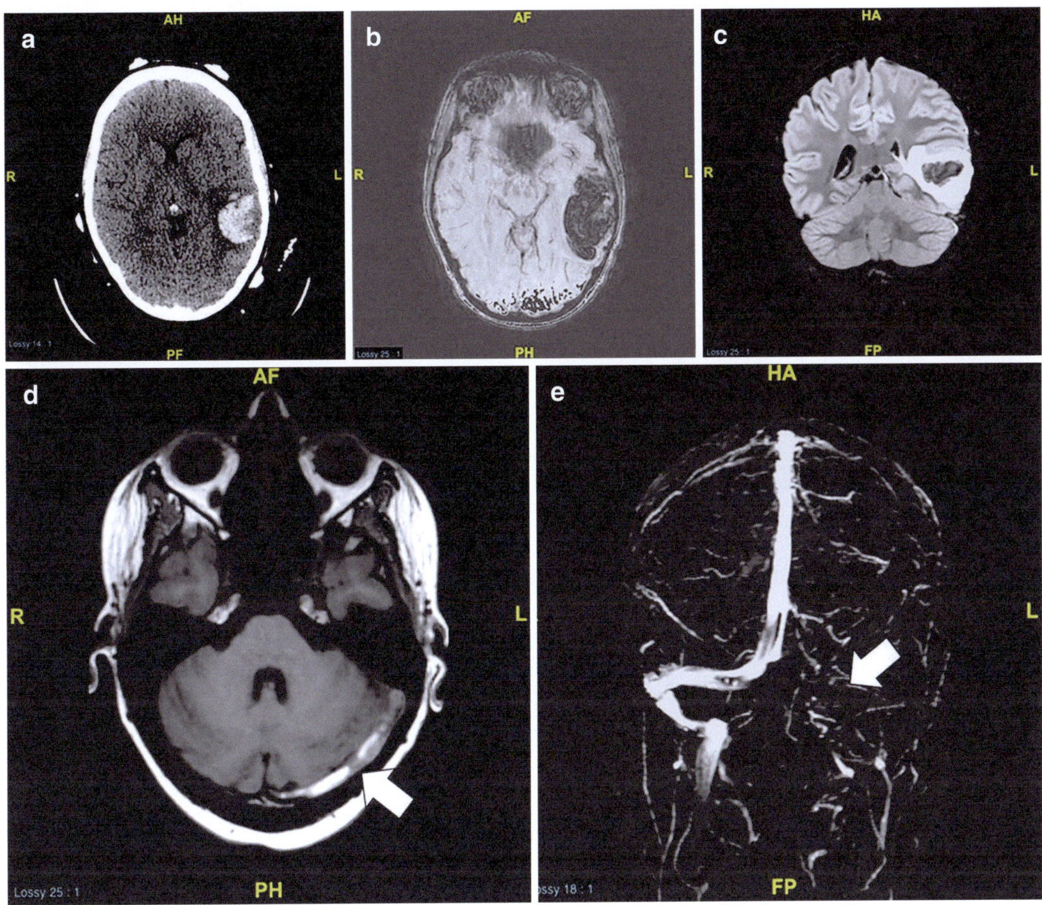

Fig. 3.2 Pregnant patient presenting with worst headache of life and confusion. (**a**) Axial CT shows hemorrhage in the left temporal lobe. (**b**) Non-contrast MRI with susceptibility weighted imaging (SWI) demonstrates marked susceptibility corresponding to the area of hemorrhage. (**c**) Coronal FLAIR image confirming temporal lobe hemorrhage and better accentuating degree of bright surrounding vasogenic edema. (**d**) Non-contrast axial T1 image shows hyperintense thrombus in the left transverse sinus. (**e**) Time-of-Flight 3D reconstruction of MR venography confirms lack of signal in the left transverse sinus (short arrow) as well as sigmoid sinus and internal jugular vein, consistent with dural venous sinus thrombosis

parietal-occipital distribution, with partial or asymmetric expression of these primary patterns possible. Involvement in the posterior parietal and occipital lobes in most common, encompassing more than 90% of cases. MRI with T2 and FLAIR sequences confirm edema without associated infarction, noting its eventual reversibility and resolution is the hallmark of PRES. Punctate infarcts characterized as bright DWI and dark ADC signal can be seen within confluent areas of vasogenic edema. Likewise, punctate parenchymal hemorrhage is seen in up to 15% of PRES cases. Persistence and progression of edema is rare, occurring in 3–6% of patients. Larger areas of infarction, significant subarachnoid or parenchymal hemorrhage, PRES development in the setting of sepsis or chemotherapy, or edema and infarct development in atypical areas including the deep brain nuclei, brainstem, and spinal cord portend to poorer prognosis (Fig. 3.3) [60]. Preeclampsia, eclampsia, and PRES are discussed in detail in Chap. 12.

Reversible Cerebral Vasoconstriction Syndrome (RCVS)

Reversible cerebral vasoconstriction syndrome (RCVS)—also known as Call–Fleming syndrome or migranous vasospasm—presents as severe headaches in the setting of reversible constriction of cerebral arteries. This is an important reversible cause of the thunderclap headache presentation. RCVS is also most commonly associated with pregnancy even without eclampsia, occurring in women between ages 20 and 50. The pathophysiology is not exactly known, but the innervation of sensory afferents from the V1 branch of the trigeminal nerve and dorsal root of C2 are thought to explain the anatomic basis of both the sensation of headache and vasoconstriction. Moreover, the presence of transient neurovascular changes and edema in both RCVS and PRES suggests that there is some overlap in their pathophysiology. Although RCVS clinical symptoms are self-limited with a typically favorable prognosis, recurrences and complications throughout life are reported depending on devel-

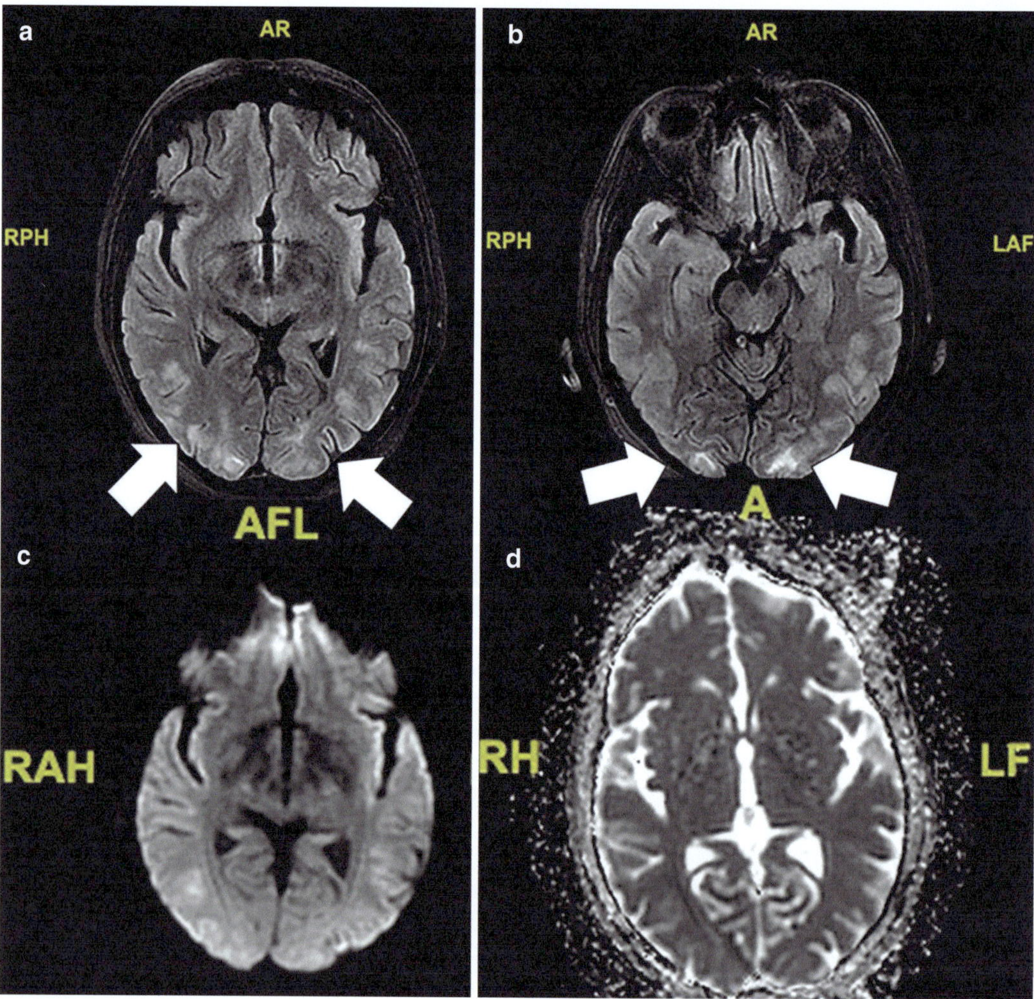

Fig. 3.3 Pregnant patient with eclampsia, hypertension, and visual disturbances. (**a, b**). Axial FLAIR images demonstrate abnormal signal in the bilateral medial occipital lobes centered in the subcortical white matter and gray-white junctions (arrows). (**c, d**) Axial diffusion weighted and accompanying ACD mapping confirming no infarction in these areas of abnormal signal. (**e, f**) Repeat MRI performed 6 days later demonstrate resolution/marked improvement in previously seen signal abnormality related to PRES

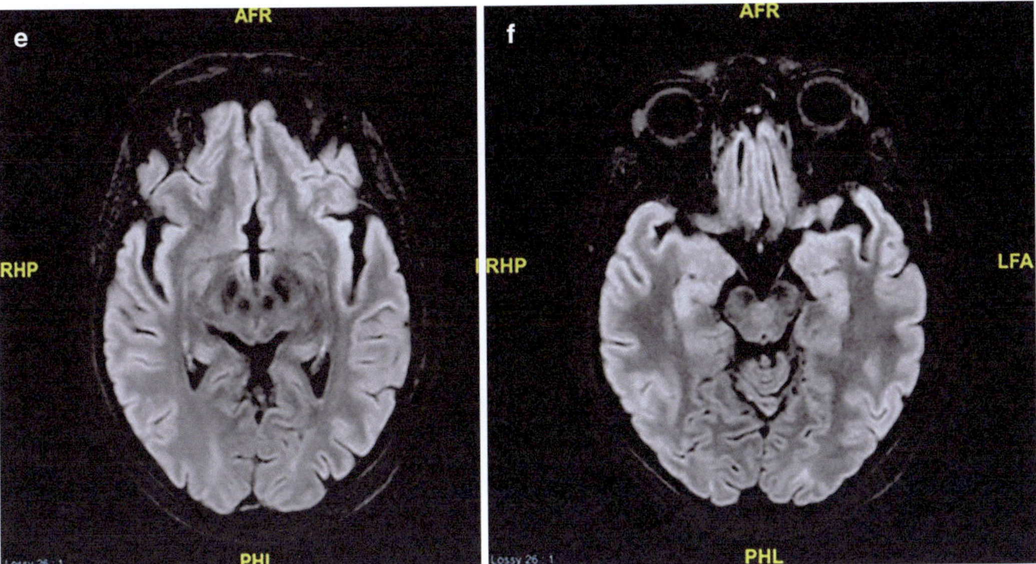

Fig. 3.3 (continued)

opment of ischemia, hemorrhage, or seizure at the time of initial presentation [60].

Neuroimaging of RCVS features are best appreciated on either CT or MR angiographic examinations, with catheter angiography remaining the gold standard of diagnosis. Vessel wall imaging with thin-section fat suppressed contrast enhanced MR with accompanying high-resolution thin section T2 weighted imaging to has been useful in differentiating RCVS (typically no wall enhancement or edema) from vasculitis (typically possess vessel wall enhancement and edema). However, its widespread utilization in the non-academic setting is less frequent given potential discrepancies in its accuracy. RCVS results in vasoconstriction of dominant central and peripheral cerebral arterial branches in a waxing and waning distribution, noting vasoconstriction with a minimum of two areas of narrowing within the same artery or on two different cerebral arteries with expected resolution by 3 months of initial detection. Unlike PRES, resultant hemorrhage of the subarachnoid type and infarcts are more common, occurring in up to 1/3rd of patients (Fig. 3.4) [60]. RCVS and its variant postpartum cerebral angiopathy are discussed in detail in Chaps. 13 and 14.

Cerebral Aneurysm, Subarachnoid Hemorrhage, and AVM

SAH in the setting of aneurysmal rupture during pregnancy is the fourth leading cause of non-obstetrical maternal death with up to 40% mortality rate, noting that its occurrence and management has been reported in the literature as early as 1965 [61, 62]. Literature suggests there is an up to 600% increase in the prevalence of aneurysmal SAH during the peripartum period, most likely as a result of pregnancy-related hormonal and physiologic changes impacting cerebral autoregulation and overall hemodynamic stability. In the absence of critical clinical grade, immediate operative or endovascular intervention is typically necessary given re-rupture occurrence in 33%–50% of cases with associated mortality rates between 50% and 68% [63]. Despite iodinated radiation exposure, CTA is typically initially performed in the pregnant patient in the setting of higher clinical grades, noting that the balance of maternal health with theoretical scatter radiation despite adequate abdominal shielding is either discussed with the patient, the healthcare proxy, or emergently agreed upon by the providing physician(s). If

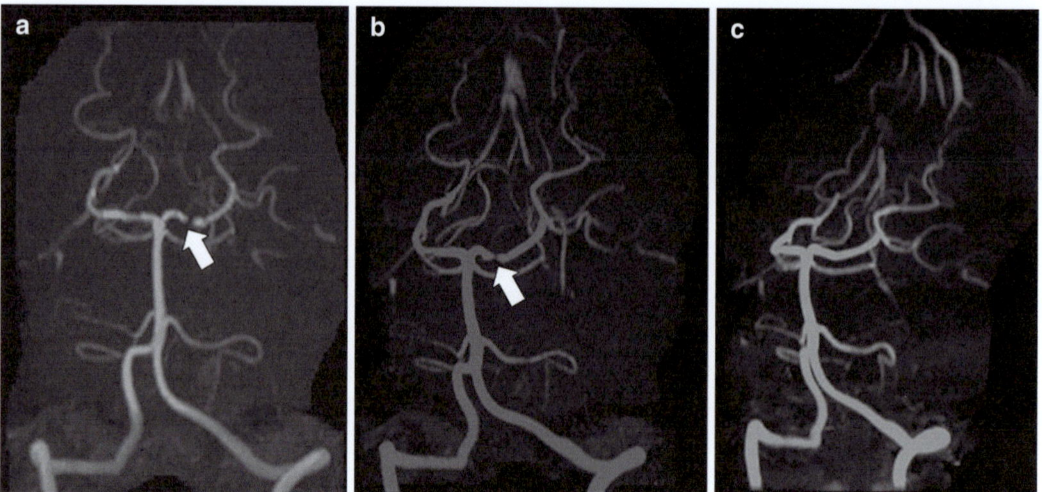

Fig. 3.4 Pregnant patient with dizziness. (**a**) Time of flight MRA 3D reconstruction of basilar circulation demonstrates focal short-segment critical stenosis of the left P1 segment of the posterior cerebral artery (arrow). (**b**) This persisted on MRA examination performed 2 weeks later. (**c**) Follow-up MRA performed 3 months latera demonstrated interval resolution of previously seen critical stenosis, in keeping with the reversible nature of RCVS

low volume SAH with maintained clinical-examination or hemorrhage distribution more suggestive of post-traumatic, venous, or perimesencephalic SAH, evaluation may still be performed with CTA, noting that non-contrast MRA with time-of-flight acquisitions can provide cerebral arterial evaluation with comparable efficacy [64]. Catheter angiography remains the gold standard for diagnosis and potential endovascular-guided treatment of aneurysms amenable to such therapy. Coil embolization efficacy is comparable to that of surgical microclipping and maybe favored in the acutely ruptured state [65–67]. Stent-assisted coiling of wide neck aneurysms may not be possible or less desired in either a ruptured aneurysm or pregnant patient for whom long-term antiplatelet therapy is not desired by either the referring providers, patient, or respective proxy [68, 69]. The advent of aneurysm intrasaccular flow disrupter devices such as the Woven Endoluminal Bridge (WEB) have widened the inclusion criteria of wide-neck aneurysms now amenable to endovascular-guided embolization [70].

Aneurysms may also be seen in the setting of underlying high-flow intracranial vascular anomalies such as arteriovenous malformations (AVMs). These are high-flow arteriovenous connections without an interweaving capillary network, instead encompassed by abnormal tangles of immature communicating vessels referred to as an AVM nidus. The prevalence of AVM is approximately 0.01%–0.5%, typically first manifesting in patients 20–40 years of age [71]. These anomalies can increase in size and possess aneurysms either within the nidus or the remaining intracranial circulation secondary to increased hemodynamic effects. These can be further exacerbated in the pregnant state due to a combination of hormone induced angiogenesis, vascular changes, and an overall increased hemodynamic state related to pregnancy itself. Although prior research has not suggested a clear link between pregnancy and an increased AVM hemorrhage risk, recent research re-examining this relationship has suggested otherwise. An observational study in 2020 of over four million pregnant women, 568 of whom had AVM,

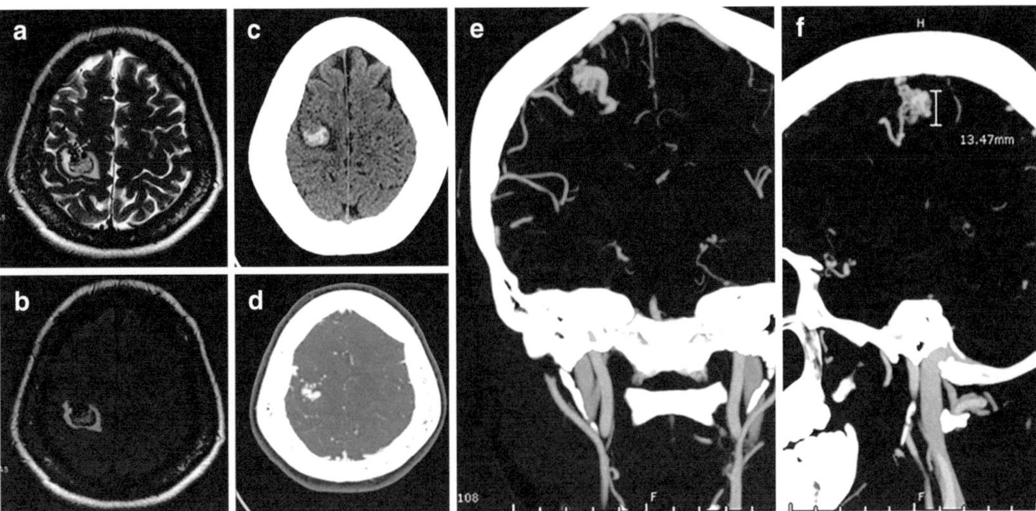

Fig. 3.5 Pregnant patient with worst headache of life and decreased left upper extremity strength. (**a, b**) Axial T2 and FLAIR MRI images demonstrate abnormal signal with edema and flow void prominence in the right frontal lobe precentral gyrus. (**c**) Non-contrast head CT demonstrates focal hemorrhage in this location. (**d**) Given hemorrhage presence, despite pregnant status, contrast administered given the underlying neurosurgical emer-gency. Axial CTA confirms abnormal tangle of vessels consistent with AVM nidus. (**e, f**) Coronal and sagittal MIPs redemonstrating right frontal AVM with superficial venous drainage and nidus measuring approximately 1.5 cm tall. Small size of AVM with less than 3 cm nidus and location in eloquent cortex result in this being a Spetzler-Martin grade 2 AVM. Rupture of an intranidal aneurysm resulted in parenchymal hemorrhage

found that the risk hemorrhage increased 3.27-fold (95% CI of 1.67–6.43) during pregnancy and the puerperium period compared with a non-pregnant period. Thus, caution is taken when caring for patients with known AVM to present rupture (Fig. 3.5) [72]. Cerebral aneurysm, SAH, and AVMs in pregnancy are discussed in detail in Chaps. 8 and 9.

Neoplasms

Intracranial neoplasms are rare in the pregnant patient when compared with the incidence of breast or lung carcinoma. Annual incidence is 2–3.2 cases per 100,000 of reproductive-aged women between 20 and 38 years of age regardless of race. However, despite its low incidence, resultant mortality is estimated between 0.5 and 1.1 deaths per 100,000 women of reproductive age,

leading to this being the nineth most common cause of cancer-related death in this age group. Presenting symptoms can be nonspecific, ranging from headache, visual disturbance, seizures, or motor and sensory deficits depending on a combination of tumoral location, size, and resultant sequalae of mass effect or shift on surrounding eloquent areas of brain parenchyma. Such non-specificity can lead to difficulty in initial diagnosis or clinical consideration. Any new neurological deficit warrants neurological consultation and potential dedicated neuroimaging [73].

Unifying these nonspecific clinical symptoms is the typical presence of elevated intracranial pressure (ICP) due to a combination of the tumor's presence itself and the overall hypervolemic state of pregnancy. The most common initial presenting symptom is headache, occurring in 36%–90% of pregnant patients with intracranial neoplasms. Headaches worse in the morning and exacerbated with maneuvers elevating intracranial pressure such as Valsalva, laying down, physical exertion, or coughing are indicators suggesting the need for further evaluation. Additional signs of elevated ICP include nausea and vomiting, occurring in 25% of patients. Though presence of these symptoms can be confounded by the typically similar hormonally mediated symptoms of the first trimester of pregnancy, development or persistence of such symptoms during the second or third trimesters may provide a stronger indication for further evaluation [73].

Imaging is performed with either CT or MRI. MRI is preferred in the pregnant patient given no ionizing radiation exposure to gestation from use, improved resolution and soft tissue characterization over CT. CT utility stems from its rapid acquisition relative to MR and ability to triage accordingly if a patient has a suspicious mass warranting further imaging. To date, research has not shown conclusive evidence of complications different from those that occur in non-pregnant patients from the use of contrast agents such as gadolinium. However, contrast enhancement with MRI is generally not utilized given the potential for crossing of the placental barrier, though its implementation is ultimately up to the discretion of the approving radiologist and receiving patient [43].

Meningiomas are frequently encountered benign intracranial neoplasms that grow dramatically in the pregnant state due to hemodynamic changes and hormone induced effects from progesterone and estrogen (between 33% and 38% have estrogen receptors and 70%–90% have progesterone receptors). They are extra-axial in location and can be detected on noncontrast CT depending on their size, mass effect, and resultant edema. MRI is more sensitive in their evaluation, characteristically demonstrating their dural origin ("dural tail"). If contrast is utilized, these masses are known for their avid enhancement (Fig. 3.6) [73].

The most common primary parenchymal brain tumors are gliomas arising from glial cells and present more frequently during the first and second trimesters. If lower grade (such as oligodendroglioma or astrocytoma), resection maybe delayed until following deliver, with steroids or anti-epileptic medications given accordingly to reduce tumoral edema and seizure frequency if present. Higher-grade gliomas (such as anaplastic astrocytomas and glioblastoma multiformes) can rapidly progress with resultant clinical deterioration. Therefore, tumoral debulking and surgery are performed even during pregnancy, with subsequent adjuvant chemoradiation held until after pregnancy. Early fetal deliver via induction or caesarian section may be considered if the gestation is advanced in age. As with meningioma detection, MRI is most sensitive and specific in its identification and staging of intracranial tumoral extent. Given their glial origin, tumors are distinguished from normal brain parenchyma via their asymmetric appearance relative to normal parenchyma and accompanying cortical and white matter track irregularity. Enhancement and edema may or may not be present and depend on a combination of tumoral stage of disease and size [73].

Other masses with increased prevalence in pregnancy due to hormonally induced growth include acoustic neuromas, pituitary neoplasia, and colloid cysts. Several other masses have also been described in the pregnant patient—though to a lesser frequency—ranging from dysembryoplastic neuroepithelial tumor, primary meningeal sarcoma, paraganglioma, CNS lymphoma, medulloblastoma, pineal region tumor, craniopharyngioma, hemangioblastoma, and ependymoma [73]. Intracranial neoplasms and sellar lesions are discussed in detail in Chaps. 36 and 37, respectively.

Noninflammatory and Inflammatory Demyelination

Hyperemedis gravidarum is characterized as severe vomiting typically occurring in the first trimester leading to dehydration, electrolyte imbalances, and weight loss. The resultant elec-

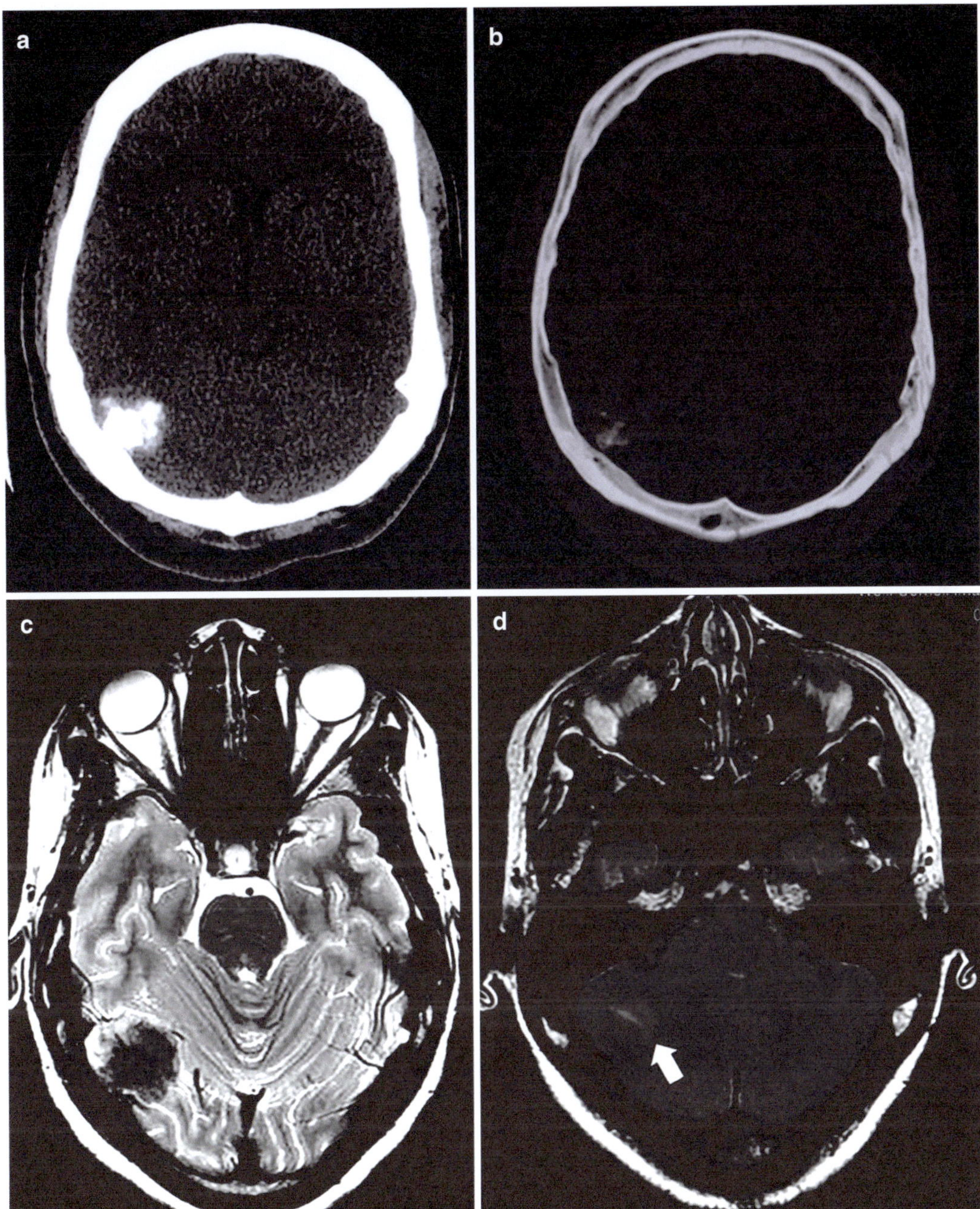

Fig. 3.6 (**a**, **b**) Head CT 2 years prior to pregnancy in soft tissue (**a**) and bone (**b**) windows demonstrate a densely calcified extra-axial meningioma along the right temporo-occipital calvarium. (**c**, **d**) Second-trimester of pregnancy MRI images demonstrating slight interval growth in the meningioma with minimal surrounding edema in the right cerebellar hemisphere (arrow). (**e**, **f**) Post-pregnancy pre-operative MRI demonstrates increased right cerebellar edema (short arrow) and further increase in size of meningioma, noting its avid enhancement and extra-axial dural origin on coronal post-contrast enhanced imaging (long arrow)

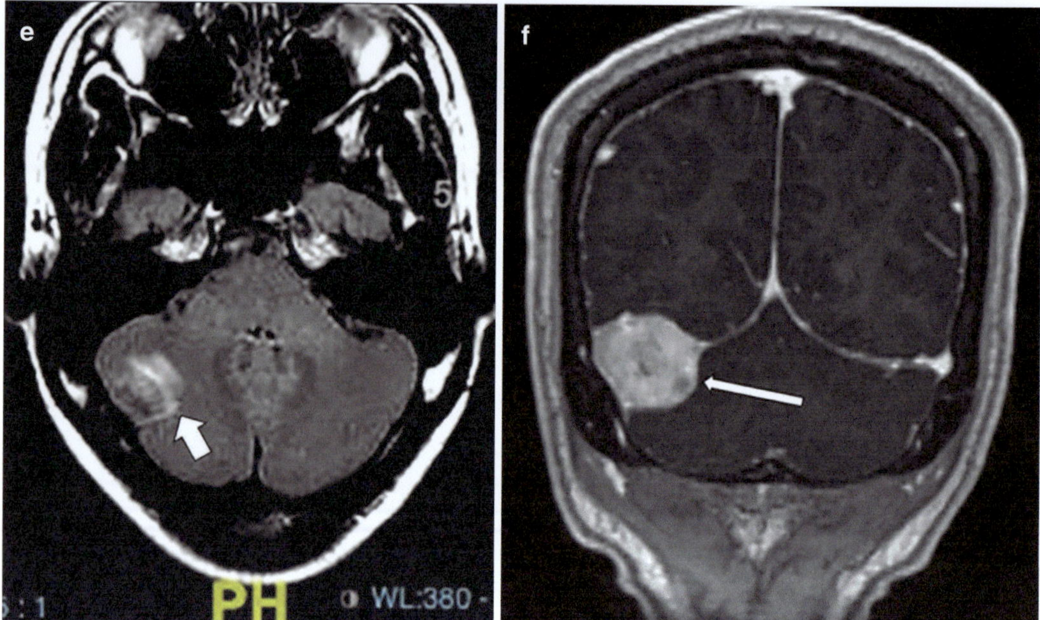

Fig. 3.6 (continued)

trolyte disturbances or management of such may result in detrimental neurological complications that can be detected with imaging. Osmotic demyelination syndrome is a non-inflammatory demyelination either involving the pons or other areas (extra-pontine) of the central nervous system that characteristically occurs following the rapid correction of serum sodium less than 135 millimole per liter (mmol/L), a state referred to as hyponatremia. Rapid hyponatremia correction is defined as sodium correction with infusion rates of more than 10–12 mmol/L (typically greater than 18 mmol/L correction in first 48 h), or consistent rates of increase measuring more than 8 mmol/L within any 24-h window [74]. However, it has been reported occurring even with slow correction if simultaneous alternate electrolyte disturbances—notably hypokalemia—are present [75, 76]. The most common sites of extra-pontine involvement include the cerebellum, lateral geniculate body, extreme capsule, external capsule, putamen, hippocampi, thalami, caudate nuclei, and generalized cerebral cortex or subcortical regions. Rarely are the internal capsules, claustrum, midbrain, maxillary bodies, medulla, or internal medullary lamella affected. MRI is most sensitive in detection of this entity, with T2 and FLAIR imaging showing characteristic expansion and edema related to fluid accumulation within either the pons or extra-pontine structures noted above. Given an overlap of this distribution with numerous other infectious/inflammatory entities, clinical history is of vital importance [77, 78].

Inflammatory demyelinating disorders such as multiple sclerosis (MS) are most commonly seen in young childbearing women between the ages of 20 and 45 years. This demographic is virtually identical to the pregnant patient, with a relationship between these conditions and pregnancy expected and subsequently explored throughout the literature. Interestingly, the incidence of an initial demyelinating episode or relapse of known diagnosis is typically lowered during third trimester and late stages of pregnancy, while the majority of either new or relapsing demyelination episodes tend to occur more in the postpartum period. The specific reasons for this relationship are unclear, though both the abrupt lowering of serum estrogen levels immediately following delivery alongside the loss of the immunosuppressive state of pregnancy play a role in this pattern. There is also emerging evidence that different cytokine profiles, specifically of proteins such as Activin A, are associated with MS activity during both pregnancy and in the postpartum period [79, 80].

MRI is most sensitive in the evaluation of demyelination relative to other white matter afflicting conditions, with diagnostic criteria including the number, location, and shape of lesions aiding in diagnosis. A variety of MS subtypes exist, most common of which are the relapsing-remitting (70% of cases) and primary-progressive (15% of cases) subtypes. MS subtypes are defined by a combination of clinical course and evolution of lesions detected over the span of a patient's life, with updated 2017 McDonald Criteria reviewing these criteria [81]. All MS subtypes share common features of T2 or FLAIR bright lesions >3 mm long axis dimension classically seen in the corpus callosum, juxtacortical and periventricular white matter, infratentorial white matter (brainstem, cerebellar peduncles or cerebellum), or spinal cord. Acute lesions are diagnosed via a combination of clinical history, detection of new lesions compared to prior imaging, and presence of intra-lesion restricted diffusion on DWI pulse sequence (Fig. 3.7) [38, 82].

The central-vein sign is an MRI finding specific to perivenous inflammatory demyelination classically seen in patients with an established diagnosis of Multiple Sclerosis and its "Radiologically Isolated Syndrome" corollary (syndrome name used to identify asymptomatic individuals with parenchymal white-matter findings with features highly suspicious for multiple sclerosis in clinically non-diagnosed patients) [83, 84]. This is a centrally prominent vein within white-matter possessing characteristic linear-bands of dark signal on susceptibility weighted imaging (SWI) corresponding to prominent draining veins within the lesion center [85]. Enhancement is not a useful diagnostic criterion for acute lesions in pregnant patient given infrequent gadolinium-based contrast administration in this population. The absence of peripheral rim of signal on SWI and more specifically the recently described Quantitative Susceptibility Mapping (QSM) sequence (hemosiderin margin presence) is also more specific to chronic lesions relative to acute [38, 82]. The approach to evaluation and management of MS is discussed in detail in Chap. 21.

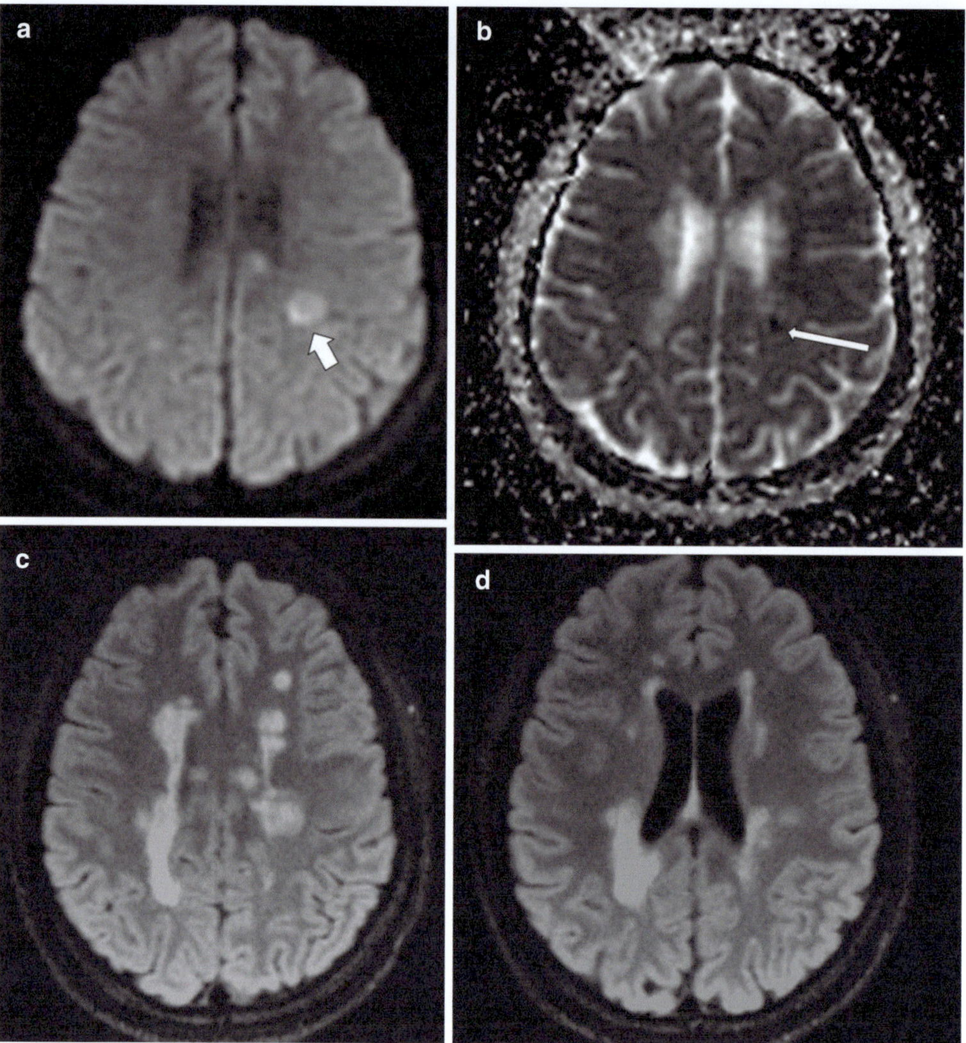

Fig. 3.7 Pregnant patient with history of multiple sclerosis presenting with acute alteration in gait disturbance different from baseline generalized weakness. (**a, b**) Diffusion weighted imaging (DWI) shows focal true restricted diffusion (short arrow) in the left periventricular white matter with accompanying dark signal on the ADC map (long arrow). Findings are consistent with acute demyelination in this patient with history of multiple sclerosis. (**c, d**) Axial FAIR images show additional chronic white matter disease changes in the bilateral centrum semi ovale and corona radiata white matter tracts related to long standing multiple sclerosis effects. (**e, f**) MRI of the cervical spine demonstrates additional chronic white matter lesions along the length of the cervical right-sided hemi-cord on sagittal (**e**) and axial (**f**) planes of imaging

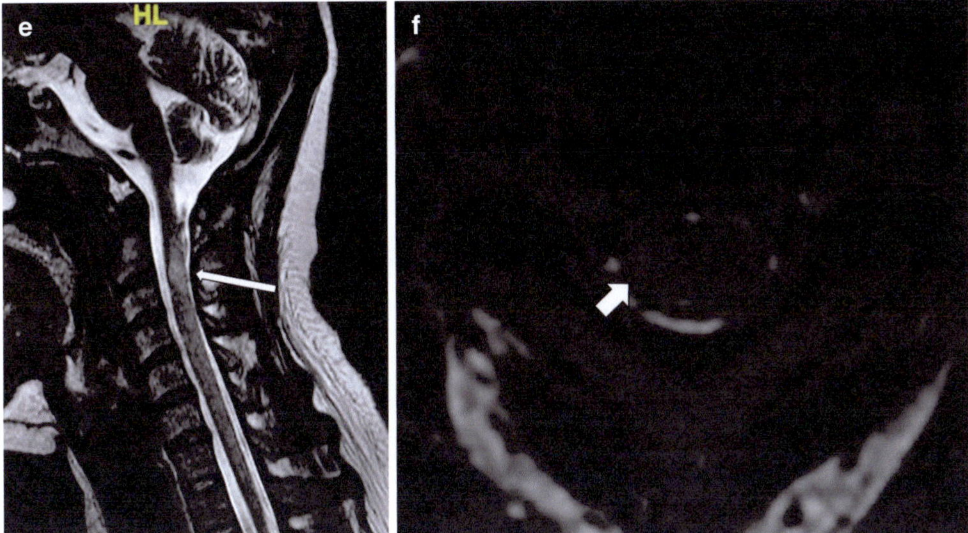

Fig. 3.7 (continued)

Section 3: Pre-natal Neuroimaging

Ultrasound and fetal MRI have vastly improved the ability to detect a variety of neuropathologic conditions in the growing gestation prior to delivery. The following section will highlight key pathologies diagnosed either during the second or third trimester via ultrasound and fetal MRI examination.

Ventriculomegaly

Microcephaly is defined as head circumference measuring more than two standard deviations below mean age. Similarly, macrocephaly is defined as head circumference measuring more than two standard deviations above mean age. Classification is made based on a combination of biparietal diameter (BPD) and occipitofrontal diameter (OFD). In the prenatal patient, ventriculomegaly is defined as a lateral ventricular size greater than 10 mm at the level of the atria, with or without dilation of the third or fourth ventricles. It is the most common diagnosed fetal brain anomaly in the prenatal setting, with prevalence estimates in the reported literature ranging from 1 in 50 to 1 in 1600 gestations. Following measurement of lateral ventricle atrial widths, severity is graded as mild (10–12 mm), moderate (13–15 mm), or severe (>15 mm).

Etiologies of ventriculomegaly spans from physiological extremes of normal variation, obstructive or non-obstructive ventricular system pathology, overproduction or increased volume of CSF, atrophy or poor brain parenchymal development with associated prominence of ventricular system, or fetal infection. For instance, congenital aqueductal stenosis is a type of non-communicating hydrocephalus in which partial or complete obstruction of CSF flow at the cerebral aqueduct (also known as the aqueduct of Sylvius) leads to upstream dilation of the lateral ventricular and third ventricular systems. Specific findings on fetal MRI aside from varying degrees of lateral and third ventricle enlargement include enlargement of the inferior recess of the third ventricle and presence of lateral ventricular diverticula. Given the focality of this process, prenatal diagnosis allows for earlier intervention with techniques such as third ventriculostomy creation to prevent further progression of hydrocephalus and its resultant effects on parenchymal development and maturation (Fig. 3.8) [86].

Ventriculomegaly is often not a condition in itself, but rather a sign indicating the need to con-

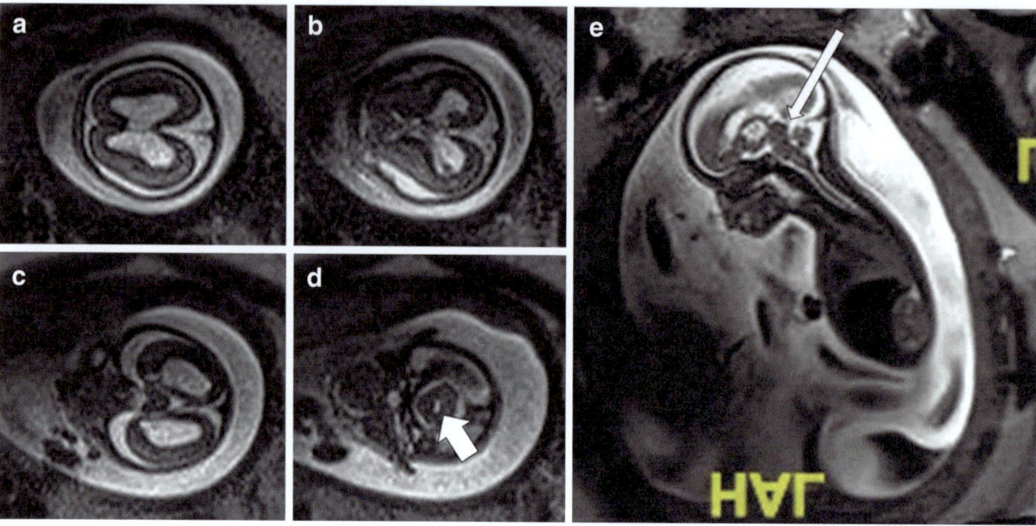

Fig. 3.8 20-week gestation with hydrocephalus noted on second trimester fetal ultrasound. Axial T2 images from fetal MRI (**a–d**) demonstrate ventriculomegaly of the lateral ventricles and third ventricle. The fourth ventricle (short arrow) caliber is within normal limits. Sagittal T2 image from same fetal MRI exam (**e**) points to the level of suspected stenosis in the cerebral aqueduct. This pattern of ventriculomegaly is highly suggestive of congenital stenosis of the aqueduct of Sylvius with associated upstream hydrocephalus

sider a broad differential diagnosis including the above-mentioned etiologies. Identification of ventriculomegaly should thus prompt a thorough evaluation including amniocentesis, detailed fetal ultrasonographic assessment, and testing for fetal infection. Adjunct performance of multiplanar fetal MRI has allowed for the detection of an underlying ventriculomegaly etiology following screening sonography regardless of severity. Meta-analyses have demonstrated the diagnosis of additional brain abnormalities alongside ventriculomegaly in as many as 19% of fetuses. Following initial suspicion on prenatal sonography, a combination of T2 weighted single shot images and T1 weighted gradient images of multiplanar fetal MRI can further characterize the type of ventriculomegaly present and readily identify contributory abnormalities if present [87].

Malformations of Cortical Development and Migrational Anomalies

Cortical maturation occurs in three steps: (1) neuronal precursor proliferation and differentiation; (2) migration of immature neurons; and (3) cortical maturation via laminar organization and development of synaptic connections. Given their alterations in spatial-temporal orientation during development, these gray matter progenitor cells are referred to as transient fetal layers. Neurons originating in the ventricular zone (also known as germinal matrix) migrate towards the pial surface of the developing cortex, utilizing radially oriented glial cells as scaffolds during their ascent. Migration occurs in waves, resulting in a laminar pattern of cell throughout the first and second trimester. The start of the third trimester (28th gestational age week) typically marks the start of germinal matrix regression, which continues until disappearance at full term (37 weeks gestational age). Errors in one or more of the cortical maturation phases lead to uniquely named malformations of cortical development, ranging from conditions of incomplete to dysmorphic cortical development. All of these malformations predispose the fetus to seizure disorders in postnatal life. Gyri with a broad flattened appearance with associated cortical thickening are referred to as pachygyria. In contrast, numerous small gyri with excessive small convolutions or any abnormal folding of one or more cortical layers are referred to as polymicrogyria. The distribution of polymicrogyria may vary, ranging from focally isolated in any one specific lobe to multifocal

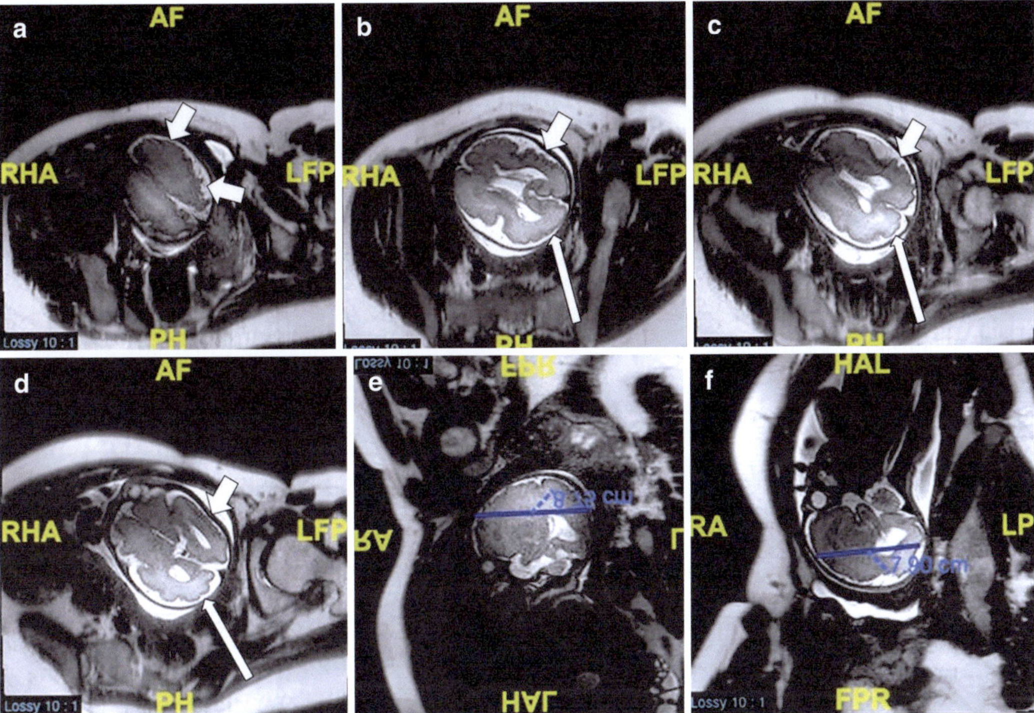

Fig. 3.9 31-year-old woman with 29-week gestation. Axial T2 images (**a–d**) demonstrate asymmetric small size of left cerebral hemisphere compared to right with several areas of clumped, polymicrogyria lining the convexities of the smaller left cerebral hemisphere (short arrows). This is compared to the relatively normal size and cortical architecture of the right cerebral hemisphere (long arrows). Sagittal T2 image of the right cerebral hemisphere (**e**) demonstrates asymmetric increase in size of the right compared to the left (**f**). Constellation of findings are consistent with unilateral cerebral hemispheric polymicrogyria with ipsilateral cerebral hemiatrophy

involvement of an entire cerebral hemisphere with resultant unilateral cerebral atrophy secondary to maldevelopment (Fig. 3.9) [88, 89].

The gray-matter structures of the cerebral hemispheres originate from the ventricular layer (germinal matrix) of the developing hemisphere, and the neurons and glia migrate outwards to their final position in either the cerebral cortex or the deep gray structures. Barkovich and coauthors classified gray matter disorders into failure of cerebral cortex neuronal/glial proliferation in the ventricular zone, failure of migration, and failure of cortical organization [90]. An abnormality in an earlier process is likely to interfere with the related later process. For instance, an abnormal neuronal formation is likely to have a deleterious impact on both neuronal migration and cortical formation. Abnormalities of cortical formation, therefore, are classified by the developmentally earliest event that is known to be defective [91–93].

Gray matter remaining in the subependymal lining of the ventricles are referred to as subependymal gray matter heterotopias (SHE). While these can be sporadic in occurrence, they are noted in as high as 30% of patients with the Chiari 2 deformity. Awareness of this entity is important, as up to 80% of patients with this develop epilepsy during lifetimes, with associated disorders of cognition ranging from 20% to 60% in the post-natal life. A recent review of fetal MRI imaging in 95 fetuses with Chiari 2 showed that although only 22 of the patients (23% of cohort) were suspected as having subependymal heterotopia, only 11 of these cases (50% of cohort) possessed actual heterotopia on post-natal MRI. Similarly, while 27 of the 95 patients (28% of cohort) were found to have true heterotopias on post-natal imaging, only 11 of these patients (41% of cohort) were suspected of possessing it on pre-natal MRI. Several factors can result in reduced detection accuracy on fetal

MRI, including fetal motion image degradation and small size of neuroanatomy relative to postnatal life. As such, because its pre-natal imaging detection can be challenging, closer scrutiny for its evaluation is warranted especially in the setting of Chiari 2 [94].

Bands of heterotopic gray matter between the ventricular lining and cortical mantle characterize subcortical band heterotopia, also known as double cortex syndrome. The overlying cortex ranges from having a normal appearance, possessing pachygyria, or possessing near-complete lack of cortical gyration referred to as lissencephaly. Lissecephaly has traditionally been categorized into types 1 and 2. Type 1 is the classic type with smooth brain surface in the setting of agyria. Type 2 is characterized by the cobblestone brain surface appearance in the spectrum of pachygyria. The type 2 subtype is typically associated with syndromes of muscular dystrophy such as muscle-eye brain (MEB) disease, Walker-Warburg syndrome, and Fukuyama syndrome [95]. New spectrums of lissencephaly classification continue to emerge based on a combination of genetic markers, patterns of agyria to pachygyria, presence or absence of band heterotopias, cortical thickness measurements, and presence of associated parenchymal abnormalities such as corpus callosal dysgenesis and cerebellar hypoplasia [96]. Co-existence of band heterotopia with polymicrogyria is rare, noting scattered case reports in the literature (Fig. 3.10) [97, 98].

Hemimegaloencephaly is characterized as a focal, nonneoplastic failure of neuronal/glial proliferation. Specifically, there is a unilateral overproduction of neurons and glia, resulting in an increased volume of the affected cerebral hemisphere. As the increased numbers of cells are embryologically immature, their migration and cortical organization are faulty. This results in the associated pachygyria, polymicrogyria, and heterotopia that are a classically a part of this entity. Ventriculomegaly is present without accompanying volume loss or sequalae of post-obstructive etiology. Midline shift of the enlarged cerebral hemisphere may occur; notably occipital lobe

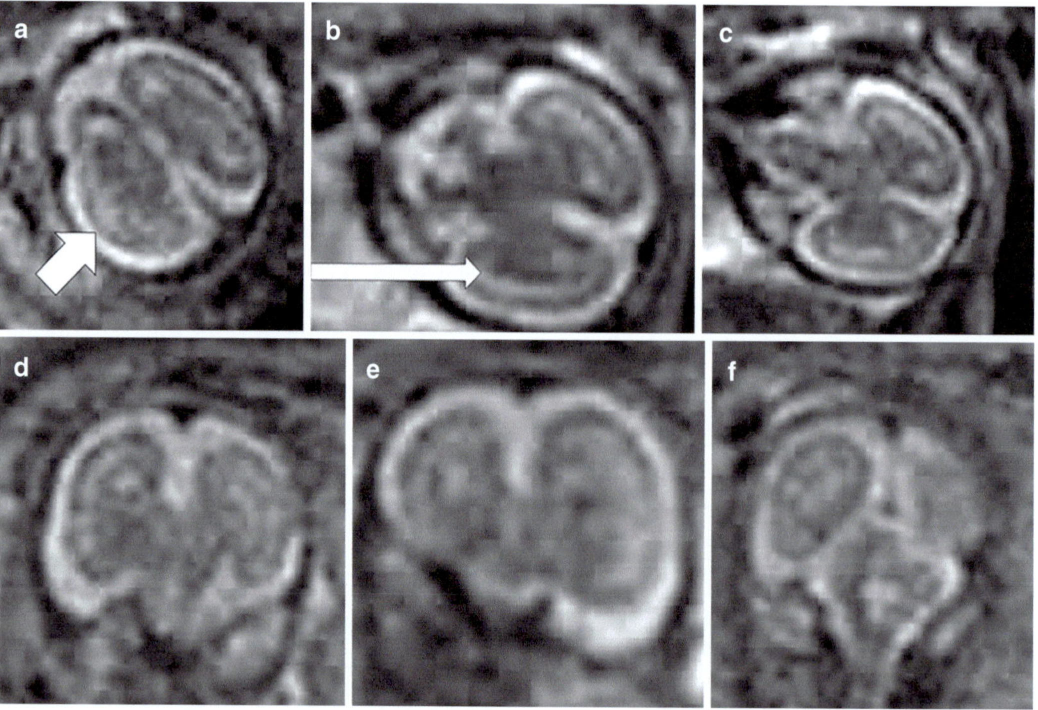

Fig. 3.10 Axial T2 MR images (**a–c**) demonstrating markedly smooth cortical surface, atypical for patient's gestational age (short arrow). Underlying band heterotopia is also present (long arrow). These findings are similarly made on coronal T2 images (**d–f**). Constellation of findings are consistent with lissencephaly

extension beyond the cerebral falx level is frequently present. There is disruption of the transient layers, best appreciated on DWI. In the fetal brain, the cell rich and cell sparse in transient structures have characteristic appearances on DWI. High diffusion coefficients are seen in the cell-sparse zones, while restricted diffusion is present in the cell rich regions with high nuclear to cytoplasmic ratios. As such, DWI is useful in detecting areas of restricted diffusion related to cellularity in areas of abnormal cortical formation in transient layers [91–93].

Post-ischemic Spectrum of Parenchymal Injury

Neuraxis insults can still occur during fetal growth in the second and third trimesters despite successful first trimester development. Causes include states of maternal-fetal infection, inflammation, placenta previa and abruption, polyhydramnios (excess amniotic fluid) associated intrauterine growth restrictions, altered maternal hemodynamics in the setting of eclampsia, seizures, trauma, and drugs such as cocaine. Resultant effects range from generalized injury of sensitive critical structures (hypoxic-ischemic spectrum and periventricular leukomalacia), unifocal and multifocal walled-off encephalomalacic zones known as porencephalic cyst(s), or global atrophy corresponding to major vascular territories (hydranencephaly) [99].

The subplate and intermediate zones are precursors of neonatal white matter. The subplate zone is particularly important in neuronal migration and axon guidance and connectivity. However, the subplate zone is vulnerable to ischemic or hypoxic effects in preterm injury [91].

Patterns of prenatal brain injury are related to the vascular distributions of brain parenchyma that are affected by the specific insult. The severity of insult can be characterized as mild, moderate, or severe depending on their imaging and clinical manifestations such as acid-base status, EEG, MRI patters, Apgar score, and overall clinical exam.

Periventricular leukomalacia or germinal matrix hemorrhage occurs as a result of hypoxic

ischemic injury in the early third trimester. This occurs as a result of hypoperfusion injury, regardless of severity or fetal location (intrauterine or extrauterine preterm). Their detection in prenatal imaging can be challenging, as imaging findings are more subtle as compared to their pronounced cystic appearance on postnatal imaging. The presence of increased periventricular echogenicity in the third trimester is specific for future PVL development in postnatal life [100]. Other pathologies can lead to similar periventricular increased echogenicity however (ranging from edema, TORCH infection, early choroid plexus and subependymal cysts, or early porencephaly). This is in contrast to fetuses in the late third trimester and term infants, as these later stage gestations succumb to watershed zone infarcts between the border zones and within the anterior—middle cerebral and middle—posterior cerebral artery territories. Severe hypotension in either the early or late third trimester additionally affects the thalami, brainstem, and cerebellum, noting increased echogenicity on prenatal ultrasound with corresponding increased T2 signal on fetal MRI (Fig. 3.11) [101].

Multifocal encephalomalacia can result in pockets of walled off cystic encephalomalacia referred to as porencephalic cysts. These may or may not be in communication with the ventricular system depending on their location. They are distinguished from regions of open-lip schizencephaly by their lack of intact gray matter lining their peripheral aspects [102, 103].

Hydranencephaly is the most severe entity in this spectrum, characterized by bilateral cerebral cortical destruction as a result of bilateral internal carotid artery territory infarcts. Classic imaging demonstrates absences of the bilateral cerebral hemispheres supplied by the anterior and middle cerebral artery territories, noting only sparing of the vertebrobasilar circulation supplied posterior fossa elements and brainstem. Variable amounts of residual cerebral parenchyma may be present depending on potential preservation of ICA territory branches. Given absence of dominant forebrain components, there can be difficulty in distinguishing this entity from alobar holoprosencephaly and severe ventriculomegaly (Fig. 3.12) [104].

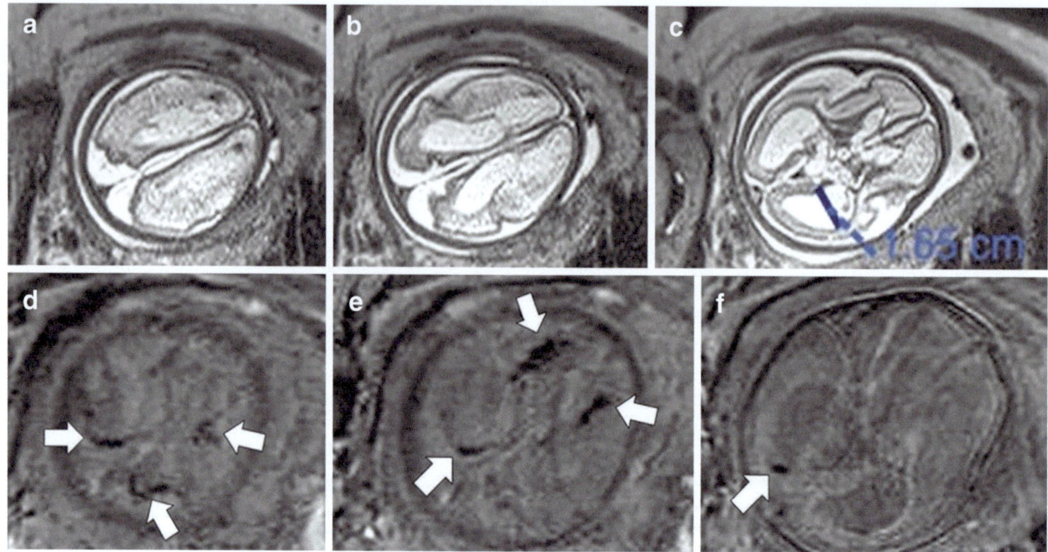

Fig. 3.11 Axial T2 images (**a–c**) demonstrate ventriculomegaly secondary to periventricular leukomalacia (PVL). Axial SWI images (**d–f**) demonstrate combination of periventricular/subependymal chronic blood products and calcifications. This combination of findings suggest sequalae of the TORCH pre-natal spectrum of diseases (in this case prenatal exposure to Rubella)

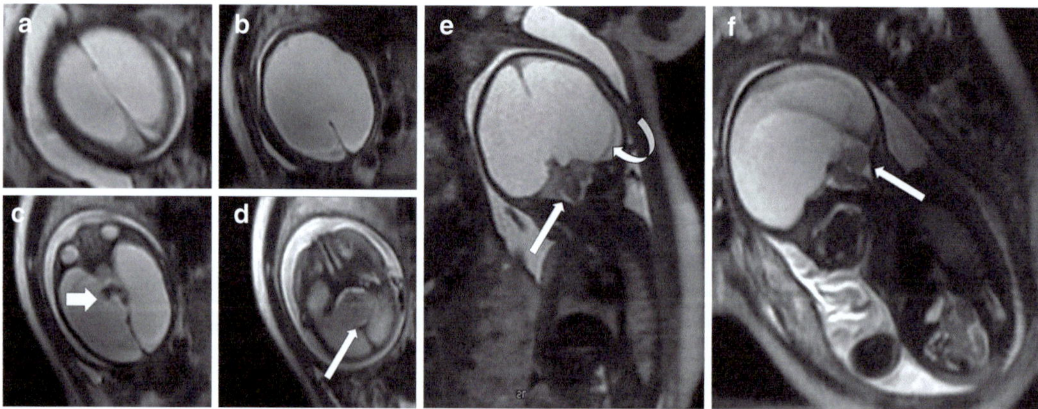

Fig. 3.12 Axial T2 (**a–d**), coronal T2 (**e**), and sagittal T2 (**f**) fetal MRI images demonstrate the presence of hydranencephaly. Note the lack of supratentorial brain parenchyma secondary to sequalae of intrauterine insult, resultant hydrocephalus secondary to surrounding global cortical and parenchymal atrophy (curved arrow pointing to marking of lateral ventricle in **e**), minimal residual midbrain (short arrow in **c**), and otherwise preserved posterior fossa anatomy (long arrows in **d–f** pointing to cerebellum and intact posterior fossa structures)

In alobar holoprosencephaly, which will be readdressed in a separate section, there are errors in primary neurulation with subsequent lack of forebrain element formation. As a result, there is incomplete separation of midline brain elements, notably the thalami and deep gray nuclei ('fused thalami' appearance of alobar holoprosencephaly). In hydranencephaly, the thalami and posterior fossa elements are formed within normal limits, remaining separate accordingly. In severe ventriculomegaly, a thin rim of peripherally located forebrain parenchyma remains as the apparent empty appearance of the cranial vault is related to central to peripheral expansion from ventricular system enlargement rather than a direct absence of brain parenchyma from destruction [104].

Abnormalities of the Corpus Collosum

The corpus callosum is the dominant supratentorial commissure connecting bilateral cerebral hemispheres arising from the lamina reunions of His and developing between weeks 8 and 20 of gestational age, and best detected on fetal MRI by 18–20 weeks. Development starts in the genu, continues dorsally along the body, and then extends from the isthmus to the splenium. The rostrum, the most ventrally located portion of the corpus callosum located anteroinferior to the genu, is the last part to be formed. Agenesis of the corpus callosum (ACC) is detected during prenatal sonography via a combination of sonographic findings, including widening of the interhemispheric fissure, absence of the cavum septum pellucidum, high-riding third ventricle, and colpocephaly. The condition classically produces a steer horn appearance to the frontal horns with associated separation of both cerebral hemispheres and elevation of the third ventricle.

Fetal MRI allows for confirmation of true agenesis. This is opposed to dysgenesis (DCC), in which parts of the callosal tract are incompletely formed rather than complete agenesis. This can occur either as a result of post-formation acquired insult or due to interruption development, both of which can be differentiated depending on which portions of the callosal tract remain intact. Maintenance of the rostrum with otherwise absent portions of the genu, body, isthmus, or splenium indicate acquired insult leading to lack of formation rather than incomplete development since the final portion of corpus callosum formation—the rostrum—remains intact. Commonly associated brain abnormalities include sulcation and posterior fossa abnormalities. Abnormalities and delays of sulcation are detectable in as early as 19 weeks gestational age (though sulcation patterns are more characteristically evaluated beginning 30 weeks of age) with fetal MRI and seen in up to 50% of fetuses with ACC. Sulcation delays are common in fetuses with ACC, suggesting that delay is a manifestation of global white matter dysgenesis rather than its own separate abnormality. Gyral malformations are frequently encountered and include polymicrogyria, lissencephaly, pachygyria, and schizencephaly. Posterior fossa abnormalities are also frequently detected, ranging from cerebellar hemispheric and vermian abnormalities, some of which are mentioned in their respective subsection. Callosal abnormalities are also included in the spectrum of findings part of numerous syndromes ranging from Aicardi syndrome, Walker-Warburg syndrome, and MASA syndrome. Following initial detection or suspicion on prenatal sonography, a combination of T2 weighted single shot images and T1 weighted gradient images of multiplanar fetal MRI can detect agenesis or dysgenesis of the corpus callosum, sulcation abnormalities, and alternate corollary abnormalities if present (Fig. 3.13) [105].

Abnormalities of the Cavum Septum Pellucidum

The septum pellucidum is identified as the midline interventricular septum separating both right and left lateral ventricles. The septum pellucidum unit is composed of an anterior (septum pellucidum) and posterior component (septum vergae), with persistent cavum formation in each known as cavum septum pellucidum (CSP) and cavum vergae (CV). CSP and CV describe the presence of a CSF-filled central cavity within these portions of the septum. This appearance is normal in the first and second trimesters, with closure of the leaflets from front to back starting around 6 months gestational age. CSP persistence into post-natal life is a common normal variant, whereas nearly all term infants have closure of the CV. Septum formation is intricately associated with development of the limbic system fornices and forebrain commissures. Originating from the lamina reuniens—tissue connecting the telencephalon near midline—this forms the upper border of the lamina terminalis at 7 weeks gestational age. At 9 weeks of age, hippocampal-septal fibers and the anterior commissure form within this lamina reuniens, with these hippocampal-septal fibers crossing midline in the posterior aspect of the lamina reuniens at

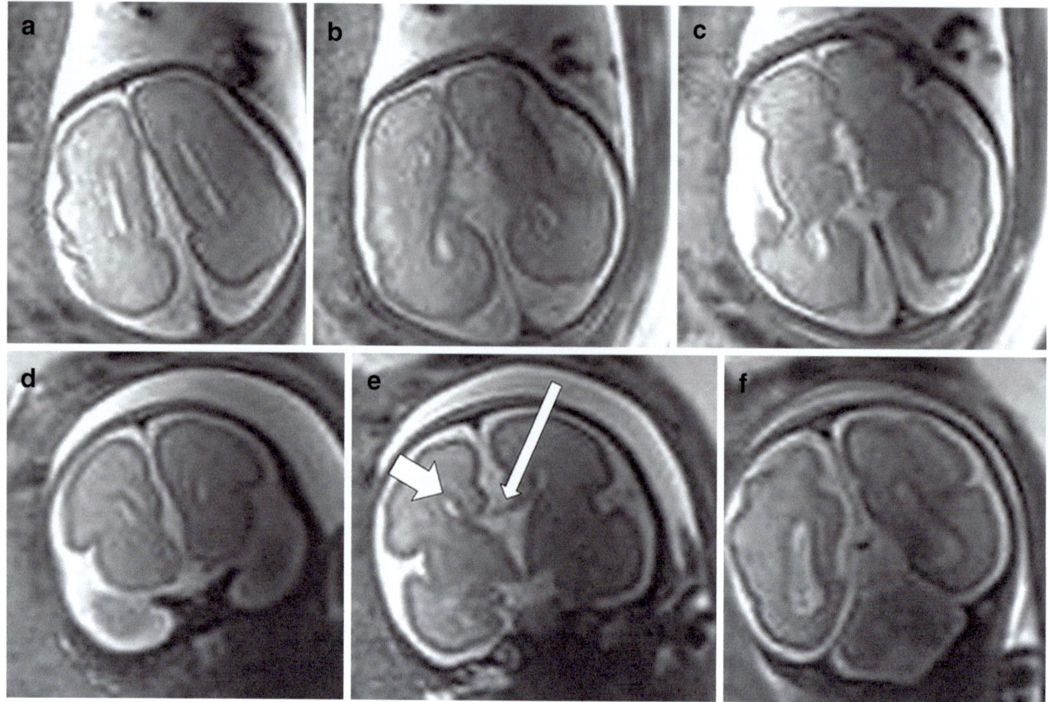

Fig. 3.13 34-year-old woman with 27-week gestation. Axial T2 (**a–c**) and Coronal T2 (**d–f**) images of the brain demonstrate complete separation of the bilateral cerebral hemispheres without evidence of a corpus collosum. There is a steer horn appearance to the frontal horns espe-cially noted on the coronal plane of imaging (**d**), with the horns simulated by the lateral ventricles (short arrow) and elevated third ventricle roof simulating the top of the steer horn's head (long arrow). Findings are consistent with agenesis of the corpus collosum

week 11. At week 12, the interhemispheric fissure—also named the sulcus medianus telecephali medii based on its origin structures—divides the lamina reuniens with its lateral walls forming the leaves of the CSP. The CSP further acts as a pivot point for the formation of the corpus callosum by allowing cingulate fibers to cross anteriorly and hippocampal commissure fibers to cross posteriorly, noting that the corpus callosum trajectory creates the roof the velum interpositum. Further development of connecting forebrain commissures continues to stretch the fornices and leaves of the CSP accordingly [106].

Given this embryologic background and close association in the development of important forebrain structures and commissures, identifying the presence or absence of the CSP is an important screening portion of the sonographic fetal anatomic survey. If the CSP is absent, fetal MRI can be considered with its combination of multiplanar T2-weighted single shot images and T1 weighted gradient images better able to detect for associated parenchymal abnormalities. Fetal MRI findings made alongside absent CSP alert practitioners to the following potential pathologies: (1) Associated incomplete separation of the cerebral hemispheres suggests holoprosencephaly spectrum; (2) Small frontal horns with colpocephaly suggest corpus callosal anomalies; (3) Severe ventriculomegaly suggests a wide differential ranging from obstructive hydrocephalus secondary to Aqueductal Stenosis, Chiari 2 malformation, Cephalocele, injury secondary to hemorrhage with resultant cystic changes and volume loss, or hydranencephaly (near-complete absence of hemispheres); and (4) Normal frontal horns suggest hypoplastic optic nerve syndrome or isolated septal deficiency. These respective differentials have either been touched upon or will be addressed in upcoming subsections (Fig. 3.14) [106].

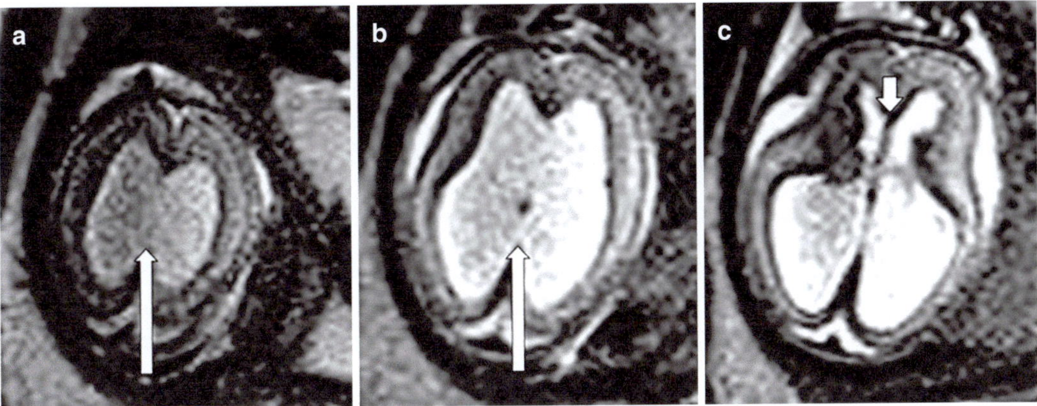

Fig. 3.14 31-year-old woman with 22-week gestation fetus. Axial T2 images demonstrate absence of the septum pellucidum (long arrows) (**a**, **b**) with maintenance of the interhemispheric fissure (short arrow) (**c**). Ventriculomegaly in this case is related to congenital aqueductal stenosis otherwise not shown on the provided images

Holoprosencephaly

Holoprosencephaly (HPE) is the most common congenital forebrain developmental abnormality and stems from abnormal separation of the prosencephalon. The prosencephalon consists of the cerebral hemispheres (telencephalon), thalamus and other deep brain structures, hypothalamus (diencephalon), and optic bulb and tracts. This embryologic separation—referred to cleavage plane formation—occurs at 5–6 weeks gestation age. Errors in forebrain cleavage typically occur as result of genetic irregularities, including chromosome anomalies (Trisomy 13), syndromic single gene mutations (CDON gene → Steinfeld syndrome, FDFR1 gene → Hartsfield syndrome, CENPF → Stromme syndrome, DHCR7 → Smith-Lemli-Opitz syndrome), and non-syndromic single gene mutations (SHH → 6% of all nonsyndromic HPE; ZIC2 → 5% of all nonsyndromic HPE; SIX3 → 3% of all nonsyndromic HPE; TGIF1 → <1% of all nonsyndromic HPE). Errors occurring in early, midway, or delayed stages of cleavage plane development result in unique neuroanatomic appearances with associated functional and neurocognitive complications. The three classic HPE subtypes are as follows [107, 108].

- Alobar HPE: There is a single "monoventricle" with no separation of the cerebral hemispheres. This is the most severe form and encompasses about 40% of cases. The range of findings include cyclopia (single eye or partially divided eye) in single orbit with a proboscis above the eye, cyclopia without proboscis, ethmocephaly (significantly closely spaced eyes with separate orbits and proboscis between eyes), cebocephaly (closely spaced eyes with single-nostril nose), closely spaced eyes, anophthalmia or microophthalmia, premaxillary agenesis with median cleft lip, depressed nasal ridge, and bilateral cleft lip (Fig. 3.15) [107, 108].

- Semilobar HPE: The left and right frontal and parietal lobes are fused and the interhemispheric fissure is only present posteriorly. This is the intermediate in severity form and encompasses another 40% of cases. The range of findings include closely spaced eyes, anophthalmia/microophthalmia, depressed nasal ridge, absent nasal septum, flat nasal tip, bilateral cleft lip with median process representing the philtrum-premaxilla anlage, midline cleft (lip and/or palate), and relatively normal facial appearance [107, 108].

- Lobar HPE: Most of the right and left cerebral hemispheres and lateral ventricles are separated. However, the frontal lobes and most superior aspect of the telencephalon are fused, especially ventrally. This least severe form encompasses the remaining 20% of cases. The range of findings include bilateral cleft lip with median process, closely spaced eyes,

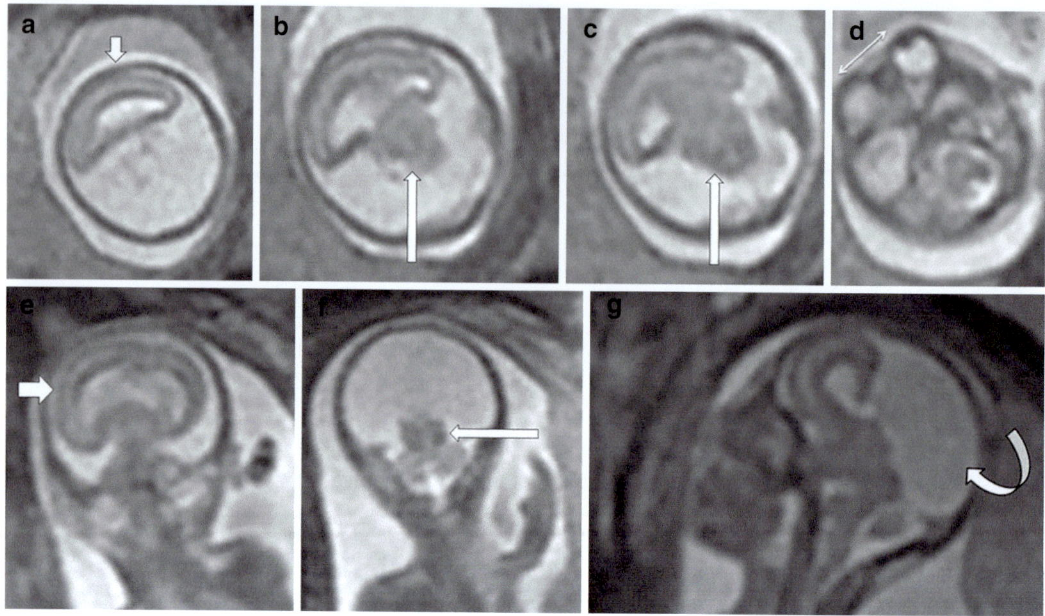

Fig. 3.15 21-year-old woman with 19-week gestation. Fetal MRI was performed given findings seen on prenatal sonography. (**a–d**) are axial T2 images. (**e, f**) are coronal T2 images. (**g**) is a sagittal T2 image. There is a boomerang-shaped monoventricle (short arrow) with a large dorsal cyst occupying two-thirds of the calvaral cavity (curved arrow). The thalami and midbrain are fused (long arrow). There is severe hypotelorism with both eyes otherwise present (double arrow). There is no sylvian fissure, no corpus callosum and most of the cerebral hemispheres are missing with only the anterior frontal lobes identified. This constellation of findings are consistent with alobar holoprosencephaly

depressed nasal ridge, and relatively normal facial appearance (Fig. 3.16) [107, 108].

Other rarer entities in this HPE spectrum include septo-optic dysplasia, middle interhemispheric variant, and microforms of HPE [107, 108].

Septopreoptic type: Nonseparation is restricted to the septal and preoptic regions, with remainder of intracranial contents otherwise within normal limits. This is also referred to as septo-optic dysplasia in the literature [107, 108].

Middle interhemispheric fusion variant (also known as syntelencephaly): The posterior frontal and parietal lobes fail to separate. There is varying lack of separation of the basal ganglia and thalami with absence of the body of the corpus callosum. However, the genu and splenium of the corpus callosum are present. The range of findings includes: closely spaced eyes, depressed nasal bridge, narrow nasal bridge, and relatively normal facial appearance [107, 108].

Microforms of HPE (also termed "microform HPE") are clinical subtypes of HPE defined by the presence of HPE-related craniofacial anomalies without structural brain defects on imaging. They may occur in simplex HPE (i.e., a single occurrence of HPE in a family) or in relatives of probands with classic forms of HPE. Their clinical spectrum includes the following: microcephaly, single central maxillary incisor, closely spaced eyes, anosmia/hyposmia (resulting from absence of olfactory tracts and bulbs), various ophthalmologic anomalies including refractive errors, ptosis, microcornea, and coloboma, sharp and narrow nasal bridge, absent superior labial frenulum, midface retrusion, congenital nasal pyriform aperture stenosis, and developmental delay (variably present) [107, 108].

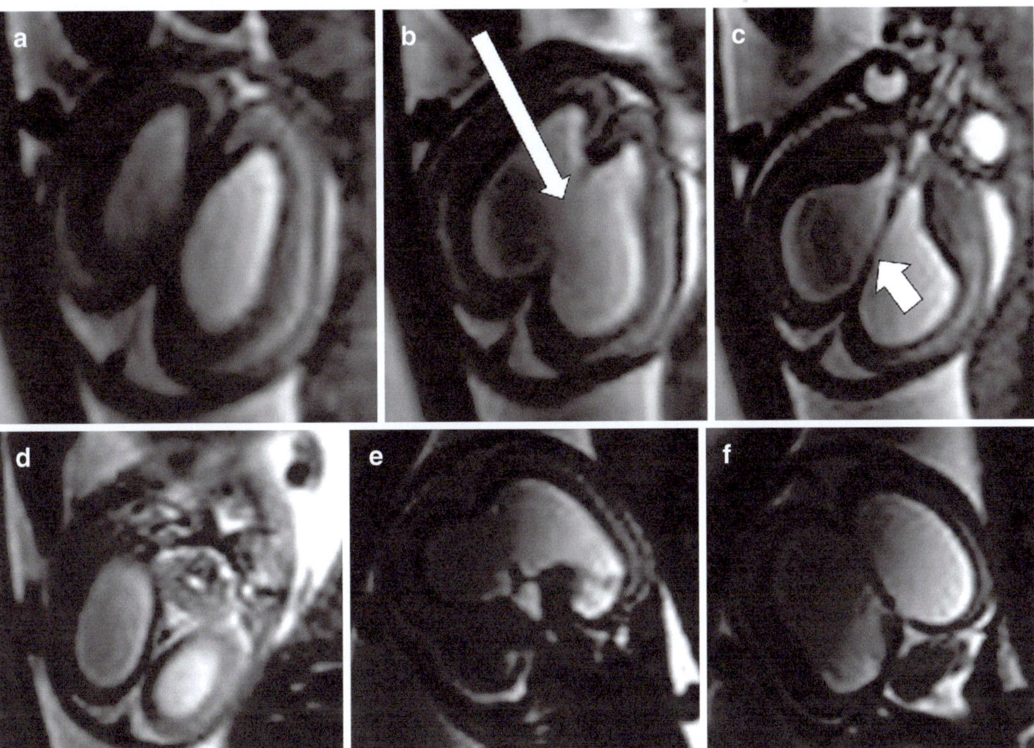

Fig. 3.16 33-year-old pregnant woman with 21-week gestation. (**a–d**) are axial T2 images of the brain. (**e, f**) are coronal T2 images of the brain. Although there is no cavum septum pellucidum, there is absence of the septum pellucidum anteriorly with fusion of the frontal horns of the lateral ventricles (long arrow). The septum is otherwise present posteriorly (short arrow). Remaining forebrain structures are within normal limits, noting that there is limitation in fine evaluation of the ocular pathways and sellar region on fetal MRI alone. Findings were suspected to be on the basis of lobar holoprosencephaly. Given lack of complete cerebral hemispheric separation, this suggests presence of a corpus collosum, noting that it is thinned in this case. Also, as the lateral and third ventricles are enlarged with an otherwise normal caliber fourth ventricle, a superimposed congenital aqueductal stenosis was diagnosed

Posterior Fossa Anomalies

Dandy-walker malformation, vermian hypoplasia/agenesis, and mega cisterna magna are the dominant pathologies comprising the otherwise heterogonous group of conditions known as posterior fossa anomalies (PFA). These occur in every 1 of 5000 live births. Fetal MRI best separates between the various PFAs given different prognoses for each. MRI also allows for whole body evaluation to assess for associated extracranial anomalies, including facial (26%), renal (28%), extremity (28%), intraventricular system (32%), and cardiac (38%) anomalies [109].

Nevertheless, ultrasound remains the test of choice for initial screening of PFAs. Specifically, the shape and contour of cerebellar hemispheres, vermis, and cisterna magna are carefully evaluated in axial, coronal, and sagittal planes. The coronal plane in helpful in differentiating the cerebellar hemispheres and vermis, facilitating the diagnosis of vermian hypoplasia/agenesis. The median sagittal plan is considered the most important plane of evaluation given the ability to evaluate the brainstem elements (including pontine diameter), midline vermis (its height, anterior-posterior measurements, and presence or absence of upward rotation), assess size and continuity of the fourth ventricle and its fastigium (roof of fourth ventricle), the primary fissure of the vermis which should be identified in all cases after 24 weeks of gestation (the fissure divides vermis into superior and inferior components, noting that the size ratio of its superior to inferior portions is typically 1:2), cisterna magna shape and diameter, and tentorial position (particularly useful in cystic malformation evaluation, as will be discussed later) [110].

Reference charts exist with regard to size ranges of the fetal intracranial contents considered to be within normal limits. It is important to note that slight variability may exist in measurements performed on prenatal ultrasound compared to MRI simply due to variations between the technologies and protocols used [111–113]. Systematic cerebellar measurements include the transcerebellar diameter (measurement of maximal cerebellum width across both hemispheres) and vermis height (measured either in sagittal or coronal plane). Vermian hypoplasia is characterized by a small vermis with an otherwise intact morphology (including preserved 1:2 ratio of superior to inferior portions separated by the primary fissure). Given its small size, there is absence or flattening of the fastigium angle and communication between the fourth ventricle and cisterna magna. Vermian agenesis refers to the complete absence of the cerebellar vermis. This is seen in Joubert syndrome, an autosomal recessive disorder characterized by abnormal behavior, ataxia, mental retardation, and vermian agenesis [110].

The Blake's pouch cyst is characterized as an apparent communication between the cisterna magna and fourth ventricle with upward rotation of the vermis. In normal development, Blake's pouch (also known as the rudimental fourth ventricular tela choroidea) is a transient structure that gradually regresses by the 12th week of gestational development to begin the formation of the foramen of Magendie. Some consider this cyst the sequalae of delayed fourth ventricle closure and within normal limits rather than a pathologic entity, as, aside from vermian orientation, its size and fastigium are within normal limits as is tentorial position (Fig. 3.17) [110].

A combination of findings characterize the Dandy-Walker malformation. Cystic dilation of the fourth ventricle with communication between the fourth ventricle and cisterna magna is the hallmark finding. What distinguishes this from the Blake's pouch cyst is absence or flattening of the fastigium angle alongside upward rotation with elevation of the tentorium seen in the setting of vermian agenesis or hypoplasia. These are typically accompanied by other malformations, including the corpus callosum agenesis/dysgenesis spectrum and interhemispheric cysts (Fig. 3.18) [110].

Mega-cisterna magna describes the condition of an enlarged cisterna magna with transverse diameter ≥10 mm in the setting of an otherwise

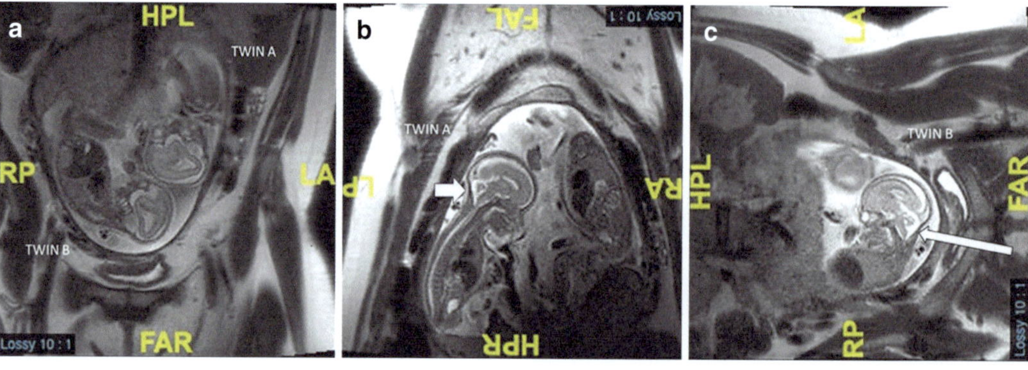

Fig. 3.17 (**a**) 30-year-old woman with 20-week twin gestations. Coronal whole body T2 MRI demonstrates a monochorionic monoamniotic twin. In this study, twin A is located above twin B. In (**b**), the posterior fossa of twin A is within normal limits, noting normal sized fourth ventricle, cerebellar vermis, and cisterna magna (short arrow). In (**c**), there is a slightly expanded cisterna magna communicating with the fourth ventricle without torcula elevation. The cerebellar vermis is intact, as is the fourth ventricle fastigium. There is otherwise preserved architecture of the posterior fossa contents. Findings are suggestive of a mega cisterna magna versus small Blake's pouch cyst (long arrow)

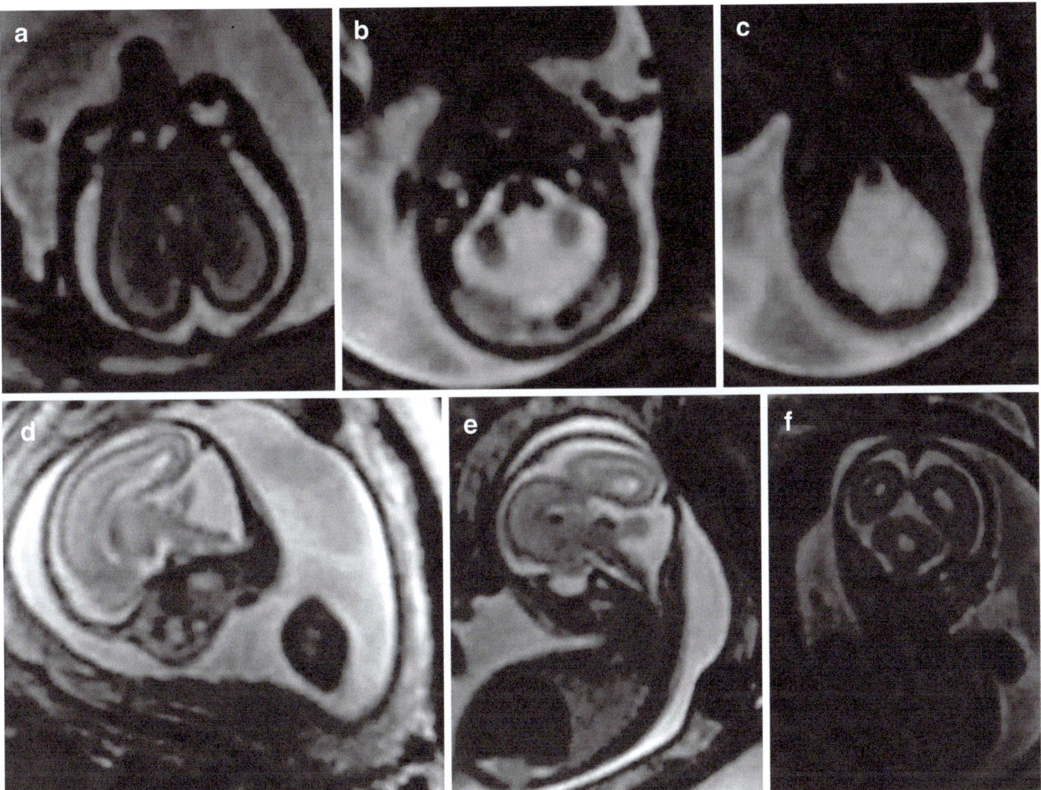

Fig. 3.18 Axial T2 images demonstrate a supratentorial compartment within normal limits (**a**), absence of the cerebellar vermis (**b**), and expansion of the posterior fossa (**c**). Sagittal T2 images show an absent cerebellar vermis with expansion of posterior fossa and tentorial elevation (**d**) and communication between fourth ventricle and cisterna magna secondary to vermian absence (**e**), noting that the cerebellar diameter is otherwise within normal limits (**f**). This constellation of findings are in keeping with Dandy Walker Malformation

normal posterior fossa anatomic evaluation. Specifically, no communication between the fourth ventricle and cisterna magna is present [110].

Rhombencephalosynapsis is characterized as fusion of the bilateral cerebellar hemispheres with characteristic triangular shape, noting fusion is present given associated vermian hypoplasia/agenesis. The key finding is identification of cerebellar hemispheric foliations demonstrating continuity is the midline without vermian interruption, best appreciated on the coronal plane of imaging (Fig. 3.19) [110].

Once cisterna magna size, fourth ventricle caliber, and vermis identification are identified to be within normal limits, remaining PFAs pertain to varying degrees of cerebellar parenchymal abnormalities. Differential considerations include cerebellar hypoplasia (smaller than normal cerebellum with diameter below tenth percentile for gestational age, noting small cerebellar size artificially can make cisterna magna appear falsely enlarged), pontocerebellar hypoplasia (small cerebellum along with flattened/thin pons, Fig. 3.20), and unilateral cerebellar lesions (partial or complete destruction of cerebellar components, typically related to prenatal insults ranging from infarction, infection, or hemorrhage) [110].

TORCH Spectrum of Infections

TORCH is a widely used acronym referring to the complex of infectious agents that possess a

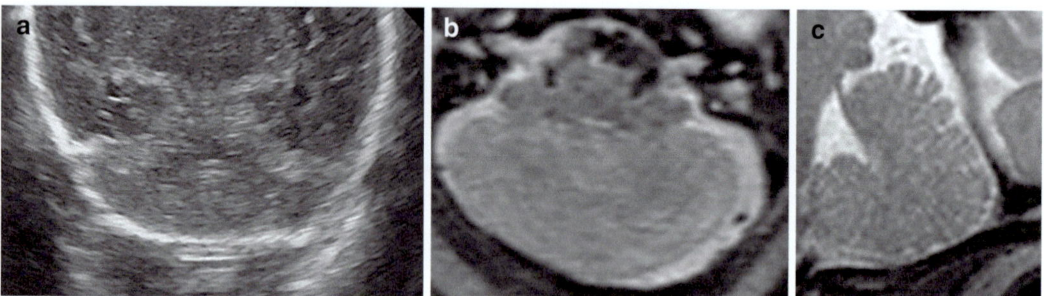

Fig. 3.19 Coronal ultrasound (**a**), axial T2 (**b**), and sagittal T2 (**c**) all demonstrate absence of the cerebellar vermis with fusion of the bilateral cerebellar hemispheres and resultant continuity of the hemispheric white matter tracts. Findings are consistent with Rhombencephalosynapsis

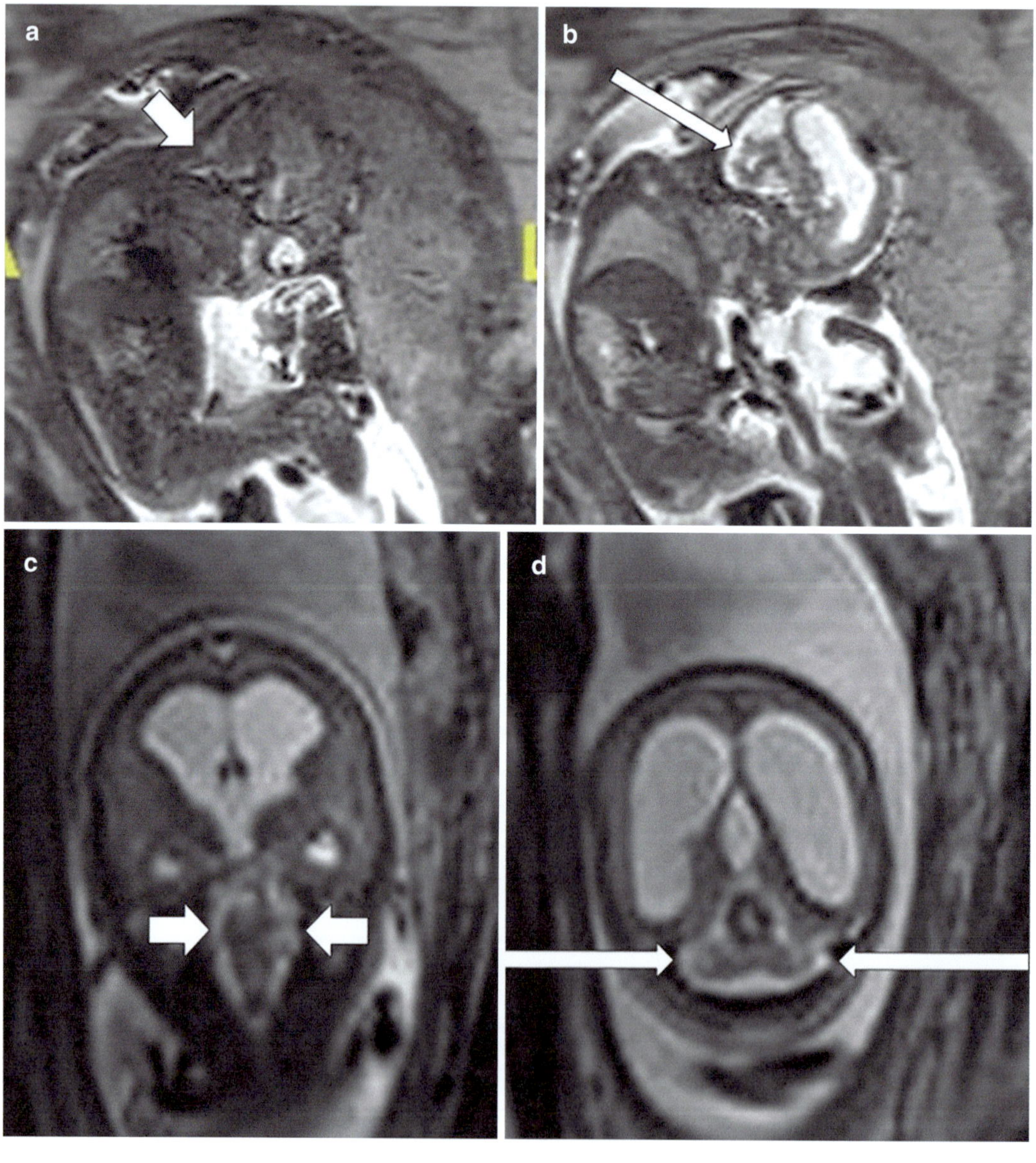

Fig. 3.20 Pontine hypoplasia (**a**, **c**). Cerebellar volume loss with small vermis (**b**, **d**). Associated ventriculomegaly. Otherwise no elevation of tentorium or torcula. Findings consistent with cerebello-pontine hypoplasia

predisposition towards induction of neurodevelopmental alterations in intrauterine gestations, particularly during the first and second trimesters of pregnancy. These agents include toxoplasmosis (TO), rubella (R), cytomegalovirus (C), and herpes-simplex 2 (H). Zika is not part of the TORCH acronym, yet their presence has also been shown to affect neuroanatomic development in characteristic ways leading to clinical sequelae such as microcephaly, hypertonia, hyperreflexia, seizures, arthrogryposis, and ventriculomegaly.

The human cytomegalovirus (CMV) is widely prevalent throughout the population, with seroprevalence reported between 40% and 100% of the general adult population. Its ubiquity stems from its predominance of either mild flu-like symptoms to asymptomatic clinical manifestations. If acquired during fetal development—referred to as congenital CMV—10–20% of exposed infants symptomatic at birth demonstrate neurodevelopmental deficits and sensorineural hearing loss, with long-term sequalae extending well into post-natal growth in 40–60% of symptomatic survivors. Highly specific fetal MR findings include polymicrogyria/spectrum of cortical malformations (blurred gray-white matter junctions on T2 weighted imaging) and periventricular calcifications (low T2 and high T1 foci signal with periventricular location highly specific for congenital CMV, with deep gray and white matter involvement next common). The presence of periventricular cysts/pseudocysts is also highly

specific for congenital CMV infection (Fig. 3.21). Widespread brain parenchymal findings indicating CMV infection include scattered white matter hyperintense signal (with temporal lobe involvement connoting worse prognosis), ventriculomegaly, ventriculitis, intraventricular septations/adhesions (most commonly in the occipital horns), clefts related to schizencephaly (true transmantle cleft lined by cortex hypointense on T2) and potencephaly (encephalomalacic cleft without true cortical lining hyperintense on T2), cerebellar hypoplasia/dysplasia (as described in prior subsection), hippocampal dysplasia (maybe difficult to appreciate on fetal MRI given limitations in modality), and lenticulostriate vasculopathy (susceptibility with low T2 signal in the basal ganglia) [114].

Congenital toxoplasmosis stems from transplacental spread of infection by the protozoan Toxoplasma gondii. Common sources of infection include the ingestion or handling of infected meat products or exposure to excrements from domestic pets, notably cats. Areas of highest prevalence include the Latin American countries. Although frequency of maternal to fetal spread is increased in the third trimester, resultant delays in neurodevelopment are more prevalent if transmission occurs during the first two trimesters. Diagnosis is made in the prenatal setting via a combination of routine screening of pregnant patients and ultrasound examination demonstrating classic findings, with adjunct fetal MRI used to primarily corroborate sonographic findings.

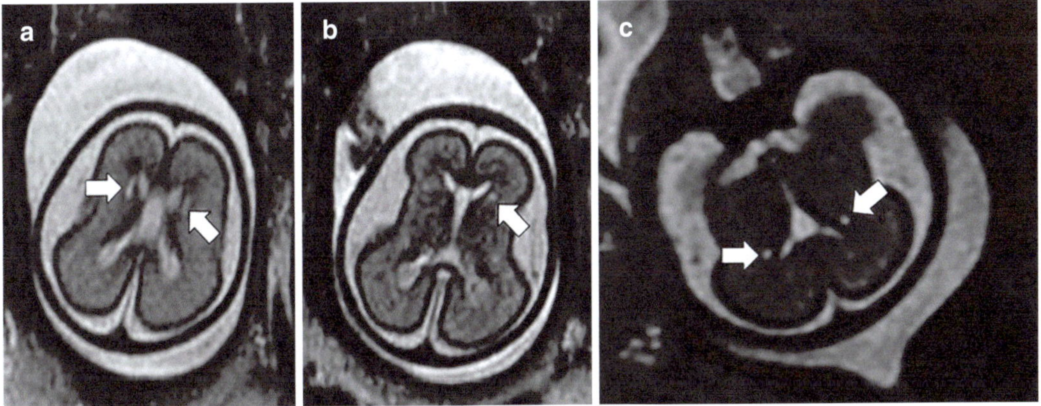

Fig. 3.21 (**a–c**) Axial T2 images demonstrate scattered periventricular cysts (arrows) in the setting of congenital TORCH exposure

Infectious deposits with or without cystic formation are seen as echogenic nodules on ultrasound or T2 hypointense foci on MRI in a random distribution, though trends toward increased identification in the periventricular gray-white junctions and caudothalamic groove are often noted. Afflicted pre-natal gestations most commonly exhibit varying degrees of encephalomalacia and cerebral/cerebellar volume loss with associated ventriculomegaly and hydrocephalus. Parenchymal chunky calcifications are common, specifically in the basal ganglia. White matter disease reflecting a combination of edema and encephalomalacia are both focal or diffuse depending on extent of protozoan deposits and extent of spread in the brain [115].

Rubella is member of the togaviridae family of viruses known for its highly contagious mechanism of spread via either direct or droplet contact with an afflicted patient's respiratory secretions. Following vaccine introduction in 1971, the virus was eliminated from the USA in 2000. However, rubella resurgence in the USA has once again occurred in the twenty-first century due to a combination of viral importation of cases from other countries with persistent outbreaks and vaccine hesitancy with an associated rise of occurrence in under-immunized communities [116]. Postnatal infection—also known as German measles—is typically self-limited and results in mild symptoms ranging from low-grade fever, lymphadenopathy and rash [117]. In contrast to its post-natal counterpart, congenital rubella transmitted via direct transplacental spread results in significant neuroanatomic changes. Microcephaly is frequently present. The most commonly seen parenchymal findings stem from the effects of post-infectious vasculopathy, with resultant ischemic changes as severe as hydranencephaly—with associated high T2 signal changes on fetal MRI indicating white matter changes—and ventriculomegaly. Cataracts, though anecdotally described as congenital, are detected more on postnatal rather than prenatal imaging given viral dormancy in the vitreous chambers well into childhood development. Periventricular calcifications can be seen, though they are less commonly seen relative to the other TORCH infections (Fig. 3.11) [118].

Herpes simplex virus is a member of the Herpesviridae family characteristically acquired in the population via either sexual transmission or direct skin-to-skin contact with genital or anal afflicted surfaces. Following primary infection, viral loads move to the sensory ganglia and limbic system elements consisting of the amygdala, hippocampus, thalamus, hypothalamus, basal ganglia, and cingulate gyrus. The virus lays in dormant with prolonged periods of latency, reactivating in times of either immunosuppression or global systemic disturbances [119]. Two distinct viral subtypes exist, type 1 (HSV-1) and type 2 (HSV-2), with HSV-1 more likely to cause oral and labial lesions and HSV-2 more likely to cause genital lesions. Neonatal herpes transmission is common, estimated in 1 of 3200 deliveries. While peripartum transmission encompasses 85% of case and postnatal transmission encompasses 10% of cases, prenatal or in utero transmission of HSV is rare, encompassing only 5% of cases [120]. The HSV-2 subtype encompasses the majority of prenatal herpes cases [121, 122]. Given its rarity, patterns of distribution have been primarily described in various case reports. Apart from the presence of calcifications commonly seen in all the TORCH infections, the most frequently reports intracranial manifestations of prenatal HSV were volume loss, multifocal encephalomalacia, porencephaly, and hydranencephaly appearing related to sequalae of both hemorrhagic and non-hemorrhagic infarcts [123, 124]. Fetal ventriculomegaly related to underlying herpes encephalitis has also been described [125].

Neuroimaging manifestations of the Zika virus came to light in late 2015 given the dramatic rise of its prevalence in South and Central America and the Caribbean. In a 2019 prospective study following 82 pregnant women with clinical criteria for probable Zika infection over the course of their pregnancy to delivery, the vast majority of fetuses (79 of 82, 96%) possessed sequentially normal neuroimaging exams, noting the absence of prolonged maternal viral load did not predict association with normal fetal imaging. However, in the small number of positive studies (3 of 82, 4%), findings were severely abnormal. Along with migration abnormalities spanning the spectrum of gray matter heterotopias, callosal and cerebellar malformations, and ventriculomegaly, resultant microcephaly, brainstem dysplasias, and encephaloceles with Chiari 2 deformity were neuroimaging features strikingly apparent in cases severely affected by the disease [126].

Twin-Twin Transfusion in Relation to Neurodevelopment

Monochorionic twin pregnancies are at risk of significant neurodevelopmental complications in one twin relative to the other. Such risks stem from the concept of twin-twin transfusion, the phenomena of blood shunting from one twin gestation to the other via arteriovenous communications in the shared placenta of monochorionic gestations that may occur in the second trimester of pregnancy.

Such excesses in vascular shunting can lead to detrimental states of anemia and growth cessation in the donor twin. The resultant effects of profound anemia manifest intracranially with ischemic changes in the white matter surrounding the ventricular margins, also known as periventricular leukomalacia. Deep parenchymal structures in fetuses less than 32 weeks of gestational age are supplied in a peripheral to central distribution by choroidal vessels and penetrating branches of the middle cerebral artery and posterior communicating vessels. As the periventricular white matter tracts are deepest and most distally supplied in the premature brain, this region is most susceptible to the effects of hypoxic-ischemic damage, which in this case is related to global anemia.

In the larger recipient twin, polycythemia and systemic volume over-loaded states are often encountered. In addition to the development of fetal hydrops, the effects of brain parenchymal hemorrhages with resultant volume loss and atrophy are often seen as a result of the volume-overloaded state, with their mechanism of development presumably related to inability to maintain fluid balances between the intracellular and extracellular compartments. Similar to periventricular leukomalacia development in the donor twin, germinal matrix hemorrhages are also frequently encountered in the recipient twin given their deep location and susceptible-to-insult friability of the germinal matrix in prenatal patients. Death can result both the recipient and donor twins as a result of these combined effects [127, 128].

Spinal Dysraphisms, Anencephaly, and Neurulation

Spinal dysraphisms are a class of disorders characterized by aberrancies and cessations in neural tube development that result in the varying appearance and location of spinal cord elements. They are classified by the location of their underlying neural progenitor cells with respect to their location in the meninges and osseous boundaries of the spinal canal and posterior elements. The spectrum of posterior element deficits is referred to as spina bifidas. The closed-type of dysraphism is characterized by defects in posterior element formation (spina bifida spectrum) with the neural tube elements otherwise remaining within the central confines of the meninges. This leads to herniation of neuraxis elements through the posterior element defect with preserved subcutaneous coverage (with or without an associated subcutaneous mass). Meanwhile, the open-type of dysraphism is characterized by extension of neuraxis elements through similar posterior element defects without a preserved subcutaneous coverage, resulting in communication of neural elements with the external environment. In order to understand the development of these pathologies, an embryological discussion is necessary [129–131].

Neuraxis development takes place across three stages during the early first trimester: gastrulation (between second and third weeks of gestation), primary Neurulation (between third and fourth weeks of gestation), and secondary Neurulation (between fifth and sixth weeks of gestation). In brief, gastrulation describes the conversion of the fertilized epiblast into a trilaminar embryo composed of the ectoderm, mesoderm, and endoderm. The primitive streak is a band of thickened progenitor epiblast cells that starts at the caudal aspect of the embryo and grows cranially. While the majority of the primitive streak goes on to differentiate further into various elements of the body and neural axis (including the neural plate and notochord), a small cluster of primitive streak cells remain and go on to form neurogenic components inferior to the S2 during secondary neurulation, as will be described shortly. Meanwhile, elements superior to the S2 level are formed during continued differentiation of primitive streak elements in the primary neurulation stage [129–131].

During primary neurulation, the neuraxis superior to the S2 level is derived from infolding of ectoderm elements and separation of the neural plate into the cranial placode, neural crest, and neural tube (in order of peripheral to central extent). The notochord—which is located deep to all of these—is derived from midline mesoderm and initiates the stages of neurulation via interaction with the overlying ectoderm. The notochord eventually regresses to become the nucleus pulposus of the spinal vertebral bodies. The cephalic portions of the neural tube becomes the prosencephalon (forebrain), mesencephalon (midbrain) and rhombencephalon (hindbrain). The remaining mid to caudal portions of the neural tube become the spinal canal (including posterior elements) and spinal cord. The neural crest cells differentiate into the meningeal layers (dura, arachnoid, and pia), neural elements of the peripheral nervous system, neurons dedicated to the enteric system, and other special structures ranging from smooth muscles, melanocytes, cartilage, and craniofacial bones. The cranial placodes—also referred to as neural placodes in embryological literature—are specialized areas of thickened epithelium in the cranial ectodermal layer that forms all the cranial nerves and other neural networks dedicated to the head (such as the pituitary and lens of eyes) [129–131].

The elements of the sacral canal formed during secondary neurulation are derived from a group of tightly packed cells known as the tail bud (or caudal cell mass) derived from the caudal portion of the primitive streak. These cells centrally burrow and fuse to level of the central canal of the primary neural tube, typically at the S2 level. Through the process of retrogressive dif-

ferentiation, these cells differentiate from a solid cord into individual nerve roots of the sacral foramina, with the filum terminale representing the remainder of the initial sacral cord. Similarly, the ventriculus terminalis represent the residual central canal of the sacral cord [129–131].

Neural tube defects (NTDs) affect approximately 1 of every 1000 pregnancies worldwide, with prevalence ranging from 0.2 to 10 per 1000 in certain geographical locations. Along with genitourinary defects and congenital heart anomalies, NTDs continue to rank the most common of birth defects. The human neural tube begins to close discontinuously at 17–18 days post fertilization. The exact sequence of human neural tube closure remains controversial to this day, with several models postulated. Studies of chicken and mouse models have demonstrated that cranioraschisis, open spina bifida, and anencephaly result from primary neurulation failure. As alluded to earlier, skin-covered spinal dysraphisms proximal to S2 result from disjunction abnormalities during primary neurulation, whereas lesions distal to S2 are caused by secondary neurulation defects (Fig. 3.22) [132].

Many genes have been identified that play critical roles in primary neurulation, rhombomere development, and subsequent cerebellar growth. The planar cell polarity pathway is particularly associated with pathologic cranial neurulation, due to its significant effect on cytokinetics and failure to initiate neural tube closure. Components in this pathway include cordon bleu (cobl), which is involved in midline differentiation of the node and its derivatives including the notochord, dorsal foregut and part of the floor plate of the primary neural tube. It also interacts with Vangl2 for midbrain neurulation [133–137].

Activation of certain isoforms of protein kinase C (PKC) is required for closure of the neural tube, and inhibition leads to open neural tube defects (NTDs). These NTDs are usually at the caudal neural tube as a result of deficient hindgut development. Similarly, mutations in the transcription factors Pax-3, Gli3 and Grhl3 work through distinct mechanisms to cause NTDs along the posterior neuropore. Both excessive and inadequate apoptotic cell death can also

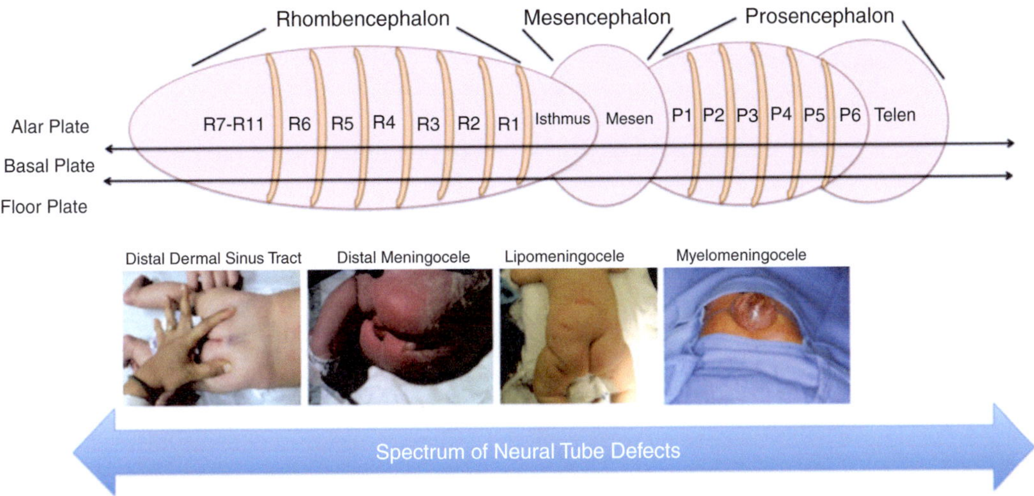

Fig. 3.22 Vertebrate neural axis and potential spectrum of neural tube defects (Telen = telencephalon; Mesen = mesencephalon). (Photographs of spinal dysraphisms courtesy of Dr. Rachana Tyagi, Westchester Medical Center, New York, USA)

cause defects in neural development in chick and mice models, particularly affecting morphogenetic processes. Intact methylation is one of the basic processes involved in gene regulation; thus folate deficiency is a well-known and studied cause of open NTDs, and its replacement and supplementation has been shown to reduce the incidence of NTDs. Methylation inhibition also reduces mesenchymal density, which Dunlevy theorized may lead to ethionine-induced exencephaly [138–142].

Although the phrase "neural placode" is used both in the above embryological discussion as well as throughout the embryological literature to describe constituents of the cranial placode and its ectodermal source in the stages of primary neurulation, physicians often use the phrase "neural placode" to describe elements of the neuraxis that are exposed in the various spinal dysraphisms. While this can be confusing, in order to maintain similar consistency with clinical and imaging reporting used by physicians, the same phrase of neural placode will be used in a similar manner to describe these meningeal-covered components of the neuraxis [129, 143].

Anencephaly is characterized as an absence of the cerebral and cerebellar hemispheres with maintenance of the hindbrain elements. This arises from neural tube closure failure during the third and fourth weeks of development. Many studies have shown this condition to be uniformly lethal. In a case series of 26 patients with fetuses with anencephaly, 6 of the 26 women (23%) had pre-labor intrauterine fetal deaths, 9 of the 26 (35%) of women had intrapartum deaths, and the remaining women who delivered their fetuses demonstrated a range of neonatal survival between 10 min and 8 days of antenatal life [144]. Developmentally, following disruption of forebrain development, what remains are areas of flattened disorganized brain tissue admixed with ependymal, choroid plexus, and meningothelium. The defect is only covered by an angiomatous stroma (referred to as the area cerebrovasculosa). This falls within the spectrum of other cranial vault entities that may be seen on pre-natal imaging, ranging from exencephaly, acalvaria, and acrania (Fig. 3.23) [145].

All open spinal dysraphisms have an abrupt tapering between the transitions of the flanking subcutaneous layer with the component of neural placode exposed to the outside environment. Closed spinal dysraphsisms demonstrate a smooth gradual tapering with otherwise preserved consistency of the flanking subcutaneous layer covering the neural placode extending through the defect [143].

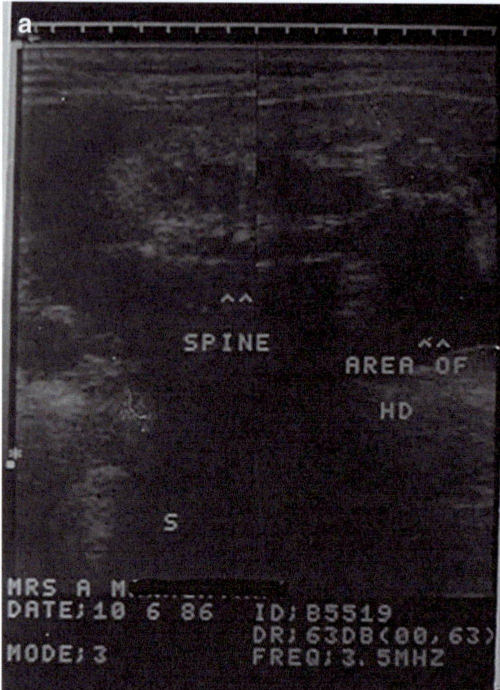

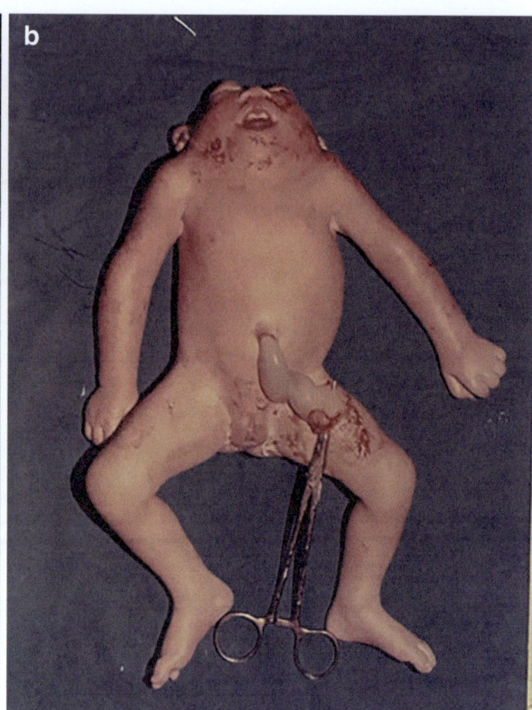

Fig. 3.23 Fetal ultrasound (**a**) demonstrates an empty cranial vault secondary to absence of the cerebral and cerebellar hemispheres (referred to as 'Area of HD' in image). Findings were consistent with the diagnosis of anencephaly. (**b**) following delivery of the fetus demonstrates the characteristic appearance of anencephaly, noting the markedly shrunken head and lack of calvarial margins due to lack of cerebral and cerebellar development. This infant passed away minutes following deliver, a common clinical end-result of this entity. (Images are courtesy of Dr. Geetha Arjun, E.V. Kalyani Medical Center, Chennai, India, Dr. S. Suresh, Mediscan Centre, Chennai, India, and Dr. Subha Sundararajan, Red Bank Gastroenterology, Redbank, New Jersey, USA)

Myelomeningoceles and myeloceles are the two most common types of open spinal dysraphisms, with myelomeningoceles encompassing 98% of all open spinal dysraphisms. Myelomeningoceles and myeloceles both possess open exposure of intramedullary nerve roots and cord elements covered by a bulging meningeal sac. What differentiates the two is the level of contact with the skin surface. Myeloceles, although open, remain flush to the skin surface. Myelomeningoceles, on the other hand, protrude prominently away from the body cavity and skin surface (Fig. 3.24) [129, 143].

The closed spinal dysraphisms are either associated or not associated with a subcutaneous mass. Those with a subcutaneous mass are the meningocele, lipomyelocele, lipomyelomeningocele, and terminal myelocystocele [129, 143].

Meningoceles are an extension of meninges alone without accompanying intramedullary cord or nerve roots that extend through a defect in the posterior elements (referred to as spina bifida occulta given defect focality without any clinical symptoms associated with it) [129, 143].

Lipomyeloceles and lipomyelomeningoceles are similarly named according to their open spinal dysraphism counterparts with regard to their relationship with the skin surface. The exception is that rather than being open dysraphisms, there is an intervening lipoma separating the neural placode from the external environment in each of these conditions. Specifically, lipomyeloceles possess an intervening lipoma in the location of the posterior element deficit, with the neural placode-lipoma complex otherwise not extending beyond the boundaries of the posterior element defect. In contrast, lipomyelomeningoceles also

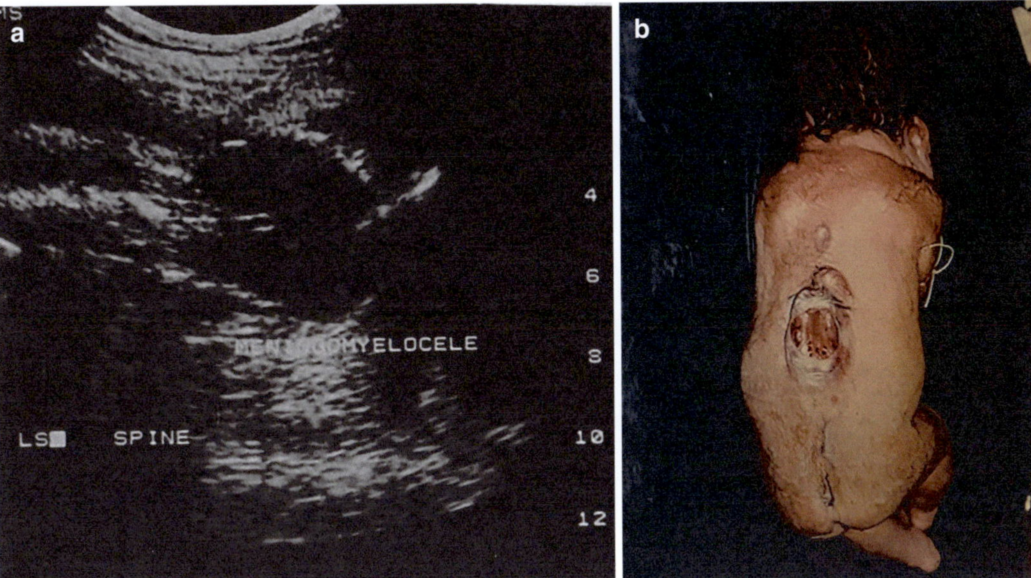

Fig. 3.24 Fetal ultrasound image demonstrating an anechoic sac continuing neural elements in contiguity with the lower thoracolumbar spine, in keeping with spinal dysraphism of the myelomeningocele type (**a**). Photograph of same fetus in post-natal life (**b**), demonstrating presence of the neural placode protruding through the patient's dorsal posterior spinal elemental defect with lack of skin covering. (**a**: ultrasound and **b**: photograph images are courtesy of Dr. Geetha Arjun, E.V. Kalyani Medical Center, Chennai, India, Dr. S. Suresh, Mediscan Centre, Chennai, India, and Dr. Subha Sundararajan, Red Bank Gastroenterology, Redbank, New Jersey, USA)

possess an intervening lipoma in the location of the posterior element deficit, though the complex of the neural placode and lipoma extend beyond the margins of the defect and protrude into the overlying subcutaneous layer. The terminal myelocystoceleis is a unique entity characterized by terminal cord syrinx formation with resultant extension of this syrinx into a meningocele meningocele extending through a prominent posterior spinal defect. There are usually associated systemic anomalies belonging to the OEIS constellation (*O*mphalocele, *E*xstrophy of the cloaca, *I*mperforate anus, and *S*pinal anomalies) [129, 143].

The closed spinal dysraphisms without a subcutaneous mass are the dermal sinus, tight filum terminale, fibrolipoma of the filum terminale, and intradural lipoma [129, 143].

The dermal sinus is a thin tract lined by epithelial cells communicating between the skin to either the neural placode elements or to an overlying soft tissue mass such as lipoma or teratoma. The tract is dark on T1 weighted imaging, although they may be difficult to visualize on

fetal MRI given their small size (Fig. 3.25) [129, 143].

A tight filum terminale is characterized as a filum with greater than 2 mm thickness in the setting of a low-lying conus medullaris (located below the inferior endplate of L2). The constellation of a tight filum terminale, low-lying conus, and clinical symptomology of bladder dysfunction, and pain in the lower back and pain suggests tethered cord syndrome. While these can be detected on post-natal MRI examinations, assessment on fetal MRI maybe limited due to lack of clinical signs and the small size of the filum in the prenatal stage [129, 143].

A fibrolipoma of the filum terminale is characterized as a focal fat in the filum of variable size. If sizable, this can be detected on fetal MRI as bright T1 signal in the caudal aspect of the terminal cord corresponding to the filum location. The conus is otherwise normal in position and the filum is of normal thickness, unlike the tight filum terminale [129, 143].

Intradural lipomas are fat-containing lesions along the dorsal midline margin of the spinal

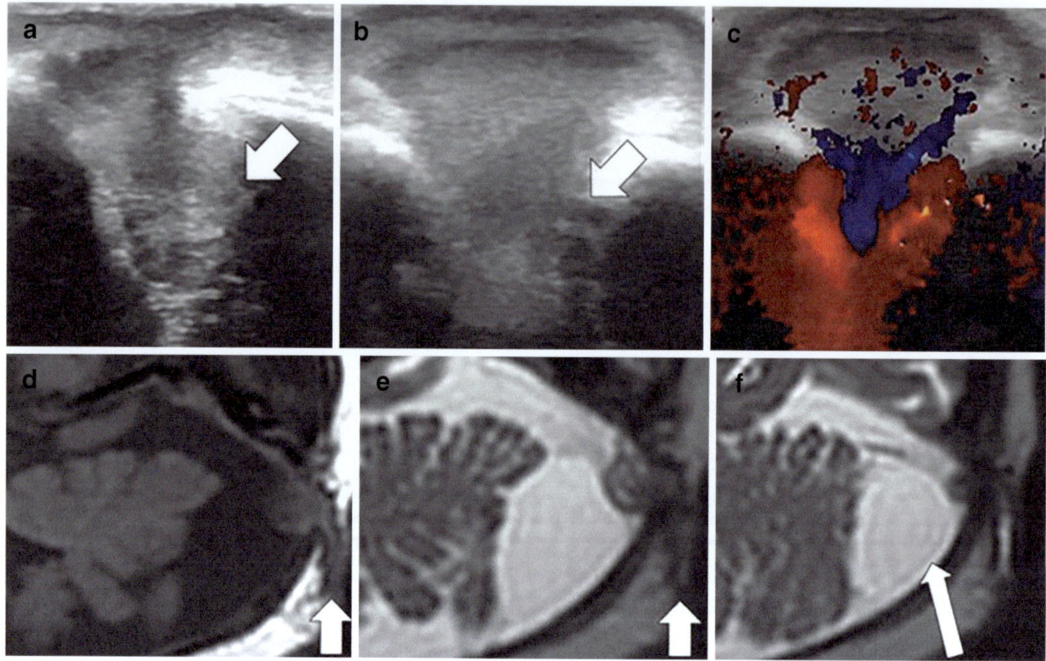

Fig. 3.25 Fetus with abnormal mound of increased echogenicity in the occiput region on ultrasound evaluation (**a**, **b**, short arrows), without increased color doppler flow to suggest this is vascular in etiology (**c**). MRI was performed, confirming a tract from the occipital scalp to the level of the torcula (**d–f**, short arrows), noting combination of T1 isointense soft tissue (**d**, **e** short arrows) and T2 bright fluid (**f**, short arrow) are seen in the cleft. Findings are consistent with a dermal sinus tract in the spectrum of cephalocele formation given communication with the intracranial compartment. No brain parenchyma or meninges is seen in this tract to call it an encephalocele or meningocele respectively. Note is made of an incidental retro-cerebellar arachnoid cyst with mid indentation of the cerebellar parenchyma anteriorly (**f**, long arrow)

canal that remain within the spinal column, purely bounded by the meningeal layers of the neural placode. As opposed to the other closed dysraphisms, defects in the posterior elements are not commonly associated with this entity. However, even if there is an associated spina bifida defect, there is rarely extension of the lipoma through the spina bifida defect. They are more commonly located in the thoracic spine in adults and the cervical spine in children. When detected on fetal MRI, a T1 bright lesion contained within the spinal canal and intradural compartment are classically seen [129, 143, 146].

Post-neurulation Errors and Cephaloceles

A congenital herniation of intracranial contents through skull defects is broadly characterized as a cephalocele, with a spectrum of cephaloceles possible. A meningocele describes meningeal herniation containing only CSF. A meningoencephalocele describes meningeal herniation containing CSF and brain parenchyma. A gliocele describes herniation of a glial-lined cyst filled with CSF. An atretic parietal cephalocele describes herniation of meninges and fibrous tissue.

Cephaloceles are named according to their location of herniation, typically occurring through the midline anterior, basal, or posterior aspects of the calvarium, with the nasoethmoidal subtype being the most commonly encountered cephalocele. Rarer cephalocele subtypes include herniation of intracranial contents along the lateral calvarial convexities and cephalocele through the clivus (Figs. 3.26 and 3.27) [147–149].

Although aberrancies in pathways leading to primary and secondary neurulation contribute to

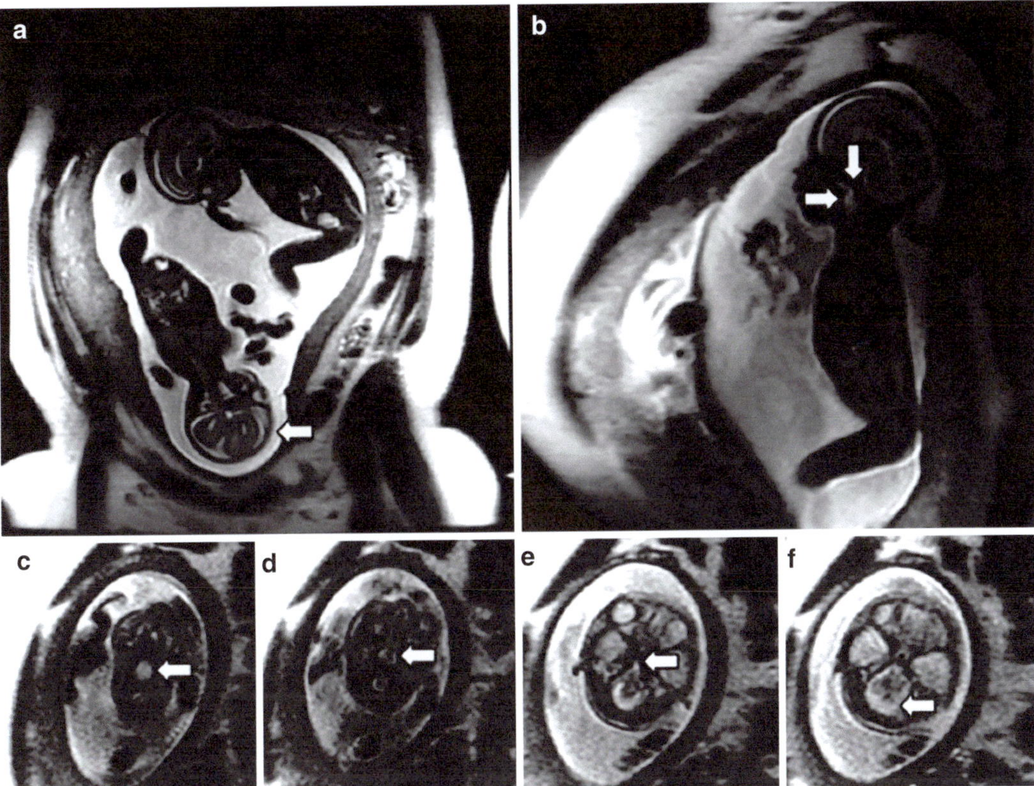

Fig. 3.26 Fetal MRI of twin gestation (**a**) with sagittal (**b**) and axial images (**c–f**) of fetus in vertex position. Fluid in oropharynx originally thought to represent oral secretions (**b–d**). Left greater than right cerebellar maldevelop- ment again noted, with prominence of posterior fossa thought to represent mega cisterna magna (**f**). In retrospect, there is suggestion of the midline clival defect with traversing CSF (**b–e**)

NTDs, cephalocele formation can occur in the post-neurulation stage. Occipital meningoencephaloceles are commonly part of the Meckel-Gruber syndrome, a rare ciliopathic genetic disorder also characterized by renal cystic dysplasia, polydactyly, hepatic developmental defects, and pulmonary hypoplasia secondary to oligohydramnios. Several genes have been described as contributing to this disorder, including CEP290, RPGRIP1L, TMEM67, TNEM216, and MKS1. Notably, MKS proteins are pivotal in the function and structure of primary cilia. Such cilia are essential for numerous signaling pathways—including downstream hedgehog proteins. However, a specific link between ciliary development and cephalocele formation has yet to be determined [132, 150].

Errors in Notochord Induction and Formation (Caudal Regression Syndrome, Vertebral Anomalies, Diastematomyelia, and Neurenteric Cysts)

As noted in the spinal dysraphisms section, the notochord is derived from midline mesoderm and initiates the stages of neurulation via interaction with the overlying ectoderm. The notochord eventually regresses to become the nucleus pulposus of the spinal vertebral bodies.

Caudal regression is characterized by abnormal development of the caudal aspect of the vertebral column and spinal cord. Its incidence is approximately 0.1–0.25 cases per 10,000 normal pregnancies. It is important to note,

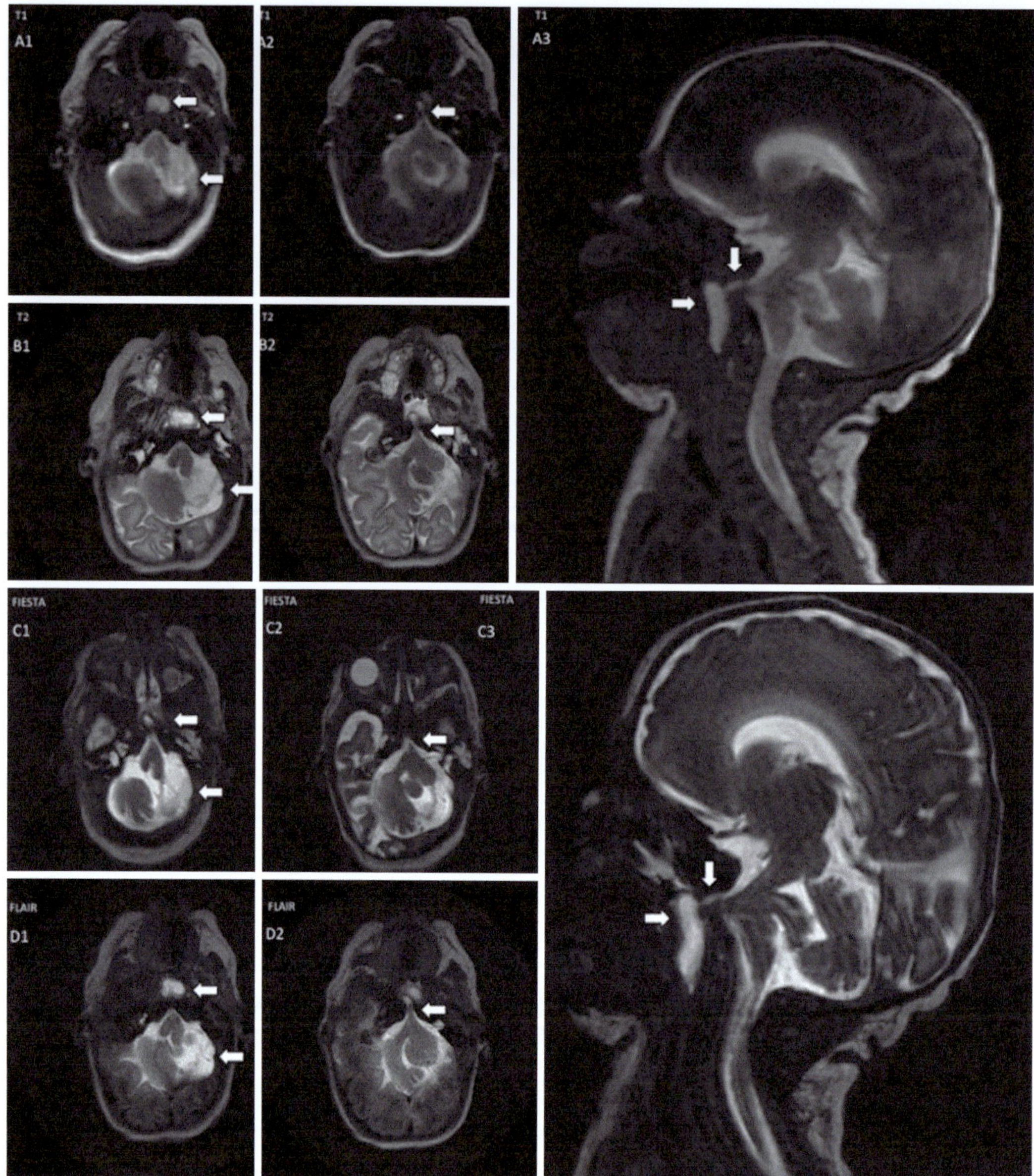

Fig. 3.27 Post myelography MRI images of the brain following delivery, with T1 (**a1–a3**), T2 (**b1, b2**), FIESTA (**c1–c3**) and FLAIR (**d1, d2**) demonstrate left cerebellar atrophy, brainstem maldevelopment, midline clival defect, and pontine extension through defect. Note myelographic contrast extending through the midline defect into the oropharyngeal collection, consistent with meningoencephalocele through the clivus

however, that the incidence rises to as high as 1 in 350 in pregnancy when the mother is diabetic, which corresponds to a 200 times increased risk. There is a male predominance relative to females of 2.7–1. There are significant neurological deficits stemming from bowel and bladder functional abnormalities to severe sensory and motor deficits of the lower extremities. Although the majority of cases are sporadic, maternal hyperglycemia is the most commonly associated risk factor, occurring in up to 1% of all pregnancies with maternal diabetes. Twenty-two percent of caudal regression cases are associated with Type 1 or 2 maternal diabetes. Prenatal ultrasound and fetal MRI are both useful in assessing for its presence and are characterized by abrupt termination in visualization of lumbar elements.

On imaging, the level of atresia or dysgenesis is typically below the L1 level and limited to the sacrum. There is blunt termination of the spinal cord with accompanying marked narrowing of the spinal above the last intact vertebral level. VACTERL is a congenital malformation syndrome that occurs in 1 in 10,000–40,000 live births, and is associated with caudal regression (falling under the *Vertebral anomalies and Atresia* portions of the acronym). The remaining entities of VACTERL include *Cardiac anomalies, Traceho-esophageal fistula, Renal anomalies, and Limb abnormalities*. Caudal regression is also associated with the Currarino Triad, an autosomal condition composed of sacral agenesis, anorectal malformation, and presacral mass (such as teratoma, anterior meningocele, or enteric cyst) [151–154].

Fetal vertebrae develop between the sixth and eighth weeks of gestational age, during which lateral chondrification centers join to form the primary ossification center of the vertebral body. Disruptions in this process may lead to either failures of vertebral formation (portions of vertebrae fail to form with incomplete presence of osseous elements) or failures in segmentation (failure of intervertebral disc formation leading to alterations in vertebral numbering, scoliosis, and varying degrees of fusion). The mechanism for their occurrence is unknown, though vascular supply disruptions during vertebra and disc formation have been postulated. Errors in vertebral formation and segmentation often occur in multiple locations and can be associated with additional anomalies of the pulmonary, cardiac, gastrointestinal, and genitourinary system. Sonography can detect errors in vertebra numbering and appearance (including hemivertebrae and wedge vertebrae) as early as the 12th week of gestational age. Assessing architectural osseous details of the spine may be less apparent on fetal MRI. However, resultant kyphoscoliosis of spinal alignment can be readily detected, allowing one to carefully inspect around the level of scoliosis for associated vertebral and segmentation malformations [155].

Separate from the neural tube, notochord, and notochordal canal is a persistent neurenteric canal. Persistence of the neurenteric canal during the third week of embryogenesis prevents complete separation of the endoderm and notochord. This can lead to either a neurenteric cyst with endodermal tissue present in an extra-axial location or a split cord malformation known as diastematomyelia if the midline cleft persists through neurulation [32].

Neurenteric cysts are rare type of foregut duplication cyst that is endodermal in origin. They can be found either within the intracranial or spinal compartments. In the spine, they are most commonly seen ventrally in the thoracic spine and are typically intradural extramedullary in location. Histopathologically, they can be categorized into Types A, B, and C cysts based on the classification schema formulated by Wilkins and Odom [156]. Type A cysts possess either columnar or cuboidal cells, with ciliated and non-ciliated components sitting atop a basal membrane composed of type IV collagen. Type B cysts include all of the features of type A along with additional tissue such as bone, cartilage, lymphatic tissue, fat, or glandular components. Type C cysts possess the features of type A as well as ependymal or glial tissue. Although this classification scheme has been used to categorize histological subtypes, there is no correlation between cyst subtype and the site, extent, or outcome after cyst resection. Cysts are typically isointense on T1 and hyperintense on T2, though signal properties are variable depending on the amount of proteinaceous or alternate complex material composition. Depending on their size, they can result in significant mass effect with flattening of underlying brain parenchyma if intracranial or in the spinal cord if intraspinal. A close inspection for associated spinal anomalies is warranted following neurenteric cyst detection, as up to 50% of cases are seen alongside a spinal dysraphism, scoliosis, spina bifida, split cord malformation, and/or Klippel-Feil syndrome [157, 158].

Diastematomyelia is a specific type of split cord malformation that typically occurs between the T9 to S1 levels, with each hemicord possessing their own ventral and doseal cord horns and central canals. They are classified according to the presence of absence of a splitting fibrous or bony spur and whether or not there is duplication of the encompassing thecal sac. Type 1 malformations possess a duplicated thecal sac, possess a midline spur, and are usually more symptomatic in postnatal life. Type 2 malformations possess a single thecal sac, contain both hemicords, and are usually less symptomatic in postnatal life [159].

Chiari Spectrum of Deformities

Chiari deformities—also referred to as Arnold-Chiari malformations—are a spectrum of disorders affecting the posterior fossa and hindbrain contents, notably the medulla oblongata, pons, and cerebellum. The deformity spectrum ranges from cerebellar tonsillar descent, full herniation, or cerebellar absence associated with either intracranial or extracranial deficits such as spinal dysraphisms, encephaloceles, syrinx formation, or hydrocephalus. The assessment of cerebellar tonsil position either above or below the foramen magnum is best appreciated on the sagittal plane, though the coronal and axial planes of imaging can be used to detect tonsil position as well. Its location is conventionally described in reference to the McRae Line, a line drawn from the basion to the opisthion. Such morphologic changes and anatomic defects of these structures are often diagnosed with imaging, noting that prenatal imaging via ultrasound and MRI continue to play a role in the earlier detection of these conditions [160].

The Chiari 1 deformity is least severe most commonly encountered entity in the spectrum. There is a slight female predominance (1.3 females to 1 male) with 0.5%–3.5% of the general population possessing this deformity. Chiari 1 is characterized by either a single or bilateral cerebellar tonsils demonstrating a pointed (non-rounded) configuration projecting ≥5 mm below the foramen magnum. This can lead to an outflow obstruction of CSF from the foramen magnum due to impairment of drainage from the

fourth ventricle's foramina of Magendie and Luschka. The resultant outflow obstruction in turn may result in syringomyelia (also known as syringobulbia) development in the brainstem and spinal cord. Syrongomyelia is recognized by the presence of a midline fluid-filled cavity (known as syrinx) [160].

The origin of this syrinx arises from post-obstructive enlargement of the central canal, an embryologic channel extending from the caudal angle of the fourth ventricle to the conus medullaris of the terminal thoracolumbar cord. The central canal is derived from neural canal of the neural tube during neurulation in the fourth week of gestational development. Following central infolding with closure of its rostral and caudal openings, the remaining patent neural canal continues to form the intraventricular system while its closed portions caudal to the fourth ventricle become lined with a single layer of columnar ependymal cells that usually remain regressed during the remainder of prenatal and postnatal life [161]. Mild prominence of the central canal to less than 5 mm is considered normal variation related to incomplete closure during development. The combination of cavity dilation greater than 5 mm and spread of extent either in a continuous manner or skipped manner has a high specificity of identifying pathologic syrinx formation in the setting of Chiari 1 [162].

Prenatal diagnosis of Chiari 1 is extremely rare in the literature, with diagnosis in postnatal life, childhood, and young adulthood being much more common. This is likely related to disease manifestation being a factor of future growth and development. That is, the prenatal intracranial fetal vault still possesses ample room for CSF drainage despite a potential future tendency for tonsillar descent below the foramen magnum. Mild nonspecific ventriculomegaly with otherwise normal posterior fossa configuration and cord evaluation can be seen in fetuses that eventually develop the Chiari 1 deformity in postnatal life [163].

Chiari 2 is characterized by more striking neuroanatomic alterations compared to its Chiari 1 counterpart. Approximately 0.44 of every 1000 births possess the Chiari 2 spectrum of findings.

Unlike Chiari 1, its incidence is without gender predominance and is lowered with folate replacement therapy taken by the pregnant patient. Chiari 2 is characterized by whole brainstem and cerebellar inferior herniation that occurs as a result of the negative pressure effects of a spinal dysraphism, with most commonly encountered spinal dysraphism in the Chiari 2 deformity being the open-type myelomeningocele. The characteristic imaging findings all stem from this common pathway of inferior descent of posterior fossa structures. These include: (1) small size of posterior fossa with low-lying torcula and tentorial attachment points; (2) elongated low-lying fourth ventricle and "pulled-down" appearance of brainstem; (3) "tectal beaking" appearance of inferior colliculi elongation with posterior tilt as a result of brainstem herniation; (4) hydrocephalus secondary to brainstem herniation-mediated angulation of the aqueduct of Sylvius and resultant aqueductal stenosis; and (5) whole cerebellar displacement below the foramen magnum—including tonsils and vermis. Chiari 2 can be seen alongside other malformations of parenchymal formation, including the dysgenesis of corpus collosum spectrum (Fig. 3.28) [160, 163].

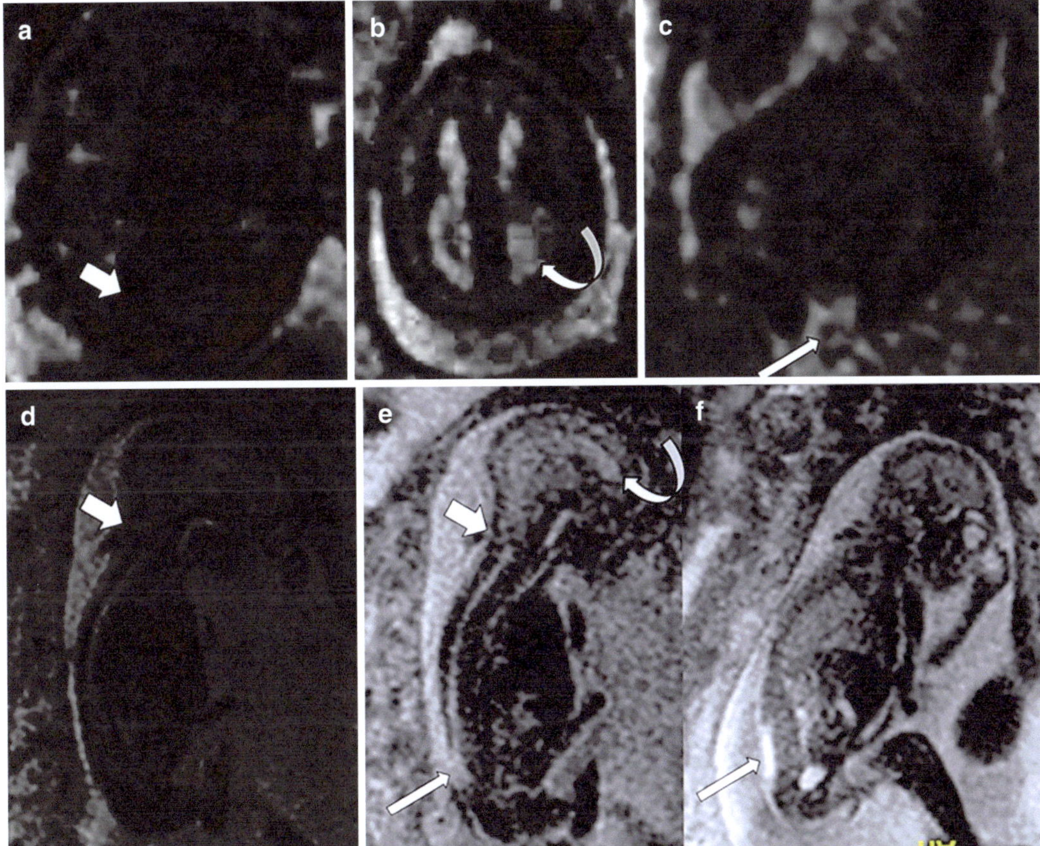

Fig. 3.28 Axial (**a–c**) and sagittal (**d–f**) T2 weighted images from fetal MRI examination in a pregnant patient with abnormal prenatal ultrasound examination. There is inferior herniation of hindbrain contents with marked reduction in space about the foramen magnum and posterior fossa (short arrows in **a**, **d**, and **e**). There is fetal ventriculomegaly related to marked narrowing of the fourth ventricle and posterior fossa CSF outflow tracts as a result of hindbrain herniation (curved arrows in **b** and **e**). There is an open spinal dysraphism, specifically the myelomeningocele in the lumbosacral spine, noting the broad lack of posterior elements and external extension of the neural placode without skin covering into the amniotic cavity (long arrows in **c**, **e**, and **f**). Findings are consistent with the Chiari 2 deformity and associated myelomeningocele.

Congenital Vascular Anomalies

The vascular anomalies spectrum is broad with the potential for each anomaly to affect anywhere in the human body. The International Society for the Study of Vascular Anomalies (ISSVA) has categorized its various constituents into specifically defined vascular malformations and vascular tumors [164]. This section will review congenital vascular anomalies affecting the neur-axis of an intrauterine gestation that can be detected on either prenatal ultrasound or fetal MRI examination.

Congenital hemangiomas are fully formed tumors present at the time of birth with nearly no growth after their birth. They are negative for the GLUT1 receptor staining, a key biochemical distinguishing factor when compared to its counterpart infantile hemangioma. There two types of congenital hemangiomas, the Rapidly Involuting Congenital Hemangioma (RICH) and the Non Involuting Congenital Hemangioma (NICH). Both RICH and NICH can appear similar macroscopically, as both are violaceous gray vascular tumors with prominent overlying veins and telangiectasias extending beyond their periphery. Imaging features are also identical on prenatal imaging, with prominent vascularity with Doppler evaluation during ultrasound examination and mixtures of both high T1 and low T2 signal related to a combination of blood products, mineralization, and vascular flow voids. The ability to distinguish a RICH from a NICH is a retrospective one. RICH tumors involute by 12 months of age, though their resultant skin changes may require future interventions. NICH tumors only partially involute hence requiring surgery for both aesthetic purposes and to improve resultant functional impairments [165–167].

Kaposiform hemangioendothelioma (KHE) is a rare aggressive vascular tumor which is typically present at the time of birth. Its cells form slit-like lumens containing erythrocytes that resemble Kaposi's sarcoma. Distinguishing features of this mass compared to a congenital hemangioma include identification of its destructive and infiltrative growth pattern and the presence of multiple arterial feeders. On prenatal sonogra-phy, the mass is solid with ill-defined borders, variable echogenicity, and prominent Doppler flow. Its infiltrative and destructive features are best appreciated on MRI, noting transpatial spread across skin, subcutaneous fat, muscle, and even bone. Urgent management via combination of surgical resection, chemotherapy, and/or endovascular-mediated embolization is warranted given the tendency of these tumors to sequester red blood cells and platelets with resultant thrombocytopenia and anemia. This pathologic process of a consumptive coagulopathy in combination with such a vascular tumor is referred to as the Kasabach-Merritt phenomenon [165–167].

Syndromes with predisposition for development of infantile hemangiomas include PHACES (*P*osterior fossa brain malformations, *H*emangiomas, *A*rterial anomalies, *C*oarctation of the aorta and *C*ardiac defects, *E*ye abnormalities, *S*ternal defects) and LUMBAR (*L*ower body segmental hemangioma, *U*rogenital anomalies and *U*lceration, *M*yelopathy, *B*ony abnormalities, *A*norectal and/or *A*rterial anomalies, *R*enal anomalies). Although these hemangiomas are not congenital and therefore unlikely to be present on prenatal imaging, awareness of their association with additional malformations more notable on screening ultrasound and fetal MRI is important and aides in the appropriate recommendation of post-natal imaging followup [165–167].

Vascular malformations are congenital vascular maldevelopments present prenatally and since birth. These are lined with mature, mitotically quiet cells, unlike the congenital vascular tumors mentioned previously. This results in a slow, proportional growth to the patient, noting sudden alterations in size maybe attributable to hormonal and hemodynamically driven changes. These lesions do not spontaneously regress over the course of life. Despite their presence since birth, VMs can remain dormant for an indefinite period of time, with variable presentation in prenatal and postnatal life. Recognizing their primary vessel constituent and speed of flow allows for an appropriate classification of the malformation type as recommended by the ISSVA guidelines. Slow flow malformations consist of venous malformations, lymphatic malformations, and capillary malformations. Fast flow malformations consist primarily of arteriovenous malformations. Complex malformations with mixed slow and fast features include venolymphatic malformations and cavernous-arteriovenous malformations [165–167].

Venous malformations (VM) are the most common type of vascular malformation. However, their detection on prenatal imaging is rare unless located in functionally important regions or of sufficient size for detection on initial evaluation. As these lesions are more common in the mid-late postnatal childhood presentation, their features of being compressible, blue, and soft alongside enlargement with gravity and Valsalva are not helpful in prenatal detection. Large-enough hemangiomas may be present in the developing vertebral bodies of the spine on fetal MRI, noting that these are actually venous malformations with GLUT1 receptor positivity. If large enough and present in the soft tissues of the head, neck or spine, they can infiltrate multiple tissue planes and extend within muscle groups alongside nerves, major arteries, or major veins. They are categorized according to the Puig system, which organizes VMs by the presence or absence of draining veins. Type 1 VMs are isolated vascular pouches without systemic venous drainage, type 2 VMs drain into normal caliber veins, type 3 VMs drain into abnormal caliber dysplastic veins, and type 4 VM lesions themselves possess significant venous ectasia and drain into abnormal caliber dysplastic veins. Although these lesions are somewhat difficult to evaluate on prenatal sonography, they would appear as tubular hypoechoic structures with low Doppler velocity. MRI allows for full depth evaluation of VMs if apparent enough at this young age, and would be characterized by T2 bright T1 intermediate to bright serpiginous structures with fat and muscle identification between their channels (due to their infiltrative nature). While phleboliths (calcifications) are a common feature of VMs in the postnatal state—seen as T2 dark foci—their appearance on fetal MRI is less likely given patient young age and limited time for development [165–167].

Previously known as cystic hygromas or lymphangiomas, lymphatic malformations (LMs) are the most common prenatally diagnosed vascular malformation. They are broad, low-flow lesions with characteristic transspatial spread, insinuating through subcutaneous, fascial, and intramuscular planes with ease. These malformations represent dilated cystic spaces filled with chylous lymphatic material. They can grow to considerable sizes, with a combination of their size and local-regional mass effect capable of disrupting physiologic function and affecting proportional growth depending on their location. Seventy-five percent of LMs are located in the head and neck regions (most frequently in the nuchal region) and 20% of LMs are found in the axilla with spread to the chest or lower neck. The remaining 5% are found systemically in the body [168]. LMs can be characterized as macrocystic, microcystic, or mixed, noting these subgroups sometimes share overlapping imaging features. On prenatal ultrasound, these lesions are largely anechoic or hypoechoic with layering echogenicities related to fluid-fluid lymphatic levels. As they are known for their lack of Doppler flow, if minimal flow is identified, it is related to small traversing arteries or veins interspersed through the malformation. On fetal MR, they are typically bright on T2 weight imaging and variable on T1 (dark if purely lymphatic fluid versus isointense to bright on T1 weighted imaging if mixed fat or blood containing, Fig. 3.29) [165–167].

Capillary malformations are essentially never detected on prenatal imaging given their superficial location and the ability to diagnose them clinically usually following direct visual inspection. They are classically red-pink flame shaped areas that darken with age, hence earning the names of "nevus flammeus" and "port-wine stains," respectively. Although bony overgrowth does occur alongside proportional capillary malformation growth, this is not commonly seen in the prenatal setting [165–167].

If capillary malformations are distributed in the fifth cranial nerve distribution however, evaluation for Sturge-Weber is indicated. The intracranial sequalae of Sturge-Weber are more readily identified on prenatal imaging compared

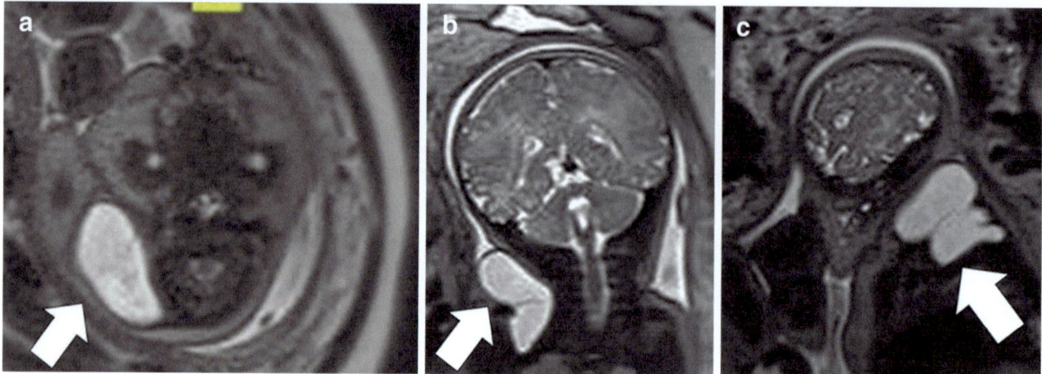

Fig. 3.29 31-year-old woman with 40-week gestation, found to have an abnormal cystic-appearing structure in the right neck soft tissues on pre-natal ultrasound. Axial (**a**), coronal (**b**), and sagittal (**c**) plane T2 weighted fetal MRI images demonstrate a broad-cystic structure in the right neck soft tissue with areas of infolding and septation extending from the suboccipital level to the supraclavicular fossa. Findings are consistent with a trans-spatial broad congenital lymphatic malformation

to the detection of capillary malformations. Sturge-Weber syndrome is caused by somatic mutation in the GNAQ gene that is involved in the regulatory development of blood vessels. This leads to the dysplasia of leptomeningeal vasculature with progressive cerebral damage, subsequent atrophy, and underlying encephalomalacia. Scattered cortical and subcortical calcifications are seen as echogenic foci on ultrasound and dark signal foci on T2 weighted imaging in fetal MRI. Depending on the gestational age of onset, the degree of resultant cortical atrophy is highly variable. The syndrome is also associated with polymicrogyria and similar gray-matter heterotopias. While continuous "tram-track" cortical and subcortical calcifications are classically associated with this entity, this extent of calcifications is usually seen in postnatal fetal imaging given the time to develop [169, 170].

Arteriovenous malformations (AVM) are fast-flow lesions with dominant arterial to venous communications intertwined by a nidus of abnormal interweaving vessels comprised of dysplastic arterioles and venules. They are characterized by their lack of a capillary transition. If large enough, they can be detected on prenatal sonographic or fetal ultrasound imaging. These lesions commonly tend to present later in postnatal life during periods of rapid growth or healing, including early childhood, puberty, pregnancy, trauma, and

surgery. Presentation characteristics for intracranial AVMS reported in the literature are more reflective of the postnatal patient, as that their incidence in prenatal imaging is either completely incidental or detected/evaluated for in the setting of a known syndrome with predisposition to formation of AVMs. Parkes Weber syndrome—also known as capillary malformation-arteriovenous malformation syndrome—is characterized by multiple small capillary malformations either in the face and limbs, noting that there are also associated AVMs in varying body parts including the brain and spine. Other AVM syndromes include Osler-Weber-Rendu and Bannayan-Riley-Ruvalcaba [169, 170].

Several findings regarding AVM characterization and subsequent prognosis are difficult to ascertain from prenatal imaging given both the field of view and difficulty in assessing for flow-related aneurysms, number of arterial feeders, nidus relative to passage vessels, or number and exact localization of draining veins.

Vein of Galen pathologies are a unique type of congenital vascular anomaly in the prenatal patient and can be characterized as either Vein of Galen varix formation, Vein of Galen aneurysmal dilation (VGAD), or Vein of Galen malformations (VGAM) [171, 172].

Dilations of the vein of Galen without the presence of an underlying intracranial arteriovenous shunt are referred to as varices. A transient type of varix formation may exist in the setting of cardiac failure of nonspecific etiology or alternate fluid-overloaded state with corresponding venous congestion. A non-transient varix of the vein of Galen can persist if there is a tendency for central drainage through the deep venous system as opposed to peripheral drainage via the venous sinuses. The term VGAD, in contrast, is used to describe dilation of a fully formed vein of Galen in the setting of an intracranial high-flow arteriovenous shunt or AVM. Given association with intracranial AVM, these are persistent regardless of alternate systemic conditions seen in association with typical findings of an AVM on prenatal imaging [171, 172].

Vein of Galen aneurysmal malformations (VGAM) are rare congenital abnormalities seen in 1:25,000 births. Although they only comprise 1% of all intracranial vascular anomalies encountered in postnatal life, they encompass 30% of all intracranial vascular anomalies in the pediatric population [173]. The Vein of Galen originates from the posterior aspect of the median prosencephalic vein of Markowski during embryological development noting the internal cerebral veins arise from the anterior median prosencephalic vein. Incomplete development of the vein of Galen due to a combination of aberrancies in angiogenesis and arteriovenous communication results in this characteristic venous aneurysm. Remaining venous drainage is variable, with the straight sinus absent in virtually all cases and small falcine dural channels draining the large venous aneurysm into the posterior superior sagittal sinus (Fig. 3.30) [171, 172].

The arteriovenous fistulous communications of VGAM arise within the choroidal fissure and extend superiorly from the interventricular foramen to the atria laterally. Their arterial inflow is supplied by choroidal arteries arising from the anterior cerebral artery A1 segment, the subependymal network of vessels arising from the dorsal circle of Willis elements, and the persistent limbic arterial arch bridging the anterior choroidal artery and posterior cerebral artery. Nidus location is midline, with all arterial branches either merging into the large dilated median prosencephalic venous pouch (poor patient prognosis, high flow related cardiac failure in prenatal or early postnatal life) or draining into separate ectatic venous pouches along the lining of the median prosencephalic vein (relatively better patient prognosis, less rapid development of high output cardiac failure, patients grow into early childhood before presentation). VGAMs are not directly supplied by paramedian arterial branches of the posterior cerebral artery P1 segment (also known as mesencephalic arteries), noting that visualization of these transmesencephalic arterial

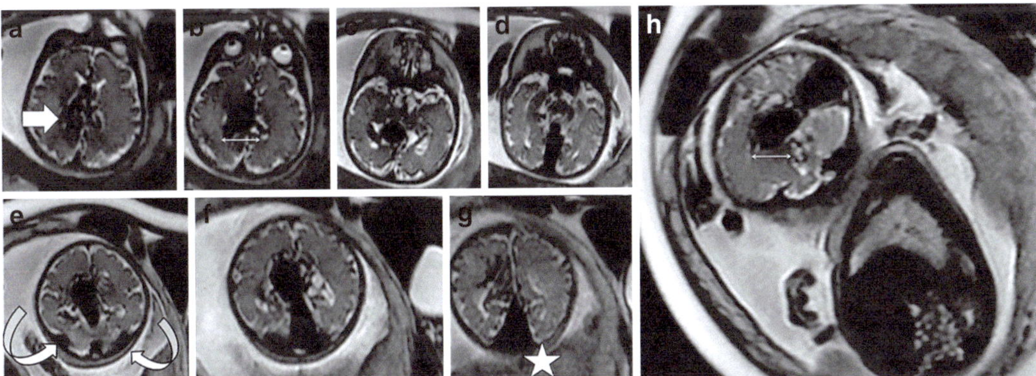

Fig. 3.30 Axial T2 (**a–d**), coronal T2 (**e–g**), and sagittal T2 (**h**) fetal MRI images demonstrate the presence of a Vein of Galen malformation. There is a dilated persistent median prosencephalic vein (double arrows in **b** and **h**) with arterial feeders primarily originating from the bilateral choroidal arteries (short arrow in **a**), to a lesser extent posterior cerebral arteries. There is associated enlargement of the torcula (star) and bilateral transverse sinuses (curved arrows). Constellation of findings are consistent with Vein of Galen Malformation

branches as primary feeders rule out VGAM and favor VGAD presence. On fetal MRI, aneurysmal dilation of the median prosencephalic vein, compensatory enlargement of the transverse and sigmoid sinuses, and enlargement of the limbic arch and bilateral anterior and posterior choroidal arteries would be seen as correlating regions of prominent T2 hypointense flow voids [171, 172].

Craniofacial Malformations

Craniofacial development occurs as a result of orderly and rapid growth of mesodermal and cranial neural crest cells. The first and second branchial arches are formed from these cell types, with errors in their development resulting in various craniofacial malformations. The term cheiloschisis is used to specify the presence of clef lip alone. Palatoschisis is the term used to specify the presence of cleft lip and cleft palate [174]. Malformation type can be categorized by Tessier's classification, a numerical classification system that specifies craniofacial anatomic locations as 0–14 while relying on the orbit as a fixed reference point. These 15 subtypes fall under broader categories of midline clefts (vertical across face through midline), paramedian clefts (vertical across face away from midline), orbital clefts (any involvement of orbit), and lateral clefts (horizontal across face) [175]. The Van de Meulen classification schema may also be implemented in assessing craniofacial malformation type. This schema categorizes malformations according to the stage in embryogenesis within which disruption and subsequent cleft formation occurs. They are broadly categorized according to location of developmental arrest in the internasal, nasal, nasalmaxillary, and maxillary regions [176]. Micrognathia is the term used to describe an undersized mandible, with the lower jaw being shorter or smaller relative to the remaining face. The Jaw Index provides a normal range of mandibular diameters based on gestational age and biparietal diameter, and can be used to support the diagnosis of micrognathia [177].

Fetal MRI is highly accurate in the detection of craniofacial malformations, regardless of fetal age before or after 24 weeks gestation. Micrognathia (size discrepancy of lower mandible relative to remainder of facial elements) can be assessed for well on the sagittal plane of imaging. The axial plane of imaging is useful in detection of cleft lip (with T2 weighted images showing T2 bright fluid signal separating cleft elements) and the sagittal and coronal planes are useful in detection of cleft palate (loss of T2 hypointense soft palate continuity and premaxillary protrusion presence) [178]. Specifically, the premaxillary protrusion is a characteristic finding of cleft palate that ventrally extends between the cleft palate elements. This is echogenic on sonography and isointense on T2-weighted imaging of fetal MRI. The presence of this protrusion is due to uninhibited growth of premaxilla alveolar and gingival given the lack of bony, gingival, and lip boundaries (Fig. 3.31) [179, 180].

Encephaloceles can occur in the setting of cleft lip and palate deformities. Some form as a result of direct lack of cranial vault congruity with the cleft defect itself (such as frontoethmoidal or sphenoethmoidal encephalocele development in the setting of midline facial clefts) [181, 182]. Others form in the setting of cleft deformity presence alongside other remote malformations (such as occipital encephalocele formation in the setting of separate cleft lip and palate) [183]. Their presence alongside cleft deformities can be initially detected on sonography, with subsequent confirmation readily achieved on fetal MRI [184].

Congenital Intracranial Tumors

Intracranial congenital tumors can be divided into teratomas and nonteratomas. Teratomas are tumors characterized by their presence of elements of all three germ layers and immature neuronal and glial cells. They are the most common brain tumor detected on pre-natal imaging, encompassing 62% of all congenital intracranial tumors. Diagnosis is typically made during the second and third trimesters of pregnancy, with first trimester diagnoses being extremely rare. Aside from size variability, imaging features are

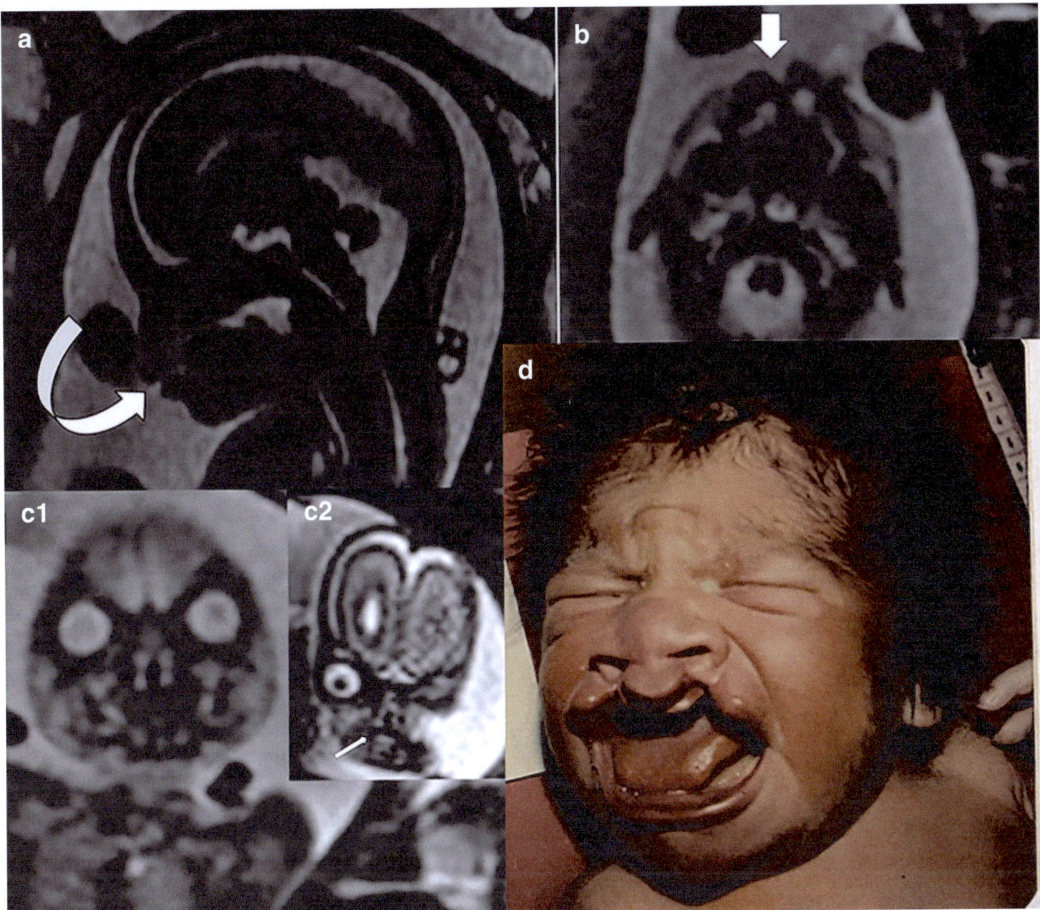

Fig. 3.31 Images demonstrating bilateral cleft lip and palate. Sagittal T2 image (**a**) demonstrates ventral extension of the premaxillary protrusion between the cleft palate elements (curved arrow). Axial T2 image (**b**) demonstrates presence of cleft lip (short arrow). Coronal T2 image demonstrates absence of the hypointense band of signal intensity corresponding to the hard palate (long arrow in **c1**). The long arrow in **c2** points to the normal hypointense palate in a separate patient for comparison. (**d**) a separate post-natal infant with bilateral cleft lip and palate. (**d** is courtesy of Dr. Geetha Arjun, E.V. Kalyani Medical Center, Chennai, India, Dr. S. Suresh, Mediscan Centre, Chennai, India, and Dr. Subha Sundararajan, Red Bank Gastroenterology, Redbank, New Jersey, USA)

heterogeneous with varying levels of vascularity owing to the amount and distribution of respective cellular layer elements. Given their rapid growth, associated cranial and systemic findings include macrocrania, secondary obstructive hydrocephalus, hemorrhage in setting of tumor, and various fluid-overladed states ranging from polyhydramnios and hydrops to high output cardiac failure [185].

The nonteratomas are less common, and include various neuroepithelial tumors (choroid plexus papilloma, medulloblastoma, astrocytoma), mesenchymal tumors types (such as cra-

niopharyngioma), or alternate cell types such as lipomas of the corpus collosum or tuberous sclerosis related tubers alongside non-neural axis tumors (like cardiac rhabdomyoma) [185].

Choroid plexus papillomas (CPP) are benign tumors composed of epithelial cells lining the ventricular choroid plexus. They correspond to 0.4–0.6% of all intracranial pre-natal tumor and are most often detected in the third trimester. CPPs can develop in the lateral ventricles, third ventricle, and/or fourth ventricle. Their combination of CSF production and obstructive locations lead to unilateral or bilateral ventriculomegaly.

On ultrasound, they are significantly echogenic, confounding their appearance with that of similarly appearing intraventricular hemorrhage on grey scale sonography. The use of Color Doppler would reveal increased vascularity within the echogenic mass, aiding in its distinction from intraventricular hemorrhage. Fetal MRI demonstrates an intraventricular mass of variable signal intensity within the ventricular system and associated hydrocephalus [185].

Craniopharyngiomas are benign extra-axial intracranial tumors encompassing 2%–5% of all congenital CNS neoplasms. They arise from squamous cells of the Rathke's pouch, an ectodermal diverticulum arising from the superior lining of the oropharynx. They are most often detected in the suprasellar location. Despite benign history, extra-axial neoplastic expansion leads to parenchymal destruction and associated hydrocephalus. These masses are difficult to distinguish from teratomas or other tumors such as astrocytomas and hamartomas. However, fetal MRI may better characterize lesion location and subsequently tailor the differential diagnosis accordingly [185].

Sacrococcygeal Teratomas and Mimics

Sacrococcygeal teratomas (SCT) are the most common fetal neoplasm with an incidence of 1 in every 35,000–40,000 live births. They are more common in female gestations and arise within the sacrococcygeal region from the primitive node (referred to as 'Henson's node' in original chick embryo literature). Some of these pluripotent stem just caudal to the coccyx escape inductive stimulation and instead grow uncontrollably into masses of nonspecific cell types of varying size. Fetal morbidity and mortality arises from alterations in fetal position and size [186].

SCTs can be classified based on location and imaging appearance. As established by the American Academy of Pediatrics Surgery Section (AAPSS), Type 1 SCTs develop strictly outside of the fetus and comprise approximately 47% of all teratomas making them the most prevalent

overall. Type II SCTs have extra-fetal components with intra-pelvic pre-sacral extension whereas Type III SCTs are extra-fetal but include abdomino-pelvic extension. Type IV SCTs develop completely within the fetal pelvis [187]. Furthermore, on imaging, SCTs can be classified by their content: A solid teratoma contains only tissues, a cystic teratoma contains only pockets of fluid or semi-fluid such as cerebrospinal fluid, sebum, or fat. A mixed teratoma contains both solid and cystic parts. Of these, cystic teratomas are the least prevalent, composing less than 15% of teratomas [186, 188].

Other lesions must also be considered in the differential when assessing cystic and solid masses in the spinal axis of neonates. These lesions include lymphatic malformation, myelomeningocele, and anterior meningocele. Macrocystic lymphatic malformation, also referred to as cystic lymphangioma or cystic hygroma, is considered a benign congenital vascular malformation that results from failure to establish normal lymphatic channel anatomy during development. This was described in a prior subsection. Sonographic images typically reveal a sharply marginated uni- or multilocular cystic lesion with internally increased echogenicity in the presence of infection or hemorrhage. Fetal MRI better depicts the anatomic extent and soft tissue contrast of the lesion and often show masses with attenuation similar to that of water and with thin, often contrast-enhanced walls and septa. Cystic lymphatic malformations appear as areas of homogeneous high signal intensity on T2-weighted images and have the signal intensity of fluid on T1-weighted images [168, 189].

Myelomeningoceles (MMCs) are largely found in the lumbosacral region, thus placing them on the differential diagnosis for suspected SCT. This was also described in a prior subsection. On sonographic imaging, MMCs appear in the posterior spinal region as a complex lesion containing neural elements, the actual neural placode, nerve roots, meninges, and cerebrospinal fluid. In comparison to these lesions, plain film imaging of SCT may show calcification of a mass projecting from the lower pelvic region. Ultrasound imaging reveals anechoic components of more cystic masses and echogenic components of solid tumors. MRI assists in evaluating mass effect of the lesion by demonstrating colonic displacement, ureteric dilation, and intraspinal extension [190].

An anterior meningocele of the sacrum is defined as herniation of the meningeal sac into the presacral retroperitoneal space via a congenital defect in the sacrum or through widened anterior sacral foramina. This is an extremely rare condition, with data on its incidence not readily available, as its presence has primarily been noted in scattered case reports or case series. This entity can be seen as part of the Currarino syndrome, which includes the presence of presacral mass such as meningocele, sacral osseous abnormality, and associated anorectal malformation. While prenatal sonography and fetal MRI can be used to raise suspicion of its presence, post-natal imaging is often needed to corroborate its presence and exclude alternate cloacal (i.e., rectum, vagina, urethra) abnormalities, enteric duplications cyst, or even hydrometrocolpos in the setting of imperforate hymen [191, 192].

Aside from diagnosis of SCT, accompanying complications must be considered. The mortality rate for infants with prenatally diagnosed SCT is worse than those diagnosed at birth. As seen in this particular patient presentation, the location and size of SCT may contribute to anatomical displacement of normal abdomino-pelvic structures resulting in signs and symptoms of obstruction—the bladder, ureters, or intestine may be constricted via mass effect and presenting physical exam findings and patient history should prompt further investigation. Other clinical complications include high output cardiac failure secondary to arteriovenous shunting and possible resultant hydrops fetalis. Bilateral hydronephrosis, spinal cord involvement, urinary and fecal incontinence, and nerve compression may also result from mass effect. Premature delivery, dystocia, tumor rupture, anemia, and fetal exsanguination are other clinical issues that can evolve secondary to SCT. Prognosis is not related solely to the size of the mass, but rather its content and extent. Solid hypervascular masses present a poorer prognosis than purely cystic masses. The

risk of malignant transformation increases with age; external masses are more readily identified on prenatal imaging and consequently result in a lesser risk of malignant transformation [186, 193].

Although the majority of SCTs are histologically benign, they are associated with significant morbidity and mortality due to their secondary effects, as discussed above. The prognosis for cure is generally good after successful complete resection of the mass and coccyx [194]. Potential surgical complications include hemorrhage and coagulopathy, with hemorrhage being the most common cause of death among neonates with SCTs. The mortality in the neonatal period is approximately 16% [186]. Features that correlate with an increased risk of hemorrhage include polyhydramnios, large-size lesions, and fetal distress. Other poor prognostic features include congestive heart failure, placentomegaly, and hydrops fetalis. These latter three findings have been associated with 100% mortality [195].

Closing

Given the extent and severity of various neurological conditions possible in the pregnant patient and their underlying gestation, a broad differential diagnosis must be considered when reviewing the neuroimaging of these special patient populations. Healthcare providers caring for pregnant patients and their respective fetuses should be aware of the background information and clinical entities discussed in this chapter given their unique predilection of manifesting as specific imaging findings in the neuraxis. Note that certain topics pertaining to these populations that providers are equally charged with being aware of are not included in this chapter. Specifically, the imaging features of conditions without uniquely described associations found beyond the pregnant patient and intrauterine gestation were not reviewed given the targeted nature of the intended chapter. This includes post-traumatic findings beyond acquired pre-natal insults in the neurovascular and neuroanatomic developmental pathways, infectious/inflammatory conditions that develop incidentally in pregnant patients with otherwise similar likelihood in the general population (excluding conditions with unique neuroanatomic findings and established clinical associations in either the pregnant patient or gestation), and pre-existing metabolic and developmental conditions independently associated with the state of pregnancy or more pertinent to the post-natal fetus (such as the various leukodystrophies seen in post-natal imaging).

References

1. Donald I, Macvicar J, Brown TG. Investigation of abdominal masses by pulsed ultrasound. Lancet. 1958;1(7032):1188–95.
2. Campbell S. A short history of sonography in obstetrics and gynaecology. Facts Views Vis Obgyn. 2013;5(3):213–29.
3. Hangiandreou NJ. AAPM/RSNA physics tutorial for residents. Topics in US: B-mode US: basic concepts and new technology. Radiographics. 2003;23(4):1019–33.
4. Shriki J. Ultrasound physics. Crit Care Clin. 2014;30(1):1–24, v.
5. Kollmann C, ter Haar G, Doležal L, Hennerici M, Salvesen K, Valentin L. Ultrasound emissions: thermal and mechanical indices. Ultraschall Med. 2013;34(5):422–31; quiz 432–424.
6. Şen T, Tüfekçioğlu O, Koza Y. Mechanical index. Anatol J Cardiol. 2015;15(4):334–6.
7. Fatahi Asl J, Farzanegan Z, Tahmasbi M, Birgani SM, Malekzade M, Yazdaninejad H. Evaluation of the scan duration and mechanical and thermal indices applied for the diagnostic ultrasound examinations. J Ultrasound Med. 2021;40:1839.
8. Abramowicz JS, Barnett SB, Duck FA, Edmonds PD, Hynynen KH, Ziskin MC. Fetal thermal effects of diagnostic ultrasound. J Ultrasound Med. 2008;27(4):541–59; quiz 560–543.
9. Ter Haar G. HIFU Tissue ablation: concept and devices. Adv Exp Med Biol. 2016;880:3–20.
10. AIUM-ACR-ACOG-SMFM-SRU Practice parameter for the performance of standard diagnostic obstetric ultrasound examinations. J Ultrasound Med. 2018;37(11):E13–e24.
11. Ratnapalan S, Bona N, Chandra K, Koren G. Physicians' perceptions of teratogenic risk associated with radiography and CT during early pregnancy. Am J Roentgenol. 2004;182(5):1107–9.
12. Lee CI, Haims AH, Monico EP, Brink JA, Forman HP. Diagnostic CT scans: assessment of patient, physician, and radiologist awareness of radiation dose and possible risks. Radiology. 2004;231(2):393–8.
13. Han B, Bednarz B, Xu XG. A study of the shielding used to reduce leakage and scattered radiation to the fetus in a pregnant patient treated with a 6-MV external X-ray beam. Health Phys. 2009;97(6):581–9.
14. Council NR. Health risks from exposure to low levels of ionizing radiation: BEIR VII Phase 2. Washington, DC: The National Academies Press; 2006.
15. Sensakovic W, Royall I, Hough M, Potrebko P, Grekoski V, Vicenti R. Fetal dosimetry at CT: a primer. Radiographics. 2020;40(4):1061–70.
16. Sidorov EV, Feng W, Caplan LR. Stroke in pregnant and postpartum women. Expert Rev Cardiovasc Ther. 2011;9(9):1235–47.
17. Bourjeily G, Chalhoub M, Phornphutkul C, Alleyne TC, Woodfield CA, Chen KK. Neonatal thyroid function: effect of a single exposure to iodinated contrast medium in utero. Radiology. 2010;256(3):744–50.
18. Ahmet A, Lawson ML, Babyn P, Tricco AC. Hypothyroidism in neonates post-iodinated contrast media: a systematic review. Acta Paediatr. 2009;98(10):1568–74.
19. Brenner DJ, Hall EJ. Computed tomography--an increasing source of radiation exposure. N Engl J Med. 2007;357(22):2277–84.
20. McNitt-Gray MF. AAPM/RSNA physics tutorial for residents: topics in CT. Radiation dose in CT. Radiographics. 2002;22(6):1541–53.
21. Tamm EP, Rong XJ, Cody DD, Ernst RD, Fitzgerald NE, Kundra V. Quality initiatives: CT radiation dose reduction: how to implement change without sacrificing diagnostic quality. Radiographics. 2011;31(7):1823–32.
22. Siegel JA, Brooks AL, Fisher DR, et al. A critical assessment of the linear no-threshold hypothesis: its validity and applicability for use in risk assessment and radiation protection. Clin Nucl Med. 2019;44(7):521–5.
23. Chodick G, Kim KP, Shwarz M, Horev G, Shalev V, Ron E. Radiation risks from pediatric computed tomography scanning. Pediatr Endocrinol Rev. 2009;7(2):29–36.
24. Schmidt CW. CT scans: balancing health risks and medical benefits. Environ Health Perspect. 2012;120(3):A118–21.
25. Radiology MSC-oAfO-EIiC, Safety MSCoOR. Implementation of the principle of as low as reasonably achievable (ALARA) for medical and dental personnel: recommendations of the National Council on Radiation Protection and Measurements. Bethesda, MD: NCRP; 1990.
26. Jackson HA, Panigrahy A. Fetal magnetic resonance imaging: the basics. Pediatr Ann. 2008;37(6):388–93.
27. Hailey D. Open magnetic resonance imaging (MRI) scanners. Issues Emerg Health Technol. 2006;92:1–4.
28. Enders J, Rief M, Zimmermann E, et al. High-field open versus short-bore magnetic resonance imaging of the spine: a randomized controlled comparison of image quality. PLoS One. 2013;8(12):e83427.

29. Victoria T, Jaramillo D, Roberts TP, et al. Fetal magnetic resonance imaging: jumping from 1.5 to 3 tesla (preliminary experience). Pediatr Radiol. 2014;44(4):376–86; quiz 373–375.

30. Krishnamurthy U, Neelavalli J, Mody S, et al. MR imaging of the fetal brain at 1.5T and 3.0T field strengths: comparing specific absorption rate (SAR) and image quality. J Perinat Med. 2015;43(2):209–20.

31. Saleem SN. Fetal MRI: an approach to practice: a review. J Adv Res. 2014;5(5):507–23.

32. Jacobs MA, Ibrahim TS, Ouwerkerk R. AAPM/ RSNA physics tutorials for residents: MR imaging: brief overview and emerging applications. Radiographics. 2007;27(4):1213–29.

33. Plewes DB, Kucharczyk W. Physics of MRI: a primer. J Magn Reson Imaging. 2012;35(5):1038–54.

34. Currie S, Hoggard N, Craven IJ, Hadjivassiliou M, Wilkinson ID. Understanding MRI: basic MR physics for physicians. Postgrad Med J. 2013;89(1050):209–23.

35. Neelavalli J, Krishnamurthy U, Jella PK, et al. Magnetic resonance angiography of fetal vasculature at 3.0 T. Eur Radiol. 2016;26(12):4570–6.

36. Kim DH, Chung S, Vigneron DB, Barkovich AJ, Glenn OA. Diffusion-weighted imaging of the fetal brain in vivo. Magn Reson Med. 2008;59(1):216–20.

37. Drake-Pérez M, Boto J, Fitsiori A, Lovblad K, Vargas MI. Clinical applications of diffusion weighted imaging in neuroradiology. Insights Imaging. 2018;9(4):535–47.

38. Wang Y, Spincemaille P, Liu Z, et al. Clinical quantitative susceptibility mapping (QSM): biometal imaging and its emerging roles in patient care. J Magn Reson Imaging. 2017;46(4):951–71.

39. Tocchio S, Kline-Fath B, Kanal E, Schmithorst VJ, Panigrahy A. MRI evaluation and safety in the developing brain. Semin Perinatol. 2015;39(2):73–104.

40. Weisstanner C, Gruber GM, Brugger PC, et al. Fetal MRI at 3T-ready for routine use? Br J Radiol. 2017;90(1069):20160362.

41. Mervak BM, Altun E, McGinty KA, Hyslop WB, Semelka RC, Burke LM. MRI in pregnancy: indications and practical considerations. J Magn Reson Imaging. 2019;49:621–31.

42. Shellock FG, Kanal E. Safety of magnetic resonance imaging contrast agents. J Magn Reson Imaging. 1999;10(3):477–84.

43. Webb JA, Thomsen HS, Morcos SK. The use of iodinated and gadolinium contrast media during pregnancy and lactation. Eur Radiol. 2005;15(6):1234–40.

44. Negro A, Delaruelle Z, Ivanova TA, et al. Headache and pregnancy: a systematic review. J Headache Pain. 2017;18(1):106.

45. Whitehead MT, Cardenas AM, Corey AS, et al. ACR Appropriateness Criteria® Headache. J Am Coll Radiol. 2019;16(11s):S364–s377.

46. Sandoe CH, Lay C. Secondary headaches during pregnancy: when to worry. Curr Neurol Neurosci Rep. 2019;19(6):27.

47. Markey KA, Uldall M, Botfield H, et al. Idiopathic intracranial hypertension, hormones, and 11β-hydroxysteroid dehydrogenases. J Pain Res. 2016;9:223–32.

48. Dinkin MJ, Patsalides A. Venous sinus stenting for idiopathic intracranial hypertension: where are we now? Neurol Clin. 2017;35(1):59–81.

49. Patsalides A, Oliveira C, Wilcox J, et al. Venous sinus stenting lowers the intracranial pressure in patients with idiopathic intracranial hypertension. J Neurointervent Surg. 2019;11(2):175–8.

50. Sivasankar R, Pant R, Indrajit IK, et al. Imaging and interventions in idiopathic intracranial hypertension: a pictorial essay. Indian J Radiol Imaging. 2015;25(4):439–44.

51. Sundararajan SH, Ramos AD, Kishore V, Michael M, Doustaly R, DeRusso F, Patsalides A. Am J Neuroradiol. 2021;42(2):288–96.

52. Dinkin MJ, Patsalides A. Venous sinus stenting in idiopathic intracranial hypertension: results of a prospective trial. J Neuroophthalmol. 2017;37(2):113–21.

53. Gurney SP, Ramalingam S, Thomas A, Sinclair AJ, Mollan SP. Exploring the current management idiopathic intracranial hypertension, and understanding the role of dural venous sinus stenting. Eye Brain. 2020;12:1–13.

54. Toscano S, Lo Fermo S, Reggio E, Chisari CG, Patti F, Zappia M. An update on idiopathic intracranial hypertension in adults: a look at pathophysiology, diagnostic approach and management. J Neurol. 2020;268:3249.

55. Struble E, Harrouk W, DeFelice A, Tesfamariam B. Nonclinical aspects of venous thrombosis in pregnancy. Birth Defects Res C Embryo Today. 2015;105(3):190–200.

56. Kashkoush AI, Ma H, Agarwal N, et al. Cerebral venous sinus thrombosis in pregnancy and puerperium: a pooled, systematic review. J Clin Neurosci. 2017;39:9–15.

57. Roth J, Deck G. Neurovascular disorders in pregnancy: a review. Obstet Med. 2019;12(4):164–7.

58. Walecki J, Mruk B, Nawrocka-Laskus E, Piliszek A, Przelaskowski A, Sklinda K. Neuroimaging of cerebral venous thrombosis (CVT) - old dilemma and the new diagnostic methods. Pol J Radiol. 2015;80:368–73.

59. Gibson PS, Powrie R. Anticoagulants and pregnancy: when are they safe? Cleve Clin J Med. 2009;76(2):113–27.

60. Pilato F, Distefano M, Calandrelli R. Posterior reversible encephalopathy syndrome and reversible cerebral vasoconstriction syndrome: clinical and radiological considerations. Front Neurol. 2020;11:34.

61. Mossa A, de Souza AZ, Souen JS, Netto Cde G, Netto Cde S, Grabert H. [Subarachnoid hemorrhage and intracerebral aneurysm in the pregnancy-puerperium cycle]. Revista de Ginecologia e d'obstetricia. 1965;116(6):294–303.

62. Pool JL. Treatment of intracranial aneurysms during pregnancy. JAMA. 1965;192(3):209–14.

63. Beighley A, Glynn R, Scullen T, et al. Aneurysmal subarachnoid hemorrhage during pregnancy: a comprehensive and systematic review of the literature. Neurosurg Rev. 2021;44:2511.

64. Yanamadala V, Sheth SA, Walcott BP, Buchbinder BR, Buckley D, Ogilvy CS. Non-contrast 3D time-of-flight magnetic resonance angiography for visualization of intracranial aneurysms in patients with absolute contraindications to CT or MRI contrast. J Clin Neurosci. 2013;20(8):1122–6.

65. Hirohata M, Abe T, Fujimura N, Takeuchi Y, Morimitsu H, Shigemori M. Clinical outcomes of coil embolization for acutely ruptured aneurysm: comparison with results of neck clipping when coil embolization is considered the first option. Interv Neuroradiol. 2004;10(2 Suppl):49–53.

66. Molyneux A, Kerr R, Stratton I, et al. International Subarachnoid Aneurysm Trial (ISAT) of neurosurgical clipping versus endovascular coiling in 2143 patients with ruptured intracranial aneurysms: a randomised trial. Lancet. 2002;360(9342):1267–74.

67. Derdeyn CP, Barr JD, Berenstein A, et al. The International Subarachnoid Aneurysm Trial (ISAT): a position statement from the executive committee of the American Society of Interventional and Therapeutic Neuroradiology and the American Society of Neuroradiology. Am J Neuroradiol. 2003;24(7):1404–8.

68. Liu P, Lv X, Li Y, Lv M. Endovascular management of intracranial aneurysms during pregnancy in three cases and review of the literature. Interv Neuroradiol. 2015;21(6):654–8.

69. Barbarite E, Hussain S, Dellarole A, Elhammady MS, Peterson E. The management of intracranial aneurysms during pregnancy: a systematic review. Turk Neurosurg. 2016;26(4):465–74.

70. Pierot L, Arthur AS, Fiorella D, Spelle L. Intrasaccular flow disruption with WEB device: current place and results in management of intracranial aneurysms. World Neurosurg. 2019;122:313–6.

71. Lv X, Li Y. The clinical characteristics and treatment of cerebral AVM in pregnancy. Neuroradiol J. 2015;28(4):385–8.

72. Lee S, Kim Y, Navi BB, et al. Risk of intracranial hemorrhage associated with pregnancy in women with cerebral arteriovenous malformations. J Neurointerv Surg. 2021;13:707.

73. Molina-Botello D, Rodríguez-Sanchez J, Cuevas-García J, Cárdenas-Almaraz B, Morales-Acevedo A, Mejía-Pérez S, Ochoa-Martinez E. Pregnancy and brain tumors; a systematic review of the literature. J Clin Neurosci. 2021;86:211–6.

74. Rondon-Berrios H. Therapeutic relowering of plasma sodium after overly rapid correction of hyponatremia. What is the evidence? Clin J Am Soc Nephrol. 2020;15(2):282–4.

75. Koul PA, Khan UH, Jan RA, et al. Osmotic demyelination syndrome following slow correction of hyponatremia: possible role of hypokalemia. Indian J Crit Care Med. 2013;17(4):231–3.

76. Lohr JW. Osmotic demyelination syndrome following correction of hyponatremia: association with hypokalemia. Am J Med. 1994;96(5):408–13.

77. Corona G, Simonetti L, Giuliani C, Sforza A, Peri A. A case of osmotic demyelination syndrome occurred after the correction of severe hyponatraemia in hyperemesis gravidarum. BMC Endocr Disord. 2014;14:34.

78. Sánchez-Ferrer ML, Prieto-Sánchez MT, Orozco-Fernández R, Machado-Linde F, Nieto-Diaz A. Central pontine myelinolysis during pregnancy: pathogenesis, diagnosis and management. J Obstet Gynaecol. 2017;37(3):273–9.

79. Cuello JP, Martínez Ginés ML, Tejeda-Velarde A, et al. Cytokine profile during pregnancy predicts relapses during pregnancy and postpartum in multiple sclerosis. J Neurol Sci. 2020;414:116811.

80. Laura Airas ME, Maghzi A-H. Pregnany and multiple sclerosis. In: Minager A, editor. Neurological disorders and pregnancy. London: Elsevier Inc.; 2011. p. 1–11.

81. Thompson AJ, Banwell BL, Barkhof F, et al. Diagnosis of multiple sclerosis: 2017 revisions of the McDonald criteria. Lancet Neurol. 2018;17(2):162–73.

82. Wattjes MP, Steenwijk MD, Stangel M. MRI in the diagnosis and monitoring of multiple sclerosis: an update. Clin Neuroradiol. 2015;25(Suppl 2):157–65.

83. Suthiphosuwan S, Sati P, Guenette M, et al. The central vein sign in radiologically isolated syndrome. AJNR Am J Neuroradiol. 2019;40(5):776–83.

84. Mistry N, Abdel-Fahim R, Samaraweera A, et al. Imaging central veins in brain lesions with 3-T T2*-weighted magnetic resonance imaging differentiates multiple sclerosis from microangiopathic brain lesions. Mult Scler. 2016;22(10):1289–96.

85. Suh CH, Kim SJ, Jung SC, Choi CG, Kim HS. The "Central Vein Sign" on T2*-weighted images as a diagnostic tool in multiple sclerosis: a systematic review and meta-analysis using individual patient data. Sci Rep. 2019;9(1):18188.

86. Heaphy-Henault KJ, Guimaraes CV, Mehollin-Ray AR, et al. Congenital aqueductal stenosis: findings at fetal MRI that accurately predict a postnatal diagnosis. AJNR Am J Neuroradiol. 2018;39:942.

87. Di Mascio D, Sileo FG, Khalil A, et al. Role of magnetic resonance imaging in fetuses with mild or moderate ventriculomegaly in the era of fetal neurosonography: systematic review and meta-analysis. Ultrasound Obstet Gynecol. 2019;54(2):164–71.

88. Guerrini R, Dobyns WB. Malformations of cortical development: clinical features and genetic causes. Lancet Neurol. 2014;13(7):710–26.

89. Severino M, Geraldo AF, Utz N, et al. Definitions and classification of malformations of cortical development: practical guidelines. Brain. 2020;143(10):2874–94.

90. Barkovich AJ, Kuzniecky RI, Jackson GD, Guerrini R, Dobyns WB. A developmental and genetic classification for malformations of cortical development. Neurology. 2005;65(12):1873–87.

91. Choi JJ, Yang E, Soul JS, Jaimes C. Fetal magnetic resonance imaging: supratentorial brain malformations. Pediatr Radiol. 2020;50(13):1934–47.

92. Laifer-Narin SL, Ayyala R, Coletta J, Miller RS. EP03.06: Fetal MRI of hemimegalencephaly: a report of 4 cases. Ultrasound Obstet Gynecol. 2015;46(S1):192–3.

93. Williams F, Griffiths PD. The diagnosis of hemimegalencephaly using in utero MRI. Clin Radiol. 2014;69(6):e291–7.

94. Nagaraj UD, Peiro JL, Bierbrauer KS, Kline-Fath BM. Evaluation of subependymal gray matter heterotopias on fetal MRI. AJNR Am J Neuroradiol. 2016;37(4):720–5.

95. Pilz DT, Quarrell OW. Syndromes with lissencephaly. J Med Genet. 1996;33(4):319–23.

96. Di Donato N, Chiari S, Mirzaa GM, et al. Lissencephaly: expanded imaging and clinical classification. Am J Med Genet A. 2017;173(6):1473–88.

97. Nagaraj UD, Hopkin R, Schapiro M, Kline-Fath B. Prenatal and postnatal evaluation of polymicrogyria with band heterotopia. Radiol Case Rep. 2017;12(3):602–5.

98. Momen AA, Momen M. Double cortex syndrome (subcortical band heterotopia): a case report. Iran J Child Neurol. 2015;9(2):64–8.

99. Ahearne CE, Boylan GB, Murray DM. Short and long term prognosis in perinatal asphyxia: an update. World J Clin Pediatr. 2016;5(1):67–74.

100. Yamamoto N, Utsu M, Serizawa M, et al. Neonatal periventricular leukomalacia preceded by fetal periventricular echodensity. Fetal Diagn Ther. 2000;15(4):198–208.

101. Chao CP, Zaleski CG, Patton AC. Neonatal hypoxic-ischemic encephalopathy: multimodality imaging findings. Radiographics. 2006;26(Suppl 1):S159–72.

102. Abergel A, Lacalm A, Massoud M, Massardier J, des Portes V, Guibaud L. Expanding porencephalic cysts: prenatal imaging and differential diagnosis. Fetal Diagn Ther. 2017;41(3):226–33.

103. Griffiths PD. Schizencephaly revisited. Neuroradiology. 2018;60(9):945–60.

104. Ghosh PS, Reid JR, Patno D, Friedman NR. Fetal magnetic resonance imaging in hydranencephaly. J Paediatr Child Health. 2013;49(4):335–6.

105. Society for Maternal-Fetal Medicine (SMFM), Rotmensch S, Monteagudo A. Agenesis of the corpus callosum. Am J Obstet Gynecol. 2020;223(6):B17–22.

106. Nagaraj UD, Calvo-Garcia MA, Kline-Fath BM. Abnormalities associated with the cavum septi pellucidi on fetal MRI: what radiologists need to know. Am J Roentgenol. 2018;210(5):989–97.

107. Kousa YA, du Plessis AJ, Vezina G. Prenatal diagnosis of holoprosencephaly. Am J Med Genet C: Semin Med Genet. 2018;178(2):206–13.

108. Tekendo-Ngongang C, et al. Holoprosencephaly overview. In: GeneReviews®. Seattle, WA: University of Washington; 1993.

109. Schlatterer SD, Sanapo L, du Plessis AJ, Whitehead MT, Mulkey SB. The role of fetal MRI for suspected anomalies of the posterior fossa. Pediatr Neurol. 2021;117:10–8.

110. Milani HJF, Barreto EQS, Ximenes RLS, Baldo CAR, Araujo Júnior E, Moron AF. Fetal posterior fossa malformations: review of the current knowledge. Radiol Bras. 2019;52(6):380–6.

111. Cignini P, Giorlandino M, Brutti P, Mangiafico L, Aloisi A, Giorlandino C. Reference charts for fetal cerebellar vermis height: a prospective cross-sectional study of 10605 fetuses. PLoS One. 2016;11(1):e0147528.

112. Vinkesteijn AS, Mulder PG, Wladimiroff JW. Fetal transverse cerebellar diameter measurements in normal and reduced fetal growth. Ultrasound Obstet Gynecol. 2000;15(1):47–51.

113. Parkar AP, Olsen ØE, Gjelland K, Kiserud T, Rosendahl K. Common fetal measurements: a comparison between ultrasound and magnetic resonance imaging. Acta Radiol. 2010;51(1):85–91.

114. Diogo MC, Glatter S, Binder J, Kiss H, Prayer D. The MRI spectrum of congenital cytomegalovirus infection. Prenat Diagn. 2020;40(1):110–24.

115. Malinger G, Werner H, Rodriguez Leonel JC, et al. Prenatal brain imaging in congenital toxoplasmosis. Prenat Diagn. 2011;31(9):881–6.

116. Feemster KA, Szipszky C. Resurgence of measles in the United States: how did we get here? Curr Opin Pediatr. 2020;32(1):139–44.

117. Parkman PD. Togaviruses: rubella virus. In: Baron S, editor. Medical microbiology. 4th ed. Galveston, TX: University of Texas Medical Branch at Galveston; 1996.

118. Yazigi A, De Pecoulas AE, Vauloup-Fellous C, Grangeot-Keros L, Ayoubi JM, Picone O. Fetal and neonatal abnormalities due to congenital rubella syndrome: a review of literature. J Matern Fetal Neonatal Med. 2017;30(3):274–8.

119. Fa F, Laup L, Mandelbrot L, Sibiude J, Picone O. Fetal and neonatal abnormalities due to congenital herpes simplex virus infection: a literature review. Prenat Diagn. 2020;40(4):408–14.

120. James SH, Sheffield JS, Kimberlin DW. Mother-to-child transmission of herpes simplex virus. J Pediatr Infect Dis Soc. 2014;3(Suppl 1):S19–23.

121. Barefoot KH, Little GA, Ornvold KT. Fetal demise due to herpes simplex virus: an illustrated case report. J Perinatol. 2002;22(1):86–8.
122. Freij BJ, Sever JL. Herpesvirus infections in pregnancy: risks to embryo, fetus, and neonate. Clin Perinatol. 1988;15(2):203–31.
123. Duin LK, Willekes C, Baldewijns MM, Robben SG, Offermans J, Vles J. Major brain lesions by intrauterine herpes simplex virus infection: MRI contribution. Prenat Diagn. 2007;27(1):81–4.
124. Marquez L, Levy ML, Munoz FM, Palazzi DL. A report of three cases and review of intrauterine herpes simplex virus infection. Pediatr Infect Dis J. 2011;30(2):153–7.
125. Sloan JK, Cawyer CR, Drever NS. Fetal ventriculomegaly and herpes encephalitis following primary maternal herpes simplex infection. Baylor Univ Med Center Proc. 2017;30(4):463–4.
126. Mulkey SB, Bulas DI, Vezina G, et al. Sequential neuroimaging of the fetus and newborn with in utero zika virus exposure. JAMA Pediatr. 2019;173(1):52–9.
127. Sutton D, Miller R. Neurologic outcomes after prenatal treatment of twin-twin transfusion syndrome. Clin Perinatol. 2020;47(4):719–31.
128. Sato H, Murata H, Sato K, Kawaharamura K, Hamanishi S, Hirose M. Encephalomalacia in surviving twin after single fetal death diagnosed at 18 weeks of gestation in monochorionic twin pregnancy. Am J Case Rep. 2013;14:341–4.
129. Acharya UV, Pendharkar H, Varma DR, Pruthi N, Varadarajan S. Spinal dysraphism illustrated; embroyology revisited. Indian J Radiol Imaging. 2017;27(4):417–26.
130. Catala M. Embryology of the spine and spinal cord. In: Rossi A, editor. Pediatric neuroradiology. Berlin: Springer; 2015. p. 1–53.
131. Catala M. Embryology of the brain. In: Tortori-Donati P, Rossi A, editors. Pediatric neuroradiology: brain. Berlin: Springer; 2005. p. 1–20.
132. Copp AJ, Stanier P, Greene ND. Neural tube defects: recent advances, unsolved questions, and controversies. Lancet Neurol. 2013;12(8):799–810.
133. Copp AJ. Neurulation in the cranial region--normal and abnormal. J Anat. 2005;207(5):623–35.
134. Curtin JA, Quint E, Tsipouri V, et al. Mutation of Celsr1 disrupts planar polarity of inner ear hair cells and causes severe neural tube defects in the mouse. Curr Biol. 2003;13(13):1129–33.
135. Gustavsson P, Greene ND, Lad D, et al. Increased expression of Grainyhead-like-3 rescues spina bifida in a folate-resistant mouse model. Hum Mol Genet. 2007;16(21):2640–6.
136. Pryor SE, Massa V, Savery D, Greene ND, Copp AJ. Convergent extension analysis in mouse whole embryo culture. Methods Mol Biol. 2012;839:133–46.
137. Carroll EA, Gerrelli D, Gasca S, et al. Cordon-bleu is a conserved gene involved in neural tube formation. Dev Biol. 2003;262(1):16–31.
138. Cogram P, Hynes A, Dunlevy LP, Greene ND, Copp AJ. Specific isoforms of protein kinase C are essential for prevention of folate-resistant neural tube defects by inositol. Hum Mol Genet. 2004;13(1):7–14.
139. Copp AJ. Genetic models of mammalian neural tube defects. CIBA Found Symp. 1994;181:118–34; discussion 134–143.
140. Massa V, Savery D, Ybot-Gonzalez P, et al. Apoptosis is not required for mammalian neural tube closure. Proc Natl Acad Sci U S A. 2009;106(20):8233–8.
141. Fleming A, Copp AJ. Embryonic folate metabolism and mouse neural tube defects. Science. 1998;280(5372):2107–9.
142. Dunlevy LP, Burren KA, Mills K, Chitty LS, Copp AJ, Greene ND. Integrity of the methylation cycle is essential for mammalian neural tube closure. Birth Defects Res A Clin Mol Teratol. 2006;76(7):544–52.
143. Aertsen M, Verduyckt J, De Keyzer F, et al. Reliability of MR imaging-based posterior fossa and brain stem measurements in open spinal dysraphism in the era of fetal surgery. AJNR Am J Neuroradiol. 2019;40(1):191–8.
144. Obeidi N, Russell N, Higgins JR, O'Donoghue K. The natural history of anencephaly. Prenat Diagn. 2010;30(4):357–60.
145. Sharif A, Zhou Y. Fetal MRI characteristics of exencephaly: a case report and literature review. Case Rep Radiol. 2016;2016:9801267.
146. Blount JP, Elton S. Spinal lipomas. Neurosurg Focus. 2001;10(1):e3.
147. David DJ. Cephaloceles: classification, pathology, and management--a review. J Craniofac Surg. 1993;4(4):192–202.
148. Puvabanditsin S, Malik I, Garrow E, Francois L, Mehta R. Clival encephalocele and 5q15 deletion: a case report. J Child Neurol. 2015;30(4):505–8.
149. Sepulveda W, Wong AE, Andreeva E, Odegova N, Martinez-Ten P, Meagher S. Sonographic spectrum of first-trimester fetal cephalocele: review of 35 cases. Ultrasound Obstet Gynecol. 2015;46(1):29–33.
150. Fleming A, Copp AJ. A genetic risk factor for mouse neural tube defects: defining the embryonic basis. Hum Mol Genet. 2000;9(4):575–81.
151. Warner T, Scullen TA, Iwanaga J, et al. Caudal regression syndrome-a review focusing on genetic associations. World Neurosurg. 2020;138:461–7.
152. Boruah DK, Dhingani DD, Achar S, et al. Magnetic resonance imaging analysis of caudal regression syndrome and concomitant anomalies in pediatric patients. J Clin Imag Sci. 2016;6:36.
153. Caro-Domínguez P, Bass J, Hurteau-Miller J. Currarino syndrome in a fetus, infant, child, and adolescent: spectrum of clinical presentations and imaging findings. Can Assoc Radiol J. 2017;68(1):90–5.
154. Kanagasabai K, Bhat V, Pramod GK, Patil SJ, Kiranmayi S. Severe caudal regression syndrome with overlapping features of VACTERL complex: antenatal detection and follow up. BJR Case Rep. 2016;3(2):20150356.

155. Passias PG, Poorman GW, Jalai CM, et al. Incidence of congenital spinal abnormalities among pediatric patients and their association with scoliosis and systemic anomalies. J Pediatr Orthop. 2019;39(8):e608–13.

156. Wilkens R, Odom G. Tumors of the spine and spinal cord, Part II. Handbook of clinical neurology. Amsterdam: Elsevier; 1976.

157. Menezes AH, Dlouhy BJ. Neurenteric cysts at foramen magnum in children: presentation, imaging characteristics, and surgical management-case series and literature review. Childs Nerv Syst. 2020;36(7):1379–84.

158. Teufack S, Campbell P, Moshel YA. Intracranial neuroenteric cysts: two atypical cases and review of the literature. JHN J. 2011;6(1):6.

159. Cheng B, Li FT, Lin L. Diastematomyelia: a retrospective review of 138 patients. J Bone J Surg Br. 2012;94(3):365–72.

160. Hidalgo JA, Tork CA, Varacallo M. Arnold Chiari malformation. Treasure Island, FL: StatPearls; 2020. https://www.ncbi.nlm.nih.gov/books/NBK431076/.

161. Saker E, Henry BM, Tomaszewski KA, et al. The human central canal of the spinal cord: a comprehensive review of its anatomy, embryology, molecular development, variants, and pathology. Cureus. 2016;8(12):e927.

162. Strahle J, Muraszko KM, Garton HJ, et al. Syrinx location and size according to etiology: identification of Chiari-associated syrinx. J Neurosurg Pediatr. 2015;16(1):21–9.

163. Righini A, Parazzini C, Doneda C, et al. Fetal MRI features related to the Chiari malformations. Neurol Sci. 2011;32(Suppl 3):S279–81.

164. ISSVA. Classification of vascular anomalies. Milwaukee, WI: ISSVA; 2018. https://www.issva.org/classification. Accessed 31 May 2020.

165. Putra J, Al-Ibraheemi A. Vascular anomalies of the head and neck: a pediatric overview. Head Neck Pathol. 2021;15:59. https://doi.org/10.1007/s12105-020-01236-x.

166. Tekes A, Koshy J, Kalayci TO, et al. S.E. Mitchell vascular anomalies flow chart (SEMVAFC): a visual pathway combining clinical and imaging findings for classification of soft-tissue vascular anomalies. Clin Radiol. 2014;69(5):443–57.

167. Blei F, Bittman M. Congenital vascular anomalies: current perspectives on diagnosis, classification, and management. J Vasc Diagn Intervent. 2016;4:23–37.

168. Oliver ER, Coleman BG, DeBari SE, et al. Fetal lymphatic malformations: more variable than we think? J Ultrasound Med. 2017;36(5):1051–8.

169. Martini S, Toni F, Paoletti V, Corvaglia L, Cordelli DM. Teaching neuroimages: neurovascular features of suspected antenatal-onset Sturge-Weber syndrome without skin involvement. Neurology. 2020;95(22):e3070–1.

170. Sturge-Weber syndrome. 2020. https://ghr.nlm.nih.gov/condition/sturge-weber-syndrome. Accessed 31 May 2020.

171. Kortman H, Navaei E, Raybaud CA, et al. Deep venous communication in vein of Galen malformations: incidence, Imaging, and Implications for treatment. J Neurointerv Surg. 2021;13(3):290–3.

172. Zhou LX, Dong SZ, Zhang MF. Diagnosis of Vein of Galen aneurysmal malformation using fetal MRI. J Magn Reson Imaging. 2017;46(5):1535–9.

173. Doyle NM, Mastrobattista JM, Thapar MK, Lantin-Hermoso MR. Perinatal pseudocoarctation: echocardiographic findings in vein of Galen malformation. J Ultrasound Med. 2005;24(1):93–8; quiz 99.

174. Arangio P, Manganaro L, Pacifici A, Basile E, Cascone P. Importance of fetal MRI in evaluation of craniofacial deformities. J Craniofac Surg. 2013;24(3):773–6.

175. Tessier P. Anatomical classification facial, craniofacial and latero-facial clefts. J Maxillofac Surg. 1976;4(2):69–92.

176. Van Der Meulen CHJ. Oblique facial clefts: pathology, etiology, and reconstruction. Plast Reconstr Surg. 1985;76(2):212–24.

177. Paladini D, Morra T, Teodoro A, Lamberti A, Tremolaterra F, Martinelli P. Objective diagnosis of micrognathia in the fetus: the jaw index. Obstet Gynecol. 1999;93(3):382–6.

178. Laifer-Narin S, Schlechtweg K, Lee J, et al. A comparison of early versus late prenatal magnetic resonance imaging in the diagnosis of cleft palate. Ann Plast Surg. 2019;82(4S Suppl 3):S242–s246.

179. Nyberg DA, Hegge FN, Kramer D, Mahony BS, Kropp RJ. Premaxillary protrusion: a sonographic clue to bilateral cleft lip and palate. J Ultrasound Med. 1993;12(6):331–5.

180. Dabadie A, Quarello E, Degardin N, et al. Added value of MRI for the prenatal diagnosis of isolated orofacial clefts and comparison with ultrasound. Diagn Intervent Imag. 2016;97(9):915–21.

181. König M, Due-Tønnessen B, Osnes T, Haugstvedt J-R, Meling TR. Median facial cleft with a fronto-ethmoidal encephalocele treated with craniofacial bipartition and free radial forearm flap: a case report. Skull Base. 2010;20(2):119–23.

182. Wexler MR, Benmeir P, Umansky F, Weinberg A, Neuman R. Midline cleft syndrome with spheno-ethmoidal encephalocele: a case report. J Craniofac Surg. 1991;2(1):38–41.

183. Ganapathy A, Sadeesh T, Swer MH, Rao S. Occipital meningoencephalocele with cleft lip, cleft palate and limb abnormalities - a case report. J Clin Diagn Res. 2014;8(12):AD03–5.

184. Gonçalves LF, Lee W, Mody S, Shetty A, Sangi-Haghpeykar H, Romero R. Diagnostic accuracy of ultrasonography and magnetic resonance imaging for the detection of fetal anomalies: a blinded case-control study. Ultrasound Obstet Gynecol. 2016;48(2):185–92.

185. Feygin T, Khalek N, Moldenhauer JS. Fetal brain, head, and neck tumors: prenatal imaging and management. Prenat Diagn. 2020;40(10):1203–19.
186. Herman TE, Siegel MJ. Cystic type IV sacrococcygeal teratoma. J Perinatol. 2002;22(4):331–2.
187. Avni FE, Guibaud L, Robert Y, et al. MR imaging of fetal sacrococcygeal teratoma. Am J Roentgenol. 2002;178(1):179–83.
188. Kocaoglu M, Frush DP. Pediatric presacral masses. Radiographics. 2006;26(3):833–57.
189. Nosher JL, Murillo PG, Liszewski M, Gendel V, Gribbin CE. Vascular anomalies: a pictorial review of nomenclature, diagnosis and treatment. World J Radiol. 2014;6(9):677–92.
190. Nagaraj UD, Bierbrauer KS, Peiro JL, Kline-Fath BM. Differentiating closed versus open spinal dysraphisms on fetal MRI. AJR Am J Roentgenol. 2016;207(6):1316–23.
191. Sumi A, Sato Y, Kakui K, Tatsumi K, Fujiwara H, Konishi I. Prenatal diagnosis of anterior sacral meningocele. Ultrasound Obstet Gynecol. 2011;37(4):493–6.
192. Braczynski AK, Brockmann MA, Scholz T, Bach J-P, Schulz JB, Tauber SC. Anterior sacral meningocele infected with Fusobacterium in a patient with recently diagnosed colorectal carcinoma – a case report. BMC Neurol. 2017;17(1):212.
193. Danzer E, Hubbard AM, Hedrick HL, et al. Diagnosis and characterization of fetal sacrococcygeal teratoma with prenatal MRI. AJR Am J Roentgenol. 2006;187(4):W350.
194. Sheth S, Nussbaum AR, Sanders RC, Hamper UM, Davidson AJ. Prenatal diagnosis of sacrococcygeal teratoma: sonographic-pathologic correlation. Radiology. 1988;169(1):131–6.
195. Murphy JJ, Blair GK, Fraser GC. Coagulopathy associated with large sacrococcygeal teratomas. J Pediatr Surg. 1992;27(10):1308–10.

Fareed Jumah, Michael S. Rallo,
Sanjeev Sreenivasan, Jonathan Lowenthal,
Sudipta Roychowdhury, Gaurav Gupta,
and Anil Nanda

Introduction

Rates of medical litigation in the USA have reached rampant proportions in the last two decades. In 2013 alone, the total cost of malpractice payout was 3.7 billion USD [1]. Obstetrics, neurology, and neurosurgery are in the top league of high-risk medical specialties. Obstetrics has the highest litigation settlement payments among medical specialties [2]. Up to 85% of obstetricians and gynecologists have been named in a lawsuit; 24% were sued once and 62% two to five times [3], and it is estimated that 74% will face a claim by the age of 45 [4]. Similarly, 19.1% of neurosurgeons face a malpractice claim each year, the highest percentage among all specialties, with indemnities averaging $350,000 [4]. A 2019 report shows that 62% of neurologists have been involved in at least 1 lawsuit [5]. These daunting trends pose a significant psychological and financial burden on physicians and the healthcare system as a whole. The constant fear of litigation has given rise to the practice of "defensive medicine," which raises the healthcare expenditure by estimates of $60 billion each year [6].

There is considerable overlap between the childbearing years and the time of onset of many female-predominant neurological diseases. Due to the complex nature of pregnancy, owing mainly to the mother-infant dyad, and its dynamic interplay with neurologic disease, certain medicolegal issues may arise. As these issues may be further compounded by the high-risk nature of neurological and obstetrical care [4, 7], it is imperative that physicians be knowledgeable and vigilant when dealing with such cases, and take the steps necessary to avoid litigation.

This chapter is divided into three sections. The first outlines some of the medicolegal principles that physicians need to be familiar with, such as

F. Jumah · M. S. Rallo
Robert Wood Johnson University Hospital,
New Brunswick, NJ, USA

S. Sreenivasan
Cerebrovascular & Endovascular Neurosurgery,
Robert Wood Johnson Medical School, Rutgers
University, New Brunswick, NJ, USA

J. Lowenthal
Department of Radiology, Rutgers Robert Wood
Johnson Medical School, New Brunswick, NJ, USA

S. Roychowdhury
Neuroradiology, University Radiology,
New Brunswick, NJ, USA

G. Gupta (✉)
Neurosurgery, Rutgers Robert Wood Johnson
Medical School, New Brunswick, NJ, USA
e-mail: guptaga@rutgers.edu

A. Nanda
Neurosurgery, Robert Wood Johnson University
Hospital, New Brunswick, NJ, USA

G. Gupta et al. (eds.), *Neurological Disorders in Pregnancy*,
https://doi.org/10.1007/978-3-031-36490-7_4

the physician's duty of care and informed consent. These principles will serve as precursors to understanding the process of litigation that ensues once a lawsuit has been filed, and the elements which underpin a court's determination that medical negligence has occurred. The two sections that follow outline various medicolegal and ethical aspects in selected neurological disorders in the pregnant or childbearing woman (section "Medicolegal and Ethical Issues in Selected Neurological Disorders in Pregnancy"), as well as in the fetus and the newborn (section "Medicolegal Issues in the Fetus and the Newborn"). The work presented in this chapter is intended solely for educational purposes and is by no means all-inclusive or a replacement for formal legal counsel.

General Principles

The Physician's Duty of Care

Pregnancy holds an interesting dynamic with neurologic disease. It can affect the natural history of a disease by alleviating or worsening it. Conversely, the course of pregnancy, delivery, or labor can in turn be jeopardized by pre-existing neurological conditions. Similarly, drugs used to treat neurologic disease may affect a woman's fertility, contraceptive use and efficacy, and the fetus' prenatal development. In order to achieve optimal patient care and minimize medical errors, physicians in neurology and neurosurgery should familiarize themselves with disease management in the setting of obstetric and perinatal care, and similarly, obstetricians should have a neurological background sufficient to achieve the same goal.

Nevertheless, regardless of the specialty, the responsibility of the physician remains universal: to act with "due care," that is to provide medical care according to the accepted standards. A physician is also obligated to provide information necessary so that the patient may fully understand the impact of their medical condition in order to make an informed decision about their care [8].

The potential for legal liability against a physician depends on several important factors. First, the plaintiff must prove in court the existence of a doctor–patient relationship. Although physicians are under no obligation to treat a patient unless they choose to (with certain exception like emergencies), a relationship is established when an action is taken in a patient's care by examining, diagnosing, treating, or agreeing to do so [9]. Importantly, the physician might be unaware that a relationship had been established, putting themselves at risk of liability. This is shown in *Mead v. Adler's* case in Oregon when an on-call neurosurgeon was consulted for a patient with low back pain. The surgeon advised that the patient did not need surgery. Four days later, the patient suffered permanent disability which could have been prevented by surgical intervention. The physician's decision to give an opinion regarding the patient's care inferred the formation of a doctor–patient relationship which, in this case, held the physician legally liable [10].

After proving that a doctor–patient relationship existed, it must be shown that, in providing medical care, the physician breached the duty of care. The standard of care by which this breach is judged is specialty-specific, but is usually determined by how a "reasonably prudent" physician would have acted in the given situation, which requires the plaintiff to provide the court with a testimony from an expert. Medical negligence can be in the form of poor medical care, breach of confidentiality, or failure to obtain informed consent. Lastly, the plaintiff must demonstrate the nature and magnitude of the damaged incurred, and that this damage was a result of the physician's negligence [8, 11].

Informed Consent

Obtaining a patient's informed consent is one of the key components in providing high-quality, ethical medical care. Doctors have a legal obligation to obtain informed consent to medical treatments, and the patient in turn has the right to gain information and ask questions which would allow them to make independent, well-studied healthcare decisions. The process of obtaining consent must take into account discussing the benefits and risks of the medical treatment and all of its reasonable alternatives, including the option of non-treatment and its outcomes. Clear communication between the physician and the patient is key to developing trust in the doctor–patient relationship and to mitigating medicolegal risk. In fact, studies have shown that the strongest reason for filing medical lawsuits against a physician is inadequate explanation of the potential impact of a treatment and the treatment alternatives to a patient [12].

At the same time, this does not mean doctors have to disclose every single risk no matter the likelihood, but only those that are *material* and are commonly known to the medical community. For example, when counseling a multiple sclerosis patient considering pregnancy, the doctor is not legally obligated to share the slightly increased risks of intrauterine growth restriction or caesarian section [13]. Although it varies between jurisdictions, a *material* risk is defined as that which a reasonably prudent patient would want to know in order to adequately assess the risks and benefits of the medical treatment at hand [8, 11]. Therefore, a physician might unknowingly fail to disclose a particular risk because they perceive the risk as arbitrary, putting themselves in jeopardy of liability further down the line. Therefore, perhaps a more prudent approach would be to share as much reasonable information with the patient and allow them to judge for themselves.

Medicolegal and Ethical Issues in Selected Neurological Disorders in Pregnancy

The following discussion outlines certain medicolegal and ethical considerations involved in selected neurological diseases in pregnancy. The medicolegal risks that will be discussed fall under one of the following four general themes. As discussed previously, the concept of informed consent is of particular importance, especially in cases where the mother lacks the capacity to make informed decisions. In other situations, legal liability may arise if the physician fails to diagnose a neurological disorder that develops

during pregnancy. Medicolegal claims may also result from failure to anticipate and properly counsel the patient about the potential effects of pregnancy on a pre-existing neurological condition, or vice versa. Similarly, negligence or ignorance can result in failure to avoid the teratogenic effects of certain medications used in treating neurological diseases.

Seizures and Epilepsy

Women with epilepsy have an increased risk of obstetric and perinatal complications compared to that of the general population. Seizures can lead to maternal and/or fetal injury by several pathways such as trauma, hypoxia, or the effects of antiepileptic drugs (AEDs) during gestation and breastfeeding. Although the majority of adverse events are not due to medical malpractice [14], clinicians that are involved with this subset of patients, including obstetricians, neurologists and neurosurgeons, are often faced with the possibility of a lawsuit if an adverse outcome should occur.

Antiepileptic treatments can pose certain medicolegal risks during a female's reproductive years. It is well recognized that no AED is entirely safe during pregnancy. However, some drugs are highly teratogenic and should be prescribed with caution in a female of childbearing potential. Besides the physician's duty to ensure optimal seizure control, they must also anticipate the possibility of pregnancy, especially an unplanned one. When optimizing a treatment regimen, the physician must thoroughly discuss the available treatment options, with the benefits and risks of each, including the option of non-treatment. If a medication with high teratogenicity, such as valproate, is prescribed, contraception and often folic acid supplements should be recommended to the patient [11, 15]. Proper documentation of the informed consent and verification of the patient's understanding are paramount to avoiding liability.

Informed consent is not always mandated, however. For example, while administering AEDs in a pregnant patient with status epilepticus might carry risks to the fetus, treatment of emergent, life-threatening conditions overrides the need to obtain informed consent in such scenarios. Therefore, it would not put the physician at risk of liability given that the protocols had been followed appropriately.

When a patient presents with convulsions, psychogenic non-epileptic seizures (PNES) should be on the list of differential diagnoses. Although they are uncommon, PNES are one of the primary seizure mimics and pose unique diagnostic and medicolegal challenges [16]. A prolonged PNES may resemble a status epilepticus, leading to unnecessary administration of teratogenic AEDs. On the other hand, suspicion of PNES can result in withdrawal of AEDs, which is sometimes necessary to establish the diagnosis. Little is known about the optimal approach to these cases given their rarity and the difficulty in capturing this patient population. Nevertheless, proper recognition of clinical clues (e.g., post-ictal state, history of conversion disorder) and video-electroencephalography monitoring can aid in diagnosis.

Sudden unexpected death in epilepsy (SUDEP) is another controversial aspect of epilepsy management. It is estimated that SUDEP is responsible for 2–18% of deaths in epilepsy [17–21]. This raises the ethical and legal question as to whether or not a pregnant patient should be told about the risk of SUDEP. A national survey in London showed that 72% of patients wished to be informed of the risk of SUDEP early on in their diagnosis [22]. Others argue that disclosing this information is not preferable, unless the patient has risk factors for SUDEP, such as a young age at onset, frequent generalized tonic–clonic seizures, intractable epilepsy, and, most importantly, medication non-compliance [23]. In such cases, it would be appropriate to disclose the patient's risk of SUDEP, and emphasize the importance of adhering to treatments and avoiding behaviors that increase seizure risk.

Clinical aspects pertaining to the management of epilepsy and prescribing of AEDs are discussed in Chap. 28.

Multiple Sclerosis

The incidence of multiple sclerosis (MS) peaks during a female's childbearing years, with a mean age of onset of 30 years. Currently, there are no unanimous guidelines that recommend for or against pregnancy in MS. However, when counseling an MS patient who is considering pregnancy, a number of issues must be taken into account. The patient should be made aware that although the activity of MS tends to decrease during pregnancy, the chances of relapse are higher after delivery, especially in the first 3 months postpartum [24, 25]. MS also appears to increase the risk of complications during gestation and in the peripartum period. For example, studies have shown a slightly increased risk of intrauterine growth restriction, as well as an increased likelihood of undergoing cesarian delivery, induction of labor, and operative interventions during delivery [13, 26]. Inversely, pregnancy in itself does not affect the long-term morbidity caused by MS [27–29]. However, patients considering in-vitro fertilization should be warned of the potential of worsening MS activity that is caused by assisted reproductive techniques [30]. In the context of breastfeeding, MS is not a contraindication, and mothers who are able to forego disease-modifying drugs can breastfeed safely [31].

The considerations for evaluation and management of MS during pregnancy are reviewed in a unique question-answer format in Chap. 21.

Headaches

Headaches are highly common in females of childbearing age, and include a wide differential diagnosis. The medicolegal concerns surrounding headaches in pregnancy are no different from those discussed previously. For instance, the failure to catch a serious diagnosis during pregnancy (e.g., pituitary apoplexy) or the prescription of a contraindicated medication (e.g., ergotamine for migraine) are two examples which can create a dangerous situation for the patient. Chapter 27 outlines the approach to headaches in pregnancy in detail, however, a few important points from a medicolegal perspective are discussed herein.

All headaches in pregnancy require careful investigation. Any headache presenting after 20 weeks gestation must be promptly evaluated for pre-eclampsia, especially in the presence of hypertension. Delays in diagnosis and treatment could precipitate seizures, which would have catastrophic consequences on the mother and fetus. Certain presentations may require consulting a neurologist or neurosurgeon, such as focal neurologic deficits or persisting headaches after the exclusion of pre-eclampsia. It is important to keep in mind that not all headaches are directly related to pregnancy. For example, clues such as the sudden onset of the headache should raise suspicion of subarachnoid hemorrhage, one of the main culprits of maternal death in hypertensive emergencies.

Migraines, another cause of headaches in pregnancy, are extremely common in women of reproductive age, reaching up to 41% in some reports [32]. Although most cases are diagnosed before pregnancy, migraines could commence during pregnancy in a minority of patients, typically during the first trimester [33]. Pregnancy tends to alleviate migraines, with up to 70% of patients reporting symptom improvement [34]. Physicians should counsel their patients about the possibility of postpartum deterioration and encourage breastfeeding, which can aid in migraine control [33, 35]. Although migraines are relatively benign compared to pre-eclampsia and SAH, the literature on the optimal pharmacotherapy during pregnancy and lactation is scarce [32]. A study of 401 pregnant/postpartum migraineurs in Norway showed that two-thirds of patients reported their migraine to be suboptimally treated, and expressed frustration regarding inconsistent information found in the patient educational materials [36]. Unfortunately, due to limited evidence, there are currently no medications that are "legally safe" for use during pregnancy and lactation [32]. This creates a pressing need for standardized guidelines on the treatment of migraines during pregnancy and lactation.

Brain Tumors

While pregnancy in itself is not a risk factor for developing brain tumors, it can affect the course of some tumors such as meningiomas, vestibular schwannomas, and certain pituitary adenomas. At the same time, management of a new or pre-existing brain tumor could impact the outcome of pregnancy. Therefore, proper patient counseling and education is key to avoiding complications and legal liability. Several important issues should be discussed during prepregnancy counseling. For example, brain tumors can often enlarge during pregnancy either due to increased peritumoral edema due to fluid retention, or hormone-mediated cellular proliferation [37, 38]. Additionally, depending on the size and location of a brain tumor, labor can be affected as well. Because intracranial CSF pressure can rise dangerously during uterine contractions and labor, the patient should be made aware of the possibility of resorting to a cesarian section with general anesthesia [39]. Medical malpractice may also occur due to failure to anticipate or diagnose a brain-tumor related complaint. A classic example is a pregnant woman presenting with headache and visual loss due to pituitary apoplexy. Thus, a high index of suspicion must be maintained, especially in patients with pre-existing pituitary adenomas, and an MRI should be obtained in any trimester to rule out this possibility.

On the other hand, gliobastoma multiforme (GBM) is rarely diagnosed in pregnant women, mainly because GBM patients are rendered infertile secondary to the chemoradiotherapy [40, 41]. However, when a GBM is discovered during pregnancy, in addition to the complex management decisions involved, an ethical dilemma ensues [42, 43]. While chemotherapy and radiation treatments are the only hope of improving maternal outcome in such a grim diagnosis, they can simultaneously be detrimental to the fetus, especially during the first trimester. The teratogenic effects are broad and can include congenital anomalies, organ dysfunction, neurocognitive impairments as well as carcinogenesis [44, 45]. Therefore, the management of these delicate cases requires a multidisciplinary team approach along with elaborate and documented discussions with the patient and family in attempt to balance the potential benefits to the mother against the risks to the fetus [45].

Chapters 32 and 33 provide detailed discussion of the clinical aspects pertaining to evaluation and management of brain and pituitary-region tumors, respectively.

Brain Death in Pregnancy

The topic of brain death in pregnancy involves multiple ethical and legal dilemmas. While determining brain death and cessation of organ support can be ethically and legally complex, the matter becomes much more challenging in the setting of pregnancy. Advances in medicine and critical care now allow a fetus to be kept viable throughout an artificially-sustained pregnancy following maternal death. This procedure of maternal somatic support is, however, an extremely rare scenario. In a study of 252 brain deaths, only 5 (2.8%) occurred during pregnancy [46]. Nevertheless, physicians must be familiar with the various medical, ethical, and legal aspects involved in managing brain death in pregnancy.

Brain death in pregnancy is most commonly caused by subarachnoid hemorrhage, hypertensive intracranial hemorrhage, and anoxic brain injury secondary to cardiac arrest [47, 48]. Delivery of a viable fetus through maternal somatic support is governed by important factors such as the gestational age at the time of brain death and the duration of maternal cardiac arrest [49, 50]. Additionally, fetal well-being may be affected by a potpourri of complications during somatic support such as hemodynamic and metabolic disturbances, acid-base imbalances, panhypopituitarism, coagulopathy, infections, and terminal cardiac rhythms, to name a few [46, 51–56].

On the same front, ethical and legal questions arise when dealing with these cases. For example, are the mother and fetus considered one or two separate entities? [48, 52] And if they are separate, whose wishes should be honored? Should the child of a dead mother be delivered and suffer physical, social, and psychological consequences later in life? [49, 51, 54, 57] In cases where the mother has an advanced directive, the decision might be clearer, however, this is rarely the case. If the mother's wishes are unknown, who is responsible for deciding the fate of the fetus? Understanding the ethical concepts involved herein is crucial in order to analyze the various factors involved in this complex decision-making process.

Various obstetric organizations have worked towards addressing some of these issues. The American College of Obstetricians and Gynecologists Ethics Committee and the International Federation of Gynecology and Obstetrics both consider the mother, not the fetus, the primary patient whose wishes take precedence over consequences to the fetus [48, 54]. In the absence of an advanced directive, the FIGO recommends the most relevant surrogate make the decision whether to continue maternal somatic support, whether it be the spouse, adult child, or other next of kin. In cases of disagreement between family members, the final verdict is delegated to court. Once the maternal wishes have been decided, the likelihood of fetal survival should be determined based on the aforementioned factors [54, 58].

Almost 60% the USA have established laws that protect the fetuses in cases of maternal injury, however, none address maternal brain death [57]. There are, however, a limited number of institutional brain-death policies address the issue of pregnancy [58]. Therefore, developing statutes that address the social and ethical challenges surrounding brain death in pregnancy is important for guiding clinical decision-making and protecting physicians against medicolegal liability.

Considerations for neurocritical care of the expectant with brain death or others forms of altered consciousness are discussed in detail in Chap. 16.

Medicolegal Issues in the Fetus and the Newborn

Hypoxic-Ischemic Encephalopathy

Hypoxic-ischemic encephalopathy (HIE) is the most common reason for medical litigation among pediatric lawsuits, with an average indemnity of $524,047 [1]. The general notion is that brain damage is caused by hypoxia during birth, which results in cerebral palsy (CP) or neurodevelopmental delay. However, lawsuits involving HIE account for some of the most complex and challenging cases in the legal arena for a multitude of reasons. First, establishing the timing and duration of asphyxia is of utmost importance. However, the ability to prove the time of occurrence of neonatal asphyxia remains elusive, and is limited by non-specific markers such as non-reassuring fetal heart activity, low scalp pH and diminished fetal movements. Indeed, the plaintiffs will try to prove that that asphyxia occurred intrapartum, while the defendant will claim that it occurred prenatally or after birth. The duration of the hypoxic insult is another critical factor. A window of 10–25 min is usually the standard in medicolegal cases [59]. In addition to the aforementioned points, even if intrapartum asphyxia did occur, the absence of studies which establish the correlation between asphyxia and CP continues to plague these scenarios. Therefore, our understanding is remains based on observational [60–66] and animal studies [67, 68]. This is mainly due to the unfeasibility of performing studies on human fetuses. Moreover, the advent of therapeutic hypothermia for neuroprotection following HIE has opened the door for more lawsuit cases, such as claiming delayed initiation of hypothermic therapy [69].

As such, a number of practices can be adopted to help mitigate malpractice litigation in these cases [1]. The newborn's status at birth should be documented in detail, including the degree of neonatal depression, muscular tone, reflexes, and the need for resuscitation. Recording the infant's umbilical cord gases and the presence of microcephaly can also be supportive. A joint task force between the American Academy of Pediatrics and the American College of Obstetricians and Gynecologists developed a checklist that aids in establishing a rational link between an intrapartum asphyxia and the resultant neurologic injury [70]. Furthermore, it is important that physicians be aware of the facility's lack of hypothermic capabilities, and if needed, coordinate with centers that could provide this therapy in a timely manner.

Imaging evaluation of neonatal hypoxic ischemic injury may be achieved through both intracranial ultrasound and MRI, both of which can assist physicians in determining the onset of the initial injury as well as predicting overall prognosis. Neonatal ultrasound is often the initial imaging study such situations due to its portability, low cost, and ability to easily be repeated, thus making it the practical first line choice for fragile neonates being monitored in intensive care settings [71–73]. The delay of approximately 24–48 h between the injury itself and the appearance of detectable brain edema on ultrasound is one means by which physicians can attempt to time the initial injury [71, 73–76]. Some studies have even extended this time frame, suggesting that it may take up to 72 h for findings of HII to become apparent on ultrasound [76]. Thus most sources recommend obtaining an initial neonatal ultrasound within 24 h of birth, as this maximizes the ability to differentiate between hypoxic ischemic injuries that occurred in the prenatal period and those that occurred during the birth itself. For instance, positive findings on an ultrasound obtained at 12 h suggest that the injury occurred at least 24 h prior, and thus in utero rather than during the birth process.

However, ultrasound can be limited a comparatively low sensitivity for subtle findings of hypoxic ischemic injury as well as inter-operator variability [77, 78]. Magnetic resonance imaging represents the most sensitive imaging modality for evaluating hypoxic ischemic injury, and is thus the gold standard in this setting [71, 73, 79]. It is also another means by which physicians can attempt to differentiate between prepartum and intrapartum injuries—specifically, by evaluating findings on conventional T1/T2 MRI sequences and diffusion weighted imaging. It is important to keep in mind that for this technique to be effective, MRI must be obtained after 24 h but within the first week of life. Specifically, the American College of Obstetricians and Gynecologists recommends an initial MRI for the purposes of timing the injury within the first 24–96 h of life, with a second MRI obtained later on at 7–21 days for purely prognostic purposes [80]. Some sources recommend obtaining an MRI at 3–5 days if only one MRI is to be performed, as this timeframe provides the best opportunity to obtain both timing and prognostic data in a single study [78, 81]. Despite this, many physicians choose to delay performing an initial MRI until after the first week, possibly due to a reluctance to transport such fragile neonates outside the strictly controlled environment of the intensive care unit. Nevertheless, this hesitancy should be weighed again the fact that delaying MRI may result in a loss of valuable diagnostic information, which can have important legal implications in the setting of a lawsuit. While some hospitals have begun implementing MRI machines in their neonatal ICU units, the practice has yet to become widespread [71].

Prognostic evaluation through both ultrasound and MRI is predicated on the fact that the brain preferably shunts oxygenated blood to highly metabolic deep brain structures when confronted with hypoxic ischemic injury, at the expense of more peripheral watershed zones [77, 78]. In severe hypoxic ischemic injury, these protective mechanisms are overcome, and deep brain structures are unable to escape being damaged. Multiple studies have demonstrated that imaging patterns with involvement of these deep brain structures (including the basal nuclei, thalami, and brainstem) indicate that a more severe hypoxic ischemic injury has occurred, and patients with such imaging patterns invariably demonstrate a poorer outcome [72, 75, 77, 80, 82–87].

Cerebral Palsy

Cerebral palsy (CP) is one of the most common reasons behind obstetrician malpractice litigation in the USA, and 60% of obstetric malpractice insurance premiums are dedicated to CP allegations [88, 89]. A diagnosis of CP puts a significant emotional and financial burden on the family and child. It has been estimated that the lifetime care of a patient with CP in 2003 cost $921,000 (approximately $1.2 million after adjustment for inflation) [90], which is one of the main motives behind seeking malpractice lawsuits. Typically, the plaintiff would attempt to prove, through expert testimonials, that the brain injury was caused by intrapartum asphyxia, and would have been prevented by timely cesarian delivery. However, that school of thought was replaced by studies showing that lack of oxygen during delivery causes only a minority of CP cases [91–94] and that prematurity, low birth weight, fetal stroke, and intrauterine infections are more important risk factors [95, 96]. Furthermore, none of these factors have a causal relationship with CP, rendering the etiology of CP in most legal cases undetermined. In addition, no evidence currently exists that immediate delivery upon discovering any of the aforementioned stressors does, in fact, prevent or ameliorate CP [96–99]. While less than 10% of plaintiffs are awarded compensation, the process of malpractice litigation is extremely stressful and cumbersome, and the constant fear of litigation has driven many obstetricians to restrict their practice to gynecology or even leave the field [100], jeopardizing access to obstetrical care [101].

A number of solutions can help solve the problem of CP litigation. In the article *"Who Will Deliver Our Grandchildren? Implications of Cerebral Palsy Litigation"* McLennan et al. outline a number of proposed solutions including hospital self-policing, establishment of special health courts and no-fault compensation systems, and increasing public awareness [99].

Spina Bifida

Spina bifida (SB) is a neural tube defect that occurs due to failure of neural tube closure by 28 days of gestation. It can take one of three forms. Spina bifida occulta, the most common type, involves a defect within the vertebral bodies without exposure of neural tissue underlying intact skin. Hydrocephalus and hindbrain malformation are usually absent, and neurological symptoms minimal. On the other hand, the bony defect in spina bifida aperta is accompanied by herniation of the meninges (meningocele) or the meninges and spinal cord (myelomeningocele). Myelomeningocele is the most common neural tube defect. Depending on the level of the lesion, patients usually suffer motor and sensory deficits as severe as complete paralysis and urinary and fecal incontinence. Chiari II malformation is a classic association, accompanied with varying degrees of hydrocephalus [102]. Importantly, studies have shown that the neurological deficits associated with spina bifida worsen throughout pregnancy [103, 104]. The "two-hit" hypothesis posits that the worsening neurological symptoms are a result of the neural tube defect itself combined with the neurotoxic effect of the amniotic fluid in utero [102, 105–107]. Fortunately, maternal fetal surgery (MFS) which has been practiced for the past two decades has offered hope to these patients and their families [108]. Results from the 2011 MOMS trial showed that earlier repair of the spina bifida carries better outcomes than postnatal repair [109].

The diagnosis of spina bifida carries significant psychological and social distress to the family, and more so to the child later in life. A myriad of medicolegal and ethical issues arise when dealing with such cases. For example, missing an antenatal diagnosis of spina bifida may cause the family to seek claims. In rare cases, children born with developmental disabilities due to missed prenatal diagnoses that could have been otherwise aborted, can sue the physician for a "wrongful life." Such legal cases have been honored in countries like the USA, France, and the Netherlands [110]. The notion of the fetus being a "potential person" independent from its mother is a topic of ongoing legal and philosophical debate to this day. Although parents cannot refuse treatment for a child, the mother in this instance cannot be forced to receive treatment to her fetus [111]. Furthermore, open MFS carries considerable maternal morbidity even in healthy mothers. The procedure poses risks not only during sur-

gery, but can jeopardize the course of the current and possibly future pregnancies as well. Due the complex nature that the decision-making process entails in these situations, it is extremely important to conduct thorough, in-depth counseling with the family in a non-directive manner. This should be done by a multidisciplinary specialty team of obstetricians, pediatric neurologists, neurosurgeons, psychologists and physiotherapists who are experienced in the field of spina bifida [110, 112]. Counselling should cover detailed discussions of the natural history of the condition, management options such as open fetal surgery or termination of pregnancy, and the risks of the maternal fetal surgery.

The success of fetal and early postnatal care for patients with spina bifida has increased the number of individuals with these conditions seeking to become pregnant. This presents a unique clinical scenario which is discussed in detail in Chap. 35.

Conclusion

The presence of a neurological disorder or injury during pregnancy presents a precarious situation in which treating obstetricians, neurosurgeons, neurologists, and other providers must carefully balance maternal and fetal well-being. The potential for ethical or legal concerns to arise is extremely high in these scenarios owing to the profound morbidity and mortality of neurological ailments and the desire for delivery of a healthy newborn. Multidisciplinary collaboration, detailed communication with the patient and their family, and consultation with institutional ethics boards are imperative to promoting positive outcomes and mitigating the risk of litigation.

References

1. Donn SM, Chiswick ML, Fanaroff JM. Medico-legal implications of hypoxic–ischemic birth injury. In: Seminars in Fetal and Neonatal Medicine. Amsterdam: Elsevier; 2014.

2. Chandra A, Nundy S, Seabury SA. The growth of physician medical malpractice payments: evidence from the national practitioner data bank: the growth of malpractice payments is less than previously thought. Health Aff. 2005;24(Suppl 1):W5-240–9.

3. Sandra Levy LK. Medscape Ob/Gyn malpractice report 2017: real physicians. Real Lawsuits. 2017. https://www.medscape.com/slideshow/2017-obgyn-malpractice-report-6009316#2.

4. Jena AB, et al. Malpractice risk according to physician specialty. N Engl J Med. 2011;365(7):629–36.

5. Martin KL. Medscape neurologist malpractice report 2019. Medscape. 2019. https://www.medscape.com/slideshow/2019-malpractice-report-neuro-6012448#2.

6. Smith TR, et al. Defensive medicine in neurosurgery: does state-level liability risk matter? Neurosurgery. 2015;76(2):105–14.

7. Studdert DM, et al. Claims, errors, and compensation payments in medical malpractice litigation. N Engl J Med. 2006;354(19):2024–33.

8. Finucane AK. Legal issues in neurology and pregnancy: the physician's duty of care. Neurol Clin. 1994;12(3):637–53.

9. Blake V. When is a patient-physician relationship established? Virtual Mentor. 2012;14(5):403–6. https://doi.org/10.1001/virtualmentor.2012.14.5.hlaw1-1205.

10. Mead v Adler. 231 Or App 451, 220 P3d 118 (Or 2009). 2009.

11. Kass JS. Epilepsy and pregnancy: a practical approach to mitigating legal risk. Continuum. 2014;20(1):181–5.

12. Hickson GB, et al. Factors that prompted families to file medical malpractice claims following perinatal injuries. JAMA. 1992;267(10):1359–63.

13. Kelly VM, Nelson LM, Chakravarty EF. Obstetric outcomes in women with multiple sclerosis and epilepsy. Obstet Gynecol Surv. 2010;65(3):156–8.

14. Brennan TA, et al. Incidence of adverse events and negligence in hospitalized patients: results of the Harvard Medical Practice Study I. N Engl J Med. 1991;324(6):370–6.

15. Harden C, et al. Practice parameter update: management issues for women with epilepsy—focus on pregnancy (an evidence-based review): vitamin K, folic acid, blood levels, and breastfeeding: report of the Quality Standards Subcommittee and Therapeutics and Technology Assessment Subcommittee of the American Academy of Neurology and American Epilepsy Society. Neurology. 2009;73(2):142–9.

16. Dworetzky BA, et al. A clinically oriented perspective on psychogenic nonepileptic seizure–related emergencies. Clin EEG Neurosci. 2015;46(1):26–33.

17. Mu J, et al. Causes of death among people with convulsive epilepsy in rural West China: a prospective study. Neurology. 2011;77(2):132–7.

18. Hughes JR. A review of sudden unexpected death in epilepsy: prediction of patients at risk. Epilepsy Behav. 2009;14(2):280–7.

19. Ficker DM. Sudden unexplained death and injury in epilepsy. Epilepsia. 2000;41:S7–S12.

20. Mohanraj R, et al. Mortality in adults with newly diagnosed and chronic epilepsy: a retrospective comparative study. Lancet Neurol. 2006;5(6):481–7.

21. Walczak TS, et al. Incidence and risk factors in sudden unexpected death in epilepsy: a prospective cohort study. Neurology. 2001;56(4):519–25.

22. Keddie S, et al. Discussing sudden unexpected death in epilepsy: are we empowering our patients? A questionnaire survey. JRSM Open. 2016;7(9):2054270416654358.

23. Brodie MJ, Holmes GL. Should all patients be told about sudden unexpected death in epilepsy (SUDEP)? Pros and Cons. Epilepsia. 2008;49:99–101.

24. Finkelsztejn A, et al. What can we really tell women with multiple sclerosis regarding pregnancy? A systematic review and meta-analysis of the literature. BJOG Int J Obstet Gynaecol. 2011;118(7):790–7.

25. Confavreux C, et al. Rate of pregnancy-related relapse in multiple sclerosis. N Engl J Med. 1998;339(5):285–91.

26. Dahl J, et al. Pregnancy, delivery, and birth outcome in women with multiple sclerosis. Neurology. 2005;65(12):1961–3.

27. Runmarker B, Andersen O. Pregnancy is associated with a lower risk of onset and a better prognosis in multiple sclerosis. Brain. 1995;118(1):253–61.

28. Ramagopalan S, et al. Term pregnancies and the clinical characteristics of multiple sclerosis: a population based study. J Neurol Neurosurg Psychiatry. 2012;83(8):793–5.

29. Verdru P, et al. Pregnancy and multiple sclerosis: the influence on long term disability. Clin Neurol Neurosurg. 1994;96(1):38–41.

30. Voskuhl RR. Assisted reproduction technology in multiple sclerosis: giving birth to a new avenue of research in hormones and autoimmunity. Ann Neurol. 2012;72(5):631.

31. Kieseier BC, Wiendl H. Postpartum disease activity and breastfeeding in multiple sclerosis revisited. Neurology. 2010;75(5):392–3.

32. Calhoun AH. Migraine treatment in pregnancy and lactation. Curr Pain Headache Rep. 2017;21(11):46.

33. Sances G, et al. Course of migraine during pregnancy and postpartum: a prospective study. Cephalalgia. 2003;23(3):197–205.

34. MacGregor EA. Headache in pregnancy. Neurol Clin. 2012;30(3):835–66.

35. Wall VR. Breastfeeding and migraine headaches. J Hum Lact. 1992;8(4):209–12.

36. Amundsen S, et al. Use of antimigraine medications and information needs during pregnancy and breastfeeding: a cross-sectional study among 401 Norwegian women. Eur J Clin Pharmacol. 2016;72(12):1525–35.

37. Carroll RS, Zhang J, Black PM. Expression of estrogen receptors alpha and beta in human meningiomas. J Neuro-Oncol. 1999;42(2):109–16.

38. Michelsen JJ, New P. Brain tumour and pregnancy. J Neurol Neurosurg Psychiatry. 1969;32(4):305.
39. Ng J, Kitchen N. Neurosurgery and pregnancy. J Neurol Neurosurg Psychiatry. 2008;79(7):745–52.
40. Preusser M, et al. Pilot study on sex hormone levels and fertility in women with malignant gliomas. J Neuro-Oncol. 2012;107(2):387–94.
41. McGrane J, Bedford T, Kelly S. Successful pregnancy and delivery after concomitant temozolomide and radiotherapy treatment of glioblastoma multiforme. Clin Oncol. 2012;24(4):311.
42. Policicchio D, et al. Ethical and therapeutic dilemmas in glioblastoma management during pregnancy: two case reports and review of the literature. Surg Neurol Int. 2019;10:41.
43. Al-Rasheedy IM, Al-Hameed FM. Advanced case of glioblastoma multiforme and pregnancy: an ethical dilemma. Neurosciences. 2015;20(4):388.
44. Lew PS, et al. Dilemmas in management of brain tumours in pregnancy. Annal Acad Med. 2010;39(1):64–5.
45. Jayasekera BA, Bacon AD, Whitfield PC. Management of glioblastoma multiforme in pregnancy: a review. J Neurosurg. 2012;116(6):1187–94.
46. Suddaby EC, et al. Analysis of organ donors in the peripartum period. J Transpl Coord. 1998;8(1):35–9.
47. FIoGa, O. Ethical issues in obstetrics and gynecology by the FIGO Committee for the Study of Ethical Aspects of Human Reproduction and Women's Health. London: FIGO; 2012.
48. Burkle CM, Tessmer-Tuck J, Wijdicks EF. Medical, legal, and ethical challenges associated with pregnancy and catastrophic brain injury. Int J Gynecol Obstet. 2015;129(3):276–80.
49. Ramsay G, Paglia M, Bourjeily G. When the heart stops: a review of cardiac arrest in pregnancy. J Intensive Care Med. 2013;28(4):204–14.
50. Soar J, et al. European Resuscitation Council guidelines for resuscitation 2005: Section 7. Cardiac arrest in special circumstances. Resuscitation. 2005;67:S135–70.
51. Farragher RA, Laffey JG. Maternal brain death and somatic support. Neurocrit Care. 2005;3(2):99–106.
52. Esmaeilzadeh M, et al. One life ends, another begins: management of a brain-dead pregnant mother-a systematic review. BMC Med. 2010;8(1):74.
53. Fadel HE. Postmortem and perimortem cesarean section: historical, religious and ethical considerations. J IMA. 2011;43(3):194.
54. Dickens B. Brain death and pregnancy: FIGO Committee for the Ethical Aspects of Human Reproduction and Women's Health. Int J Gynecol Obstet. 2011;115(1):84–5.
55. Wawrzyniak J. Continuation of pregnancy in a woman with critical brain injury. Anaesthesiol Intens Ther. 2015;47(1):40–4.
56. Powner DJ, Bernstein IM. Extended somatic support for pregnant women after brain death. Crit Care Med. 2003;31(4):1241–9.
57. Gostin LO. Legal and ethical responsibilities following brain death: the McMath and Muñoz cases. JAMA. 2014;311(9):903–4.
58. Lewis A. Contentious ethical and legal aspects of determination of brain death. In: Seminars in neurology. Stuttgart: Thieme Medical Publishers; 2018.
59. Baxter P. Markers of perinatal hypoxia–ischaemia and neurological injury: assessing the impact of insult duration. Dev Med Child Neurol. 2020;62(5):563–8.
60. Kodama Y, et al. Intrapartum fetal heart rate patterns preceding terminal bradycardia in infants (> 34 weeks) with poor neurological outcome: a regional population-based study in Japan. J Obstet Gynaecol Res. 2015;41(11):1738–43.
61. Kayani SI, Walkinshaw SA, Preston C. Pregnancy outcome in severe placental abruption. BJOG Int J Obstet Gynaecol. 2003;110(7):679–83.
62. Katz VL, Dotters DJ, Droegemueller W. Perimortem cesarean delivery. Obstet Gynecol. 1986;68(4):571–6.
63. Rutherford M, et al. Athetoid cerebral palsy with cysts in the putamen after hypoxic-ischaemic encephalopathy. Arch Dis Child. 1992;67(7 Spec No):846–50.
64. Thomson AJ, Searle M, Russell G. Quality of survival after severe birth asphyxia. Arch Dis Child. 1977;52(8):620–6.
65. Murray DM, et al. Fetal heart rate patterns in neonatal hypoxic-ischemic encephalopathy: relationship with early cerebral activity and neurodevelopmental outcome. Am J Perinatol. 2009;26(8):605–12.
66. Barkovich AJ. MR and CT evaluation of profound neonatal and infantile asphyxia. Am J Neuroradiol. 1992;13(3):959–72.
67. Inder TE, Volpe JJ. Hypoxic-ischemic injury in the term infant: clinical-neurological features, diagnosis, imaging, prognosis, therapy. In: Volpe's Neurology of the Newborn. Amsterdam: Elsevier; 2018. p. 510–563.e15.
68. McAdams RM, et al. Long-term neuropathological changes associated with cerebral palsy in a nonhuman primate model of hypoxic-ischemic encephalopathy. Dev Neurosci. 2017;39(1–4):124–40.
69. Shankaran S, et al. Whole-body hypothermia for neonates with hypoxic–ischemic encephalopathy. N Engl J Med. 2005;353(15):1574–84.
70. Obstetricians, A.C.o., Gynecologists, and A.A.o. Pediatrics. Neonatal encephalopathy and neurologic outcome. Itasca, IL: American Academy of Pediatrics; 2014.
71. Hwang M. Gray-scale ultrasound findings of hypoxic-ischemic injury in term infants. Pediatr Radiol. 2021;51(9):1738–47.
72. Rutherford MA. The asphyxiated term infant. In: MRI of the neonatal brain. Philadelphia, PA: W.B. Saunders; 2022.
73. Thakkar H, Sanone S, Khodke R. Transcranial ultrasound in evaluation of hypoxic-ischemic encephalopathy and bleed in preterm neonates. Int J Sci Stud. 2019;7(4):27–38.

74. Salas J, et al. Head ultrasound in neonatal hypoxic-ischemic injury and its mimickers for clinicians: a review of the patterns of injury and the evolution of findings over time. Neonatology. 2018;114(3):185–97.

75. de Vries LS, Groenendaal F. Patterns of neonatal hypoxic-ischaemic brain injury. Neuroradiology. 2010;52(6):555–66.

76. Annink KV, et al. The development and validation of a cerebral ultrasound scoring system for infants with hypoxic-ischaemic encephalopathy. Pediatr Res. 2020;87(Suppl 1):59–66.

77. Huang BY, Castillo M. Hypoxic-ischemic brain injury: imaging findings from birth to adulthood. Radiographics. 2008;28(2):417–39; quiz 617.

78. Ghei SK, et al. MR imaging of hypoxic-ischemic injury in term neonates: pearls and pitfalls. Radiographics. 2014;34(4):1047–61.

79. Rana L, et al. MR imaging of hypoxic ischemic encephalopathy - distribution patterns and ADC value correlations. Eur J Radiol Open. 2018;5:215–20.

80. Executive summary: Neonatal encephalopathy and neurologic outcome, second edition. Report of the American College of Obstetricians and Gynecologists' Task Force on Neonatal Encephalopathy. Obstet Gynecol. 2014;123(4):896–901.

81. Fineschi V, et al. A controversial medicolegal issue: timing the onset of perinatal hypoxic-ischemic brain injury. Mediat Inflamm. 2017;2017:6024959.

82. Chao CP, Zaleski CG, Patton AC. Neonatal hypoxic-ischemic encephalopathy: multimodality imaging findings. Radiographics. 2006;26(Suppl 1):S159–72.

83. Heinz ER, Provenzale JM. Imaging findings in neonatal hypoxia: a practical review. AJR Am J Roentgenol. 2009;192(1):41–7.

84. Bano S, Chaudhary V, Garga UC. Neonatal hypoxic-ischemic encephalopathy: a radiological review. J Pediatr Neurosci. 2017;12(1):1–6.

85. Martinez-Biarge M, et al. Predicting motor outcome and death in term hypoxic-ischemic encephalopathy. Neurology. 2011;76(24):2055–61.

86. Martinez-Biarge M, et al. Outcomes after central grey matter injury in term perinatal hypoxic-ischaemic encephalopathy. Early Hum Dev. 2010;86(11):675–82.

87. Rutherford M, et al. Assessment of brain tissue injury after moderate hypothermia in neonates with hypoxic-ischaemic encephalopathy: a nested substudy of a randomised controlled trial. Lancet Neurol. 2010;9(1):39–45.

88. Obstetricians, A.C.o. and Gynecologists. Survey on professional liability. Washington, DC: ACOG; 2003.

89. Freeman J, Freeman A. No-fault birth-related neurologic injury compensation: perhaps its time has come, again. In: Harv Risk Manage Found Forum. 2003.

90. Honeycutt AA et al. Economic costs of mental retardation, cerebral palsy, hearing loss, and vision impairment. Using survey data to study disability: results from the National Health Interview Survey on Disability. 2003;3:207–28.

91. Ellenberg JH, Nelson KB. The association of cerebral palsy with birth asphyxia: a definitional quagmire. Dev Med Child Neurol. 2013;55(3):210–6.

92. Hankins GD, Speer M. Defining the pathogenesis and pathophysiology of neonatal encephalopathy and cerebral palsy. Obstet Gynecol. 2003;102(3):628–36.

93. Nelson KB. What proportion of cerebral palsy is related to birth asphyxia? J Pediatr. 1988;112(4):572–4.

94. Perlman JM. Intrapartum hypoxic-ischemic cerebral injury and subsequent cerebral palsy: medicolegal issues. Pediatrics. 1997;99(6):851–9.

95. Drougia A, et al. Incidence and risk factors for cerebral palsy in infants with perinatal problems: a 15-year review. Early Hum Dev. 2007;83(8):541–7.

96. Kuban KCK, Leviton A. Cerebral palsy. N Engl J Med. 1994;330(3):188–95.

97. Gibbs RS. Management of clinical chorioamnionitis at term. Am J Obstet Gynecol. 2004;191(1):1–2.

98. Nelson KB. Can we prevent cerebral palsy? Waltham, MA: Massachusetts Medical Society; 2003.

99. MacLennan A, et al. Who will deliver our grandchildren?: implications of cerebral palsy litigation. JAMA. 2005;294(13):1688–90.

100. MacLennan AH, Spencer MK. Projections of Australian obstetricians ceasing practice and the reasons. Med J Aust. 2002;176(9):425–8.

101. Robinson P, et al. The impact of medical legal risk on obstetrician–gynecologist supply. Obstet Gynecol. 2005;105(6):1296–302.

102. Copp AJ, et al. Spina bifida. Nat Rev Dis Prim. 2015;1(1):1–18.

103. Meuli M, et al. Creation of myelomeningocele in utero: a model of functional damage from spinal cord exposure in fetal sheep. J Pediatr Surg. 1995;30(7):1028–33.

104. Sival D, et al. Perinatal motor behaviour and neurological outcome in Spina bifida aperta. Early Hum Dev. 1997;50(1):27–37.

105. McLone DG, Dias MS. The Chiari II malformation: cause and impact. Childs Nerv Syst. 2003;19(7–8):540–50.

106. Joyeux L, et al. Fetoscopic versus open repair for spina bifida aperta: a systematic review of outcomes. Fetal Diagn Ther. 2016;39(3):161–71.

107. Heffez DS, et al. The paralysis associated with myelomeningocele: clinical and experimental

data implicating a preventable spinal cord injury. Neurosurgery. 1990;26(6):987–92.

108. Sutton LN, Sun P, Adzick NS. Fetal neurosurgery. Neurosurgery. 2001;48(1):124–44.

109. Adzick NS, et al. A randomized trial of prenatal versus postnatal repair of myelomeningocele. N Engl J Med. 2011;364(11):993–1004.

110. Van Calenbergh F, Joyeux L, Deprest J. Maternal-fetal surgery for myelomeningocele: some thoughts on ethical, legal, and psychological issues in a Western European situation. Childs Nerv Syst. 2017;33(8):1247–52.

111. Deprest J, et al. The fetal patient–ethical aspects of fetal therapy. Facts Views Vis ObGyn. 2011;3(3):221.

112. Sacco A, et al. Fetal surgery for open spina bifida. Obstetr Gynaecol. 2019;21(4):271.

Cardiovascular and Cerebrovascular Changes During Pregnancy

5

Manan Shah and Kiwon Lee

Introduction

Pregnancy is a dynamic process associated with significant physiologic, and mostly reversible, changes in the cardiovascular and cerebrovascular systems. The maternal cardiovascular system has to adapt to growing demands of both maternal and dynamic fetal circulations. Failure to meet these hemodynamic changes can result in maternal and fetal morbidity, as seen in pre-eclampsia and intrauterine growth restriction. The adaptation of cerebral circulation in pregnancy is unique from other vascular beds because of the need for a constant blood supply and the relative intolerance to increase in blood volume. Compared with other organs, we have a limited understanding of the adaptation of the cerebral circulation to pregnancy and the underlying mechanisms that drive it. While the adaptation of the cerebral circulation to pregnancy provides for relatively normal cerebral blood flow and blood–brain barrier (BBB) properties in the face of substantial cardiovascular changes and high levels of circulating factors, under pathologic conditions, these adaptations appear to promote greater brain injury, including edema formation during acute hypertension, and greater sensitivity to bacterial endotoxin [1]. This chapter aims to shed light on the critical maternal cardiovascular and cerebrovascular adaptations during different stages of pregnancy. The sound understanding of these physiologic adaptations will also provide insight into the unified pathogenesis behind several cerebrovascular complications of pregnancy, discussed later in the chapter.

Cardiovascular Changes

The goal of the cardiovascular changes that occur during pregnancy is to provide adequate utero-placental perfusion for fetal development without compromising maternal function. These changes are the result of complex interplay between the nervous system, circulating humoral factors, and functional and structural alterations that occur in the heart and the vascular tissue. The cardiovascular adaptations in pregnancy begin early, persist postpartum, and appear to be enhanced by a subsequent pregnancy [2].

The major hemodynamic changes during pregnancy are outlined in Table 5.1. These changes begin as early as 4–5 weeks of gestation and tend to plateau during the end of the second or early third trimesters [3]. Major hemodynamic

M. Shah (✉)
Department of Neurology, Medical College of Georgia at Augusta University, Augusta, GA, USA
e-mail: mashah1@augusta.edu

K. Lee
Department of Neurology, Rutgers, The State University of New Jersey, Robert Wood Johnson Medical School, New Brunswick, NJ, USA
e-mail: kiwon.lee@rutgers.edu

Table 5.1 Cardiovascular changes during pregnancy

Parameter	Adaptation	Peak effect	Time of peak adaptation	Comment
Blood pressure	↓	(−)10 mm	24 weeks	↓↓DBP > ↓SBP
SVR	↓↓	(−)20–30%	16–20 weeks	–
Blood volume	↑↑↑↑	(+)40–60%	28–34 weeks	Affected by RAAS activation, circulating pregnancy hormones
Plasma volume	↑↑↑↑	(+)40–60%	28–34 weeks	–
RBC volume	↑↑	(+)20–30%	Term	↑ Erythropoietin production, physiologic anemia of pregnancy
Cardiac output	↑↑↑↑↑	(+)50%	24 weeks	Altered by maternal positioning during third trimester, ↑ during labor and immediate postpartum due to autotransfusion
Stroke volume	↑↑	(+)25–30%	16–24 weeks	↑ Preload
Heart rate	↑↑	(+)10–20 beats/min	32 weeks	–
Ventricular mass	↑↑↑↑		Term	–
Left		(+)52%,		
Right		(+)40%		
Contractility	↔	–	–	↔ejection fraction

DBP diastolic blood pressure, *RAAS* Renin-Angiotensin-Aldosterone system, *SBP* systolic blood pressure, *SVR* systemic vascular resistance. ↑/(+) suggests relative increase, ↓/(−) suggests relative decrease and ↔ suggests no change in parameters from their pre-pregnancy values

changes include changes in blood pressure (BP), systemic vascular resistance (SVR), total blood volume (TBV), plasma volume, red blood cell (RBC) volume, cardiac output (CO), stroke volume (SV), heart rate (HR), and cardiac contractility.

Blood Pressure

Arterial pressures reach a nadir during the second trimester with the average mean arterial pressure (MAP) drop being about 10 mmHg, the majority of which occurs early in pregnancy (6–8 weeks of gestational age) [4]. In general, diastolic blood pressure (DBP) and MAP decline more than systolic blood pressure (SBP) during pregnancy. The reduction in blood pressure is thought to be related to the vasodilatory effect of nitric oxide (NO) as well as hormonal and other factors such as prostacyclin and relaxin that mediate a decrease in peripheral vascular resistance [5].

Arterial pressures start to increase during third trimester and return close to pre-pregnancy values during the postpartum period. Although the majority of studies have reported similar changes in BP during pregnancy, some have instead reported increase in blood pressure throughout gestation [6].

Systemic Vascular Resistance

The reduction in SVR begins as early as 5 weeks of gestation and reaches a nadir by the middle of the second trimester (16–20 weeks) with subsequent plateau or slight increase for the remainder of pregnancy [7]. There is about 20–30% reduction in SVR from baseline. The SVR increases significantly postpartum, however, it may not return to its pre-pregnancy value until 1-year postpartum [2]. The decreased vascular resistance is due to softening of collagen fibers and hypertrophy of smooth muscle, systemic vasodilatation due to circulating progesterone and prostaglandins, and the addition of low-resistance utero-placental circulation [3, 5, 8].

Total Blood Volume, Plasma Volume, and Red Blood Cell Volume

Total blood volume (TBV) is a combination of plasma volume and RBC volume. All three parameters undergo significant increase during pregnancy [9, 10]. The increase in circulating TBV begins by 6 weeks of gestation, increases rapidly by mid-pregnancy and then rises more slowly during the later half. Peak TBV is approached between 28 and 34 weeks, following which it plateaus or decreases slightly to term. Plasma volume contributes to about 75% of total blood volume. The increase in plasma volume parallels that of TBV with both increasing by 40–60% of their respective nonpregnancy values [5, 8].

Both blood and plasma volume changes are influenced by circulating hormone effects, NO mediated vasodilatation, mechanical factors (blood flow in utero-placental vessels) and changes in the renal system leading to alterations in fluid and electrolyte homeostasis. In a normal pregnancy, there is substantial activation of the renin-angiotensin-aldosterone system (RAAS). The enhanced activity of RAAS occurs early in pregnancy, with increases in plasma volume starting at 6–8 weeks and rising progressively until 28–30 weeks. This activation maintains blood pressure and helps retain salt and water throughout gestation [11]. Furthermore, during pregnancy, relaxin stimulates increased vasopressin secretion and thirst, resulting in enhanced water retention. Despite the increase in exchangeable sodium, overall plasma osmolality is reduced and the hyponatremic hypervolemia of pregnancy ensues [12].

Red blood cell production and thus volume increases throughout pregnancy to a level that is 20–30% higher than nonpregnant values. The change in RBC volume is mediated by increased production of maternal erythropoietin, which itself is stimulated by circulating progesterone,

prolactin and placental lactogen [13]. The expansion of plasma volume, however, outpaces RBC volume expansion, causing hemodilution and resultant physiologic anemia of pregnancy with hemoglobin values as low as 11 g/dl [7].

Cardiac Output, Stroke Volume, and Heart Rate

Changes in HR and SV are reported as early as 5 and 8 weeks of gestation, respectively. SV reaches its peak value of 25–30% above prepregnant values by 16–24 weeks of gestation [5, 14]. SV subsequently declines during the third trimester and returns to the prepregnant range at term. The changes in SV are likely due to increased ventricular muscle mass and end-diastolic volume changes. Unlike other cardiovascular parameters, HR increases progressively throughout the pregnancy by 10–20 beats per minute, reaching a maximum in the third trimester at around 32 weeks of gestation [4, 7]. HR becomes a dominant factor in determining cardiac output during the later half of pregnancy.

CO, the product of SV and HR, is one of the most significant cardiovascular changes encountered during pregnancy. CO measurements are typically made with the mother in the left lateral decubitus position to avoid positional variation. CO is significantly increased during the first trimester, with 125% of the pre-pregnancy values occurring by 8 weeks of gestation. It peaks to about 50% above the pre-pregnancy values by 24 weeks of gestation [2, 15]. The third trimester has been associated with significant discrepancies in the pattern of CO adaptation, with either a continual increase, decrease or plateau within the final weeks of gestation [16]. A recent large meta-analysis in 2016 distilled this data and showed that peak CO is achieved in the early third trimester, followed by a decrease towards term. One explanation for this pattern could be that compression of the inferior vena cava (IVC) as a result of considerable and progressive fetal growth occurring during the third trimester negatively affects venous return. In addition, blood flow to the utero-placental circulation is at its peak (approximately 12% of total CO) during the late third trimester in order to meet fetal metabolic demands [17, 18]. Both factors could contribute to a reduced cardiac preload and, therefore, a drop in CO during the late third trimester [19]. Change in maternal body position (especially in the third trimester) causes marked fluctuation in CO, with a 25–30% drop noted after a change from the left lateral decubitus to supine positioning. This drop is due to marked compression of the IVC by the gravid third trimester uterus, which causes a decrease in venous return, SV, and thus CO. A progressive rise in CO is seen during the intrapartum period, peaking to 50% above pregnancy values during the second stage of labor. This increase in CO is caused by increases in both HR and SV, contributed to by (1) sympthathetic stimulation induced by pain and exertion, (2) uterine contraction causing enhanced venous return, and (3) increased circulating blood volume. Overall, CO increases approximately 60–80% above prelabor values immediately after delivery, caused by relieved IVC compression and autotransfusion (of up to 500 ml blood) from the utero-placental circulation during placental separation. Cardiac output remains elevated for at least 48 h postpartum and gradually decreases to nonpregnant values by 6–12 weeks in the majority of women [5, 20].

Cardiac Remodeling and Contractility

During pregnancy, TBV expansion leads to an increase in ventricular preload and compensatory structural changes in the left ventricle (LV). Left ventricular wall thickness and wall mass increase by up to 28% and 52% of nonpregnant values, throughout the pregnancy, respectively [21]. Similarly, right ventricular (RV) mass seems to increase by 40% of nonpregnant values as measured by newer cardiac magnetic resonance imaging (MRI) techniques [22]. Progesterone has been shown to increase protein synthesis in cardiac muscle and can cause cardiomyocyte hypertrophy [23]. Physiologic hypertrophy of the ventricle is supported by coronary angiogenesis which is driven by placenta-derived vascular

endothelial growth factor (VEGF) [24]. Interestingly, in spite of the significant alteration in multiple cardiovascular parameters, myocardial contractility and LV/RV ejection fractions do not seem to change during pregnancy [22].

Overall, the cardiovascular adaptations during pregnancy begin early, peak by the end of the second trimester and persist through the puerperium. Notably, these adaptations appear to be enhanced during subsequent pregnancies, suggesting the possibility of sustained improved compliance of the cardiovascular system from pregnancy [2]. It remains to be seen if this alteration in compliance has any long-term beneficial effects on the cardiovascular health of multiparous women.

Cerebrovascular Changes

The cerebrovascular changes during pregnancy are unique among all of the systemic hemodynamic changes associated with this period. The brain has a relatively narrow capacity to tolerate changes in ion and water balance, and blood flow [25]. Being enclosed in the rigid container that is the skull, the brain is intolerant of any significant volume change. Therefore, any increase in vascular permeability or volume could result in detrimentally elevated intracranial pressure (ICP) that can cause serious neurological symptoms, brain herniation, and even death. Therefore, it is imperative that the cerebrovascular system adapts throughout pregnancy to maintain relatively normal blood flow and water flux in the face of a 40–60% increase in plasma volume and cardiac output. Unfortunately, there is a lack of robust information regarding cerebrovascular adaptations during pregnancy due to limitations in performing studies on cerebral blood flow (CBF) and cerebrovascular structure in human pregnant subjects. As such, animal models have been the primary source of data for characterizing the adaption of the cerebral circulation to pregnancy. Throughout this chapter, the effect of pregnancy on several aspects of the cerebral circulation will be discussed, including hemodynamics, cerebral autoregulation, and structure of the cerebral vasculature and BBB. This comprehensive review of

Table 5.2 Summary of cerebrovascular changes during pregnancy

	Adaptations
Cerebral blood flow	Probably unchanged
Cerebral autoregulation	Enhanced autoregulation, bi-directional extension of autoregulatory curve
Cerebral vascular resistance	Decreased
Vascular structural changes	Increased pial arterial reactivity to vasodilatation, outward hypotrophic remodeling of parenchymal arterioles and cerebral veins, increased capillary density
Blood brain barrier	No change in permeability, increased expression of efflux transporter protein

physiologic adaptations will lay the foundation for our understanding of several cerebrovascular complications encountered during pregnancy (Table 5.2).

Cerebral Blood Flow and Cerebral Autoregulation

The measurement of CBF in pregnant patients poses a unique challenge, as gold standard techniques including single photo emission computerized tomography (SPECT), positron emission tomography, stable xenon computerized tomography, and/or xenon 133 clearance techniques, employ ionizing radiation and therefore cannot be used. The non-invasive transcranial Doppler (TCD) has been increasingly used to estimate blood flow velocity, as a correlate for CBF, in human pregnancy studies [26–31]. Unfortunately, the results of these studies are of limited value since the correlation between blood flow velocities and CBF is not linear, especially during pregnancy where vascular tone is lower than in nonpregnant women. Some studies have used angle-independent dual-beam ultrasound with digital doppler to measure blood flow volume (BFV) in the internal carotid artery (ICA), as a correlate for CBF in the corresponding hemisphere. One such study found an increase in cor-

responding CBF values from 44.4 ml/100 g/min in the first trimester to 51.8 ml/100 g/min in third trimester [32]. More recently, velocity-encoded phase contrast MRI has been used for accurate determination of absolute blood flow in the intracranial, renal, and cardiopulmonary circulations [33–36]. Zeeman et al. found a ~20% decrease in CBF using this imaging technique for the middle cerebral (MCA) and posterior cerebral arteries (PCA) in ten pregnant women [37]. One very recent study using TCD showed lower blood flow velocity prior to delivery which increased to nonpregnant values a day after delivery [38]. The discrepancy in CBF values, reported in these studies, highlight the difficultly in measuring CBF in pregnant women. Several animal studies have shown absolute changes in CBF during pregnancy using invasive microsphere techniques [39–41]. One animal study in sheep showed decrease in CBF during late-pregnancy, [39] while another study in rats found little change in CBF at late-gestation compared with their nonpregnant counterparts [41]. Overall, CBF values show no to minimal changes during pregnancy.

This phenomenon may be explained by cerebral autoregulation, an important mechanism that ensures relatively constant blood supply during fluctuation in cerebral perfusion pressure (CPP), the parameter which closely follows MAP changes during pregnancy [Recall: CPP = MAP − ICP]. In normotensive adults, CBF is ~50 ml/100 g/min provided that cerebral perfusion pressure is between ~60 and 160 mmHg [42, 43]. CBF becomes dependent on perfusion pressure linearly, above and below these CPP limits. The autoregulatory capacity can be assessed by using a combination of TCD and continuous non-invasive blood pressure measurement, and it is often expressed as the autoregulation index (ARI), with 0 being absent and 9 being perfect cerebral autoregulation [44]. Cerebral autoregulation appears to remain intact during normal pregnancy [45, 46]. In fact, a recent study by Van et al. showed further enhanced autoregulation capacity during the second half of pregnancy compared with nonpregnant women [47]. In this case, pregnancy appears to extend both the upper and the lower limits of the CBF autoregula-

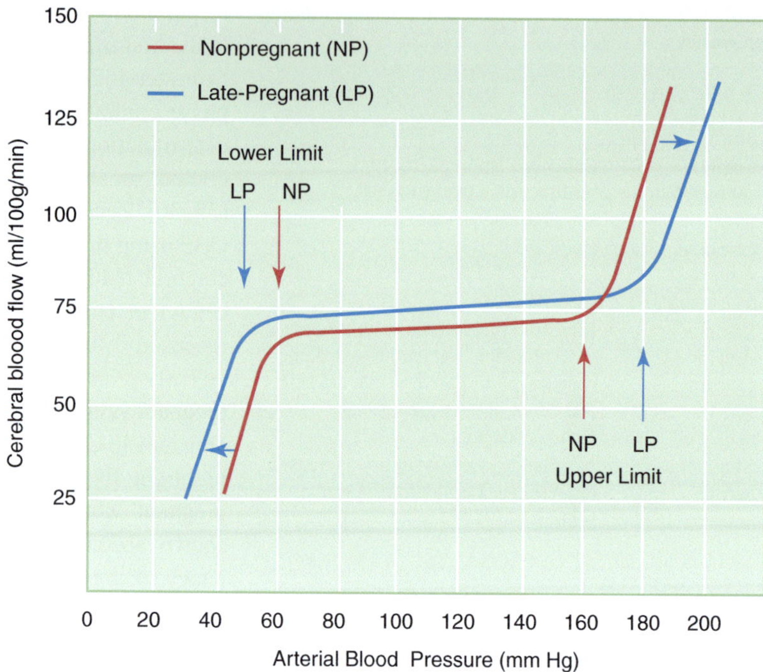

Fig. 5.1 Cerebral autoregulation curve in normal and pregnant states. (Johnson AC, Cipolla MJ. The Cerebral Circulation During Pregnancy: Adapting to Preserve Normalcy. Physiology. 2015 Mar;30(2):139–47)

tory curve (Fig. 5.1). This effect on the autoregulatory curve is confirmed in animal studies by inducing hypotension through controlled hemorrhage or hypertension by phenylephrine infusion in pregnant rats, coupled with continuous CBF measurements using laser Doppler flowmetry [48, 49]. This bi-directional extension of the autoregulatory curve is designed to provide protection against acute hypotension or hypertension episodes, especially those associated with parturition [50]. One explanation for the observed maintenance and/or enhancement of cerebral autoregulation during pregnancy might be the increasing concentrations of estrogen and progesterone, which have important protective effects on endothelial function and cerebrovascular health [51, 52]. For example, estrogens are shown to increase cerebrovascular reactivity, [52] and have a direct vasodilator effect on the microvasculature. Other factors that might be involved in the enhancement of autoregulatory capacity might include the RAAS [53], perivascular innervation, vascular structure, or cytokines. Interestingly, all of these factors are known to be altered in preeclampsia, a condition characterized by impaired cerebrovascular regulation during pregnancy [1].

Cerebral Vascular Resistance and Vascular Structural Changes

Cerebral vascular resistance is an important factor that drives changes in CBF and thus influences cerebral autoregulation during pregnancy. Pregnant women appear to have higher diastolic velocity and lower cerebrovascular resistance in small-diameter cerebral arterioles, but not in larger cerebral arteries [54]. This selective change is related to different degrees of myogenic and chemical adaptations in arteries, arterioles, and capillary beds.

Cerebral pial arteries undergo minimal structural changes during pregnancy. They appear to have no change in basal myogenic tone during pregnancy, however, they do show enhanced myogenic response to changes in intravascular pressure. Relatedly, cerebral arteries from pregnant rats had an exaggerated vasodilatation response to decreased intravascular pressure [48]. This exaggerated response is driven by increased sensitivity to nitric oxide (NO) and/or increased expression of inducible nitric oxide synthase (iNOS) on cerebral arteries during pregnancy [55].

The cerebral vasculature, like many other organ systems, undergo structural remodeling to accommodate physiologic adaptations of pregnancy, albeit in a selective manner. Only brain parenchymal arterioles that branch off pial arteries and perfuse the brain tissue, undergo outward hypotrophic remodeling during pregnancy, resulting in a larger vascular lumen and thinner vessel wall than in the nonpregnant state [41]. This selective remodeling is driven by increased peroxisome proliferator-activated receptor gamma (PPARγ) activation by circulating hormone relaxin. Relaxin, produced by the placenta during pregnancy, crosses the BBB and is thought to activate PPARγ on astrocytes and neurons, which in turn exert a paracrine effect on parenchymal arterioles to drive outward remodeling. This does not occur in pial vessels as they are not in direct contact of parenchymal cells [56]. The same mechanism is also linked to an increase in capillary density in the posterior cerebral cortex [41].

In conclusion, the combination of structural remodeling of parenchymal arterioles and increased capillary density coupled with physiologic anemia of pregnancy lead to decreased cerebral vascular resistance and potential for increased CBF. However, pial vessels resist any structural alteration and act as gate keeper in maintaining physiologic CBF. The enhanced reactivity of these vessels to vasodilatation is important for protecting the brain against hypotensive insults, especially those that may be encountered during parturition.

The Cerebral Veins

Unlike the arterial side of the vasculature, in which blood is constantly in transit, 70–80% of cerebral blood volume resides on the venous side [57]. Therefore, changes in venous outflow can significantly affect cerebral blood volume and intracranial pressure. However, how pregnancy changes cerebral veins in addition to its effect on the coagulation cascade remain largely unknown. A recent study investigated the vein of Galen during pregnancy and found a decreased level of basal tone in the smooth muscle layer of the vein during pregnancy compared to the nonpregnant state. The veins also seem to undergo outward hypotrophic remodeling, similar to arterioles [58]. The combined effect of the above-described changes may promote venous pooling or stasis. The venous stasis and hypercoagulable state of pregnancy are responsible for the increased incidence of complications such as cerebral venous thrombosis, venous infarct, and intracerebral hemorrhage.

Blood–Brain Barrier Alteration

The BBB, formed by a unique capillary endothelium expressing high levels of tight junctions that is encircled by astrocytic end-feet and pericytes, is a complex interface that protects the delicate cerebral milieu by tightly regulating passage of molecules, including water. BBB permeability is modulated by limiting paracellular and transcellular passage across the capillary endothelium owing to its unique properties such as high electrical resistance tight junctions, lack of fenestrations, and low rate of pinocytosis [59, 60]. Notably, BBB permeability does not increase during pregnancy nor does pregnancy seem to affect expression of mRNA encoding tight junction proteins [41]. Moreover, hydraulic conductivity, referring to water movement through the vessel wall in response to hydrostatic pressure, is maintained very low within the CNS and remains unchanged during pregnancy [61].

Pregnancy is, however, associated with a marked increase in circulating permeability factors to which the cerebral vasculature must become adapted. For example, VEGF and placental growth factor (PlGF), which are critical factors required for successful pregnancy, are secreted in large amounts by the placenta [62,

63]. Both are potent vasodilators and increase peripheral vascular permeability to serum protein and macromolecules, in preparation for angiogenesis. The prevention of these permeability factors from altering BBB integrity is, therefore, a critical adaptation to ensure maintenance of brain homeostasis. Interestingly, despite elevated circulating VEGF and PlGF during pregnancy, exposure of cerebral vessels to pregnant plasma or serum does not increase BBB permeability. In fact, plasma from late-gestation rats prevents VEGF-induced increases in BBB permeability, [64] likely due to increased levels of soluble fms-like tyrosine kinase 1 (sFlt-1). The selective binding of VEGF and PlGF to sFlt-1 is important for regulating their bioavailability, thus limiting the permeability-promoting effects at the BBB during pregnancy [65]. Additionally, increased expression of efflux transporter proteins such as *p*-glycoprotein during pregnancy prevents passage of circulating factors.

In addition to increased circulating factors, pregnancy is associated with production of large amounts of hormones and pro-inflammatory cytokines that have seizure-provoking potential. For example, neurons analyzed via in vitro slice culture studies in nonpregnant rat brains showed hyperexcitability upon exposure to serum from late-gestation rats without any seizure history [61]. Thus, preservation of BBB properties and adaptation of efflux transporters also seem to provide protection from potential seizure-inducing agents as well.

Pathophysiology of Cerebrovascular Complications During Pregnancy

Pregnancy has been considered the ultimate stress test for women. The cerebrovascular changes accompanying pregnancy represent vital protective mechanisms that ensure homeostasis of cerebral blood flow and the brain milieu in the face of adverse hemodynamic scenarios encountered throughout pregnancy and more importantly during parturition. However, these adaptations are also complicit in the pathogenesis of several cerebrovascular complications of pregnancy such as posterior reversible encephalopathy syndrome (PRES), preeclampsia/eclampsia, peripartum angiopathy (PPA), and reversible cerebral vasoconstriction syndrome (RCVS), which can lead to cerebral infarction, intracerebral hemorrhage, and/or seizures. The relationship between cerebrovascular adaptations and these pathologies are discussed briefly below and in detail in dedicated chapters of this text.

Placental Ischemia Model

The placental ischemia model is one of the widely cited theoretical models that integrates currently available clinical and basic science data to explain cerebrovascular dysfunction during preeclampsia. Cerebrovascular dysfunction, coupled with endothelial dysfunction, seem to be a central mechanism in the pathogenesis of neurologic manifestations of preeclampsia/eclampsia, including PRES. Placental ischemia, caused by impairments in spiral artery remodeling, preexisting maternal vascular disease, or other factors, leads to production of antiangiogenic factors including TNF-α and sFlt-1. These factors, especially TNF-α, can act on vascular smooth muscles and perturb myogenic tone, leading to derangement in cerebral autoregulation [66] (Fig. 5.2). This effect is confirmed in a clinical study by van Veen et al., where women with preeclampsia had impaired dynamic CBF and an overall lower dynamic cerebral autoregulatory index compared to the healthy pregnancy group [67]. Failure of cerebral blood vessels to autoregulate in response to increases in blood pressure leads to forced dilatation of cerebral arteries and increase in CPP. The outward hypotrophic remodeling of parenchymal arterioles transmits increased hydrostatic pressure further downstream causing cerebral hyperperfusion and increased BBB permeability due to increased hydraulic conductivity [41]. The elevated circulating vasoactive factors, as described by the placental ischemia model, then trigger endothelial dysfunction and widespread BBB disruption. These processes lead to cerebral vasogenic

Fig. 5.2 Postulated mechanism for cerebrovascular dysfunction in preeclampsia. *BBB* blood-brain barrier, *CBF* cerebral blood flow, *sFlt-1* soluble fms-like tyrosine kinase 1, *TNF-α* tumor necrosis factor-alpha. (Reprinted from Curr Hypertens Rep. 2019 Jul 1;21(7):1–8(66))

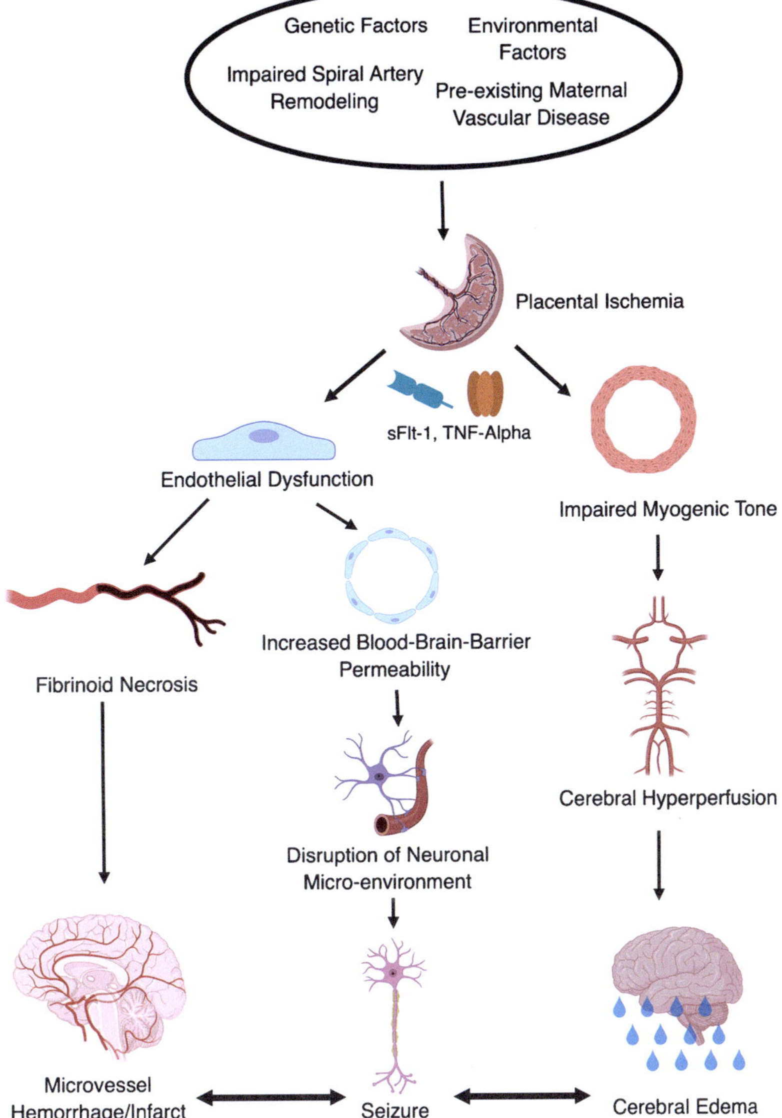

edema, encountered in states such as preeclampsia, eclampsia, and PRES.

From the cerebral perfusion standpoint, a type of cerebral hyperperfusion syndrome occurs during these disease states which lead to predominantly white matter congestion. The edema and concomitant disruption of the cerebral microenvironment may cause seizure, a common manifestation in PRES and eclampsia. An increase in peri-neural trigeminal innervation of posterior cerebral arteries (PCA) may also be related to the appearance of headache during PRES. [1, 68] Due to endothelial cell activation, fibrinoid necrosis of the vessels may occur leading to bursting of delicate microvessels with subsequent microhemorrhages, particularly in the setting of generalized tonic-clonic seizure and concomitant neurovascular coupling-mediated local vasodilation. Similarly, the absence of endothelial-derived vasodilatory factors may lead to vasospasm, resulting in cerebral ischemia. The findings of cerebral artery narrowing, similar to RCVS, on vascular imaging studies is seen in over half the patients who present with eclampsia and PRES, which further suggests a unifying disease process in these conditions [69].

Posterior Reversible Encephalopathy Syndrome

PRES was first described as reversible posterior leukoencephalopathy syndrome (RPLS) in 1996 by Hinchey et al. [70], in association with acute hypertension, eclampsia, renal disease, sepsis, and immunosuppressant therapy. The exact incidence of PRES in pregnancy remains unknown, however, multiple studies have confirmed that nearly all patients with eclampsia have clinical and radiologic findings of PRES. [71–73] PRES is, increasingly, being considered an anatomic substrate of eclampsia with overlapping clinical/radiologic findings and shared pathogenesis (described above). It is characterized by a variety of neurological symptoms, including headache, seizures, visual abnormalities, altered mental status and sometimes, focal deficits such as hemiparesis. Cases of pregnancy-related PRES usually have milder symptoms like headache and visual disturbances when compared to nonpregnancy-related PRES. [64] Multiple small studies have reported a 15–25% incidence of intracranial hemorrhage in pregnancy-related PRES, the majority of which are either multifocal intraparenchymal hemorrhage or sulcal subarachnoid hemorrhage [64, 71, 74]. Although the majority of PRES cases have a history of abrupt hypertension, 15–20% of patients with PRES are normotensive or hypotensive, and even among those who are hypertensive, less than 50% have a documented MAP above the classically quoted upper limit of CBF autoregulation [75]. Therefore, the incitement of endothelial dysfunction by vasoactive substances in preeclampsia, as described in the placental ischemia model, might explain the development of PRES in the absence of hypertension. The hallmark radiologic findings of PRES include reversible T2/FLAIR hyperintensities on brain MRI, typically located in bilateral parieto-occipital areas and subcortical white matter, suggestive of vasogenic edema.

Frontal lobe involvement has also been reportedly frequently, usually in the posterior portion of the superior frontal gyrus (anterior cerebral artery distribution) and the precentral gyrus (middle cerebral artery distribution) [76]. The predilection for edema in the subcortical white matter of the posterior circulation is thought to be due to the relatively low density of vasoconstricting sympathetic receptors in the vessels of the posterior circulation [76]. The edematous lesions in pregnancy-related PRES less commonly involve the brain stem and follow-up imaging shows resolution of edema in nearly all cases within 2 weeks. The overall clinical recovery rate tends to be better in PRES associated with pregnancy compared to that occurring in nonpregnant cohorts. Preeclampsia, eclampsia, and PRES are discussed in detail in Chaps. 23 and 33.

Conclusion

Cardiovascular and cerebrovascular changes are arguably the most important physiologic adaptations occurring within the maternal body, after utero-placental circulation. While the majority of cardiovascular parameters increase through the pregnancy and are aimed to accommodate growing maternal and fetal needs, the cerebrovascular changes tend to preserve normalcy of cerebral blood flow in order to protect the brain microenvironment. Knowledge of these physiologic changes is essential to achieving a better understanding of several cardiac and neurological complications that can result in substantial maternal-fetal morbidity and mortality.

References

1. Cipolla MJ. The adaptation of the cerebral circulation to pregnancy: mechanisms and consequences. J Cereb Blood Flow Metab. 2013;33:465–78.
2. Clapp JF, Capeless E. Cardiovascular function before, during, and after the first and subsequent pregnancies. Am J Cardiol. 1997;80:1469.
3. Fu Q, Levine BD. Autonomic circulatory control during pregnancy in humans. Semin Reprod Med. 2009;27(4):330–7.

4. Mahendru AA, Everett TR, Wilkinson IB, Lees CC, McEniery CM. A longitudinal study of maternal cardiovascular function from preconception to the postpartum period. J Hypertens. 2014;32(4):849–56.

5. Blackburn S. Maternal, fetal, & neonatal physiology. 4th ed. Elsevier; 2012.

6. Nama V, Antonios TF, Onwude J, Manyonda IT. Mid-trimester blood pressure drop in normal pregnancy: myth or reality? J Hypertens. 2011;29(4):763–8.

7. Sanghavi M, Rutherford JD. Cardiovascular physiology of pregnancy. Circulation. 2014;130(12):1003–8.

8. Monga M. Maternal cardiovascular, respiratory, renal adaptation to pregnancy in Maternal–fetal medicine: principles and practice. 6th ed. Creasy R, Resnik R, Iams JD, Lockwood C, Moore TR, editors. Elsevier; 2009.

9. Pritchard JA. Changes in the blood volume during pregnancy and delivery. Anesthesiology. 1965;26:393–9.

10. Chesley LC. Plasma and red cell volumes during pregnancy. Am J Obstet Gynecol. 1972;112(3):440–50.

11. Lumbers ER, Pringle KG. Roles of the circulating renin-angiotensin-aldosterone system in human pregnancy. Am J Physiol Regul Integr Comp Physiol. 2014;306:91–101.

12. Brunton PJ, Arunachalam S, Russell JA. Control of neurohypophysial hormone secretion, blood osmolality and volume in pregnancy. J Physiol Pharmacol. 2008;59:27.

13. Jepson JH, Montreal MA. Endocrine control of maternal and fetal erythropoiesis. Can Med Assoc J. 1968;98:844.

14. Roberts J, Cunningham F, Lindheimer M. Chesley's hypertensive disorders in pregnancy. 2nd ed. NewYork: Appleton and Lange; 1999.

15. Robson SC, Hunter S, Boys RJ, Dunlop W. Serial study of factors influencing changes in cardiac output during human pregnancy. Am J Physiol. 1989;256(4):H1060.

16. Bader RA, Bader ME, Rose DJ, Braunwald E. Hemodynamics at rest and during exercise in normal pregnancy as studied by cardiac catheterization. J Clin Invest. 1955;34(10):1524–36.

17. Thaler I, Manor D, Itskovitz J, Rottem S, Levit N, Timor-Tritsch I, et al. Changes in uterine blood flow during human pregnancy. Am J Obstet Gynecol. 1990;162(1):121–5.

18. Dowell R, Kauer C. Maternal hemodynamics and uteroplacental blood flow throughout gestation in conscious rats. Methods Find Exp Clin Pharmacol. 1997;19:613–25.

19. Meah VL, Cockcroft JR, Backx K, Shave R, Stöhr EJ. Cardiac output and related haemodynamics during pregnancy: a series of meta-analyses. Heart. 2016;102(7):518–26.

20. Abbas AE, Lester SJ, Connolly H. Pregnancy and the cardiovascular system. Int J Cardiol. 2005;98:179–89.

21. Robson SC, Dunlop W, Moore M, Hunter S. Haemodynamic changes during the puerperium: a Doppler and M-mode echocardiographic study. BJOG. 1987;94(11):1028–39.

22. Ducas RA, Elliott JE, Melnyk SF, Premecz S, Dasilva M, Cleverley K, et al. Cardiovascular magnetic resonance in pregnancy: insights from the cardiac hemodynamic imaging and remodeling in pregnancy (CHIRP) study. J Cardiovasc Magn Reson. 2014;16(1):1.

23. Goldstein J, Sites CK, Toth MJ. Progesterone stimulates cardiac muscle protein synthesis via receptor-dependent pathway. Fertil Steril. 2004;82(2):430–6.

24. Umar S, Nadadur R, Iorga A, Amjedi M, Matori H, Eghbali M. Cardiac structural and hemodynamic changes associated with physiological heart hypertrophy of pregnancy are reversed postpartum. J Appl Physiol. 2012;113(8):1253–9.

25. Siegel GJ, Albers RW, Brady ST, Price DL. Basic neurochemistry: molecular, cellular, and medical aspects. Am J Neuroradiol. 2006;27(2):465.

26. Belfort M, Giannina G, Herd JA. Transcranial and orbital Doppler ultrasound in normal pregnancy and preeclampsia. Clin Obstet Gynecol. 1999;42(3):479.

27. Belfort MA, Tooke-Miller C, Allen JC, Saade GR, Dildy GA, Grunewald C, et al. Changes in flow velocity, resistance indices, and cerebral perfusion pressure in the maternal middle cerebral artery distribution during normal pregnancy. Acta Obstet Gynecol Scand. 2001;80(2):104–12.

28. Williams K, MacLean C. Transcranial assessment of maternal cerebral blood flow velocity in normal vs. hypertensive states. Variations with maternal posture. J Reprod Med. 1994;39(9):685–8.

29. Broderick J, Brott T, Zuccarello M. Management of intracerebral hemorrhage. In: Batjer HH, editor. Cerebrovascular disease. Philadelphia: Lippincott-Raven; 1997. p. 611–27.

30. Demarin V, Rundek T, Hodek B. Maternal cerebral circulation in normal and abnormal pregnancies. Acta Obstet Gynecol Scand. 1997;76(7):619–24.

31. Zunker P, Happe S, Georgiadis AL, Louwen F, Georgiadis D, Ringelstein EB, et al. Maternal cerebral hemodynamics in pregnancy-related hypertension. A prospective transcranial Doppler study. Ultrasound Obstet Gynecol. 2000;16(2):179–87.

32. Nevo O, Soustiel JF, Thaler I. Maternal cerebral blood flow during normal pregnancy: a cross-sectional study. Am J Obstet Gynecol. 2010;203:475.e1–6.

33. Marks MP, Pelc NJ, Ross MR, Enzmann DR. Determination of cerebral blood flow with a phase-contrast cine MR imaging technique: evaluation of normal subjects and patients with arteriovenous malformations. Radiology. 1992;182(2):467–76.

34. Enzmann DR, Marks MP, Pelc NJ. Comparison of cerebral artery blood flow measurements with gated cine and ungated phase-contrast techniques. J Magn Reson Imaging. 1993;3(5):705–12.

35. Hundley WG, Li HF, Hillis LD, Meshack BM, Lange RA, Willard JE, et al. Quantitation of cardiac output with velocity-encoded, phase-difference magnetic resonance imaging. Am J Cardiol. 1995;75(17):1250–5.

36. Hundley WG, Lange RA, Clarke GD, Meshack BM, Payne J, Landau C, et al. Assessment of coronary arterial flow and flow reserve in humans with magnetic resonance imaging. Circulation. 1996;93(8):1502–8.

37. Zeeman GG, Mustapha H, Twickler DM. Maternal cerebral blood flow changes in pregnancy. Am J Obstet Gynecol. 2003;189:968.

38. Batur Caglayan HZ, Nazliel B, Cinar M, Ataoglu E, Moraloglu O, Irkec C. Assessment of maternal cerebral blood flow velocity by transcranial Doppler ultrasound before delivery and in the early postpartum period. J Matern Neonatal Med. 2019;32(4):584–9.

39. Gant N. Measurement of uteroplacental blood flow in the human. Ithaca: Perinatol Press; 1989.

40. Buelke-Sam J, Nelson CJ, Byrd RA, Holson JF. Blood flow during pregnancy in the rat: I. Flow patterns to maternal organs. Teratology. 1982;26(3):269–77.

41. Cipolla MJ, Sweet JG, Chan SL. Cerebral vascular adaptation to pregnancy and its role in the neurological complications of eclampsia. J Appl Physiol. 2011;110(2):329–39.

42. Kety SS, Schmidt CF. The nitrous oxide method for the quantitative determination of cerebral blood flow in man: theory, procedure and normal values 1. J Clin Invest. 1948;27:476–83.

43. Hurn P. Overview of cerebrovascular hemodynamics. In: KMA W, Caplan LR, Reis DJ, Siesjo BK, Weir B, editors. Primer on cerebrovascular diseases. San Diego: Academic; 1997.

44. Tiecks FP, Lam AM, Aaslid R, Newell DW. Comparison of static and dynamic cerebral autoregulation measurements. Stroke. 1995;26(6):1014–9.

45. Janzarik WG, Ehlers E, Ehmann R, Gerds TA, Schork J, Mayer S, et al. Dynamic cerebral autoregulation in pregnancy and the risk of preeclampsia. Hypertension. 2014;63(1):161–6.

46. Sherman RW. Cerebral haemodynamics in pregnancy and pre-eclampsia as assessed by transcranial Doppler ultrasonography. Br J Anaesth. 2002;89:687.

47. van Veen TR, Panerai RB, Haeri S, van den Berg PP, Zeeman GG, Belfort MA. Changes in cerebral autoregulation in the second half of pregnancy and compared to non-pregnant controls. Pregnancy Hypertens. 2016;6(4):380–3.

48. Chapman AC, Cipolla MJ, Chan SL. Effect of pregnancy and nitric oxide on the myogenic vasodilation of posterior cerebral arteries and the lower limit of cerebral blood flow autoregulation. Reprod Sci. 2013;20(9):1046–54.

49. Cipolla MJ, Bishop N, Chan SL. Effect of pregnancy on autoregulation of cerebral blood flow in anterior versus posterior cerebrum. Hypertension. 2012;60(3):705–11.

50. Johnson AC, Cipolla MJ. The cerebral circulation during pregnancy: adapting to preserve normalcy. Physiology. 2015;30(2):139–47.

51. Reeves MJ, Bushnell CD, Howard G, Gargano JW, Duncan PW, Lynch G, et al. Sex differences in stroke: epidemiology, clinical presentation, medical care, and outcomes. Lancet Neurol. 2008;7:915–26.

52. Krause DN. Influence of sex steroid hormones on cerebrovascular function. Artic J Appl Physiol. 2006;101(4):1252–61.

53. Irani R, Xia Y. Renin angiotensin signaling in normal pregnancy and preeclampsia. Semin Nephrol. 2011;31(1):47–58.

54. Belfort MA, Saade GR, Snabes M, Dunn R, Moise KJ, Cruz A, et al. Hormonal status affects the reactivity of the cerebral vasculature. Am J Obstet Gynecol. 1995;172(4):1273–8.

55. Cipolla MJ, Houston EM, Kraig RP, Bonney EA. Differential effects of low-dose endotoxin on the cerebral circulation during pregnancy. Reprod Sci. 2011;18(12):1211–21.

56. Chan S, Cipolla MJ. Relaxin causes selective outward remodeling of brain parenchymal arterioles via activation of peroxisome proliferator-activated receptor-γ. FASEB J. 2011;25(9):3229–39.

57. An H, Lin W. Cerebral venous and arterial blood volumes can be estimated separately in humans using magnetic resonance imaging. Magn Reson Med. 2002;48(4):583–8.

58. Van Der Wijk AE, Schreurs MPH, Cipolla MJ. Pregnancy causes diminished myogenic tone and outward hypotrophic remodeling of the cerebral vein of Galen. J Cereb Blood Flow Metab. 2013;33(4):542–9.

59. Ueno M. Molecular anatomy of the brain endothelial barrier: an overview of the distributional features. Curr Med Chem. 2007;14(11):1199–206.

60. Zlokovic BV. The blood-brain barrier in health and chronic neurodegenerative disorders. Neuron. 2008;57:178–201.

61. Cipolla MJ, Pusic AD, Grinberg YY, Chapman AC, Poynter ME, Kraig RP. Pregnant serum induces neuroinflammation and seizure activity via TNFα. Exp Neurol. 2012;234(2):398–404.

62. Valdés G, Corthorn J. Review: the angiogenic and vasodilatory utero-placental network. Placenta. 2011;32(Suppl 2):S170–5.

63. Krauss T, Pauer H-U, Augustin HG. Prospective analysis of placenta growth factor (PlGF) concentrations in the plasma of women with normal pregnancy and pregnancies complicated by preeclampsia. Hypertens Pregnancy. 2004;23(1):101–11.

64. Liman TG, Bohner G, Heuschmann PU, Scheel M, Endres M, Siebert E. Clinical and radiological differences in posterior reversible encephalopathy syndrome between patients with preeclampsia-eclampsia and other predisposing diseases. Eur J Neurol. 2012;19(7):935–43.

65. Schreurs MPH, Houston EM, May V, Cipolla MJ. The adaptation of the blood-brain barrier to vascular endothelial growth factor and placental growth factor during pregnancy. FASEB J. 2012;26(1):355–62.

66. Younes ST, Ryan MJ. Pathophysiology of cerebral vascular dysfunction in pregnancy-induced hypertension. Curr Hypertens Rep. 2019;21(7):1–8.

67. Van Veen TR, Panerai RB, Haeri S, Griffioen AC, Zeeman GG, Belfort MA. Cerebral autoregulation in normal pregnancy and preeclampsia. Obstet Gynecol. 2013;122(5):1064–9.

68. Aukes AM, Bishop N, Godfrey J, Cipolla MJ. The influence of pregnancy and gender on perivascular innervation of rat posterior cerebral arteries. Reprod Sci. 2008;15:411–9.

69. Razmara A, Bakhadirov K, Batra A, Feske SK. Cerebrovascular complications of pregnancy and the postpartum period. Curr Cardiol Rep. 2014;16:1–8.

70. Hinchey J, Chaves C, Appignani B, Breen J, Pao L, Wang A, et al. A reversible posterior leukoencephalopathy syndrome. N Engl J Med. 1996;334(8):494–500.

71. Wen Y, Yang B, Huang Q, Liu Y. Posterior reversible encephalopathy syndrome in pregnancy: a retrospective series of 36 patients from mainland China. Ir J Med Sci. 2017;186(3):699–705.

72. Gao B, Lv C. Posterior reversible encephalopathy syndrome in 46 of 47 patients with eclampsia: beyond it. Am J Obstet Gynecol. 2014;211(1):83–4.

73. Wagner SJ, Acquah LA, Lindell EP, Craici IM, Wingo MT, Rose CH, et al. Posterior reversible encephalopathy syndrome and eclampsia: pressing the case for more aggressive blood pressure control. Mayo Clin Proc. 2011;86(9):851–6.

74. Sharma A, Whitesell RT, Moran KJ. Imaging pattern of intracranial hemorrhage in the setting of posterior reversible encephalopathy syndrome. Neuroradiology. 2010;52(10):855–63.

75. Fugate JE, Rabinstein AA. Posterior reversible encephalopathy syndrome: clinical and radiological manifestations, pathophysiology, and outstanding questions. Lancet Neurol. 2015;14:914–25. https://doi.org/10.1016/S1474-4422(15)00111-8.

76. Beausang-Linder M, Bill A. Cerebral circulation in acute arterial hypertension—protective effects of sympathetic nervous activity. Acta Physiol Scand. 1981;111(2):193–9.

Pregnancy and Ischemic Stroke

Mena Samaan, Deepika Dhawan, Linda Ye,
Ramandeep Sahni, Fawaz Al-Mufti,
and Christeena Kurian

Introduction

Ischemic stroke is a leading cause of death and long-term disability and is more common in men than in women except for in advanced age and from ages 20 to 39, where the incidence is higher in women [1]. In addition to known risk factors, such as taking oral contraceptive pills, pregnancy and puerperium contribute to the increased risk of stroke observed in the younger population. In fact, although the incidence of stroke in pregnancy and puerperium is only 11–34 per 10,000, there is a threefold increase in incidence of stroke in pregnant as compared to non-pregnant women of reproductive age [2–5].

A recent systemic review and meta-analysis demonstrated a pregnancy-related stroke incidence of 30 per 100,000 deliveries with 12.2 per 100,000 deliveries related to ischemic stroke, 12.2 per 100,000 deliveries related to hemor-

rhagic stroke, and 9.1 per 100,000 deliveries related to cerebral venous sinus thrombosis [6]. Although the overall incidence of stroke in the US population has declined in recent years, incidence of maternal stroke has increased due to increasing maternal age and rising trends in the prevalence of cardiovascular risk factors among young women [7]. In the USA, between 1994–1995 and 2006–2007, there was a 47% increase in antenatal stroke admissions and 83% increase in postpartum stroke admissions [8]. In Canada, stroke incidence increased from 10.8 per 100,000 deliveries in 2003–2004 to 16.6 per 100,000 in 2015–2016.

The highest risk for stroke occurs peripartum, from 2 days before to 1 day following delivery (relative risk = 33.8) and continues through 6 weeks postpartum [9]. Kittner et al. demonstrated that the adjusted relative risk for cerebral infarction during pregnancy was 0.7 (95% confidence interval [CI], 0.3–1.6), but increased to 8.7 (95% CI, 4.6–16.7) for the postpartum period after a live birth or stillbirth [10].

Pathophysiology

Physiologic and pathophysiologic processes related to pregnancy alter blood flow and the clotting cascade in a way that can increase the risk of stroke during pregnancy and puerperium. Physiologic changes during pregnancy include

M. Samaan · R. Sahni
Department of Neurology, Westchester Medical Center, New York Medical College,
Valhalla, NY, USA

D. Dhawan · L. Ye · C. Kurian
Department of Neurosurgery, Westchester Medical Center at New York Medical College,
Valhalla, NY, USA

F. Al-Mufti (✉)
Department of Neurology, Neurosurgery and Radiology, New York Medical College - Westchester Medical Center, Valhalla, NY, USA
e-mail: fawaz.al-mufti@wmchealth.org

© The Author(s), under exclusive license to Springer Nature Switzerland AG 2023
G. Gupta et al. (eds.), *Neurological Disorders in Pregnancy*,
https://doi.org/10.1007/978-3-031-36490-7_6

alterations in cardiovascular hemodynamics, coagulation factors, hormone levels, and vascular tone. Cardiovascular and hematologic changes accompanying pregnancy are discussed briefly below and in detail in Chap. 5.

Coagulation Factors

In preparation for the tissue disruption and trauma that can accompany childbirth, evolution favors hemostasis with various changes occurring in the coagulation cascade. These include changes in levels of procoagulant factors, coagulation inhibitors, and other mediators of clot formation and lysis, including placental production of anti-fibrinolytics. This results in a state of hypercoagulability during late pregnancy that persists through 12 weeks postdelivery.

The levels of procoagulant factors I, VII, VIII, IX, X, and XII increase during pregnancy, while levels of factors II, V, and XI show little change [11]. The coagulation inhibitor antithrombin III falls and is at its nadir in the third trimester. Total and free levels of the coagulation inhibitor cofactor protein S are significantly decreased as well. Although levels of protein C remain unchanged, almost a third of women have functional activated protein C resistance during the third trimester [9]. These changes in coagulation mediators are summarized in Table 6.1.

Table 6.1 Changes in hemostatic factors during pregnancy

Hemostatic parameter	Change at term pregnancy (% change)
Factor I (Fibrinogen)	Increases more than 100%
Factor VII	Up to 1000% increase
Factor VIII, IX, X, XII, and VWF	Increase more than 100%
D-Dimer	Up to 400% increase
Factor II and V	No change
Protein C	No change
Factor XI	Variable
Protein S	Up to 50% decrease
Factor XIII	Up to 50% decrease
Platelet count	Up to 20% decrease

Vascular Tone

In addition to normal physiologic changes in pregnancy that can induce a hypercoagulable state, pathophysiologic processes such as preeclampsia and eclampsia can induce structural changes in the vascular wall, such as endothelial dysfunction and impaired cerebrovascular autoregulation, that predispose pregnant women to hemorrhagic and ischemic stroke. Although the exact pathological mechanism of how preeclampsia/eclampsia leads to hemorrhagic stroke is not clearly delineated yet, it likely involves endothelial dysfunction leading to vasogenic edema due to the increase in permeability of blood vessels [12, 13]. Evidence suggests that placental antiangiogenic factors, specifically soluble fms-related tyrosine kinase 1 and soluble endoglin are upregulated and disrupt the maternal endothelium, which can result in hypertension, proteinuria, and glomerular endotheliosis [14]. The regulation of these antiangiogenic factors in the placenta is unknown; however, this is an area of increased interest for the development of markers to predict and diagnose preeclampsia as well as identify therapeutic targets. Other possible mechanisms include reduced placental perfusion, aberrant trophoblast (blastocyst cell) invasion into the uterus and uterine spiral arteries, and excessive intravascular inflammatory response to placental tissue [15–17]. Fluctuating blood pressure may also play a significant role as it leads to variable degrees of vasospasm and vasodilation. Additionally, disturbance to the cerebral autoregulation system because of chronic hyperventilation during pregnancy may lead to higher cerebral perfusion pressures and cause further blood vessel damage.

Risk Factors

It is important to recognize that in addition to pregnancy-related stroke risk factors, women may have pre-existing vascular risk factors that can compound their likelihood of stroke. In fact, antecedent traditional vascular risk factors can increase the risk of stroke during pregnancy. Women should be advised about the increased risk of stroke in pregnancy if they have a history of high blood pressure, smoking, migraine, arterial disease, hyperlipidemia, thrombophilia, infection, heart disease, paradoxical emboli or substance abuse. Additionally, those with maternal age over 35 years, non-white race, and migraine with aura are too at higher risk [3]. Migraine in particular increases the risk of gestational hypertension (OR 1.23–1.68) and preeclampsia (OR 1.08–3.5), and is responsible for a 15-fold increased risk of pregnancy-related stroke (OR 15.05, 95% CI 8.26–27.5) [18].

Those who acquire stroke risk factors unique to pregnancy including peripartum infection, pregnancy-induced hypertension, cesarean delivery, and multiple gestation should be counseled that they are at higher risk of stroke as well [3, 19–21]. Other conditions related to pregnancy including amniotic fluid embolus, postpartum angiopathy, and postpartum cardiomyopathy can also lead to ischemic stroke. Early identification and control of these risk factors and conditions is vital to prevent stroke related morbidity and mortality.

Etiology

Cerebral Venous Sinus Thrombosis (CVST)

CVST occurs in 9.1 per 100,000 pregnancies (95% CI of 4.3–18.9) [6]. The risk of CVST in pregnancy is increased, although pregnancy-associated CVST has a better prognosis than CVST from other etiologies. In the first trimester, the risk may be attributed to underlying thrombophilia, but the risk is most increased in the first 4–8 weeks postpartum [6]. Cerebral venous sinus thrombosis disrupts cerebral venous outflow causing dangerous congestion that can result in non-hemorrhagic or hemorrhagic ischemia or intracerebral hemorrhage. Parenchymal lesions caused by CVST display specific anatomic patterns that are determined by the site of venous

occlusion. The sites most commonly affected according to the International Study on Cerebral Venous and Dural Sinuses Thrombosis ($n = 624$) are as follows: (1) Superior Sagittal Sinus: 62%, (2) Transverse (Lateral) Sinus: 41–45%, and (3) Straight Sinus: 18% [22]. Hemorrhages are common, particularly when involving the superior sagittal sinus resulting in parasagittal "venous" infarcts. The deep venous system can also be affected in 11%, as well as internal jugular vein in 12% of patients. If the deep cerebral vein (or the draining straight sinus) is involved, infarcts can involve the globus pallidi.

The most common clinical findings in CVST include:

- Intracranial hypertension (headache in 90% of patients, and papilledema).
- Focal neurologic deficits (e.g., motor weakness, sensory deficit, aphasia).
- Encephalopathy.
- Seizures (30–50%).

Clinically, a patient with CVST presents with symptoms of increased intracranial pressure (ICP), a focal brain lesion, or both. A headache is one of the most common symptoms and in some cases, the only symptom. Other symptoms include craniofacial pain, seizures, motor weakness, visual field loss, and sensory symptoms. A focused discussion of CVST in pregnancy is provided in Chap. 11.

Hypertensive Disorders of Pregnancy

Hypertensive disorders of pregnancy are the leading cause of maternal stroke [23]. There are three different types of hypertensions that occur during pregnancy:

- *Chronic Hypertension*: High blood pressure (>140/90 mmHg) that is present before pregnancy, presents before week 20 of pregnancy, or that continues after delivery.
- *Hypertension*: High blood pressure that develops after week 20 of pregnancy and resolves

after delivery. Also referred to as pregnancy-induced hypertension (PIH).

- *Preeclampsia*: De-novo hypertension that presents after 20 weeks of gestation combined with proteinuria (>300 mg/day), other maternal organ dysfunction, such as renal insufficiency, liver involvement, neurological or hematological complications, uteroplacental dysfunction, or fetal growth restriction [24].

Elevated SBP in particular has been shown to be a more important indicator in evaluating stroke risk than DBP. Martin et al. found that in 95.8% of the patients, the SBP was at or greater than 160 mmHg right before the onset of a stroke while only 11% of patients exhibited DBP within the same severity range ($\geq$110 mmHg) [25]. This emphasizes the importance of closely monitoring and controlling SBP to mitigate stroke risk.

Preeclampsia and Eclampsia

Preeclampsia is a systemic syndrome that complicates approximately 2–5% of pregnancies. Eclampsia is a complication of 1–2% of preeclampsia cases in which the pregnant or recently delivered woman presents with new-onset seizures or coma not due to any other underlying neurological cause [26]. It is well established that women with a history of preeclampsia, chronic hypertension, and gestational hypertension are at increased risk for preeclampsia recurrence. A recent large study which included 40,673 women has identified additional risk factors associated with preeclampsia during subsequent pregnancies. These include obesity and diagnosis of gestational diabetes mellitus, which are independent from their age and inter-pregnancy interval [27]. History of preterm delivery, perinatal mortality or low birthweight also showed association with higher risk for preeclampsia in subsequent pregnancies [28]. Preeclampsia and eclampsia are described briefly below and in detail in Chap. 12.

Clinically, preeclampsia classically manifests as new onset of hypertension with systolic blood pressure (SBP) at or over 140 mmHg and diastolic blood pressure (DBP) at or over 90 mmHg on at least two occasions over a period of 4 h, and

either proteinuria (>0.3 g protein in 24 h urine specimen) or end-organ dysfunction after 20 weeks of gestation in a previously normotensive woman. Preeclampsia remains a leading cause of maternal and neonatal morbidity and mortality. The criteria for diagnosis of preeclampsia according to the American College of Obstetricians and Gynecologists (ACOG) and International Society for the Study of Hypertension in Pregnancy (ISSHP) are outlined in Table 6.2.

Systemic defects, including renal damage, are also important components of preeclampsia and eclampsia. In 2013, the ACOG removed proteinuria as an essential criterion for diagnosis of preeclampsia and included other maternal organ dysfunction (as outlined in Table 6.2). Moreover, the ISSHP endorsed that there should be no attempt to diagnose mild versus severe preeclampsia clinically as all cases may become emergencies, often rapidly [25].

Severe features of preeclampsia indicating systemic dysfunction as outlined by ACOG are the following [26]:

- Thrombocytopenia (platelet count <100 × 10⁹/L).
- Impaired liver function tests (to twice the upper limit of normal concentration) or severe persistent right upper quadrant or epigastric pain and not accounted for by alternative diagnoses.
- Renal insufficiency (Creatinine >1.1 mg/dL or doubling of Creatinine in absence of other renal disease).
- Pulmonary edema.
- New onset headache unresponsive to acetaminophen and not accounted for by alternative diagnoses or visual disturbances.

Postpartum Angiopathy (PPA)

Postpartum angiopathy is generally grouped under the overarching category of reversible cerebral vasoconstriction syndromes (RCVS) and is characterized by narrowing of the cere-

Table 6.2 Preeclampsia diagnostic criteria according to ACOG and ISSHP criteria

	ACOG (2019 revision) [29]	ISSHP (2018 revision) [26]
New onset, persistent hypertension ≥20 weeks in a woman with previously normal BP and	• SBP ≥140 mmHg or DBP ≥90 mmHg on 2 occasions ≥4 h apart or • SBP of ≥160 mmHg or DBP ≥110 mmHg confirmed within a short interval (minutes)	
Proteinuria	≥300 mg per 24-h urine collection or protein/creatinine ratio of ≥0.3 or urine dipstick reading of 2+	
Or in absence of proteinuria, new onset of:	• Renal insufficiency (serum creatinine >1.1 mg/dL or doubling of serum creatinine in absence of other renal disease) • Impaired liver function (LFTs elevated twice normal) • Thrombocytopenia (platelets <100) • New-onset headache (unresponsive to medication and not accounted for by alternative diagnoses or visual symptoms) • Pulmonary edema	• Acute kidney injury (serum creatinine >1 mg/dL) • Liver involvement (elevated LFTs with or without RUQ or epigastric pain) • Hematological complications (platelets <150K, DIC, hemolysis) • Neurological complications (eclampsia, altered mental status, blindness, stroke, clonus, severe headaches, persistent visual scotomata) • Uteroplacental dysfunction (fetal growth restriction, abnormal umbilical artery Doppler wave form analysis, or stillbirth)

RUQ right upper quadrant, *DIC* disseminated intravascular coagulation, *LFTs* liver function tests, *ACOG* American College of Obstetricians and Gynecologists, *ISSHP* International Society for the Study of Hypertension in Pregnancy

bral arteries without the presence of inflammation. Previous terms for the same disorder include benign angiopathy of the CNS, Call-Fleming syndrome, crash migraine, drug-induced arteritis, eclampsia-associated vasoconstriction, drug-induced angiitis, migraine angiitis, and CNS pseudovasculitis. PPA has a variety of clinical presentations including headache, focal neurological deficit, and seizures, but most often presents as multiple attacks of bilateral throbbing thunderclap headaches. These headaches are a presenting feature in 94% of cases over a mean period of 1 week and may occur spontaneously or be triggered by cough, exertion, or Valsalva. Visual blurring, scotomas, and blindness are also commonly associated. The cerebral vasoconstriction of PPA is additionally associated with abnormal brain imaging. Both hemorrhage and infarction are common presentations, but vasogenic edema is also seen [30].

The diagnostic criteria for RCVS include:

• Thunderclap headache(s) with or without focal neurologic deficits or seizures.
• Monophasic course without new symptoms more than 1 month after initial onset of symptoms.
• Multifocal, multi-vessel, segmental vasoconstriction of cerebral arteries.
• Absence of aneurysmal subarachnoid hemorrhage, Normal or near-normal cerebrospinal fluid (CSF); CSF Protein <100 mg/dL, CSF WBC <15 per mm^3, CSF Glucose normal.
• Complete or substantial normalization of cerebral arteries within 12 weeks of symptom onset.

When clinical suspicion for RCVS is high despite normal vasculature on angiography performed early after the onset of symptoms, repeat vascular imaging after several weeks is indicated in search of vasoconstriction. RCVS and PPA are discussed in detail in Chaps. 13 and 14, respectively.

Peripartum Cardiomyopathy (PPCM)

Cardiomyopathy is an established risk factor for cardioembolic stroke. Peripartum, or postpartum, cardiomyopathy (PPCM) is an uncommon cause of heart failure that develops during the last month of pregnancy or up to 5 months after giving birth in the absence of a pre-existing heart disease. It is estimated to occur in about 1 in 4000 pregnancies with approximately 1000–1300 women developing the condition in the U.S. each year. PPCM produces a dilated cardiomyopathy in which the heart's chambers enlarge and muscle weakens. This causes a decrease in the percentage of blood ejected from the left ventricle of the heart with each contraction and a subsequent reduction in cardiac output. Decreased ejection fraction can lead to pooling of blood and subsequent formation of cardiac thrombi. The presence of left ventricular thrombi is common in PPCM and can result in peripheral embolization of the clots to the brain, causing thromboembolic stroke [31]. PCCM may be difficult to detect because symptoms of heart failure can mimic those of third trimester pregnancy, such as shortness of breath, swelling in the feet, and legs. Echocardiogram is critical to detecting cardiomyopathy by uncovering the decreased ejection fraction.

PPCM is diagnosed when the following three criteria are met [32]:

- Heart failure secondary to left ventricular systolic dysfunction towards the end of pregnancy or within 5 months of delivery.
- Ejection fraction (EF) is reduced less than 45% (typically measured by an echocardiogram).
- No other cause for heart failure with reduced EF can be found.

PCCM is associated with high rate of recurrence so women with a previous history should be monitored closely during subsequent pregnancies.

Other Causes of Embolic Stroke

Embolic stroke can result from a number of other pregnancy-related causes including venous thrombosis, air embolism, and amniotic fluid embolism. The physiologic hypercoagulability of pregnancy underlies an increased rate of venous thrombosis while fluctuating intrathoracic pressure can increase the risk of a paradoxical embolus through a patent foramen ovale. Air embolism has been reported as a complication of obstetric procedures which frequently leads to hemodynamic collapse and death from pulmonary embolism. Management typically involves hyperbaric oxygen [33]. Finally, amniotic fluid embolism can develop during delivery or postpartum and, though rare, is associated with high mortality. This condition is associated with respiratory distress, hemodynamic collapse, disseminated intravascular coagulation, and, in some cases, seizures [34].

Diagnosis

Brain Imaging

Computed Tomography

Brain imaging is required when there is clinical suspicion for stroke. Given widespread access and rapid acquisition, non-contrast head computed tomography (CT) is typically the first diagnostic study utilized for suspected stroke. Potential risks of fetal malformation are limited to the first few weeks of gestation [30, 35, 36]. Radiation exposure to the fetus related to head CT is 0.05 rad which is considered safe as the accepted limit for cumulative fetal radiation exposure during pregnancy is 5 rad [37]. Additionally, there is no evidence suggesting adverse effects on lactation [38].

Iodinated CT contrast is FDA class B, with no evidence of teratogenicity or mutagenicity in animal studies [39]. However, conflicting reports suggest some association with neonatal hypothyroidism and thyroid testing should be performed during the first week in exposed neonates [40]. Despite lack of known fetal harm, iodinated contrast is only recommended if additional diagnostic information will affect the care of the pregnant women or fetus. Postdelivery, minimal iodinated CT contrast enters the mother's breast milk and is rarely absorbed across the normal gut; therefore, administration of iodinated contrast is not contraindicated during breastfeeding.

Magnetic Resonance Imaging

Magnetic resonance imaging (MRI) is more sensitive than CT in detecting early cerebral infarction, lacunar, and brainstem infarcts [41, 42]. There has been no evidence of adverse fetal effects with MRI exposure up to 3 T [43].

Gadolinium contrast is FDA class C and should be avoided during pregnancy. When benefits clearly outweigh risks and gadolinium is essential, no specific monitoring tests are required. During breastfeeding, gadolinium administration is not contraindicated. Based on radiology consensus, lactation after MRI with gadolinium can be resumed immediately, given less than 0.04% of contrast dose is excreted into breast milk within 24 h, and infants absorb less than 1% of that amount [39].

Evaluation for Stroke Mechanism

Cranio-Cervical Vessel Imaging

Non-invasive vessel imaging is emergently warranted if there is clinical suspicion for large vessel arterial occlusion for evaluation for emergent mechanical thrombectomy.

Carotid ultrasound, CT angiography (CTA), CT venography (CTV), MR angiography (MRA), MR venography (MRV) or digital subtraction angiography (DSA) can be used to investigate the underlying mechanism of ischemic stroke. MRA and MRV with gadolinium should be avoided in pregnancy. As an alternative to contrast injection, imaging of the arterial and venous circulation can be performed using time-of-flight sequences.

Echocardiogram

Transthoracic echocardiogram (TTE) is useful for detecting cardiac pathology. TTE non-invasively assesses cardiac structure, function, and EF. TTE with agitated saline can detect shunts such as patent foramen ovale (PFO) or atrial septal defect (ASD). If right to left shunt is present, lower extremity venous duplex and venography of the pelvis should be obtained to assess for deep venous thrombosis (DVT).

If there is continued clinical suspicion for cardiac pathology, invasive testing with transesophageal echocardiogram (TEE) may be considered if TTE is unrevealing. TEE is superior for evaluating the aortic arch, ascending aorta, left atrial appendage, valves, and atrial septum [44].

Laboratory Evaluation

Complete blood count, comprehensive metabolic panel including renal function and liver function testing should be completed. Laboratory testing for traditional modifiable risk factors for ischemic stroke should be completed including hemoglobin A1C and lipid panel.

Laboratory testing for inherited thrombophilia should be completed in all pregnant women presenting with cryptogenic stroke as pregnancy does not influence a genetic thrombophilia panel, despite physiologic changes in coagulation factors. Acquired thrombophilia work-up, which looks for the presence of sickle cell disease, anti-phospholipid syndrome, and protein C/S deficiencies, can also be pursued. Unfortunately, anti-phospholipid antibodies such as lupus anti-coagulant and anti-cardiolipin antibodies can be falsely elevated during pregnancy and should be reevaluated postpartum [45].

Management

Acute Reperfusion

IV Alteplase (tPA)

Tissue plasminogen activator (Alteplase; tPA) is not teratogenic based on animal studies and is too large as a molecule to cross the placenta. It is, however, classified as category C as no randomized controlled trial has included pregnant women.

Any risk associated with IV tPA in pregnancy is thought to be due to bleeding. IV tPA has a short half-life of 4–5 min, with 10% concentration remaining after 20 min. However, pregnancy was an exclusion criterion in all randomized controlled trials for IV tPA in stroke, therefore pregnancy classically been considered a relative contraindication to the use of IV tPA.

Data on intravenous thrombolytic therapy during pregnancy are limited (28 reported cases). Case reports and series on the pregnancy outcomes of women who received intravenous alteplase during all trimesters indicate that, generally, the mother experienced marked improvement following treatment and delivered a healthy baby, while the incidence of symptomatic intracerebral hemorrhage (sICH) was low, and comparable to non-pregnant patients. Overall, the safety profile appears similar to that of non-pregnant patient [46–56].

Treatment with thrombolytic agents in the early postpartum period (48 h) is more controversial, given the increased risk of bleeding. Akazawa and Nishida documented 13 cases where thrombolytics were given to women during this period [57]. The most common indication for treatment in this series was pulmonary embolus which usually requires a higher dose compared to stroke; only a single case of ischemic stroke was reported in this series. Blood transfusions were not required in all but one case [57]. Safety and efficacy of IV tPA within 14 days of delivery have not been well established [52, 53, 57]. The Canadian Stroke Best Practice Consensus Statement currently states that it is reasonable to give IV tPA to pregnant women with ischemic stroke whom are otherwise candidates for this intervention [58].

Mechanical Thrombectomy

Since pregnant women were excluded from large-scale clinical trials evaluating the efficacy of mechanical thrombectomy in acute ischemic stroke, there is a paucity of prospective data examining this procedure in this population. There are four reported cases of women treated with mechanical thrombectomy during pregnancy, all of which occurred during the third trimester [59, 60]. Second-generation devices were used in all cases. The maternal outcomes were good in three cases (modified Rankin Scale; mRS scores 0–1), with greater residual disability in the fourth case (mRS 2) [58]. The pregnancy was ongoing and healthy in one published report, while three women had delivered healthy babies. There were no cases of sICH.

Additionally, a recent, large, population-based analysis showed of 4590 pregnant and postpartum (within 6 weeks) women between 2011 and 2018, 3.9% (180) received mechanical thrombectomy. When compared with a matched cohort of non-pregnant women with stroke, pregnant and postpartum women experienced lower rates of ICH and were less likely to have poor functional outcome at discharge. Additionally, no pregnant patients experienced mortality or miscarriage during hospitalization. This large-scale clinical data is helpful in aiding clinical decision making, but further prospective trials are necessary [61].

For women with large vessel occlusion who are eligible for endovascular thrombectomy, proceeding directly to this treatment with or without IV alteplase, depending on the timing of onset, could be considered. Collaborative care from vascular neurology, neuro-critical care, neurosurgery, and obstetrics is critical for making treatment decisions regarding thrombolysis and/or thrombectomy. These interventions should currently be considered on a case-by-case basis.

Secondary Prevention of Ischemic Stroke

Modification of risk factors to reduce the risk of subsequent infarction is a mainstay of ischemic stroke management. This is accomplished generally through administration of antithrombotics, control of blood pressure, and management of hyperlipidemia.

Antithrombotics

Aspirin at a low dose (60–150 mg/day) is considered safe after the first trimester, but efforts should be made to avoid higher doses. The safety of ASA after the first trimester is well-established from trials of its use in the prevention of preeclampsia development in high-risk women, including those with recurrent fetal loss [62, 63]. Unfractionated heparin (UFH) or Low Molecular Weight Heparin (LMWH) are the agents of choice in cases requiring anticoagulation. Warfarin is contraindicated in the first trimester and not preferred during the rest of gestation due to its ability to cross the placenta and induce teratogenicity or promote fetal bleeding. The teratogenic risks of various antithrombotic agents are summarized in Table 6.3.

Hypertension

In the setting of preeclampsia or severe hypertension, the goal is to achieve an urgent and sustained reduction of systolic and diastolic blood pressure to less than 160/110 mmHg to reduce the risk of maternal stroke. That can be followed by titration of medications to lower pressure below 140/90 mmHg. The impact of blood pressure reduction on placental perfusion should be considered. Obstetrics/Maternal Fetal Medicine practitioners should be involved in ongoing assessments of the maternal-placental-fetal unit and decision making related to blood pressure lowering and the approach to fetal monitoring and surveillance where appropriate. Care must be taken to not cause hypotension or hypoperfusion [64, 65].

In pregnancy, first-line medications for blood pressure control are labetalol, methyldopa, and long acting nifedipine [66]. Selection of specific antihypertensive medication should consider side-effect profiles for the woman, fetus, or neonate. Angiotensin-converting enzyme inhibitors and angiotensin II receptor blockers—two common classes of medications used in stroke prevention—carry an increased risk of fetal complications (kidney injury) and low amniotic fluid, especially if used after the first trimester. These medications should be discontinued prior to pregnancy or as soon as a pregnancy is recognized. If they have been inadvertently taken, prompt referral to a regional center for detailed fetal structural ultrasound and counseling is encouraged. Atenolol, angiotensin-converting enzyme inhibitors, and renin direct renin inhibitors are contraindicated in pregnancy and should not be used *(Class III; Level of Evidence C)* [66]. Selected groups of antihypertensives are summarized in Table 6.4 with consideration of their maternal and fetal adverse effects.

Hyperlipidemia

Statins are contraindicated for use in pregnancy and lactation due to the lack of sufficient pregnancy data and concern for fetal/neonatal harm [67, 68]. There is no available information describing the effect of statins on breastfed infants or milk production. A recent systematic

Table 6.3 Teratogenic risks antithrombotic therapies

Antithrombotic drugs	Placental transfer	First trimester	Second and third trimester
Low-dose aspirin (60–150 mg/day)	Yes	Contraindicated (risk of gastroschisis)	Not contraindicated
Other antiplatelets	No data	No data	No data
Warfarin	Yes	Contraindicated (teratogenic)	Not preferred regular check of INR
UFH	No data	Not contraindicated risk of HIT	Not contraindicated risk of HIT regular check of aPTT
LMWH	No data	Not contraindicated	Not contraindicated
DOAC	Dabigaran: Yes rivaroxaban: Yes Apixaban: No data edoxaban: No data	No data	No data

Unfractionated heparin (UFH), or Low Molecular Weight Heparin (LMWH). Direct Oral Anticoagulant (DOAC). Heparin-induced thrombocytopenia (HIT)

Table 6.4 Summary of antihypertensive drugs used during pregnancy

Category	Maternal side effects	Teratogenicity or fetal-neonatal adverse effects	Class/level of evidence
ACE	Hyperkalemia	Skeletal and cardiovascular abnormalities, renal dysgenesis, pulmonary hypoplasia	III/C
		If prior use, refer to OB for fetal structural ultrasound, and counseling	
β-Blockers (Atenolol)	Headache	Associated with fetal growth restriction.	III/B
β-Blockers (Labetalol, Metoprolol)	Headache, may provoke asthma exacerbation	Animal studies have failed to reveal evidence of teratogenicity. Possible neonatal bradycardia	IIa/B
Calcium Channel Blockers (e.g., Nifedipine)	Headache, possible interaction with magnesium sulfate; may interfere with labor	No	I/A
Centrally acting α2-adrenergic agonist (e.g., Methyldopa)	Sedation, elevated LFTs, depression	No	IIa/C
Hydralazine	Reflex tachycardia, delayed hypotension	Neonatal thrombocytopenia, fetal bradycardia	III/B
Diuretics (thiazide)	Hypokalemia	No	III/B

ACE indicated angiotensin-converting enzyme. *LFTs* liver function tests

review failed to demonstrate a clear relationship between congenital anomalies and statin use in pregnancy, suggesting that they may not be teratogenic. However, the authors concluded that until more information is available, statins should still be avoided in pregnancy [67].

Disease-Specific Treatment

Cerebral Venous Sinus Thrombosis

For acute CVST occurring during pregnancy, consider treatment with full therapeutic doses of anticoagulation (UFH or LMWH) even in the presence of a hemorrhage with continuation for the remainder of pregnancy and for at least 6 weeks postpartum or until a postpartum switch to oral anticoagulation is feasible. Based on the guidelines of the European Federation of Neurological Societies (EFNS), in cases where patients are resistant to anticoagulation therapy, exhibit worsening of symptoms, do not have an intracranial hemorrhage, or are not at risk for herniation, endovascular thrombolysis and surgical thrombectomy may also be considered [69, 70].

A woman with a remote history of spontaneous CVST, not currently anticoagulated, can be considered for LMWH prophylaxis during pregnancy and for at least 6 weeks postpartum. Warfarin is potentially teratogenic and should be avoided especially between 6- and 12 weeks gestational age. There are insufficient data on the safety of direct oral anticoagulants (DOAC) (apixaban, dabigatran, edoxaban, and rivaroxaban) in pregnancy. Switching to LMWH is encouraged as soon as a pregnancy is identified or if pregnancy is planned. IV UFH could be considered in a hospitalized woman in place of LMWH if there is concern about need for urgent delivery or invasive procedures. A low dose, without bolus is the preferred dose in stroke patients including during pregnancy. Refer to Table 6.3 for data on relative risks of anticoagulants.

Anticoagulation should be suspended prior to administration of regional anesthesia or planned induction:

- If low-dose LMWH: stop at least 12 h prior to regional anesthesia or planned induction.
- If full-dose LMWH: stop at least 24 h prior to regional anesthesia or planned induction.

LMWH or UFH can be restarted at least 4–6 h after the removal of the neuraxial catheter if bleeding is well controlled and there are no neuraxial concerns. The regimen can then be continued for 6–12 weeks postdelivery.

If anticoagulation is required beyond 6–12 weeks postdelivery, LMWH and warfarin are both considered safe options during breastfeeding. The safety of DOACs in breastfeeding has not been established. The duration of anticoagulation is determined by results of a thrombophilia panel. Long-term anticoagulation therapy should be reconsidered in cases where patients have recurrent episodes of CVST or those who have an episode of CVST with "severe" thrombophilia. Anticoagulation during pregnancy is discussed in detail in Chap. 15.

Hypertensive Disorders of Pregnancy

The main goal for the treatment of preeclampsia, eclampsia, and HELLP syndrome is to stabilize the mother, prevent recurrent eclamptic seizures, and treat the severe hypertension to reduce or prevent cerebral edema and hemorrhage. First, prompt delivery is recommended as it is the definitive cure for preeclampsia, eclampsia, and HELLP. Antihypertensive therapy is also suggested women with systolic pressures over 140 mmHg and diastolic pressures over 90 mmHg. Magnesium sulfate (1–3 g/h) should be administered to prevent recurrent eclamptic seizures. Platelet transfusion should be administered in HELLP syndrome patients with maternal bleeding or platelet count of <20,000 cells/μL.

PPCM

Treatment of PPCM follows that of heart failure unrelated to pregnancy [32, 71]. Diuretic agents (e.g., loop diuretics) are the agents of choice for volume control. However, these agents can cause hypotension and impair uterine perfusion so caution is needed if used before delivery. Neurohormonal blockade with angiotensin-converting enzyme inhibitors or angiotensin receptor blockers should only be pursued in the postpartum due to fetal risks (see Table 6.4). A combination of organic nitrates and hydralazine

can be used instead during gestation. β-blockers as well as digoxin can be safely used during pregnancy, although the role of digoxin in the treatment of systolic heart failure is currently being debated [72, 73]. Antithrombotic agents with anticoagulation (with LMWH or UFH) are advisable during pregnancy and for the first 2 months postpartum given the high-risk of thromboembolism [74–77].

Intracranial Pressure (ICP) Management

In the setting of large vessel disease, rapid development of cerebral edema leads to intracranial hypertension, a phenomenon known as malignant cerebral infarction or edema. Elevated intracranial pressure and mass effect from intracranial hemorrhage can also result from CVST. Managing intracranial hypertension is critical to combat maternal morbidity and mortality and typically involves staged medical and surgical interventions.

Urgent management focuses on support of vital functions (Airway, Breathing and Circulation). Early intubation should be performed for patients with impaired arousal due to the associated risk of aspiration, hypoxemia, and hypercarbia.

Efforts to reduce intracranial pressure include the following:

- Elevation of the head of the bed to 30°.
- Osmotherapy: Mannitol 20% 0.25–0.5 g/kg every 4 h, or Hypertonic saline with goal osmolarity of 320.
  - Mannitol is assigned a pregnancy category C by FDA. Mannitol can cause maternal dehydration, which can lead to hypotension, uterine hypoperfusion, and fetal injury. Mannitol is only recommended for use during pregnancy when benefit outweighs risk.
- ICP monitor placement in patients with hydrocephalus or clinical deterioration secondary to

elevated ICP with goal ICP <20 mmHg and cerebral perfusion pressure

- (CPP) >70 mm Hg.
- External ventricular drainage (EVD) may be indicated in patients with or at risk for hydrocephalus.
- Neurosurgical evaluation for hemicraniectomy that is refractory to the above-described measures.

Preventing Secondary Brain Injury

Glucose

Due to increased red cell turnover, hemoglobin A1C is slightly lower in normal pregnancy than in normal non-pregnant women [78]. The American Diabetes Association (ADA) recommends a fasting glucose target <95 mg/dL and a 2-h postprandial glucose <120 mg/dL [78]. Although pregnant women were excluded from a recent large randomized trial, which failed to support using intensive glucose control in acute ischemic stroke [79], it is reasonable to maintain a glucose level of 140–180 mg/dL for pregnant women with ischemic stroke. Insulin is the preferred medication for treating hyperglycemia during pregnancy. Other oral and non-insulin injectable glucose-lowering medications lack long-term safety data [78].

Temperature

Fluctuations from normal temperature, including hyperthermia or hypothermia, should be avoided. To limit secondary injury related to fever, any concurrent infection including asymptomatic urinary tract infection should be treated.

Prevention of Other Medical Complications

Patients being treated for ischemic stroke may be hospitalized and/or immobile for extended periods, therefore increasing the risk of medical complications such as venous thromboembolism (VTE) or nosocomial infection. For the prevention of VTE formation and subsequent pulmonary or paradoxical emboli, mechanical prophylaxis and/or chemoprophylaxis should be considered. As described above, LMWH or UFH are the preferred agents for VTE prophylaxis during pregnancy. Preventative measures to reduce nosocomial infection should be taken such as minimizing use of indwelling catheters, weaning ventilation as soon as possible, and limiting antibiotic usage.

Prognosis

Maternal stroke has severe consequences with in-hospital mortality of 10–16%. It accounts for 7.4% maternal deaths in the USA [6, 20, 80, 81]. Non-fatal stroke in young women can lead to long-term disability, depression, and financial consequences, with half of the survivors having residual neurological deficits [80]. Pregnant women should undergo a similar rehabilitation program to those who are non-pregnant, with modifications as needed. The elements associated with improved functional outcome following a moderately disabling stroke include adequate intensity of therapy, task-oriented training, and excellent team coordination. It is important that the rehabilitation therapies be tailored to the tasks that need to be retrained and developed, as well as to the activities of the patient's choice and oriented to their social roles. The need for a highly coordinated, specialized team, who meet regularly to discuss the rehabilitation goals and progress, is also vital. Rehabilitation should start early during acute care following current standards of rehabilitation for stroke patients [82].

Stroke Secondary Prevention

Women who are postpartum and have previous history of stroke require education and monitoring, especially in the first 6 weeks after delivery when recurrent stroke risk rates have been reported to be highest. Following a pregnancy-related stroke, a women may also be at risk for complications in future pregnancies. The risk of recurrent stroke has been reported to be between 0 and 1.8% in a subsequent pregnancy and 0.5% in the future outside of pregnancy. This higher risk of stroke further strengthens the need to closely monitor future pregnancies. For example, women should be monitored for the presence of certain conditions such as thrombophilia or use of blood thinning medications such as aspirin.

Cerebral Venous Sinus Thrombosis

Guidelines for venous thromboembolism are most commonly followed (aspirin, or low molecular weight heparin, or both). Vascular neurology, hematology, and/or maternal fetal medicine consultation should be conducted prior to subsequent pregnancy.

Prevention of Preeclampsia [65]

Women with one or more of the following risk factors: history of preeclampsia, multifetal gestation, chronic hypertension, pre-gestational type 1 or 2 diabetes, renal disease, or autoimmune disease should initiate low dose aspirin (81 mg/day) starting between the 12th and 28th weeks of pregnancy and continue until delivery (*Class I; Level of Evidence A*) [62, 63, 66, 83, 84]. Calcium supplementation of ≥ 1 g/dL orally should be considered for women with low dietary intake of calcium (<600 mg/day) to prevent eclampsia [66].

Finally, preconception counseling should be offered to all women prior to a future pregnancy and should include the following:

- Counseling on healthy diet, regular exercise, achievement of healthy body weight, smoking cessation, alcohol cessation, and other lifestyle factors that may increase recurrent stroke risk during pregnancy.
- Address risk factors assessment, and pharmacological management.

- Review stroke etiology, and optimal treatment.
- Review current medications to evaluate for potential teratogenicity using available reference databases.
- Multidisciplinary approach to maternal-fetal care, including maternal-fetal medicine specialists, and stroke neurologists.

Delivery Considerations After Stroke

Delivery after pregnancy-related stroke should be guided by obstetric indications. History of stroke is not a contraindication for vaginal delivery. Valsalva-related hemodynamic changes can be minimized with an assisted second stage of labor and appropriate analgesia. Cesarean delivery has not been shown to improve outcomes and is associated with an increased risk of peripartum stroke of all types [3]. Epidural anesthesia is safe with aspirin 81 mg. A multidisciplinary approach to maternal-fetal care after stroke is recommended, including maternal-fetal medicine specialists, stroke neurologists, and obstetric anesthesiologists.

Contraceptive Options After Stroke

All hormones increase the risk of venous or arterial thromboembolism with the risk increased in women with underlying thrombogenic mutations. Although stroke risk with combined oral contraceptive is 1.7–2.0 times that of non-users, progestin-only contraception including pills, implants, injectables, and intrauterine devices did not show an increased risk. Progesterone-only pills, progesterone-only or non-hormonal intrauterine devices or barrier contraception are considered safe in women with history of stroke [70]. Further studies need to be done to understand the risk of other methods in women with prior stroke.

Summary

Understanding the various risk factors and etiologies can lead to a better approach for diagnosis and disease-specific treatment strategies to address neurological conditions in pregnant women. Additionally, further understanding will allow healthcare professionals to better assist patients as they address these neurological conditions and obstetrics. Given the role of ischemic strokes in pregnancy-related morbidity and mortality, further assessment and careful monitoring of risk factors can help guide timely and effective interventions and treatment decisions.

References

1. Persky RW, Turtzo LC, McCullough LD. Stroke in women: disparities and outcomes. Curr Cardiol Rep. 2010;12(1):6–13.
2. Petitti DB, Sidney S, Quesenberry CP Jr, Bernstein A. Incidence of stroke and myocardial infarction in women of reproductive age. Stroke. 1997;28(2):280–3.
3. James AH, Bushnell CD, Jamison MG, Myers ER. Incidence and risk factors for stroke in pregnancy and the puerperium. Obstet Gynecol. 2005;106(3):509–16.
4. Davie CA, O'Brien P. Stroke and pregnancy. J Neurol Neurosurg Psychiatry. 2008;79(3):240–5.
5. Scott CA, Bewley S, Rudd A, Spark P, Kurinczuk JJ, Brocklehurst P, et al. Incidence, risk factors, management, and outcomes of stroke in pregnancy. Obstet Gynecol. 2012;120(2 Pt 1):318–24.
6. Swartz RH, Cayley ML, Foley N, Ladhani NNN, Leffert L, Bushnell C, et al. The incidence of pregnancy-related stroke: a systematic review and meta-analysis. Int J Stroke. 2017;12(7):687–97.
7. Elgendy IY, Bukhari S, Barakat AF, Pepine CJ, Lindley KJ, Miller EC. Maternal stroke: a call for action. Circulation. 2021;143(7):727–38.
8. Kuklina EV, Tong X, Bansil P, George MG, Callaghan WM. Trends in pregnancy hospitalizations that included a stroke in the United States from 1994 to 2007: reasons for concern? Stroke. 2011;42(9):2564–70.
9. Salonen Ros H, Lichtenstein P, Bellocco R, Petersson G, Cnattingius S. Increased risks of circulatory diseases in late pregnancy and puerperium. Epidemiology. 2001;12(4):456–60.
10. Kittner SJ, Stern BJ, Feeser BR, Hebel R, Nagey DA, Buchholz DW, et al. Pregnancy and the risk of stroke. N Engl J Med. 1996;335(11):768–74.
11. Sankaran S. Creasy and Resnik's maternal–fetal medicine: principles and practice sixth edition. Obstet Med. 2012;5(2):88–9.
12. Katz D, Beilin Y. Disorders of coagulation in pregnancy. Br J Anaesth. 2015;115 Suppl 2:ii75–88.
13. Ives CW, Sinkey R, Rajapreyar I, Tita ATN, Oparil S. Preeclampsia-pathophysiology and clinical presentations: JACC state-of-the-art review. J Am Coll Cardiol. 2020;76(14):1690–702.
14. Abimanyu B. The role of angiogenic factors in preeclampsia. Pregnancy Hypertens. 2014;4(3):246.
15. Maynard SE, Karumanchi SA. Angiogenic factors and preeclampsia. Semin Nephrol. 2011;31(1):33–46.
16. Roberts JM, Lain KY. Recent insights into the pathogenesis of pre-eclampsia. Placenta. 2002;23(5):359–72.
17. Zhou Y, Damsky CH, Fisher SJ. Preeclampsia is associated with failure of human cytotrophoblasts to mimic a vascular adhesion phenotype. One cause of defective endovascular invasion in this syndrome? J Clin Invest. 1997;99(9):2152–64.
18. Miller EC, Wen T, Elkind MSV, Friedman AM, Boehme AK. Infection during delivery hospitalization and risk of readmission for postpartum stroke. Stroke. 2019;50(10):2685–91.
19. Redman CW, Sacks GP, Sargent IL. Preeclampsia: an excessive maternal inflammatory response to pregnancy. Am J Obstet Gynecol. 1999;180(2 Pt 1):499–506.
20. Lanska DJ, Kryscio RJ. Risk factors for peripartum and postpartum stroke and intracranial venous thrombosis. Stroke. 2000;31(6):1274–82.
21. Miller EC, Gallo M, Kulick ER, Friedman AM, Elkind MSV, Boehme AK. Infections and risk of peripartum stroke during delivery admissions. Stroke. 2018;49(5):1129–34.
22. Wabnitz A, Bushnell C. Migraine, cardiovascular disease, and stroke during pregnancy: systematic review of the literature. Cephalalgia. 2015;35(2):132–9.
23. Saposnik G, Barinagarrementeria F, Brown RD Jr, Bushnell CD, Cucchiara B, Cushman M, et al. Diagnosis and management of cerebral venous thrombosis: a statement for healthcare professionals from the American Heart Association/American Stroke Association. Stroke. 2011;42(4):1158–92.
24. Tranquilli AL, Dekker G, Magee L, et al. The classification, diagnosis and management of the hypertensive disorders of pregnancy: a revised statement from the ISSHP. Pregnancy Hypertens. 2014;4:97–104.
25. Brown MA, Magee LA, Kenny LC, Karumanchi SA, McCarthy FP, Saito S, et al. Hypertensive disorders of pregnancy: ISSHP classification, diagnosis, and management recommendations for international practice. Hypertension. 2018;72(1):24–43.
26. Gestational hypertension and preeclampsia: ACOG practice bulletin, number 222. Obstet Gynecol. 2020;135(6):e237–60.
27. Lo JO, Mission JF, Caughey AB. Hypertensive disease of pregnancy and maternal mortality. Curr Opin Obstet Gynecol. 2013;25(2):124–32.

28. Duckitt K, Harrington D. Risk factors for pre-eclampsia at antenatal booking: systematic review of controlled studies. BMJ. 2005;330(7491):565.
29. Bellos I, Fitrou G, Daskalakis G, Papantoniou N, Pergialiotis V. Serum cystatin-c as predictive factor of preeclampsia: a meta-analysis of 27 observational studies. Pregnancy Hypertens. 2019;16:97–104.
30. Hall EJ. Scientific view of low-level radiation risks. Radiographics. 1991;11(3):509–18.
31. Sliwa K, Skudicky D, Bergemann A, Candy G, Puren A, Sareli P. Peripartum cardiomyopathy: analysis of clinical outcome, left ventricular function, plasma levels of cytokines and Fas/APO-1. J Am Coll Cardiol. 2000;35(3):701–5.
32. Davis MB, Arany Z, McNamara DM, Goland S, Elkayam U. Peripartum cardiomyopathy: JACC state-of-the-art review. J Am Coll Cardiol. 2020;75(2):207–21.
33. Kim CS, Liu J, Kwon JY, Shin SK, Kim KJ. Venous air embolism during surgery, especially cesarean delivery. J Korean Med Sci. 2008;23(5):753–61.
34. Shamshirsaz AA, Clark SL. Amniotic fluid embolism. Obstet Gynecol Clin N Am. 2016;43(4):779–90.
35. Yamazaki JN, Schull WJ. Perinatal loss and neurological abnormalities among children of the atomic bomb. Nagasaki and Hiroshima revisited, 1949 to 1989. JAMA. 1990;264(5):605–9.
36. Otake M, Schull WJ. In utero exposure to A-bomb radiation and mental retardation; a reassessment. Br J Radiol. 1984;57(677):409–14.
37. Jain C. ACOG Committee Opinion No. 723: guidelines for diagnostic imaging during pregnancy and lactation. Obstet Gynecol. 2019;133(1):186.
38. Committee Opinion No. 723: guidelines for diagnostic imaging during pregnancy and lactation: correction. Obstet Gynecol. 2018;132(3):786.
39. Webb JA, Thomsen HS, Morcos SK. The use of iodinated and gadolinium contrast media during pregnancy and lactation. Eur Radiol. 2005;15(6):1234–40.
40. Lee SY, Rhee CM, Leung AM, Braverman LE, Brent GA, Pearce EN. A review: radiographic iodinated contrast media-induced thyroid dysfunction. J Clin Endocrinol Metab. 2015;100(2):376–83.
41. Khalid AS, Hadbavna A, Williams D, Byrne B. A review of stroke in pregnancy: incidence, investigations and management. Obstet Gynaecol. 2020;22(1):21–33.
42. Kertesz A, Black SE, Nicholson L, Carr T. The sensitivity and specificity of MRI in stroke. Neurology. 1987;37(10):1580–5.
43. Smajlović D, Sinanović O. Sensitivity of the neuroimaging techniques in ischemic stroke. Med Arh. 2004;58(5):282–4.
44. Fischer M, Schmutzhard E. Posterior reversible encephalopathy syndrome. J Neurol. 2017;264(8):1608–16.
45. Grear KE, Bushnell CD. Stroke and pregnancy. clinical presentation, evaluation, treatment and epidemiology. Clin Obstet Gynecol. 2013;56(2):350.
46. Kamphuisen PW, Eikenboom JC, Bertina RM. Elevated factor VIII levels and the risk of thrombosis. Arterioscler Thromb Vasc Biol. 2001;21(5):731–8.
47. Elford K, Leader A, Wee R, Stys PK. Stroke in ovarian hyperstimulation syndrome in early pregnancy treated with intra-arterial rt-PA. Neurology. 2002;59(8):1270–2.
48. Li Y, Margraf J, Kluck B, Jenny D, Castaldo J. Thrombolytic therapy for ischemic stroke secondary to paradoxical embolism in pregnancy: a case report and literature review. Neurologist. 2012;18(1):44–8.
49. Tversky S, Libman RB, Reppucci ML, Tufano AM, Katz JM. Thrombolysis for ischemic stroke during pregnancy: a case report and review of the literature. J Stroke Cerebrovasc Dis. 2016;25(10):e167–70.
50. Wiese KM, Talkad A, Mathews M, Wang D. Intravenous recombinant tissue plasminogen activator in a pregnant woman with cardioembolic stroke. Stroke. 2006;37(8):2168–9.
51. Tassi R, Acampa M, Marotta G, Cioni S, Guideri F, Rossi S, et al. Systemic thrombolysis for stroke in pregnancy. Am J Emerg Med. 2013;31(2):448.e1–3.
52. Landais A, Chaumont H, Dellis R. Thrombolytic therapy of acute ischemic stroke during early pregnancy. J Stroke Cerebrovasc Dis. 2018;27(2):e20–3.
53. DeKoninck PL, Pijnenborg JM, van Zutphen SW, Arnoldus EP. Postpartum stroke, a diagnostic challenge. Am J Emerg Med. 2008;26(7):843.e3–4.
54. Rønning OM, Dahl A, Bakke SJ, Hussain AI, Deilkås E. Stroke in the puerperium treated with intra-arterial rt-PA. J Neurol Neurosurg Psychiatry. 2010;81(5):585–6.
55. Johnson DM, Kramer DC, Cohen E, Rochon M, Rosner M, Weinberger J. Thrombolytic therapy for acute stroke in late pregnancy with intra-arterial recombinant tissue plasminogen activator. Stroke. 2005;36(6):e53–5.
56. Mantoan Ritter L, Schüler A, Gangopadhyay R, Mordecai L, Arowele O, Losseff N, et al. Successful thrombolysis of stroke with intravenous alteplase in the third trimester of pregnancy. J Neurol. 2014;261(3):632–4.
57. Ritchie J, Lokman M, Panikkar J. Thrombolysis for stroke in pregnancy at 39 weeks gestation with a subsequent normal delivery. BMJ Case Rep. 2015;2015:bcr2015209563.
58. Akazawa M, Nishida M. Thrombolysis with intravenous recombinant tissue plasminogen activator during early postpartum period: a review of the literature. Acta Obstet Gynecol Scand. 2017;96(5):529–35.
59. Bhogal P, Aguilar M, AlMatter M, Karck U, Bäzner H, Henkes H. Mechanical thrombectomy in pregnancy: report of 2 cases and review of the literature. Interv Neurol. 2017;6(1–2):49–56.
60. Aaron S, Shyamkumar NK, Alexander S, Babu PS, Prabhakar AT, Moses V, et al. Mechanical thrombectomy for acute ischemic stroke in pregnancy using the penumbra system. Ann Indian Acad Neurol. 2016;19(2):261–3.

61. Dicpinigaitis AJ, et al. Endovascular thrombectomy for treatment of acute ischemic stroke during pregnancy and the early postpartum period. Stroke. 2021;52(12):3796–804.

62. Rolnik DL, et al. Aspirin versus placebo in pregnancies at high risk for preterm preeclampsia. N Engl J Med. 2017;377(7):613–22.

63. Stevens W, Shih T, Incerti D, Ton TGN, Lee HC, Peneva D, et al. Short-term costs of preeclampsia to the United States health care system. Am J Obstet Gynecol. 2017;217(3):237–48.e16.

64. Butalia S, Audibert F, Côté AM, Firoz T, Logan AG, Magee LA, et al. Hypertension Canada's 2018 guidelines for the management of hypertension in pregnancy. Can J Cardiol. 2018;34(5):526–31.

65. Nerenberg KA, Zarnke KB, Leung AA, Dasgupta K, Butalia S, McBrien K, et al. Hypertension Canada's 2018 guidelines for diagnosis, risk assessment, prevention, and treatment of hypertension in adults and children. Can J Cardiol. 2018;34(5):506–25.

66. Bushnell C, McCullough LD, Awad IA, Chireau MV, Fedder WN, Furie KL, et al. Guidelines for the prevention of stroke in women: a statement for healthcare professionals from the American Heart Association/American Stroke Association. Stroke. 2014;45(5):1545–88.

67. Kazmin A, Garcia-Bournissen F, Koren G. Risks of statin use during pregnancy: a systematic review. J Obstet Gynaecol Can. 2007;29(11):906–8.

68. Karalis DG, Hill AN, Clifton S, Wild RA. The risks of statin use in pregnancy: a systematic review. J Clin Lipidol. 2016;10(5):1081–90.

69. Chan WS, Rey E, Kent NE, Chan WS, Kent NE, Rey E, et al. Venous thromboembolism and antithrombotic therapy in pregnancy. J Obstet Gynaecol Can. 2014;36(6):527–53.

70. Swartz RH, Ladhani NNN, Foley N, Nerenberg K, Bal S, Barrett J, et al. Canadian stroke best practice consensus statement: secondary stroke prevention during pregnancy. Int J Stroke. 2018;13(4):406–19.

71. Arany Z, Elkayam U. Peripartum cardiomyopathy. Circulation. 2016;133(14):1397–409.

72. Cleland JG, Cullington D. Digoxin: quo vadis? Circ Heart Fail. 2009;2(2):81–5.

73. Chaggar PS, Shaw SM, Williams SG. Is foxglove effective in heart failure? Cardiovasc Ther. 2015;33(4):236–41.

74. Altuwaijri WA, Kirkpatrick ID, Jassal DS, Soni A. Vanishing left ventricular thrombus in a woman with peripartum cardiomyopathy: a case report. BMC Res Notes. 2012;5:544.

75. Shimamoto T, Marui A, Oda M, Tomita S, Nakajima H, Takeuchi T, et al. A case of peripartum cardiomyopathy with recurrent left ventricular apical thrombus. Circ J. 2008;72(5):853–4.

76. Kharwar RB, Chandra S, Dwivedi SK, Saran RK. A pedunculated left ventricular thrombus in a women with peripartum cardiomyopathy: evaluation by three dimensional echocardiography. J Cardiovasc Ultrasound. 2014;22(3):139–43.

77. Kim DY, Islam S, Mondal NT, Mussell F, Rauchholz M. Biventricular thrombi associated with peripartum cardiomyopathy. J Health Popul Nutr. 2011;29(2):178–80.

78. American Diabetes Association. Management of diabetes in pregnancy: standards of medical care in diabetes-2020. Diabetes Care. 2020;43(Suppl 1):S183–92.

79. Johnston KC, Bruno A, Pauls Q, Hall CE, Barrett KM, Barsan W, et al. Intensive vs standard treatment of hyperglycemia and functional outcome in patients with acute ischemic stroke: the SHINE randomized clinical trial. JAMA. 2019;322(4):326–35.

80. Leffert LR, Clancy CR, Bateman BT, Cox M, Schulte PJ, Smith EE, et al. Patient characteristics and outcomes after hemorrhagic stroke in pregnancy. Circ Cardiovasc Qual Outcomes. 2015;8(6 Suppl 3):S170–8.

81. Creanga AA, Syverson C, Seed K, Callaghan WM. Pregnancy-related mortality in the United States, 2011-2013. Obstet Gynecol. 2017;130(2):366–73.

82. Hebert D, Lindsay MP, McIntyre A, Kirton A, Rumney PG, Bagg S, et al. Canadian stroke best practice recommendations: stroke rehabilitation practice guidelines, update 2015. Int J Stroke. 2016;11(4):459–84.

83. Werner EF, Hauspurg AK, Rouse DJ. A cost-benefit analysis of low-dose aspirin prophylaxis for the prevention of preeclampsia in the United States. Obstet Gynecol. 2015;126(6):1242–50.

84. Wright D, Poon LC, Rolnik DL, Syngelaki A, Delgado JL, Vojtassakova D, et al. Aspirin for evidence-based preeclampsia prevention trial: influence of compliance on beneficial effect of aspirin in prevention of preterm preeclampsia. Am J Obstet Gynecol. 2017;217(6):685.e1–5.

Pregnancy and Hemorrhagic Stroke

7

Mena Samaan, Deepika Dhawan, Linda Ye, Ramandeep Sahni, and Fawaz Al-Mufti

Introduction

Stroke is the most common cause of long-term disability and a leading cause of death. Intracranial hemorrhage during pregnancy is a rare, yet severe pathology that occurs in 0.002–0.05% of all pregnancies [1–3]. In fact, intracranial hemorrhage is responsible for 5–12% of all maternal deaths [4, 5]. Intracerebral hemorrhage, specifically, was demonstrated in a 2006 study to account for 7.1% of all pregnancy-related mortality [3, 5]. Though rare, pregnant women are more prone to developing strokes than their non-pregnant counterparts underscoring the importance of screening and controlling risk factors. This increased risk of stroke is highest during the puerperium.

Pathophysiology

A number of physiologic and pathologic changes occurring during pregnancy contribute to the elevated risk of hemorrhagic stroke. Alterations in vascular tone, coagulation factors, and cardiovascular and cerebrovascular changes are briefly discussed below. Additional information on coagulation factors and cardiovascular changes accompanying pregnancy are provided in Chaps. 20 and 5, respectively.

Vascular Tone

Changes in connective tissue during pregnancy contribute to the increased risk of hemorrhagic stroke in pregnant women. Several animal models have shown that cerebrovasculature architectural changes occur during pregnancy, leading to decreased collagen, elasticity, and distensibility [5]. Although unclear on how these changes translate to humans, the cerebral arteries may not be able to compensate for the hypervolemia and increased cardiac demands, which could theoretically lead to increased risk of hemorrhagic infarctions [6].

Additionally, disturbance in the cerebral autoregulation system because of chronic hyperventilation during pregnancy may lead to higher cerebral perfusion pressures and cause further blood vessel damage. During pregnancy, the

M. Samaan · R. Sahni
Department of Neurology, Westchester Medical Center, New York Medical College,
Valhalla, NY, USA

D. Dhawan · L. Ye
Department of Neurosurgery, Westchester Medical Center, New York Medical College,
Valhalla, NY, USA

F. Al-Mufti (✉)
Department of Neurology, Neurosurgery and Radiology, New York Medical College - Westchester Medical Center, Valhalla, NY, USA

© The Author(s), under exclusive license to Springer Nature Switzerland AG 2023
G. Gupta et al. (eds.), *Neurological Disorders in Pregnancy*,
https://doi.org/10.1007/978-3-031-36490-7_7

increased susceptibility to forced dilation of cerebral blood vessels may be due to a variety of factors. Gestation-induced changes in the smooth muscle calcium-activated potassium channels, channels that regulate the arterial tone and pressure at which forced dilation occurs, have been shown in the myometrium [7]. It is possible that the same changes occur in the cerebral circulation [7]. Another factor that may increase the susceptibility to forced dilation during pregnancy is alterations in the state of actin polymerization in cerebrovascular smooth muscle [7]. This may lower the pressure at which forced dilation occurs [7].

Preeclampsia and eclampsia, a spectrum of pregnancy-related syndromes that are major risk factors for hemorrhagic stroke, has been associated with altered cerebrovascular activity and autoregulatory failure that causes forced dilation of the cerebral arteries and arterioles [8]. Patients in late pregnancy and postpartum period have been found to have dilation of their posterior cerebral artery at much lower pressures when compared to non-pregnant patients [8]. These alterations also lead to decreased cerebrovascular resistance and hyperperfusion, which would thereby increase the pressure in the microcirculation [8]. While these changes are more prominent in eclampsia patients, normal pregnancies also exhibit progressive increase in cerebral perfusion pressure, decreased cerebrovascular resistance, and a shifted autoregulatory curve to the lower range of pressures [8].

In preeclampsia, evidence suggests that placental antiangiogenic factors, specifically soluble fms-related tyrosine kinase 1 and soluble endoglin are upregulated and disrupt the maternal endothelium, which can result in hypertension, proteinuria, and glomerular endotheliosis [9]. The regulation of these antiangiogenic factors in the placenta is unknown; however, this is an area that is currently being tested to predict and diagnose preeclampsia as well as identify therapeutic targets. Other possible mechanisms include reduced placental perfusion, aberrant trophoblast (blastocyst cell) invasion into the uterus and uterine spiral arteries, and excessive intravascular inflammatory response to placental tissue [7, 10, 11]. Fluctuating blood pressure may also play a significant role as it leads to variable degrees of vasospasm and vasodilation.

Coagulation Factors

Although the physiological changes favor the development of a hypercoagulable state, in late pregnancy these changes can contribute to that develops in late pregnancy to risk of cerebral venous sinus thrombosis which can present with hemorrhagic venous infarct. The role of the coagulation cascade in stroke in pregnancy was described in greater detail in Chap. 6: (Pregnancy and Ischemic stroke).

Cardiovascular Hemodynamics

Pregnancy is considered a stress test of the maternal cardiovascular system. Changes in cardiovascular hemodynamics include increased blood volume and cardiac output by 30–50%, lower peripheral vascular resistance due to increased compliance, and increased left ventricular mass with eccentric remodeling, in addition to changes in coagulation factors (Table 7.1) [10].

Table 7.1 Hemodynamic changes in pregnancy [12]

Hemodynamic parameter	Change at term pregnancy (% change)
Cardiac Output (L/min)	Up to 45% Increase
Systolic Blood Pressure (mmHg)	Decreased in first and second trimester, increased in third trimester
Diastolic Blood Pressure (mmHg)	Decreased up to 10% in first and second trimester, increased in third trimester
Mean Arterial Pressure (mmHg)	Decreased up to 10% in first and second trimester, increased in third trimester
Sympathetic Vasomotor Activity	Increased baroreceptor sensitivity and responsiveness to alpha-adrenergic stimulation
Renin-Angiotensin-Aldosterone System	Decreased plasma osmolality and hyponatremic hypervolemia occurs
Atrial natriuretic peptide	Increase by 40% to third trimester and 50% first week postpartum
Total Blood Volume	Average 45% increase up to 100%
Red Blood Cell Mass	Up to 40% increase
Left Ventricular Wall Thickness	Up to 28% increase
Left Ventricular Wall Mass	Up to 52% increase
Right Ventricular Wall Mass	Up to 40% increase

Risk Factors

The most common cause of subarachnoid hemorrhage (SAH) or intracerebral hemorrhage during pregnancy or the postpartum is due to either aneurysmal rupture or bleeding from an arteriovenous malformation (AVM) [5]. One recent study found that of 154 cases of intracranial hemorrhage, 77% were due to ruptured aneurysm and 23% were due to ruptured AVM. The incidence of aneurysmal ruptures increases progressively throughout the three trimesters of gestation, with the highest incidence rate during the third trimester [4, 5]. In detailing timing, it has been found that 55% of aneurysm ruptures in pregnancy happen during the third trimester, 31% in the second trimester, 6% in the first trimester, and 8% in the postpartum period [5].

The data surrounding the increased risk of aneurysm rupture during pregnancy is controversial and numerous studies have attempted to determine the cause of increased risk. Autopsy and angiographic studies have documented a higher prevalence of cerebral aneurysms in women, as well as a higher risk of rupture [13–15]. There is also a difference in the distribution of aneurysm locations in women versus men. A recent retrospective observational study found that aneurysms in women were more likely to occur at the internal carotid artery and the posterior communicating artery, while aneurysms in men most commonly occurred in the anterior cerebral artery. These data suggest an influence of hormonal factors, which could contribute to a higher hemorrhage risk [16].

Similarly, whether pregnancy and the puerperium truly increase the risk of AVM rupture is a topic of ongoing debate. Some studies have reported the odds for rupture of AVM during pregnancy and puerperium being significantly lower compared with the control period [17]. In contrast, a recent retrospective cohort reported a significant increase in the risk of AVM rupture among women with AVM who became pregnant before obliteration. In this study, the annual rate of hemorrhage was 5.7% in pregnant women compared with 1.3% in non-pregnant women [18].

Other common causes of hemorrhagic stroke in pregnant patients are preeclampsia, eclampsia, and/or HELLP syndrome [5]. Preeclampsia or eclampsia account for roughly 30% of intracranial hemorrhages during pregnancy [4].

Etiology

Aneurysms and Arteriovenous Malformations (AVMs)

Aneurysms result from the weakening of arterial walls, which leads to the enlargement or outpouching of affected vessels. Aneurysms can leak or rupture into their surroundings, leading to SAH. Aneurysmal SAH (aSAH) presents clinically with thunderclap headache, nuchal rigidity, nausea, vomiting, seizures, and decreased levels of consciousness. Patients with aSAH often have complex hospital courses with post-insult complications including hydrocephalus and vasospasm [10].

AVM is a congenital abnormality characterized by the formation of tangled, malformed vessels with bypassing of capillary networks. The direct connection of arteries and veins can result in higher pressures being transmitted to abnormally formed, weakened blood vessels which then rupture. AVMs are important causes of hemorrhagic stroke with one review demonstrating that these malformations accounted for intracerebral hemorrhage in 3 out of 14 patients [19]. It is estimated that 50% of AVMs present with intracranial hemorrhage, with prior hemorrhage being associated with a high risk of rebleeding [18]. Hemorrhage can occur within the parenchyma of the brain (intracerebral hemorrhage), in the subarachnoid space (SAH), or in the ventricles (intraventricular hemorrhage; IVH). Symptoms can be similar to that of aSAH. Notably, SAH from AVM is usually less severe than aneurysmal SAH (aSAH) and only infrequently results in vasospasm. In patients younger than 45 years old presenting with lobar hemorrhage, the most likely cause is AVM rupture. Among the 50% of patients without hemorrhage, the most common presentations are: seizures (16–53%), headache (7–48%), and focal progressive (stroke like symptoms 1–40%), deficit.

Aneurysms and AVMs in pregnancy are discussed in detail in Chaps. 8 and 9.

Cerebral Venous Sinus Thrombosis (CVST)

CVST occurs in 9.1 per 100,000 pregnancies (95% CI of 4.3–18.9) [20]. The risk of CVST in pregnancy is increased, although pregnancy-associated CVST has a better prognosis than CVST from other etiologies. In the first trimester, the risk may be attributed to underlying thrombophilia, but the risk is most increased in the first 4–8 weeks postpartum [21]. When CVST occurs,

it impedes venous outflow resulting in dangerous venous congestion and risk of non-hemorrhagic or hemorrhagic ischemia or intracerebral hemorrhage. Parenchymal lesions caused by CVST display specific anatomic patterns that are determined by the site of venous occlusion. The sites most commonly affected according to the International Study on Cerebral Venous and Dural Sinuses Thrombosis ($n = 624$) are as follows: (1) Superior Sagittal Sinus: 62%, (2) Transverse (Lateral) Sinus: 41–45%, and (3) Straight Sinus: 18% [21]. The deep venous system can also be affected in 11%, as well as internal jugular vein in 12% of patients. If the deep cerebral vein (or the draining straight sinus) is involved, infarcts can involve the globus pallidi [22–24].

The most common clinical findings of CVST include:

- Intracranial hypertension (headache in 90% of patients, and papilledema).
- Focal neurologic deficits (e.g., motor weakness, sensory deficit, aphasia),
- Encephalopathy.
- Seizures (30–50%)

Clinically, a patient with CVST presents with symptoms of increased intracranial pressure (ICP), a focal brain lesion, or both. A headache is one of the most common symptoms and in some cases, the only symptom. Other symptoms include craniofacial pain, seizures, motor weakness, visual field loss, and sensory symptoms.

CVST and ischemic stroke is discussed in Chap. 20. A detailed discussion of CVST in pregnancy is provided in Chap. 11.

Hypertensive Disorders of Pregnancy

Hypertensive disorders of pregnancy are the leading cause of maternal stroke [25]. There are three different types of hypertension that occur during pregnancy:

- Chronic Hypertension: High blood pressure (>140/90 mmHg) that is present before pregnancy, presents before week 20 in pregnancy, or that continues after delivery.

- Gestational Hypertension: High blood pressure that develops after week 20 of pregnancy and resolves after delivery. Also referred to as pregnancy-induced hypertension (PIH).
- Preeclampsia: De-novo hypertension that presents after 20 weeks of gestation combined with proteinuria (>300 mg/day), other maternal organ dysfunction, such as renal insufficiency, liver involvement, neurological or hematological complications, uteroplacental dysfunction, or fetal growth restriction [26].

Elevated SBP in particular has been shown to be a more important indicator in evaluating stroke risk than DBP. Martin et al. found that in 95.8% of the patients, the SBP was at or greater than 160 mmHg right before the onset of a stroke while only 11% of patients exhibited DBP within the same severity range (≥110 mmHg) [27]. This emphasizes the importance of closely monitoring and controlling SBP to mitigate stroke risk.

Preeclampsia and Eclampsia

Preeclampsia is a systemic syndrome that complicates approximately 2–5% of pregnancies.

It is well established that women with a history of preeclampsia, chronic hypertension and gestational hypertension are at increased risk for preeclampsia recurrence. A recent large study which included 40,673 women has identified additional risk factors associated with preeclampsia during subsequent pregnancies. These included obesity and diagnosis of gestational diabetes mellitus, which are independent from their age and inter-pregnancy interval. History of preterm delivery, perinatal mortality or low birthweight also showed association with higher risk for preeclampsia in subsequent pregnancies [25, 28]. Preeclampsia classically manifests as new onset of hypertension with systolic blood pressure (SBP) at or over 140 mmHg and diastolic blood pressure (DBP) at or over 90 mmHg on at least two occasions over a period of 4 h, and either proteinuria (>0.3 g protein in 24 h urine specimen) or end-organ dysfunction after

20 weeks of gestation in a previously normotensive woman. Preeclampsia is a leading cause of maternal and neonatal morbidity and mortality and can progress into the devastating condition, eclampsia. Guidelines for diagnosis of preeclampsia are summarized in Table 7.2.

Eclampsia is a complication of 1–2% of severe preeclampsia cases in which the pregnant or recently delivered woman presents with new-onset seizures or coma in addition to preeclampsia symptoms [27]. The frequency of hemorrhagic stroke in patients with eclampsia is high, with one studying finding that 89% of women with preeclampsia/eclampsia had hemorrhagic stroke. Eclampsia accounts for roughly one-third of all hemorrhagic strokes during pregnancy and is the main cause of intraparenchymal hemorrhages during pregnancy largely due to severe hypertension [31]. One study of 31 subjects found that eclampsia accounted for 44% of intraparenchymal hemorrhages, often with poor maternal prognosis [31]. Additionally, preeclampsia/eclampsia can be complicated by HELLP Syndrome, which involves a constellation of hemolysis, elevated liver enzymes, and low platelets from which the syndrome is named. Preeclampsia and eclampsia are described in detail in Chap. 12.

Clinical presentation of stroke during preeclampsia/eclampsia most commonly includes severe headache. It is a key symptom in the early diagnosis of stroke in the puerperium period. Impairment of consciousness is another common symptom of preeclampsia-associated hemorrhagic stroke.

In 2013, the American College of Obstetricians and Gynecologists (ACOG) removed proteinuria as an essential criterion for diagnosis of preeclampsia and included other maternal organ dysfunction (as outlined in the Table 7.2). Moreover, the International Society for the Study of Hypertension in Pregnancy (ISSHP) endorsed that there should be no attempt to diagnose mild versus severe preeclampsia clinically as all cases may become emergencies, often rapidly [30].

Severe features of preeclampsia indicating systemic dysfunction as outlined by ACOG are the following: [29]

Table 7.2 Preeclampsia diagnostic criteria from ACOG and ISSHP criteria

	ACOG (2019 Revision) [29]	ISSHP (2018 Revision) [30]
New onset, persistent hypertension ≥20 weeks in a women with previously normal BP and	• SBP ≥140 mmHg or DBP ≥90 mmHg on 2 occasions ≥4 h apart or • SBP of ≥160 mmHg or DBP ≥110 mmHg confirmed within a short interval (minutes)	
Proteinuria	≥300 mg per 24-h urine collection or Protein/Creatinine ratio of ≥0.3 or Urine Dipstick reading of 2+	
Or In absence of proteinuria, new onset of:	• Renal insufficiency (Serum Creatinine >1.1 mg/dL or doubling of serum Creatinine in absence of other renal disease)	• Acute kidney injury (Serum Creatinine >1 mg/dL)
	• Impaired liver function (LFTs elevated twice normal)	• Liver involvement (elevated LFTs with or without RUQ or epigastric pain)
	• Thrombocytopenia (Platelets < 100)	• Hematological complications (platelets <150K, DIC, hemolysis)
	• New-onset headache (Unresponsive to medication and not accounted for by alternative diagnoses or visual symptoms)	• Neurological complications (eclampsia, altered mental status, blindness, stroke, clonus, severe headaches, persistent visual scotomata)
	• Pulmonary edema	• Uteroplacental dysfunction (fetal growth restriction, abnormal umbilical artery Doppler wave form analysis, or stillbirth)

RUQ right upper quadrant, *DIC* disseminated intravascular coagulation, *LFTs* liver function tests, *ACOG* American College of Obstetricians and Gynecologists, *ISSHP* International Society for the Study of Hypertension in Pregnancy

- Thrombocytopenia (Platelet count <100 × 10⁹/L),
- Impaired liver function tests (to twice the upper limit of normal concentration) or severe persistent right upper quadrant or epigastric pain and not accounted for by alternative diagnoses.
- Renal insufficiency (Creatinine >1.1 mg/dL or doubling of Creatinine in absence of other renal disease)
- Pulmonary edema.
- New-onset headache unresponsive to acetaminophen and not accounted for by alternative diagnoses or visual disturbances.

Postpartum Angiopathy (PPA)

Postpartum angiopathy is generally grouped under the overarching category of reversible cerebral vasoconstriction syndromes (RCVS) and is characterized by narrowing of the cerebral arteries without the presence of inflammation. Previous terms for the same disorder include benign angiopathy of the CNS, Call–Fleming syndrome, crash migraine, drug-induced arteritis, eclampsia-associated vasoconstriction, drug-induced angiitis, migraine angiitis, and CNS pseudovasculitis. PPA has a variety of clinical presentations including headache, focal neurological deficit, and seizures, but most often presents as multiple attacks of bilateral throbbing thunderclap headaches. These headaches are a presenting feature in 94% of cases over a mean period of 1 week and may occur spontaneously or be triggered by cough, exertion, or Valsalva. Visual blurring, scotomas, and blindness are also commonly associated. The cerebral vasoconstriction of PPA is additionally associated with abnormal brain imaging. Both hemorrhage and infarction are common presentations, but vasogenic edema is also seen [32].

The diagnostic criteria for RCVS include the following:

- Thunderclap headache(s) with or without focal neurologic deficits or seizures.
- Monophasic course without new symptoms more than 1 month after initial onset of symptoms
- Multifocal, multi-vessel, segmental vasoconstriction of cerebral arteries.
- Absence of aneurysmal subarachnoid hemorrhage, Normal or near-normal cerebrospinal fluid (CSF); CSF Protein < 100 mg/dL, CSF WBC <15 per mm^3, CSF Glucose normal.
- Complete or substantial normalization of cerebral arteries within 12 weeks of symptom onset.

When clinical suspicion for RCVS is high despite normal vasculature on angiography performed early after the onset of symptoms, repeat vascular imaging after several weeks is indicated in search of vasoconstriction. RCVS and PPA are discussed in detail in Chaps. 13 and 14, respectively.

Posterior Reversible Encephalopathy Syndrome (PRES)

Also known as reversible posterior leukoencephalopathy (RPLE), PRES is a relatively new brain disorder that predominantly affects the cerebral white matter with edematous lesions particularly involving the posterior parietal and occipital lobes, though they may spread to basal ganglia, brain stem, and cerebellum [33]. Involvement of midline structures including the thalami, basal ganglia, and brainstem are characteristic of the Central Variant of PRES. RCVS is quite common (24%) in PRES patients. Purported causes of PRES include uncontrolled hypertension with abrupt increase in blood pressure, preeclampsia and renal failure. It classically presents with encephalopathy, headache, nausea, vomiting, visual impairment and seizures and may be associated with hydrocephalus. PRES is also discussed in Chap. 12.

Collagen Type IV, Alpha 1 (COL4A1) Associated Syndrome [34]

This syndrome is caused by mutations in the COL4A1 gene encoding the type IV collagen alpha 1 chain. It is classically associated with porencephaly and infantile hemiparesis, but has more recently been recognized as a monogenic cause of small vessel disease that can present in adulthood. Stroke is often the first presentation of the disease with a mean age of onset of 36.1 years (SD, 12.95; range, 14–49). Hemorrhages, often recurrent, have been associated with physical trauma and activity and anticoagulant therapy. Migraine (with and without aura) was reported in ten subjects, with a mean age at onset of 31.7. Systemic features are also frequent, affecting the eye (10/21, 47.6%), kidney (15.4%), and muscle (15.4%). MRI often demonstrates leukoaraiosis (63.5%), microbleeds that are usually subcortical (52.9%), lacunar infarction (13.5%), and dilated perivascular spaces (19.2%). Extensive leukoaraiosis was seen in a number of asymptomatic adult mutation carriers. Asymptomatic intracranial aneurysms were also common (44.4% of 18 with angiography).

Diagnosis

Brain Imaging

The use of computer tomography (CT) in the workup of stroke in pregnancy is described in detail in Chap. 20.

Magnetic Resonance Imaging

The use of magnetic resonance imaging (MRI) in the workup of stroke in pregnancy is described in detail in Chap. 20.

Lumbar Puncture

As SAH may be missed on CT, lumbar puncture may be used to make or confirm the diagnosis. A lumbar puncture (LP) significant for xanthochromia, a pink or yellow tint in the CSF representing hemoglobin degradation products, can be used to diagnose suspected subarachnoid patients with a normal CT scan [6]. The classic lumbar puncture findings for SAH are an elevated opening pressure, an elevated red blood cell (RBC) count, and xanthochromia. While the presence of xanthochromia may confirm the diagnosis of SAH, the absence of xanthochromia does not exclude the occurrence of SAH as xanthochromia shows up at least 2 h after blood enters the CSF [35]. Therefore, if an LP is done soon after SAH onset, xanthochromia may not be visually detected in the specimen. In addition, while differential RBC counts between tube 1 through tube 4 have been used as a distinguishing feature between traumatic puncture and aSAH, a recent study showed that even in aSAH, a 25% reduction of RBC concentration may occur between first and fourth tube. Therefore, formal evaluation for the presence of a cerebral aneurysm via cerebral angiogram is still indicated [36].

Evaluation for Hemorrhagic Stroke Mechanism

Craniocervical Vessel Imaging

CT angiography (CTA), CT venography (CTV), MR angiography (MRA), MR venography (MRV) or digital subtraction angiography (DSA) can be used to investigate the underlying mechanism of hemorrhagic stroke. MRA and MRV with gadolinium should be avoided in pregnancy. As an alternative to contrast injection, imaging of the arterial and venous circulation can be performed using time-of-flight sequences.

Diagnostic Cerebral Angiography

DSA is considered the gold standard to evaluate for vascular malformation or aneurysm in the setting of SAH. It is recommended to determine various characteristics of the lesion such as location, size, flow rate, coexisting aneurysm, and type of venous drainage [36].

Laboratory Evaluation

Complete blood count, comprehensive metabolic panel including renal function and liver function testing should be completed. Laboratory testing for inherited and acquired thrombophilia should be completed in pregnant women presenting with cerebral venous sinus thrombosis.

Management

Acute Management of Hemorrhagic Stroke

Goals for the acute management of hemorrhagic stroke include the following:

- Urgent support of vital functions (Airway, Breathing and Circulation).
- Prevention of hematoma expansion.
- Intracranial pressure management.
- Prevention of secondary brain injury.
- Prevention of medical complications.

Urgent Support of Vital Function (Airway, Breathing and Circulation)

Early intubation is essential for patients with impaired arousal due to risk of aspiration, hypoxemia, and hypercarbia.

Prevention of Hematoma Expansion

Controlling blood pressure and reversing coagulopathy is essential for preventing further hematoma expansion.

Controlling Blood Pressure

In the setting of preeclampsia or severe hypertension with neurological symptoms, the goal is to achieve an urgent and sustained reduction of SBP and DBP to less than 160/110 mmHg to reduce the risk of maternal stroke. That can be followed by titration of medications to lower pressure below 140/90 mmHg. The impact of blood pressure reduction on placental perfusion should be considered. Obstetrics/Maternal Fetal Medicine practitioners should be involved in ongoing assessments of the maternal-placental-fetal unit and decision-making related to blood pressure lowering and the approach to fetal monitoring and surveillance where appropriate. Care must be taken to not cause hypotension or hypoperfusion [37, 38].

In pregnancy, first-line medications for blood pressure control are labetalol, methyldopa, and long acting nifedipine [39]. Selection of specific antihypertensive medication should consider side-effect profiles for the woman, fetus, or neonate. Angiotensin-converting enzyme inhibitors and angiotensin II receptor blockers—two common classes of medications used in stroke prevention—carry an increased risk of fetal complications (kidney injury) and low amniotic fluid, especially if used after the first trimester. These medications should be discontinued prior to pregnancy or as soon as a pregnancy is recognized. If they have been inadvertently taken, prompt referral to a regional center for detailed fetal structural ultrasound and counseling is encouraged. Atenolol, angiotensin-converting enzyme inhibitor and renin direct renin inhibitors are contraindicated in pregnancy and should not be used (*Class III; Level of Evidence C*) [39].

Selected groups of antihypertensives are summarized in Table 7.3 with consideration of their maternal and fetal adverse effects.

Reversing Coagulopathy

In intracranial hemorrhage, evidence suggests that significant hematoma expansion usually occurs during the first 4 h after onset, making this the critical time window for a hemostatic treatment [40–42]. In patients on anticoagulation medication, such as warfarin or direct oral anticoagulants (DOAC), prothrombotic strategies are typically employed to reverse the effects of these medications and thereby decrease hemorrhage and hematoma expansion [40–43]. Administration of an effective hemostatic agent at an early stage appears to accelerate the formation of a fibrin clot, which stops the bleeding. Specifically, for reversing heparin anticoagulation, protamine is the most effective treatment. The administration of protamine can rapidly and completely normalize partial thromboplastin time (PTT) [43, 44]. Several treatment options can be considered for the reversal of warfarin anticoagulation with elevated international normalized ratio (INR) which include fresh frozen plasma (FFP), prothrombin complex concentrates (PCC), and rF-VIIa [44].

Table 7.3 Summary of antihypertensive drugs used during pregnancy

Category	Maternal side effects	Teratogenicity or fetal-neonatal adverse effects	Class/Level of Evidence
ACE	Hyperkalemia	Skeletal and Cardiovascular abnormalities, renal dysgenesis, pulmonary hypoplasia If prior use, refer to OB for fetal structural ultrasound, and counseling	III/C
β-Blockers (Atenolol)	Headache	Associated with fetal growth restriction.	III/B
β-Blockers (Labetalol, Metoprolol)	Headache, may provoke asthma exacerbation	Animal studies have failed to reveal evidence of teratogenicity. Possible neonatal bradycardia	IIa/B
Calcium Channel Blockers (e.g. Nifedipine)	Headache, possible interaction with magnesium sulfate; may interfere with labor	No	I/A
Centrally acting α2-adrenergic agonist (e.g. Methyldopa)	Sedation, elevated LFTs, Depression	No	IIa/C
Hydralazine	Reflex tachycardia, delayed hypotension	Neonatal thrombocytopenia, fetal bradycardia	III/B
Diuretics (thiazide)	Hypokalemia	No	III/B

ACE angiotensin-converting enzyme, *LFTs* liver function tests

Recent trials showed benefit of PCC over FFP where normalization of INR was achieved in 77% of patients with PCC compared to 9% with FFP [44]. Also, PCC is capable of normalizing INR within minutes while FFP may require hours [44]. Moreover, there were no differences in thrombotic complications [45–48]. Vitamin K 10 mg IV should be given for all life-threatening bleeding to reverse coagulopathy from warfarin administration and can be an adjunct to PCC reversal [45, 46]. Although there is minimal data with PCCs in pregnancy to inform decision-making regarding drug-associated maternal or fetal risk, it is classified as class "C" and should only be used if the benefits outweigh risks.

For DOAC-related Coagulopathy, typical coagulation tests (e.g., prothrombin time [PT], PTT, and INR) do not reflect the anticoagulant effect of these drugs. Specific anti-Xa assays are the preferred tests to evaluate the anticoagulant effects of factor Xa inhibitors (FXaIs), but these tests are not widely available. A recent trial evaluated reversal of rivaroxaban and apixaban by PCC and did show effective bleeding control, with few observed thromboembolic events [49]. Several novel DOAC reversal agents have been developed including idarucizumab, a monoclonal antibody fragment targeting dabigatran, and Andexanet alfa, a recombinant modified human factor Xa decoy protein that has been shown to reverse the inhibition of factor Xa [50, 51]. Unfortunately, studies evaluating these agents excluded pregnant women and many patients with severe ICH and poor prognoses. Furthermore, the reduction in anti-Xa activity associated with these agents was short-lived and returned to normal 4 h after completion of the infusion [52].

Antifibrinolytic Therapy

The use of epsilon-aminocaproic acid resulted in decreased aneurysm rebleeding from 11.4% (non-treated patients) to 2.7% (treated patients); however, there was an eightfold increase in deep venous thrombosis in the treated group [53]. Tranexamic acid treatment is believed to reduce in-hospital morality in aSAH, although a recent study failed to show any difference in clinical outcome at 6 months as measured by the modified Rankin Scale [54, 55].

Intracranial Pressure (ICP) Management

With intracerebral and subarachnoid hemorrhage, intracranial pressure (ICP) is increased given the mass effect of the clotted blood and secondary obstructive hydrocephalus that can complicate intracranial hemorrhage. Therefore, understanding how to identify and manage increased ICP is crucial.

Medical and surgical approaches to reducing ICP include: [56]

- Elevation of the head of the bed to 30°.
- Osmotherapy: Mannitol 20% 0.25–0.5 g/kg every 4 h.
  - Mannitol is assigned a pregnancy category C by FDA. Mannitol can cause maternal dehydration, which can lead to hypotension, uterine hypoperfusion, and fetal injury. Mannitol is only recommended for use during pregnancy when benefit outweighs risk.
- ICP monitor placement in patients with hydrocephalus or clinical deterioration secondary to elevated ICP with goal ICP <20 mmHg and cerebral perfusion pressure (CPP) >70 mmHg.
- External ventricular drainage (EVD) may be indicated in patients with or at risk for hydrocephalus.
- Neurosurgical evaluation
  - Many patients with hemorrhagic stroke may need neurosurgical interventions (i.e., ventriculostomy; if there is evidence of hydrocephalus and for close intracranial pressure monitoring or hematoma evacuation if there is significant mass effect).

Prevention of Secondary Brain Injury

Prevention of and Monitoring for Delayed Cerebral Ischemia (DCI)

Delayed cerebral ischemia (DCI) is a feared complication of aneurysmal SAH (aSAH) and occurs in up to 30% of aSAH patients. DCI is defined as new infarct or neurological deterioration or both within 6 weeks of aneurysm rupture, regardless of presence of angiographic vasospasm. Large vessel vasospasm has historically been thought to be the cause of DCI, but up to 70% of patients with aSAH present with angiographically evident narrowing of cerebral vessels, while only 20–30% of those patients have concomitant infarct or neurological deterioration required for diagnosis of DCI [57].

Although there have been numerous trials to find effective pharmacological interventions to prevent DCI, nimodipine is the only agent that is associated with better outcome in SAH patients [58]. The standard regimen is 60 mg every 4 h for 21 days, but caution should be used in pregnant patients because although there is minimal data in humans, it has been linked with teratogenicity in some animal experiments [59, 60]. Additionally, since nimodipine can cause hypotension, special care should be given to monitor hypoperfusion in the uteroplacental system to avoid detrimental effects on the fetus. In addition to pharmacologic intervention, patients should be maintained in a euvolemic state with normonatremia, as both hypovolemia and hyponatremia have been shown to increase the risk of development of DCI [58].

Early detection and diagnosis of DCI is vital for performing intervention and managing symptoms. Serial neurological examinations are required to monitor for presence of new-onset changes in neurological status. Transcranial doppler (TCD) can also be used to detect narrowing of cerebral blood vessels and is non-invasive and does not present any radiation exposure for mother or fetus. Additionally, multimodal monitoring using ICP monitoring and parenchymal brain tissue oxygenation ($PbtO_2$) can elucidate cerebral blood flow compromise and may be especially important in those patients who are intubated or sedated where a complete neurological exam may not be able to be performed [58]. Finally, clinical imaging to examine cerebral perfusion such CTA, CTP, or DSA should be considered and weighed with the risk of contrast and radiation exposure they present to mother and fetus. Further discussion of the risks and benefits of these imaging modalities are discussed in Diagnosis: Brain Imaging section.

Glucose

Due to increased red cell turnover, hemoglobin A1C is slightly lower in normal pregnancy than in healthy non-pregnant women. The American Diabetes Association (ADA) recommends a fasting glucose target <95 mg/dL and a 2-h postprandial glucose <120 mg/dL [61]. Although pregnant women were excluded from a recent large, randomized trial, which failed to support using intensive glucose control in acute ischemic stroke, it is reasonable to maintain a glucose level of 140–180 mg/dL for pregnant women with ischemic stroke. Insulin is the preferred medication for treating hyperglycemia during pregnancy [62]. Other oral and non-insulin injectable glucose-lowering medications lack long-term safety data [61].

Temperature

Fluctuations from normal temperature, including hyperthermia or hypothermia should be avoided. To limit secondary injury related to fever, any concurrent infection including asymptomatic urinary tract infection should be treated.

Seizure Prophylaxis

Patients with intracranial hemorrhage including SAH have an estimated 30-day risk of clinically evident seizure activity of 8%, with lobar ICH (e.g., from AVM rupture) being an independent predictor of early seizure onset. Up to 2% of intracranial hemorrhage patients will develop convulsive status epilepticus after their index event, and status will be present in up to 28% of continuously monitored stuporous or comatose patients. Although prophylactic AEDs are usually not advised in acute intracranial hemorrhage, oral levetiracetam (500–1000 mg) can be considered in pregnancy and the postpartum when indicated [63].

Prevention Other Medical Complications

Patients being treated for ischemic stroke may be hospitalized and/or immobile for extended periods, therefore increasing the risk of medical complications such as venous thromboembolism (VTE) or nosocomial infection. For the prevention of VTE formation and subsequent pulmonary or paradoxical emboli, mechanical prophylaxis and/or chemoprophylaxis should be considered. When indicated, chemoprophylaxis with low-molecular weight heparin (LMWH) or unfractionated heparin (UFH) is preferred. Chemoprophylaxis should be withheld for at least 24 h of stable hemorrhagic stroke, and ideally for 2–3 days after hematoma size is stabilized. Preventative measures to reduce nosocomial infection should be taken such as minimizing use of indwelling catheters, weaning ventilation as soon as possible, and limiting antibiotic usage.

Disease Specific Treatment

Intracranial Hemorrhage from Aneurysms and Arteriovenous Malformations (AVMs)

If the patient's neurological and overall clinical status is stable, consider deferring treatment until the postpartum period. Current data seems to support no increased risk of aneurysmal subarachnoid hemorrhage in patients with unruptured intracranial aneurysm during pregnancy, delivery, and puerperium, although this topic still remains controversial [63]. Ruptured aneurysm should be treated urgently based on accepted standards of care. Intracerebral aneurysms and AVMs are generally managed via surgery or via endovascular treatment of the lesion. Generally, treatment for symptomatic, enlarging intracerebral aneurysms and AVMs are the same for both pregnant and non-pregnant women [5].

While endovascular coiling is well described for the management of unruptured and ruptured aneurysms, surgical clipping has often preferred for aneurysms with broad necks, a low neck-to-fundus ratio, distal segment lesions, or giant aneurysms. Although these lesions were previously not considered amenable to coiling, new devices including stents and flow diverters have permitted endovascular management of previously untreatable aneurysms [5]. Regardless of the modality, stabilizing the ruptured aneurysm is essential as multiple studies have found that

interventional management of aneurysms is linked to lower maternal and fetal mortality rates compared to more conservative treatments [3, 4]. The procedure for surgical clipping is generally the same with a pregnant patient compared to a non-pregnant patient. However, additional precautions should be considered during pregnancy. The patient should be positioned supine, with her trunk rotated to the left side, on the operating table so that the fetus does not compress the inferior vena cava [4]. Compression of the inferior vena cava can lead to decreased venous return, and, therefore, hypotension and shock [4]. Considerations for evaluation and management of unruptured and ruptured aneurysms in pregnancy are discussed in Chap. 8.

Compared to aneurysms, the treatment of AVMs tend to be less clear and more individualized to each patient [4]. For symptomatic ruptured AVMs, treatment often involves surgical resection alone or staged embolization followed by surgical resection [5]. Evaluation of the malformation's angioarchitecture is typically done through non-invasive vessel imaging (CTA/MRA) or conventional catheter angiography (DSA). This is essential to delineating key features of the AVM including location of venous drainage and presence of any pre-nidal or intranidal aneurysms that might be the source of the bleed [5]. When modalities employing ionizing radiation are used (i.e., CT/CTA/DSA), shielding of the abdominopelvic region should be in place to limit fetal radiation exposure.

Decisions regarding the approach to management of an AVM, particularly one that is high-grade requiring multimodal treatment (combination of surgery, endovascular, or radiosurgery), should be made with an interdisciplinary team, including neurosurgery, neurology, radiology/radiation oncology, and specialists in maternal fetal medicine. Risks for endovascular and radiosurgical interventions include radiation and contrast exposure. Moreover, radiosurgical intervention is associated with a latency to obliteration of 1–2 years and, therefore, will not afford protection during gestation. Although surgical resection lacks radiation risk, blood loss and use of osmotic diuretics (e.g., mannitol) to reduce edema can result in both maternal and fetal compromise.

The hypertension that accompanies labor and delivery, specifically that corresponding to Valsalva in stage 2 of labor, has been considered a risk factor for aneurysm and AVM rupture. Therefore, control of hypertension and minimization in fluctuations of blood pressure is important during this time [5]. Pregnant women who have had their aneurysms and/or AVMs definitely treated may undergo traditional vaginal delivery according to obstetric indications [4, 5]. Pregnant women who have not had their aneurysms and/or AVMs definitively treated may undergo either vaginal delivery or cesarean section depending on obstetric criteria and with modifications to prevent acute hemodynamic fluctuations [4, 5]. In most cases with residual lesions, women are able to undergo vaginal delivery without worsening symptoms. However, careful monitoring and meticulous care should be employed in these cases due to the risk of rupture [63].

Cerebral Venous Sinus Thrombosis [64–66]

For acute CVST occurring during pregnancy, consider treatment with full therapeutic doses of anticoagulation (UFH or LMWH) even in the presence of a hemorrhage with continuation for the remainder of pregnancy and for at least 6 weeks postpartum or until a postpartum switch to oral anticoagulation is feasible. Based on the guidelines of the European Federation of Neurological Societies (EFNS), in cases where patients are resistant to anticoagulation therapy, exhibit worsening of symptoms, do not have an intracranial hemorrhage, or are not at risk for an herniation, endovascular thrombolysis and surgical thrombectomy may also be considered [66].

For women with a remote history of spontaneous CVST, not currently anticoagulated, it is reasonable to consider LMWH prophylaxis during pregnancy and at least 6 weeks postpartum.

Although the risk of recurring CVST in pregnancy is limited [67]. further counseling and assessment should be taken to help best evaluate individual risk in future pregnancies. Warfarin crosses the placenta, is potentially teratogenic, and can result in fetal bleeding and, therefore, should be avoided especially between 6- and 12-weeks gestational age. There are insufficient data on the safety of direct oral anticoagulants (DOAC) (apixaban, dabigatran, edoxaban, rivaroxaban) in pregnancy. Switching to LMWH is encouraged as soon as a pregnancy is identified or if pregnancy is planned.

IV UFH could be considered in a hospitalized woman in place of LMWH if there is concern about need for urgent delivery or invasive procedures. A low dose, without bolus is the preferred dose in stroke patients including during pregnancy. Table 7.4 provides a summary of relative fetal risks of anticoagulants.

Anticoagulation should be suspended prior to administration of regional anesthesia or planned induction:

- If low-dose LMWH: stop at least 12 h prior to regional anesthesia or planned induction.
- If full-dose LMWH: stop at least 24 h prior to regional anesthesia or planned induction.

Table 7.4 Teratogenic risks antithrombotic therapies

Antithrombotic drugs	Placental transfer	First trimester	Second and third trimester
Low-dose aspirin (60–150 mg/day)	Yes	Contraindicated (risk of gastroschisis)*	Not Contraindicated
Other Antiplatelets	No data	No data	No data
Warfarin	Yes	Contraindicated (Teratogenic)	Not preferred Regular check of INR
UFH	No data	Not contraindicated Risk of HIT	Not contraindicated Risk of HIT Regular check of aPTT
LMWH	No data	Not contraindicated	Not contraindicated
DOAC	Dabigaran: Yes Rivaroxaban: Yes Apixaban: No data Edoxaban: No data	No data	No data

UFH unfractionated heparin, *LMWH* low-molecular weight heparin, *DOAC* direct oral anticoagulant

LMWH or UFH can be restarted at least 4–6 h after the removal of the neuraxial catheter if bleeding is well controlled and there are no neuraxial concerns. The regimen can then be continued for 6–12 weeks post-delivery. If anticoagulation is required beyond 6–12 weeks post-delivery, LMWH, and warfarin are both considered safe options during breastfeeding. The safety of direct oral anticoagulants in breastfeeding has not been established. The duration of anticoagulation is determined by results of a thrombophilia panel. Long-term anticoagulation therapy should be reconsidered in cases where patients have recurrent episodes of CVST or those who have an episode of CVST with "severe" thrombophilia. Newer anticoagulants have also been developed, although research on their use and effects in pregnant women is limited [68]. Oral direct thrombin inhibitors and factor Xa inhibitors have been developed recently. Some research has found trace levels of a direct thrombin inhibitor in breast milk [68]. Therefore, while further evidence is obtained, these types of anticoagulants should be avoided in women who are breastfeeding.

Aspirin is considered relatively safe at low doses (60–150 mg/day) after the first trimester. The safety of ASA after the first trimester is well-established from trials of its use in prevention of preeclampsia development in high-risk women, including those with recurrent fetal loss [69, 70]. Theoretical concerns over premature closure of the ductus arteriosus have not been borne out in trials. Additionally, aspirin is not excreted into breast milk and therefore considered safe for women during breastfeeding.

Anticoagulation during pregnancy is discussed in detail in Chap. 15.

Hypertensive Disorders of Pregnancy

The main goal for the treatment of preeclampsia, eclampsia, and HELLP syndrome is to stabilize the mother, prevent recurrent eclamptic seizures, and treat the severe hypertension to reduce or prevent cerebral edema and hemorrhage. Prompt delivery is recommended as it is the only definitive cure for preeclampsia, eclampsia, and HELLP.

Antihypertensive therapy is suggested for adult pregnant women with systolic pressures over 140 mmHg and diastolic pressures over 90 mmHg. Magnesium sulfate 1–3 g/h should be administered to prevent recurrent eclamptic seizures; the only known cure is delivery of the placenta. Platelet transfusion should be administered in HELLP syndrome patients with maternal bleeding or platelet count of <20,000 cells/μL.

Prognosis

Maternal stroke has severe consequences with in-hospital mortality of 10–16%. It accounts for 7.4% maternal deaths in the USA [21, 22, 71, 72]. The prognosis of hemorrhagic stroke occurring during pregnancy or the postpartum seems to be more severe than ischemic stroke [5]. Adequate care in an intensive care environment can ensure a better prognosis [5]. Additionally, a hemorrhagic stroke during pregnancy requires the treating team to balance maternal care with considerations of fetal risk. Prognosis in the setting of maternal stroke is discussed in more depth in Chap. 20.

Stroke Secondary Prevention

- Described in greater detail in Chap. 20.

Summary

Given the role of hemorrhagic strokes in pregnancy-related morbidity and mortality, further assessment and careful monitoring of risk factors can help guide timely and effective interventions and treatment decisions.

References

1. Lynch JC, Andrade R, Pereira C. [Intracranial hemorrhage during pregnancy and puerperium: experience with fifteen cases]. Arq Neuropsiquiatr 2002;60(2-a):264–8.

2. Fairhall JM, Stoodley MA. Intracranial haemorrhage in pregnancy. Obstet Med. 2009;2(4):142–8.

3. Bateman BT, Schumacher HC, Bushnell CD, Pile-Spellman J, Simpson LL, Sacco RL, et al. Intracerebral hemorrhage in pregnancy: frequency, risk factors, and outcome. Neurology. 2006;67(3):424–9.

4. Dias MS, Sekhar LN. Intracranial hemorrhage from aneurysms and arteriovenous malformations during pregnancy and the puerperium. Neurosurgery. 1990;27(6):855–65; discussion 65–6.

5. Laadioui M, Bouzoubaa W, Jayi S, Fdili FZ, Bouguern H, Chaara H, et al. Spontaneous hemorrhagic strokes during pregnancy: case report and review of the literature. Pan Afr Med J. 2014;19:372.

6. Grear KE, Bushnell CD. Stroke and pregnancy: clinical presentation, evaluation, treatment, and epidemiology. Clin Obstet Gynecol. 2013;56(2):350–9.

7. Zhou Y, Damsky CH, Fisher SJ. Preeclampsia is associated with failure of human cytotrophoblasts to mimic a vascular adhesion phenotype. One cause of defective endovascular invasion in this syndrome? J Clin Invest. 1997;99(9):2152–64.

8. Cipolla MJ, Vitullo L, McKinnon J. Cerebral artery reactivity changes during pregnancy and the postpartum period: a role in eclampsia? Am J Physiol Heart Circ Physiol. 2004;286(6):H2127–32.

9. Maynard SE, Karumanchi SA. Angiogenic factors and preeclampsia. Semin Nephrol. 2011;31(1):33–46.

10. Roberts JM, Lain KY. Recent insights into the pathogenesis of pre-eclampsia. Placenta. 2002;23(5):359–72.

11. Redman CW, Sacks GP, Sargent IL. Preeclampsia: an excessive maternal inflammatory response to pregnancy. Am J Obstet Gynecol. 1999;180(2 Pt 1):499–506.

12. Martin NA, Doberstein C, Zane C, Caron MJ, Thomas K, Becker DP. Posttraumatic cerebral arterial spasm: transcranial Doppler ultrasound, cerebral blood flow, and angiographic findings. J Neurosurg. 1992;77(4):575–83. https://doi.org/10.3171/jns.1992.77.4.0575. PMID: 1527618.

13. Crovetto F, Somigliana E, Peguero A, Figueras F. Stroke during pregnancy and pre-eclampsia. Curr Opin Obstet Gynecol. 2013;25(6):425–32.

14. Katz D, Beilin Y. Disorders of coagulation in pregnancy. Br J Anaesth. 2015;115(Suppl 2):ii75–88.

15. Wardlaw JM, White PM. The detection and management of unruptured intracranial aneurysms. Brain. 2000;123(Pt 2):205–21.

16. Rinkel GJ, Djibuti M, Algra A, van Gijn J. Prevalence and risk of rupture of intracranial aneurysms: a systematic review. Stroke. 1998;29(1):251–6.

17. Ghods AJ, Lopes D, Chen M. Gender differences in cerebral aneurysm location. Front Neurol. 2012;3:78.

18. Liu XJ, Wang S, Zhao YL, Teo M, Guo P, Zhang D, et al. Risk of cerebral arteriovenous malformation rupture during pregnancy and puerperium. Neurology. 2014;82(20):1798–803.

19. Porras JL, Yang W, Philadelphia E, Law J, Garzon-Muvdi T, Caplan JM, et al. Hemorrhage risk of brain arteriovenous malformations during pregnancy and puerperium in a North American Cohort. Stroke. 2017;48(6):1507–13.

20. Lanska DJ, Kryscio RJ. Risk factors for peripartum and postpartum stroke and intracranial venous thrombosis. Stroke. 2000;31(6):1274–82.

21. Saposnik G, Barinagarrementeria F, Brown RD Jr, Bushnell CD, Cucchiara B, Cushman M, et al. Diagnosis and management of cerebral venous thrombosis: a statement for healthcare professionals from the American Heart Association/American Stroke Association. Stroke. 2011;42(4):1158–92.

22. Marwah S, Shailesh GH, Gupta S, Sharma M, Mittal P. Cerebral venous thrombosis in pregnancy-a poignant allegory of an unusual case. J Clin Diagn Res. 2016;10(12):Qd8–9.

23. Behrouzi R, Punter M. Diagnosis and management of cerebral venous thrombosis. Clin Med (Lond). 2018;18(1):75–9.

24. Ferro JM, Canhão P, Stam J, Bousser MG, Barinagarrementeria F. Prognosis of cerebral vein and dural sinus thrombosis: results of the International Study on Cerebral Vein and Dural Sinus Thrombosis (ISCVT). Stroke. 2004;35(3):664–70.

25. Lo JO, Mission JF, Caughey AB. Hypertensive disease of pregnancy and maternal mortality. Curr Opin Obstet Gynecol. 2013;25(2):124–32.

26. Tranquilli AL, Dekker G, Magee L, et al. The classification, diagnosis and management of the hypertensive disorders of pregnancy: a revised statement from the ISSHP. Pregnan Hyper. 2014;4:97–104.

27. Martin JN Jr, Thigpen BD, Moore RC, Rose CH, Cushman J, May W. Stroke and severe preeclampsia and eclampsia: a paradigm shift focusing on systolic blood pressure. Obstet Gynecol. 2005;105(2):246–54.

28. Duckitt K, Harrington D. Risk factors for pre-eclampsia at antenatal booking: systematic review of controlled studies. BMJ. 2005;330(7491):565.

29. ACOG. Gestational hypertension and preeclampsia: ACOG practice bulletin, number 222. Obstet Gynecol. 2020;135(6):e237–e60.

30. Brown MA, Magee LA, Kenny LC, Karumanchi SA, McCarthy FP, Saito S, et al. Hypertensive disorders of pregnancy: ISSHP classification, diagnosis, and management recommendations for international practice. Hypertension. 2018;72(1):24–43.

31. Sharshar T, Lamy C, Mas JL. Incidence and causes of strokes associated with pregnancy and puerperium. A study in public hospitals of Ile de France. Stroke in Pregnancy Study Group. Stroke. 1995;26(6):930–6.

32. Fugate JE, Ameriso SF, Ortiz G, Schottlaender LV, Wijdicks EF, Flemming KD, et al. Variable presentations of postpartum angiopathy. Stroke. 2012;43(3):670–6.

33. Fischer M, Schmutzhard E. Posterior reversible encephalopathy syndrome. J Neurol. 2017;264(8):1608–16.

34. Lanfranconi S, Markus HS. COL4A1 mutations as a monogenic cause of cerebral small vessel disease: a systematic review. Stroke. 2010;41(8):e513–8.

35. Heasley DC, Mohamed MA, Yousem DM. Clearing of red blood cells in lumbar puncture does not rule out ruptured aneurysm in patients with suspected subarachnoid hemorrhage but negative head CT findings. AJNR Am J Neuroradiol. 2005;26(4):820–4.

36. Jain C. ACOG Committee Opinion No. 723: guidelines for diagnostic imaging during pregnancy and lactation. Obstet Gynecol. 2019;133(1):186.

37. Butalia S, Audibert F, Côté AM, Firoz T, Logan AG, Magee LA, et al. Hypertension Canada's 2018 Guidelines for the management of hypertension in pregnancy. Can J Cardiol. 2018;34(5):526–31.

38. Nerenberg KA, Zarnke KB, Leung AA, Dasgupta K, Butalia S, McBrien K, et al. Hypertension Canada's 2018 Guidelines for diagnosis, risk assessment, prevention, and treatment of hypertension in adults and children. Can J Cardiol. 2018;34(5):506–25.

39. Bushnell C, McCullough LD, Awad IA, Chireau MV, Fedder WN, Furie KL, et al. Guidelines for the prevention of stroke in women: a statement for healthcare professionals from the American Heart Association/American Stroke Association. Stroke. 2014;45(5):1545–88.

40. Mayer SA. Ultra-early hemostatic therapy for intracerebral hemorrhage. Stroke. 2003;34(1):224–9.

41. Brott T, Broderick J, Kothari R, Barsan W, Tomsick T, Sauerbeck L, et al. Early hemorrhage growth in patients with intracerebral hemorrhage. Stroke. 1997;28(1):1–5.

42. Kazui S, Naritomi H, Yamamoto H, Sawada T, Yamaguchi T. Enlargement of spontaneous intracerebral hemorrhage. Incidence and time course. Stroke. 1996;27(10):1783–7. https://doi.org/10.1161/01.str.27.10.1783. PMID: 8841330.

43. Moussouttas M. Challenges and controversies in the medical management of primary and antithrombotic-related intracerebral hemorrhage. Ther Adv Neurol Disord. 2012;5(1):43–56.

44. Steiner T, Poli S, Griebe M, Hüsing J, Hajda J, Freiberger A, et al. Fresh frozen plasma versus prothrombin complex concentrate in patients with intracranial haemorrhage related to vitamin K antagonists (INCH): a randomised trial. Lancet Neurol. 2016;15(6):566–73.

45. Woo CH, Patel N, Conell C, Rao VA, Faigeles BS, Patel MC, et al. Rapid Warfarin reversal in the setting of intracranial hemorrhage: a comparison of plasma, recombinant activated factor VII, and prothrombin complex concentrate. World Neurosurg. 2014;81(1):110–5.

46. Goldstein JN, Refaai MA, Milling TJ Jr, Lewis B, Goldberg-Alberts R, Hug BA, et al. Four-factor prothrombin complex concentrate versus plasma for rapid vitamin K antagonist reversal in patients needing urgent surgical or invasive interventions: a phase 3b, open-label, non-inferiority, randomised trial. Lancet. 2015;385(9982):2077–87.

47. Sarode R, Milling TJ Jr, Refaai MA, Mangione A, Schneider A, Durn BL, et al. Efficacy and safety of a 4-factor prothrombin complex concentrate in patients on vitamin K antagonists presenting with major bleeding: a randomized, plasma-controlled, phase IIIb study. Circulation. 2013;128(11):1234–43.

48. Parry-Jones AR, Di Napoli M, Goldstein JN, Schreuder FH, Tetri S, Tatlisumak T, et al. Reversal strategies for vitamin K antagonists in acute intracerebral hemorrhage. Ann Neurol. 2015;78(1):54–62.

49. Majeed A, Ågren A, Holmström M, Bruzelius M, Chaireti R, Odeberg J, et al. Management of rivaroxaban- or apixaban-associated major bleeding with prothrombin complex concentrates: a cohort study. Blood. 2017;130(15):1706–12.

50. Pollack CV Jr, Reilly PA, van Ryn J, Eikelboom JW, Glund S, Bernstein RA, et al. Idarucizumab for dabigatran reversal - full cohort analysis. N Engl J Med. 2017;377(5):431–41.

51. Connolly SJ, Milling TJ Jr, Eikelboom JW, Gibson CM, Curnutte JT, Gold A, et al. Andexanet alfa for acute major bleeding associated with factor Xa inhibitors. N Engl J Med. 2016;375(12):1131–41.

52. Bower MM, Sweidan AJ, Shafie M, Atallah S, Groysman LI, Yu W. Contemporary reversal of oral anticoagulation in intracerebral hemorrhage. Stroke. 2019;50(2):529–36.

53. Starke RM, Kim GH, Fernandez A, Komotar RJ, Hickman ZL, Otten ML, et al. Impact of a protocol for acute antifibrinolytic therapy on aneurysm rebleeding after subarachnoid hemorrhage. Stroke. 2008;39(9):2617–21.

54. Post R, Germans MR, Boogaarts HD, Ferreira Dias Xavier B, Van den Berg R, Coert BA, et al. Short-term tranexamic acid treatment reduces in-hospital mortality in aneurysmal sub-arachnoid hemorrhage: a multicenter comparison study. PLoS One. 2019;14(2):e0211868.

55. Post R, Germans MR, Tjerkstra MA, Vergouwen MDI, Jellema K, Koot RW, et al. Ultra-early tranexamic acid after subarachnoid haemorrhage (ULTRA): a randomised controlled trial. Lancet. 2021;397(10269):112–8.

56. Tate J, Bushnell C. Pregnancy and stroke risk in women. Womens Health. 2011;7(3):363–74.

57. Sarrafzadeh AS, et al. Monitoring in neurointensive care–the challenge to detect delayed cerebral ischemia in high-grade aneurysmal SAH. Front Neurol. 2014;5:134.

58. Francoeur CL, Mayer SA. Management of delayed cerebral ischemia after subarachnoid hemorrhage. Crit Care. 2016;20:1–12.

59. Stoodley MA, Macdonald RL, Weir BKA. Pregnancy and intracranial aneurysms. Neurosurg Clin N Am. 1998;9:549–56.

60. Roman H, Descargues G, Lopes M, et al. Subarachnoid hemorrhage due to cerebral aneurysmal rupture during pregnancy. Acta Obstet Gynecol Scand. 2004;83:330–4.

61. American Diabetes Association. Management of diabetes in pregnancy: standards of medical care in diabetes-2020. Diabetes Care. 2020;43(Suppl 1):S183–s92.

62. Johnston KC, Bruno A, Pauls Q, Hall CE, Barrett KM, Barsan W, et al. Intensive vs standard treatment of hyperglycemia and functional outcome in patients with acute ischemic stroke: the SHINE randomized clinical trial. JAMA. 2019;322(4):326–35.

63. Katsuragi S, Yoshimatsu J, Tanaka H, Tanaka K, Nii M, Miyoshi T, et al. Management of pregnancy complicated with intracranial arteriovenous malformation. J Obstet Gynaecol Res. 2018;44(4):673–80.

64. Chan WS, Rey E, Kent NE, Chan WS, Kent NE, Rey E, et al. Venous thromboembolism and antithrombotic therapy in pregnancy. J Obstet Gynaecol Can. 2014;36(6):527–53.

65. Swartz RH, Ladhani NNN, Foley N, Nerenberg K, Bal S, Barrett J, et al. Canadian stroke best practice consensus statement: secondary stroke prevention during pregnancy. Int J Stroke. 2018;13(4):406–19.

66. Einhäupl K, Stam J, Bousser MG, De Bruijn SF, Ferro JM, Martinelli I, et al. EFNS guideline on the treatment of cerebral venous and sinus thrombosis in adult patients. Eur J Neurol. 2010;17(10):1229–35.

67. Mehraein S, Ortwein H, Busch M, Weih M, Einhäupl K, Masuhr F. Risk of recurrence of cerebral venous and sinus thrombosis during subsequent pregnancy and puerperium. J Neurol Neurosurg Psychiatry. 2003;74(6):814–6.

68. Tang AW, Greer I. A systematic review on the use of new anticoagulants in pregnancy. Obstet Med. 2013;6(2):64–71.

69. Rolnik DL, Nicolaides KH, Poon LC. Prevention of preeclampsia with aspirin. Am J Obstet Gynecol. 2020;226:S1108.

70. Stevens W, Shih T, Incerti D, Ton TGN, Lee HC, Peneva D, et al. Short-term costs of preeclampsia to the United States health care system. Am J Obstet Gynecol. 2017;217(3):237–48.e16.

71. Leffert LR, Clancy CR, Bateman BT, Cox M, Schulte PJ, Smith EE, et al. Patient characteristics and outcomes after hemorrhagic stroke in pregnancy. Circ Cardiovasc Qual Outc. 2015;8(6 Suppl 3):S170–8.

72. Creanga AA, Syverson C, Seed K, Callaghan WM. Pregnancy-related mortality in the United States, 2011-2013. Obstet Gynecol. 2017;130(2):366–73.

Cerebral Aneurysms in Pregnancy: Considerations for Diagnosis and Management

Michael S. Rallo, Neil Majmundar,
Sanjeev Sreenivasan, Arevik Abramyan,
Priyank Khandelwal, Ashish Sonig,
Sudipta Roychowdhury, Anil Nanda,
and Gaurav Gupta

Introduction

The management of cerebral aneurysms, both unruptured and ruptured, during pregnancy poses a unique challenge for clinicians not only in clinical decision making, but also patient counseling.

M. S. Rallo
Robert Wood Johnson University Hospital,
New Brunswick, NJ, USA

N. Majmundar · S. Sreenivasan
Department of Neurological Surgery, Rutgers Robert Wood Johnson Medical School,
New Brunswick, NJ, USA

A. Abramyan
Department of Neurosurgery, Rutgers Robert Wood Johnson Medical School, New Brunswick, NJ, USA

P. Khandelwal
Department of Neurology, Robert Wood Johnson University Hospital, New Brunswick, NJ, USA

A. Sonig
Department of Neurological Surgery, Rutgers New Jersey Medical School, Newark, NJ, USA

S. Roychowdhury
Neuroradiology, University Radiology,
New Brunswick, NJ, USA

A. Nanda
Neurosurgery, Robert Wood Johnson University Hospital, New Brunswick, NJ, USA

G. Gupta (✉)
Neurosurgery, Rutgers Robert Wood Johnson Medical School, New Brunswick, NJ, USA
e-mail: guptaga@rwjms.rutgers.edu

Cerebral aneurysms, when ruptured, represent a significant cause of morbidity and mortality in pregnant patients. This chapter focuses on (1) natural course, in particular the association of pregnancy and risk of rupture; (2) role of endocrinologic changes upon aneurysm formation and evolution; (3) management; (4) fetal risks and protective measures; and (5) mode and timing of delivery.

Pathology and Pathogenesis of Aneurysms and Subarachnoid Hemorrhage

Cerebral aneurysms are acquired, degenerative cerebrovascular lesions that arise in areas of weakness within the arterial wall. The majority of aneurysms arise sporadically under the influence of genetic, hemodynamic, inflammatory, and endocrinologic factors [1]. Polymorphisms and mutations conferring increased risk of cerebral aneurysms have been identified in genes encoding collagen, elastin, matrix metalloproteases (MMPs), vasoregulators (i.e., *ACE* and *NOS5*), and inflammatory factors (i.e., *IL6*) [2]. Cerebral aneurysms also occur in several syndromes, most notably autosomal dominant polycystic kidney disease (ADPKD) and Ehlers-Danlos [3, 4]. Endothelial dysfunction, incited by hemodynamic stress (i.e., as in hypertension) and environmental influences (i.e., ciga-

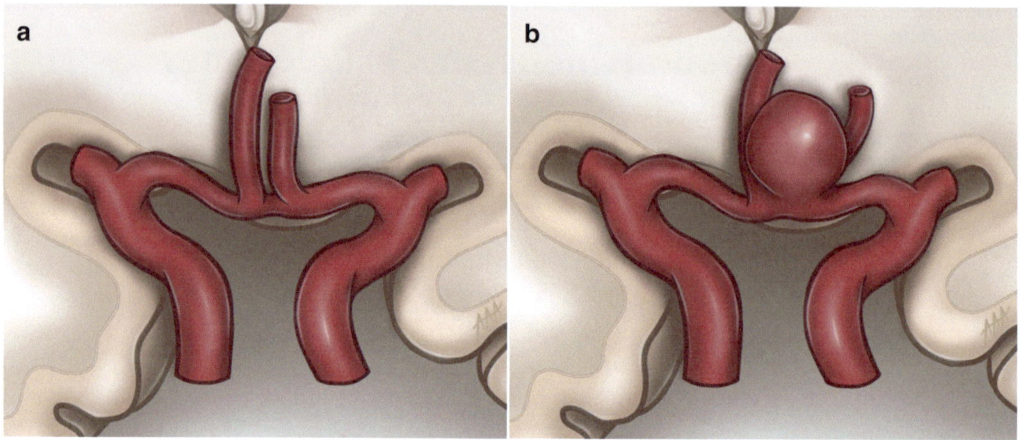

Fig. 8.1 Illustration of normal cerebrovascular anatomy (**a**) and the presence of a cerebral aneurysm in the anterior communicating artery region (**b**)

rette smoke, alcohol), is thought to be the earliest pathogenic event in aneurysm formation [5–7]. This injury invokes a coordinated inflammatory response leading to further vessel weakening, growth of the aneurysm, and rupture [8, 9]. Figure 8.1 demonstrates the appearance of a cerebral aneurysm and localization to bifurcations.

Pregnancy has been purported as a risk factor for cerebral aneurysm rupture and subsequent subarachnoid hemorrhage (SAH) [10]. The risk is hypothesized to result from the cardiovascular hemodynamic changes that accompany pregnancy, particularly the increased cardiac output and blood volume that peaks in the third trimester and enhanced cerebral blood flow resulting from estrogen [11, 12]. A similar increase in risk of rupture has been reported during vaginal delivery and is thought to result from spikes in blood pressure accompanying Valsalva in the second stage of labor [13, 14]. The notion of pregnancy and delivery increasing risk of aneurysm rupture has been opposed by more recent studies making this a topic of controversy; this will be discussed in more detail below [15].

Hormonal influence plays an important role in modulating aneurysm formation and growth across the lifespan and is thought to underly the disparity in aneurysm risk between males and females.

Epidemiologic studies have identified a female preponderance of cerebral aneurysms, particularly in women over the age of 50, suggesting that estrogen deficiency associated with menopause may influence aneurysm formation and growth [16, 17]. Focused analysis of aneurysms in cohorts of pre- and post-menopausal females has, indeed, demonstrated that the prevalence of aneurysms is higher following menopause and that menopause is associated with a trend toward increased aneurysm dome and neck size. Interestingly, aneurysms in premenopausal women displayed a trend toward a greater number of lobes [18]. Moreover, earlier age of menopause has been associated with increased incidence of aneurysms [19]. Transcriptome studies have identified differential expression of genes related to the estrogen receptor pathway in cerebral aneurysm tissue providing a molecular basis for the observations from the above described epidemiologic studies [20]. Estrogen is thought to have an important role in maintenance of cerebrovascular homeostasis and vessel wall, particularly endothelial, integrity through its antioxidant and anti-inflammatory effects [21, 22]. Relating to its role in inflammation, estrogen deficiency has been shown to increase risk of aneurysmal rupture through upregulation of IL-17A, IL-6, and circulating Th17 cells [23, 24]. This is supported by animal studies in which estrogen deficiency, induced by ovariectomy in females, increased the incidence of aneurysm formation and rupture. This effect was abrogated by administration of an estrogen receptor-β agonist, although treatment with a nitric oxide synthase inhibitor was sufficient to negate this protective effect [25, 26]. Of clinical relevance, there is evidence identifying reduced risk of aneurysmal rupture in women treated with hormonal replacement therapy, however, future research is necessary before such therapy can be adopted [27]. The conflicting reports of elevated aneurysm risk in pregnancy, a high estrogen state, and in post-menopausal women, characterized by estrogen deficiency, further highlight the need for additional scientific evaluation of the role of sex steroids in cerebrovascular disease.

Epidemiology, Presentation, and Natural Course

Scope of the Problem

The prevalence of unruptured intracranial aneurysms in the general population has been estimated to be 3.2% with a mean age of 50 years old. Female sex is an important risk factor for aneurysms, with females over the age of 50 having a twofold greater prevalence than males. Female sex is also associated with larger aneurysm size and presence of multiple aneurysms [17, 28, 29]. Based on this prevalence data, it is estimated that 1.8% of women of childbearing age harbor an unruptured intracranial aneurysm [15].

Rupture resulting in SAH is the most feared outcome of cerebral aneurysm and carries substantial morbidity and mortality [30]. The devastating consequences of aneurysmal SAH (aSAH) are reflected by the case fatality rate of 30–40% within the first 3 months following rupture [31, 32]. In addition to female sex, larger aneurysm size, location of the aneurysm in the posterior circulation, symptoms associated with the aneurysm, and older age are all associated with higher risk of rupture [33]. Early studies indicate that the incidence of aneurysm rupture during pregnancy is significantly elevated, approximately 3–11 per 100,000 pregnancies, resulting in substantial fetal mortality and maternal morbidity and mortality [10, 34, 35]. One study identified SAH resulting from aneurysm and AVM as the third leading cause of nonobstetric maternal death [35]. Another reported aSAH as the cause of nearly half of all intracranial hemorrhages during pregnancy. The lack of a control group in this study, however, limits the generalizability of the results [10]. These findings are contrasted by more recent analyses demonstrating similar rates of aneurysm rupture in women during pregnancy and delivery compared with non-pregnant women of childbearing age. Importantly, these new studies included appropriate control groups and for the larger one was substantially more powerful [15, 36]. While this data is controversial, the incidence of aneurysm rupture in late gestation is consistent with purported role for increased cardiac output, plasma volume, and blood pressure underlying rupture risk [10, 23].

Clinical Manifestations and Natural Course

Most cerebral aneurysms (approximately 85%) are located in the anterior circulation, mostly within the Circle of Willis reflecting their tendency to form at bifurcations. Interestingly, there appears to be a great deal of gender discrepancy in localization, with females more likely to develop aneurysms along the internal carotid artery (ICA), especially at the posterior communicating artery (PCOM) junction, and males more likely to develop them along the anterior cerebral artery (ACA) [37–39]. While unruptured aneurysms continue to grow under the influence of biologic and hemodynamic factors, they typically remain asymptomatic [40]. Rarely, they may produce symptoms of mass effect including headache or focal neurological deficit due to compression of surrounding structures including cranial nerves, optic or pyramidal tracts, or brain parenchyma [41–43]. Onset of new neurological deficit, especially acute, in any patient warrants neurological evaluation.

In patients whom aneurysmal rupture occurs, the classic complaint is the sudden onset of a headache which immediately reaches maximal intensity (i.e., "the worst headache of life") [44]. Other symptoms include brief loss of consciousness, nausea or vomiting, and those of meningeal irritation (meningismus), including nuchal rigidity, neck or back pain, and photophobia [45]. The clinical setting of aSAH onset may be important; there are innumerable anecdotal reports and some larger studies describing onset of the headache associated with aSAH during or following periods of moderate or severe exertion (e.g., sneezing, micturition, exercise, strenuous work, sexual intercourse, and emotional shock). These are activities primarily involving rapid increase in blood pressure, and therefore increased aneurysm wall stress, due to enhanced sympathetic tone or some form of Valsalva maneuver [46]. This is the physiological basis underlying supposed risk of rupture during childbirth.

For the 80–85% of individuals with aSAH who survive until hospitalization, the clinical course is complicated. This is especially true in the setting of pregnancy, where consideration must be given to both maternal and fetal health. The earliest, most important cause of death in aSAH patients is aneurysm rerupture (3–4% risk in first 12 h; 1–2% daily risk in first month; 3% risk in first year) [47]. Elimination of this risk is only accomplished through early intervention either by surgical clipping or endovascular occlusion [48]. Rebleeding from an untreated ruptured aneurysm is particularly concerning during pregnancy, due to hemodynamic changes, and is a significant source of maternal mortality [10, 49]. Elevations in intracranial pressure (ICP) related to the initial hemorrhage volume, hydrocephalus, cytotoxic edema, and cerebral hyperemia have been reported to occur in up to 81% of patients with SAH [50]. Hydrocephalus presenting acutely is typically obstructive (non-communicating) due to impaired CSF circulation within the ventricular system (e.g., blood clots in cerebral aqueduct or outlets of fourth ventricle) [51, 52]. Ischemic complications of aSAH results acutely due the reduction in cerebral blood flow (CBF) accompanying elevations in ICP [53, 54]. These events contributing to early brain injury in SAH are also predictive of later complications, including the classic syndrome of delayed cerebral ischemia (DCI) [55]. Outside of the nervous system, SAH may exhibit manifestations including cardiovascular, respiratory and endocrine dysfunction, hematologic and fluid/electrolyte disturbances, and gastrointestinal complications [56]. Future research is necessary to determine how the physiological changes accompanying pregnancy may modify the natural history of unruptured and ruptured cerebral aneurysms.

Diagnostic Considerations for the Pregnant Patient

Clinical Evaluation and Grading

Clinical evaluation of the pregnant patient with aSAH does not vary substantially from that of the general aSAH population. The most likely concern regarding evaluation under these circumstances is radiation exposure and the potential risk to the fetus, which will be discussed in the following neuroimaging section. Though rare, these situations provide a unique opportunity for multidisciplinary collaboration of clinicians from a variety of specialties, including neurosurgery, neurology/neurocritical care, obstetrics/gynecology, anesthesiologists, and radiology. Early consultation and evaluation by this team is crucial to establishing a plan of care that ensures maternal and fetal safety.

While headache is the most common and classical presentation of SAH, it is a relative unspecific finding. Indeed, headache is the most common neurological complaint reported by pregnant women in the emergency department and may represent a variety of conditions including pre-eclampsia, reversible cerebral vasoconstriction syndrome (RCVS), cerebral venous thrombosis [57]. It is critical for evaluating clinicians to consider SAH in all pregnant patients presenting with severe headache: this should include obtaining a noncontrast head computed tomography (CT) scan and performing a lumbar puncture if imaging is nondiagnostic but SAH is still suspected [58].

Neuroimaging

The mainstay imaging modality for the detection of suspected SAH is noncontrast CT, which typically reveals hypderdense blood in the basilar cisterns that may extend within the subarachnoid space to the sylvian fissures, interhemispheric fissure, interpeduncular fossa, and suprasellar, ambient, and quadrigeminal cisterns [59]. Of concern in the pregnant patient is the reliance of CT on ionizing radiation which poses potential fetal risk. While it may be tempting to utilize MRI in evaluation of the pregnant patient with suspected intracranial hemorrhage, the speed and sensitivity of CT, and the exclusion of the abdomen from the field of scan makes it a more appropriate choice. Of course, all precautions must be taken to reduce fetal exposure (i.e., lead shielding of abdomen and pelvis) [60, 61].

Identification of the source of bleeding through angiography is the next step in the evaluation of SAH. CT and MR angiography (CTA/MRA) are noninvasive modalities that are sensitive to the majority of aneurysms, although they are less sensitive for detecting lesions less than three millimeters [62]. The benefit of CTA is that it can be performed rapidly and easily with the patient not even being required to move following the initial noncontrast CT. However, CTA exposes the patient to ionizing radiation and iodinated contrast. MRA is typically performed utilizing a gadolinium-based contrast agent which is also known to cross the placenta and accumulate in fetal tissues. However, certain MRI sequences (i.e., time of flight, TOF) which do not require contrast have demonstrated similar sensitivity to detecting aneurysms as conventional MRA and CTA and therefore may provide an alternative in pregnant patients [63]. However, the logistical challenges associated with MR-based techniques, including scanning time and requirement for limited movement, may reduce its applicability in this setting. Conventional digital subtraction angiography (DSA) is considered the gold standard for identifying the source of bleeding due to its high resolution; DSA can identify even the smallest aneurysms and appraise their anatomic/morphologic features [58]. DSA is often required for preoperative planning and permits immediate endovascular intervention if an aneurysm is identified and considered amenable to this approach. For these reasons, at some institutions, DSA is the first line angiographic imaging technique for evaluation of SAH. However, DSA requires arterial catheterization, substantial exposure to ionizing radiation, and administration of iodinated contrast. These risks are not negligible and must be discussed with the patient or family. Despite these risks, pregnancy should not delay or deter performing DSA required for decision making or intervention. With appropriate shielding and limitation of beam time, the estimated fetal radiation well below the accepted limit [64]. Considerations for neuroradiologic imaging in the pregnant patient is reviewed extensively in a separate chapter.

Counseling and Management

The literature related to the management of pregnant patients with cerebral aneurysms is sparse consisting of single case reports or series and very few large-scale studies. There are no guidelines or consensus statements on this subject and the discussion below consists of reviews of reported cases and expert opinions.

Counseling: Patients Planning to Become Pregnant and Hereditary Concerns

Previous reports of elevated risk of SAH secondary to aneurysm rupture have led some clinicians to counsel against childbearing in women with known aneurysms. In those women who chose to become pregnant, delivery via cesarean (C)-section was recommended. This is reflected by the disproportionate incidence of C-section in women with unruptured aneurysms (70% of deliveries) compared to the general population (25% of deliveries) [15]. However, these recommendations do not appear to be supported by more recent evidence [15, 36]. Rather, an aneurysm identified in a nongravid woman should be treated based on individual risk factors for rupture. Treatment is generally safer prior to pregnancy as it limits the potential of fetal exposure to radiation in endovascular treatment or hypoxia that is risked by maintenance of reduced blood pressure in surgical clipping [65].

Counseling of women intending to become pregnant may also involve a discussion of the genetics of intracranial aneurysms as it relates to preconception screening and risk of hereditary transmission. Familial clustering of intracranial aneurysms is well described: first-degree relatives of individuals with intracranial aneurysms or sporadic SAH have a two to four-fold increased risk of developing an aneurysm compared to the general population [66, 67]. In addition, familial aneurysms rupture more frequently than sporadic aneurysms and demonstrate a tendency to rupture at younger age, often within the same decade in siblings, and at smaller sizes [68, 69]. For patients with aneurysm in the setting of ADPKD, where the incidence of aneurysm ranges from 5 to 10% throughout the lifespan, risk of rupture has been reported as high as 80% with rupture occurring before the age of 50 in 64% [70]. Screening for aneurysms by CTA or MRA in patients with family history is, generally, recommended when there are two or more affected first-degree relatives [68, 71]. Recommendations for screening in ADPKD patients currently remains limited to those at high risk, including family history of aneurysm or intracranial hemorrhage [72–74]. While no formal guidelines exists, we recommend screening according to the above guidelines prior to conception in women intending to become pregnant to facilitate preconception intervention, if neurosurgically indicated. Patients concerned for the health of their expected child should be appropriately counseled on the current data regarding familial aneurysms, indicating that the likelihood of hereditary transmission is relatively low, and reassured by modern ability to detect and treat these lesions.

Management of Unruptured Aneurysms in Pregnancy

There is minimal evidence and no formal guidelines for decision making regarding management of unruptured aneurysms identified during pregnancy. The conventional dogma regarding unruptured aneurysms in pregnancy is that they only warrant treatment if they are symptomatic or continually enlarging [75]. This is largely based on several studies of the natural history of unruptured aneurysms identifying extremely low rates of rupture and hemorrhage in small, asymptom-

atic aneurysms, including both the International Study of Unruptured Intracranial Aneurysm (ISUIA), first published in 1998, and the Unruptured Cerebral Aneurysm Study (UCAS) Japan published nearly 10 years later [76–78]. Factors associated with increased risk of rupture include: larger (>7 mm) aneurysm size, aneurysm growth, symptoms related to the aneurysm, presence of a daughter sac, localization to the posterior circulation, and previous history of SAH [77–80]. The overall conclusion of these studies has been that intervention is unlikely to alter the natural course for small, stable aneurysms without symptoms, but has the potential to result in significant complication [78, 81]. Therefore, in the pregnant patient with a diagnosed, low risk (relatively small, asymptomatic) aneurysm, it is reasonable to recommend monitoring, preferably via noncontrast MRA, to detect changes in aneurysm size during gestation. This complements recommendations for screening for growth in the general population with unruptured aneurysms [74].

Large size, aneurysm growth, or development of symptoms should warrant strong consideration of intervention [15, 75]. A recent analysis has critiqued this approach suggesting that intervention for smaller aneurysms (6 mm) may be prudent due to their higher propensity for rupture in pregnant patients [82]. The choice of intervention remains controversial: there are significant risks to both endovascular and surgical therapies and both have been reported in the pregnant population with success [83, 84]. Endovascular embolization offers shorter operating times, less anesthesia exposure, minimal impact on maternal hemodynamics, and shorter hospital stays compared to surgical clipping [82, 84]. Moreover, the reported fetal dose of radiation associated with DSA during embolization is well below the established acceptable limits, thereby reducing concerns of undue fetal radiation [64]. Furthermore, as endovascular interventions transition toward a radial first approach, further studies regarding radiation exposure to the fetus with adequate protection will be interesting to follow. For these reasons, it appears reasonable to recommend endovascular embolization for the management of unruptured intracranial aneurysms in the pregnant patient in accordance with neurosurgical indications. Delay of the procedure past the stage of organogenesis, when appropriate, may help minimize fetal risk from radiation [75, 85]. Figures 8.2, 8.3 and 8.4 summarizes these available treatment modalities. However, this should not place the patient at undue risk of rupture. As with all medical decisions, thorough discussion of the intervention and potential complications with the patient is essential. Regarding delivery, at this time there is insufficient evidence associating vaginal delivery with an increased risk of aneurysm rupture to support recommen-

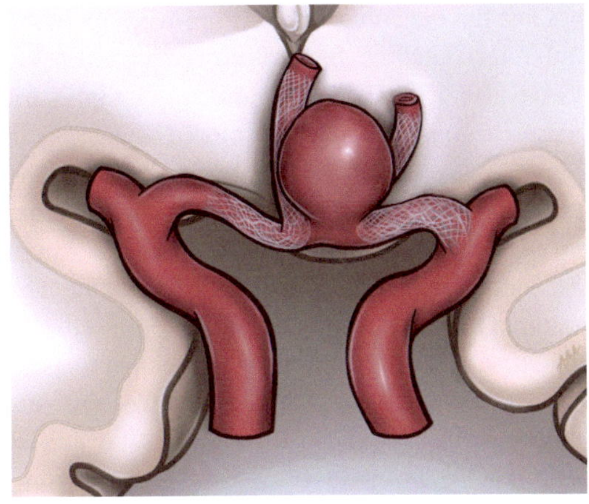

Fig. 8.4 Illustration of the employment of flow diverter devices for the treatment of a cerebral aneurysm

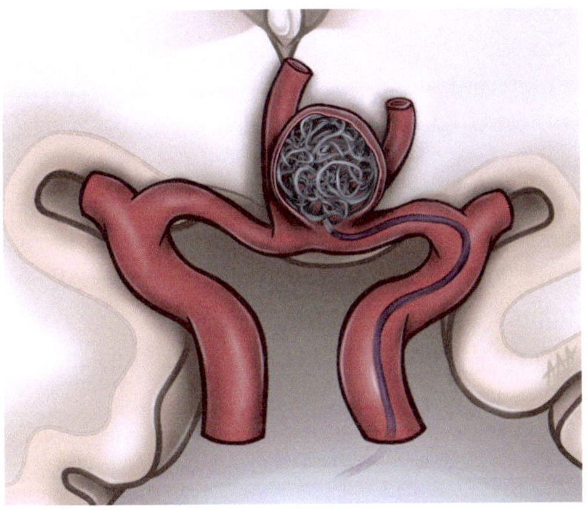

Fig. 8.2 Illustration of a coiling procedure for the treatment of a cerebral aneurysm

dation of C-section [15, 36]. However, it has been suggested that these recommendations should be stratified: women at higher risk, for example, with aneurysm and concurrent gestational hypertension, may benefit from C-section, while those at lower risk can undergo vaginal delivery [85]. Vaginal delivery should be accompanied by sufficient analgesia as to limit maternal stress and acute hemodynamic changes [86]. The decision making process regarding intervention and mode of delivery in this setting should include multidisciplinary discussion with the interventionalist, obstetrician, and anesthesiologist to ensure the safest and most effective approach is chosen.

Management of Ruptured Aneurysms in Pregnancy

The management of ruptured aneurysms and resultant aSAH is complex. This section will be limited to decision making regarding intervention with little discussion of the aspects of neurocritical care which have been described elsewhere. In general, it is regarded that care of the pregnant patient with aSAH should occur in the same way as patients who are not pregnant; that is to say that neurosurgical considerations shall take precedence over obstetric considerations in an effort to preserve maternal vitality [65]. Multiple

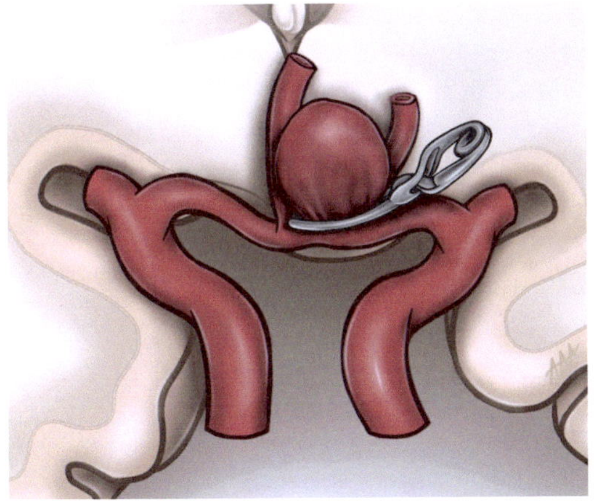

Fig. 8.3 Illustration of a microsurgical clipping procedure for the treatment of a cerebral aneurysm

studies have demonstrated improved maternal and fetal outcome in treated versus untreated aSAH [10, 15]. The two mainstay therapies for definitive management of ruptured aneurysm in the general population include surgical clipping and endovascular coil embolization. To date there have been few randomized trials directly comparing endovascular versus surgical management of ruptured aneurysms. The largest and only multicenter study, the International Subarachnoid Aneurysm Trial (ISAT), found that for patients with aneurysms suitable for either endovascular or surgical management, the endovascular arm showed significantly lower risk of disability [87]. However, endovascular management was associated with higher recurrence and rebleeding [88]. While the results of the ISAT prompted a general swing in management toward coiling in Europe, there was concern over its applicability to pregnant patients given the prolonged exposure to radiation. Importantly, it was subsequently proven that, even in relatively prolonged procedures, the amount of radiation exposure during the procedure is well below the threshold of fetal harm [64]. The general strategy for management of ruptured aneurysms in pregnancy should involve early perinatal evaluation to determine fetal viability; if delivery is feasible (i.e., rupture in late third trimester), it should be performed via C-section prior to aneurysm treatment. When delivery is feasible, there are only few cases in which aneurysm treatment is so emergent that it must be performed prior to delivery, such as those in which compressive cerebral hematoma requires emergent evacuation for reduction in ICP [89–91]. One systematic review determined that clipping was the most common method for treatment of ruptured aneurysms [15], while a subsequent review several years later identified coiling more commonly [82]. This likely reflects more general trends in management of ruptured aneurysms toward coiling. Importantly, both techniques have been performed successfully with good maternal and fetal outcome [90, 92]. While the majority of aneurysm rupture during pregnancy occurs in the third trimester, endovascular therapy may have an important role for management in cases occurring earlier in gesta-

tion where delivery is not feasible due to its shorter operative time, lower anesthetic exposure, and minimal impact on maternal hemodynamics [82].

Early medical management of aSAH focuses on airway surveillance and preservation, respiratory assistance, and circulatory control. Efforts to minimize the detrimental impact of post-rupture complications such as rebleeding, intracranial hypertension, and DCI/vasospasm are essential to limiting morbidity and mortality. Prior to definitive intervention, the occurrence of rebleeding is countered by control of acute hypertension. This must be balanced with the risk of cerebral ischemia secondary to reduced cerebral perfusion, and in the pregnant patient, with consideration of fetal sensitivity to changes in maternal blood pressure [47, 58]. Similar caution must be exercised in management of cerebral edema utilizing osmotic diuretics (i.e., mannitol) which are known to reduce cardiac output and uterine perfusion thereby posing risk of fetal hypoxia [49, 93]. Nimodipine, a calcium channel blocker thought to prevent/treat vasospasm/DCI, is associated with improved outcomes in aSAH [58]. While nimodipine has been found to be teratogenic in animal studies, a prospective, multicenter study of exposure to calcium channel antagonists in the first trimester of pregnancy showed no increase in the risk of major congenital malformations. Therefore, it is typically recommended for nimodipine to be given to all expectant women with aSAH. It may, however, be prudent to stratify treatment to patients at high risk for vasospasm (i.e., large volume of subarachnoid blood) [60]. Close fetal monitoring should be maintained to observe the impact of these interventions of fetal wellbeing and facilitate early intervention to counter fetal distress [91].

Conclusion

Intracranial aneurysms harbor the potential to result in significant morbidity and mortality upon rupture and resultant aSAH. The management of unruptured and ruptured aneurysms is complex and, in some cases, controversial; the additional concerns regarding preservation of fetal health in the setting of pregnancy make the complexity even more apparent. In general, decision making in this setting should involve multidisciplinary collaboration between the patient, family, obstetricians, and neurologists/neurosurgeons. While there is some evidence supporting pregnancy as a risk factor for aneurysm rupture, there is a general consensus that the evidence is insufficient to definitively confirm this relationship. Nor does the evidence support recommendation of C-section, a surgical procedure with its own risks, to prevent rupture during delivery. For women diagnosed with a high risk unruptured aneurysm, it is reasonable to recommend intervention prior to attempts at pregnancy. Those diagnosed with an unruptured aneurysm during pregnancy should be managed based on neurosurgical indications (i.e., risk of rupture); there may be a role for intervention in aneurysms that are not considered as high risk in the general population (i.e., smaller aneurysms) as some reports indicate an increased risk of rupture in these lesions. Mode of delivery should be based on obstetric indications in the women with a low risk unruptured aneurysm, with efforts made to reduce hemodynamic stresses during vaginal delivery. Women presenting with aSAH during pregnancy should be managed in an effort to reduce maternal and fetal morbidity and mortality; interventions taken should be in such a way as to reduce risk of fetal harm. When feasible, delivery via C-section prior to intervention is recommended in these cases to reduce the potential for fetal harm.

References

1. Hackenberg KAM, Hanggi D, Etminan N. Unruptured intracranial aneurysms. Stroke. 2018;49(9):2268–75.
2. Zhou S, Dion PA, Rouleau GA. Genetics of intracranial aneurysms. Stroke. 2018;49(3):780–7.
3. Perrone RD, Malek AM, Watnick T. Vascular complications in autosomal dominant polycystic kidney disease. Nat Rev Nephrol. 2015;11(10):589–98.
4. De Paepe A, Malfait F. The Ehlers-Danlos syndrome, a disorder with many faces. Clin Genet. 2012;82(1):1–11.
5. Draghia F, Draghia AC, Onicescu D. Electron microscopic study of the arterial wall in the cerebral aneurysms. Romanian J Morphol Embryol. 2008;49(1):101–3.
6. Jamous MA, Nagahiro S, Kitazato KT, Satoh K, Satomi J. Vascular corrosion casts mirroring early morphological changes that lead to the formation of saccular cerebral aneurysm: an experimental study in rats. J Neurosurg. 2005;102(3):532–5.
7. Jamous MA, Nagahiro S, Kitazato KT, Tamura T, Aziz HA, Shono M, et al. Endothelial injury and inflammatory response induced by hemodynamic changes preceding intracranial aneurysm formation: experimental study in rats. J Neurosurg. 2007;107(2):405–11.
8. Aoki T, Nishimura M, Matsuoka T, Yamamoto K, Furuyashiki T, Kataoka H, et al. PGE(2)-EP(2) signalling in endothelium is activated by haemodynamic stress and induces cerebral aneurysm through an amplifying loop via NF-kappaB. Br J Pharmacol. 2011;163(6):1237–49.
9. Chalouhi N, Ali MS, Jabbour PM, Tjoumakaris SI, Gonzalez LF, Rosenwasser RH, et al. Biology of intracranial aneurysms: role of inflammation. J Cereb Blood Flow Metab. 2012;32(9):1659–76.
10. Dias MS, Sekhar LN. Intracranial hemorrhage from aneurysms and arteriovenous malformations during pregnancy and the puerperium. Neurosurgery. 1990;27(6):855–65; discussion 865–6.
11. Meah VL, Cockcroft JR, Backx K, Shave R, Stohr EJ. Cardiac output and related haemodynamics during pregnancy: a series of meta-analyses. Heart. 2016;102(7):518–26.
12. Slopien R, Junik R, Meczekalski B, Halerz-Nowakowska B, Maciejewska M, Warenik-Szymankiewicz A, et al. Influence of hormonal replacement therapy on the regional cerebral blood flow in postmenopausal women. Maturitas. 2003;46(4):255–62.
13. Jaigobin C, Silver FL. Stroke and pregnancy. Stroke. 2000;31(12):2948–51.
14. Prins M, Boxem J, Lucas C, Hutton E. Effect of spontaneous pushing versus valsalva pushing in the second stage of labour on mother and fetus: a systematic review of randomised trials. BJOG. 2011;118(6):662–70.
15. Kim YW, Neal D, Hoh BL. Cerebral aneurysms in pregnancy and delivery: pregnancy and delivery do not increase the risk of aneurysm rupture. Neurosurgery. 2013;72(2):143–9; discussion 150.
16. de Rooij NK, Linn FH, van der Plas JA, Algra A, Rinkel GJ. Incidence of subarachnoid haemorrhage: a systematic review with emphasis on region, age, gender and time trends. J Neurol Neurosurg Psychiatry. 2007;78(12):1365–72.
17. Vlak MH, Algra A, Brandenburg R, Rinkel GJ. Prevalence of unruptured intracranial aneurysms, with emphasis on sex, age, comorbidity, country, and time period: a systematic review and meta-analysis. Lancet Neurol. 2011;10(7):626–36.

18. Dharmadhikari S, Atchaneeyasakul K, Ambekar S, Saini V, Haussen DC, Yavagal D. Association of menopausal age with unruptured intracranial aneurysm morphology. Interv Neurol. 2019;8(2–6):109–15.

19. Ding C, Toll V, Ouyang B, Chen M. Younger age of menopause in women with cerebral aneurysms. J Neurointerv Surg. 2013;5(4):327–31.

20. Lai PMR, Du R. Differentially expressed genes associated with the estrogen receptor pathway in cerebral aneurysms. World Neurosurg. 2019;126:e557–e63.

21. Barrow JW, Turan N, Wangmo P, Roy AK, Pradilla G. The role of inflammation and potential use of sex steroids in intracranial aneurysms and subarachnoid hemorrhage. Surg Neurol Int. 2018;9:150.

22. Tamura T, Jamous MA, Kitazato KT, Yagi K, Tada Y, Uno M, et al. Endothelial damage due to impaired nitric oxide bioavailability triggers cerebral aneurysm formation in female rats. J Hypertens. 2009;27(6):1284–92.

23. Hoh BL, Rojas K, Lin L, Fazal HZ, Hourani S, Nowicki KW, et al. Estrogen deficiency promotes cerebral aneurysm rupture by upregulation of Th17 cells and interleukin-17A which downregulates E-cadherin. J Am Heart Assoc. 2018;7(8):e008863.

24. Wajima D, Hourani S, Dodd W, Patel D, Jones C, Motwani K, et al. Interleukin-6 promotes murine estrogen deficiency-associated cerebral aneurysm rupture. Neurosurgery. 2020;86(4):583–92.

25. Tada Y, Makino H, Furukawa H, Shimada K, Wada K, Liang EI, et al. Roles of estrogen in the formation of intracranial aneurysms in ovariectomized female mice. Neurosurgery. 2014;75(6):690–5; discussion 695.

26. Tada Y, Wada K, Shimada K, Makino H, Liang EI, Murakami S, et al. Estrogen protects against intracranial aneurysm rupture in ovariectomized mice. Hypertension. 2014;63(6):1339–44.

27. Mhurchu CN, Anderson C, Jamrozik K, Hankey G, Dunbabin D, Australasian Cooperative Research on Subarachnoid Hemorrhage Study Group. Hormonal factors and risk of aneurysmal subarachnoid hemorrhage: an international population-based, case-control study. Stroke. 2001;32(3):606–12.

28. Juvela S. Risk factors for multiple intracranial aneurysms. Stroke. 2000;31(2):392–7.

29. Kaminogo M, Yonekura M, Shibata S. Incidence and outcome of multiple intracranial aneurysms in a defined population. Stroke. 2003;34(1):16–21.

30. van Gijn J, Kerr RS, Rinkel GJ. Subarachnoid haemorrhage. Lancet. 2007;369(9558):306–18.

31. Nieuwkamp DJ, Setz LE, Algra A, Linn FH, de Rooij NK, Rinkel GJ. Changes in case fatality of aneurysmal subarachnoid haemorrhage over time, according to age, sex, and region: a meta-analysis. Lancet Neurol. 2009;8(7):635–42.

32. Mackey J, Khoury JC, Alwell K, Moomaw CJ, Kissela BM, Flaherty ML, et al. Stable incidence but declining case-fatality rates of subarachnoid hemorrhage in a population. Neurology. 2016;87(21):2192–7.

33. Wermer MJ, van der Schaaf IC, Algra A, Rinkel GJ. Risk of rupture of unruptured intracranial aneurysms in relation to patient and aneurysm characteristics: an updated meta-analysis. Stroke. 2007;38(4):1404–10.

34. Daane TA, Tandy RW. Rupture of congenital intracranial aneurysm in pregnancy. Obstet Gynecol. 1960;15:305–14.

35. Barno A, Freeman DW. Maternal deaths due to spontaneous subarachnoid hemorrhage. Am J Obstet Gynecol. 1976;125(3):384–92.

36. Tiel Groenestege AT, Rinkel GJ, van der Bom JG, Algra A, Klijn CJ. The risk of aneurysmal subarachnoid hemorrhage during pregnancy, delivery, and the puerperium in the Utrecht population: case-crossover study and standardized incidence ratio estimation. Stroke. 2009;40(4):1148–51.

37. Kongable GL, Lanzino G, Germanson TP, Truskowski LL, Alves WM, Torner JC, et al. Gender-related differences in aneurysmal subarachnoid hemorrhage. J Neurosurg. 1996;84(1):43–8.

38. Park SK, Kim JM, Kim JH, Cheong JH, Bak KH, Kim CH. Aneurysmal subarachnoid hemorrhage in young adults: a gender comparison study. J Clin Neurosci. 2008;15(4):389–92.

39. Ghods AJ, Lopes D, Chen M. Gender differences in cerebral aneurysm location. Front Neurol. 2012;3:78.

40. Brisman JL, Song JK, Newell DW. Cerebral aneurysms. N Engl J Med. 2006;355(9):928–39.

41. Raps EC, Rogers JD, Galetta SL, Solomon RA, Lennihan L, Klebanoff LM, et al. The clinical spectrum of unruptured intracranial aneurysms. Arch Neurol. 1993;50(3):265–8.

42. Friedman JA, Piepgras DG, Pichelmann MA, Hansen KK, Brown RD Jr, Wiebers DO. Small cerebral aneurysms presenting with symptoms other than rupture. Neurology. 2001;57(7):1212–6.

43. Date I. Symptomatic unruptured cerebral aneurysms: features and surgical outcome. Neurol Med Chir (Tokyo). 2010;50(9):788–99.

44. Bassi P, Bandera R, Loiero M, Tognoni G, Mangoni A. Warning signs in subarachnoid hemorrhage: a cooperative study. Acta Neurol Scand. 1991;84(4):277–81.

45. Petridis AK, Kamp MA, Cornelius JF, Beez T, Beseoglu K, Turowski B, et al. Aneurysmal subarachnoid hemorrhage. Dtsch Arztebl Int. 2017;114(13):226–36.

46. Anderson C, Ni Mhurchu C, Scott D, Bennett D, Jamrozik K, Hankey G, et al. Triggers of subarachnoid hemorrhage: role of physical exertion, smoking, and alcohol in the Australasian Cooperative Research on Subarachnoid Hemorrhage Study (ACROSS). Stroke. 2003;34(7):1771–6.

47. Bederson JB, Connolly ES Jr, Batjer HH, Dacey RG, Dion JE, Diringer MN, et al. Guidelines for the management of aneurysmal subarachnoid hemorrhage: a statement for healthcare professionals from a special writing group of the Stroke Council, American Heart Association. Stroke. 2009;40(3):994–1025.

48. Rosenorn J, Eskesen V, Schmidt K, Ronde F. The risk of rebleeding from ruptured intracranial aneurysms. J Neurosurg. 1987;67(3):329–32.
49. Cho CS, Kim YJ, Cho KT, Lee SK, Park BJ, Cho MK. Temporary hidden aneurysms during pregnancy. A case report. Interv Neuroradiol. 2005;11(3):255–9.
50. Zoerle T, Lombardo A, Colombo A, Longhi L, Zanier ER, Rampini P, et al. Intracranial pressure after subarachnoid hemorrhage. Crit Care Med. 2015;43(1):168–76.
51. Saliou G, Paradot G, Gondry C, Bouzerar R, Lehmann P, Meyers ME, et al. A phase-contrast MRI study of acute and chronic hydrodynamic alterations after hydrocephalus induced by subarachnoid hemorrhage. J Neuroimaging. 2012;22(4):343–50.
52. Paisan GM, Ding D, Starke RM, Crowley RW, Liu KC. Shunt-dependent hydrocephalus after aneurysmal subarachnoid hemorrhage: predictors and long-term functional outcomes. Neurosurgery. 2018;83(3):393–402.
53. Fujii M, Yan J, Rolland WB, Soejima Y, Caner B, Zhang JH. Early brain injury, an evolving frontier in subarachnoid hemorrhage research. Transl Stroke Res. 2013;4(4):432–46.
54. Brinker T, Seifert V, Dietz H. Cerebral blood flow and intracranial pressure during experimental subarachnoid haemorrhage. Acta Neurochir. 1992;115(1–2):47–52.
55. Sehba FA, Hou J, Pluta RM, Zhang JH. The importance of early brain injury after subarachnoid hemorrhage. Prog Neurobiol. 2012;97(1):14–37.
56. Wartenberg KE, Schmidt JM, Claassen J, Temes RE, Frontera JA, Ostapkovich N, et al. Impact of medical complications on outcome after subarachnoid hemorrhage. Crit Care Med. 2006;34(3):617–23; quiz 624.
57. Bilello LA, Greige T, Singleton JM, Burke RC, Edlow JA. Retrospective review of pregnant patients presenting for evaluation of acute neurologic complaints. Ann Emerg Med. 2020;77:210.
58. Connolly ES Jr, Rabinstein AA, Carhuapoma JR, Derdeyn CP, Dion J, Higashida RT, et al. Guidelines for the management of aneurysmal subarachnoid hemorrhage: a guideline for healthcare professionals from the American Heart Association/American Stroke Association. Stroke. 2012;43(6):1711–37.
59. Suarez JI. Diagnosis and management of subarachnoid hemorrhage. Continuum. 2015;21(5 Neurocritical Care):1263–87.
60. Fairhall JM, Stoodley MA. Intracranial haemorrhage in pregnancy. Obstet Med. 2009;2(4):142–8.
61. Kanekar S, Bennett S. Imaging of neurologic conditions in pregnant patients. Radiographics. 2016;36(7):2102–22.
62. White PM, Teadsale E, Wardlaw JM, Easton V. What is the most sensitive non-invasive imaging strategy for the diagnosis of intracranial aneurysms? J Neurol Neurosurg Psychiatry. 2001;71(3):322–8.
63. Levent A, Yuce I, Eren S, Ozyigit O, Kantarci M. Contrast-enhanced and time-of-flight MR angiographic assessment of endovascular coiled intra-

cranial aneurysms at 1.5 T. Interv Neuroradiol. 2014;20(6):686–92.
64. Marshman LA, Aspoas AR, Rai MS, Chawda SJ. The implications of ISAT and ISUIA for the management of cerebral aneurysms during pregnancy. Neurosurg Rev. 2007;30(3):177–80; discussion 180.
65. Selo-Ojeme DO, Marshman LA, Ikomi A, Ojutiku D, Aspoas RA, Chawda SJ, et al. Aneurysmal subarachnoid haemorrhage in pregnancy. Eur J Obstet Gynecol Reprod Biol. 2004;116(2):131–43.
66. Raaymakers TW. Aneurysms in relatives of patients with subarachnoid hemorrhage: frequency and risk factors. MARS study group. Magnetic resonance angiography in relatives of patients with subarachnoid hemorrhage. Neurology. 1999;53(5):982–8.
67. Ronkainen A, Hernesniemi J, Puranen M, Niemitukia L, Vanninen R, Ryynanen M, et al. Familial intracranial aneurysms. Lancet. 1997;349(9049):380–4.
68. Broderick JP, Brown RD Jr, Sauerbeck L, Hornung R, Huston J III, Woo D, et al. Greater rupture risk for familial as compared to sporadic unruptured intracranial aneurysms. Stroke. 2009;40(6):1952–7.
69. Ronkainen A, Hernesniemi J, Tromp G. Special features of familial intracranial aneurysms: report of 215 familial aneurysms. Neurosurgery. 1995;37(1):43–6; discussion 46–7.
70. Schievink WI, Torres VE, Piepgras DG, Wiebers DO. Saccular intracranial aneurysms in autosomal dominant polycystic kidney disease. J Am Soc Nephrol. 1992;3(1):88–95.
71. Bor AS, Koffijberg H, Wermer MJ, Rinkel GJ. Optimal screening strategy for familial intracranial aneurysms: a cost-effectiveness analysis. Neurology. 2010;74(21):1671–9.
72. Zhou Z, Xu Y, Delcourt C, Shan J, Li Q, Xu J, et al. Is regular screening for intracranial aneurysm necessary in patients with autosomal dominant polycystic kidney disease? A systematic review and meta-analysis. Cerebrovasc Dis. 2017;44(1–2):75–82.
73. Flahault A, Trystram D, Fouchard M, Knebelmann B, Nataf F, Joly D. Screening for unruptured intracranial aneurysms in autosomal dominant polycystic kidney disease: a survey of 420 nephrologists. PLoS One. 2016;11(4):e0153176.
74. Thompson BG, Brown RD Jr, Amin-Hanjani S, Broderick JP, Cockroft KM, Connolly ES Jr, et al. Guidelines for the management of patients with unruptured intracranial aneurysms: a guideline for healthcare professionals from the American Heart Association/American Stroke Association. Stroke. 2015;46(8):2368–400.
75. Sloan MA, Stern BJ. Cerebrovascular disease in pregnancy. Curr Treat Options Neurol. 2003;5(5):391–407.
76. International Study of Unruptured Intracranial Aneurysms Investigators. Unruptured intracranial aneurysms--risk of rupture and risks of surgical intervention. N Engl J Med. 1998;339(24):1725–33.
77. Investigators UJ, Morita A, Kirino T, Hashi K, Aoki N, Fukuhara S, et al. The natural course of unruptured

cerebral aneurysms in a Japanese cohort. N Engl J Med. 2012;366(26):2474–82.

78. Wiebers DO, Whisnant JP, Huston J 3rd, Meissner I, Brown RD Jr, Piepgras DG, et al. Unruptured intracranial aneurysms: natural history, clinical outcome, and risks of surgical and endovascular treatment. Lancet. 2003;362(9378):103–10.

79. Villablanca JP, Duckwiler GR, Jahan R, Tateshima S, Martin NA, Frazee J, et al. Natural history of asymptomatic unruptured cerebral aneurysms evaluated at CT angiography: growth and rupture incidence and correlation with epidemiologic risk factors. Radiology. 2013;269(1):258–65.

80. Inoue T, Shimizu H, Fujimura M, Saito A, Tominaga T. Annual rupture risk of growing unruptured cerebral aneurysms detected by magnetic resonance angiography. J Neurosurg. 2012;117(1):20–5.

81. Kotowski M, Naggara O, Darsaut TE, Nolet S, Gevry G, Kouznetsov E, et al. Safety and occlusion rates of surgical treatment of unruptured intracranial aneurysms: a systematic review and meta-analysis of the literature from 1990 to 2011. J Neurol Neurosurg Psychiatry. 2013;84(1):42–8.

82. Barbarite E, Hussain S, Dellarole A, Elhammady MS, Peterson E. The management of intracranial aneurysms during pregnancy: a systematic review. Turk Neurosurg. 2016;26(4):465–74.

83. Weir BK, Drake CG. Rapid growth of residual aneurysmal neck during pregnancy. Case report. J Neurosurg. 1991;75(5):780–2.

84. Liu P, Lv X, Li Y, Lv M. Endovascular management of intracranial aneurysms during pregnancy in three cases and review of the literature. Interv Neuroradiol. 2015;21(6):654–8.

85. Kataoka H, Miyoshi T, Neki R, Yoshimatsu J, Ishibashi-Ueda H, Iihara K. Subarachnoid hemorrhage from intracranial aneurysms during pregnancy and the puerperium. Neurol Med Chir (Tokyo). 2013;53(8):549–54.

86. Wilson SR, Hirsch NP, Appleby I. Management of subarachnoid haemorrhage in a non-neurosurgical Centre. Anaesthesia. 2005;60(5):470–85.

87. Molyneux AJ, Kerr RS, Yu LM, Clarke M, Sneade M, Yarnold JA, et al. International subarachnoid aneurysm trial (ISAT) of neurosurgical clipping versus endovascular coiling in 2143 patients with ruptured intracranial aneurysms: a randomised comparison of effects on survival, dependency, seizures, rebleeding, subgroups, and aneurysm occlusion. Lancet. 2005;366(9488):809–17.

88. Molyneux AJ, Kerr RS, Birks J, Ramzi N, Yarnold J, Sneade M, et al. Risk of recurrent subarachnoid haemorrhage, death, or dependence and standardised mortality ratios after clipping or coiling of an intracranial aneurysm in the International Subarachnoid Aneurysm Trial (ISAT): long-term follow-up. Lancet Neurol. 2009;8(5):427–33.

89. van Buul BJ, Nijhuis JG, Slappendel R, Lerou JG, Bakker-Niezen SH. General anesthesia for surgical repair of intracranial aneurysm in pregnancy: effects on fetal heart rate. Am J Perinatol. 1993;10(2):183–6.

90. Kriplani A, Relan S, Misra NK, Mehta VS, Takkar D. Ruptured intracranial aneurysm complicating pregnancy. Int J Gynaecol Obstet. 1995;48(2):201–6.

91. Roman H, Descargues G, Lopes M, Emery E, Clavier E, Diguet A, et al. Subarachnoid hemorrhage due to cerebral aneurysmal rupture during pregnancy. Acta Obstet Gynecol Scand. 2004;83(4):330–4.

92. Piotin M, de Souza Filho CB, Kothimbakam R, Moret J. Endovascular treatment of acutely ruptured intracranial aneurysms in pregnancy. Am J Obstet Gynecol. 2001;185(5):1261–2.

93. Whitburn RH, Laishley RS, Jewkes DA. Anaesthesia for simultaneous caesarean section and clipping of intracerebral aneurysm. Br J Anaesth. 1990;64(5):642–5.

Cerebral Vascular Malformations in Pregnancy: Considerations for Diagnosis and Management

Michael S. Rallo, Neil Majmundar, Sanjeev Sreenivasan, Sudipta Roychowdhury, Anil Nanda, and Gaurav Gupta

Introduction

Vascular malformations of the nervous system comprise a diverse range of pathologies that have classically been divided into several categories: arteriovenous malformations (AVM), dural arteriovenous fistulas (DAVF), cavernous malformation (CM), developmental venous anomaly (DVA), and capillary telangiectasia [1]. Cerebral vascular malformations are complex problems and, although their occurArence in pregnancy is rare, they pose a unique challenge to clinicians seeking to balance optimal neurosurgical and obstetric care.

Stabilizing these lesions is important due to the risk of significant maternal and fetal morbidity and mortality, especially when associated with acute events such as rupture and hemorrhage. However, the natural history and indications for treatment of each type of lesion are unique and dependent on patient-specific factors. Therefore, decision making, and patient counseling require an intimate understanding of the literature and a collaborative approach between neurosurgical and obstetric providers. In this chapter, we will discuss in detail AVMs and CMs with particular attention to: (1) natural history, in particular the association of pregnancy and risk of rupture; (2) role of genetic and endocrinologic changes in malformation formation development; (3) management; (4) fetal risks and protective measures; and (5) mode and timing of delivery.

M. S. Rallo
Robert Wood Johnson University Hospital,
New Brunswick, NJ, USA

N. Majmundar · S. Sreenivasan
Department of Neurological Surgery, Rutgers Robert
Wood Johnson Medical School,
New Brunswick, NJ, USA

S. Roychowdhury
Neuroradiology, University Radiology,
New Brunswick, NJ, USA

A. Nanda
Neurosurgery, Robert Wood Johnson University
Hospital, New Brunswick, NJ, USA

G. Gupta (✉)
Neurosurgery, Rutgers Robert Wood Johnson
Medical School, New Brunswick, NJ, USA
e-mail: guptaga@rutgers.edu

Arteriovenous Malformation

Pathology and Pathogenesis of Arteriovenous Malformations

AVMs, more formally pial or parenchymal AVMs, are vascular anomalies characterized by abnormal, fistulous connections between arteries and veins bypassing the capillary network. These abnormal connections are typically tortuous in nature and form a localized cluster, termed the nidus, with a large, meningeal oriented base and a triangular, ventricular oriented apex. The lack

© The Author(s), under exclusive license to Springer Nature Switzerland AG 2023
G. Gupta et al. (eds.), *Neurological Disorders in Pregnancy*,
https://doi.org/10.1007/978-3-031-36490-7_9

of resistance, typically offered by capillary beds, results in high-flow arteriovenous shunting posing substantial risk for rupture and life-threatening hemorrhage (Fig. 9.1) [2]. The majority of AVMs are thought to be congenital lesions that arise spontaneously during development. This is supported by recent discovery of somatic mutations in genes of the Ras/MAPK pathway within AVM tissue [3, 4]. While causative germline mutations underlying these lesions have not been definitively identified, there is evidence associating polymorphisms in components of the tissue growth factor-beta (TGF-β) pathway with risk of AVM development [5, 6]. Moreover, polymorphisms in inflammation-related genes, including the interleukin-6 (IL-6) and tissue necrosis factor-alpha (TNF-α), correspond to the increased risk of AVM hemorrhage [7]. Familial cases of AVMs have also been described; however, it is unclear if these cases are coincidental, owing to the relative rarity of these lesions, or truly inherited [8, 9]. Finally, despite the widely held view that AVMs represent congenital lesions owing to dysfunctional processes during development, there is

accumulating evidence implicating insults to the brain, such as stroke, injury, infection, and even surgery, as a cause of de novo AVMs [10, 11]. In a minority (2–5%) of AVM patients the lesion can be syndromic in origin. AVMs are most often associated with hereditary hemorrhagic telangiectasia (HHT), capillary malformation-arteriovenous malformation (CM-AVM) syndrome and, less commonly, Wyburn-Mason syndrome [2, 12, 13]. Screening guidelines for syndromic AVMs will be discussed in the "Counseling and Management of Arteriovenous Malformations" section.

Influence of Pregnancy and Sex Hormones on Arteriovenous Malformation Pathogenesis

The maternal cardiovascular and hemodynamic changes accompanying pregnancy include a 40–50% increase in plasma volume, a comparable increase in cardiac output, and a significant reduction in systemic vascular resistance and blood pressure. These changes are critical for placental-fetal development and begin early in gestation, reaching a nadir during the second

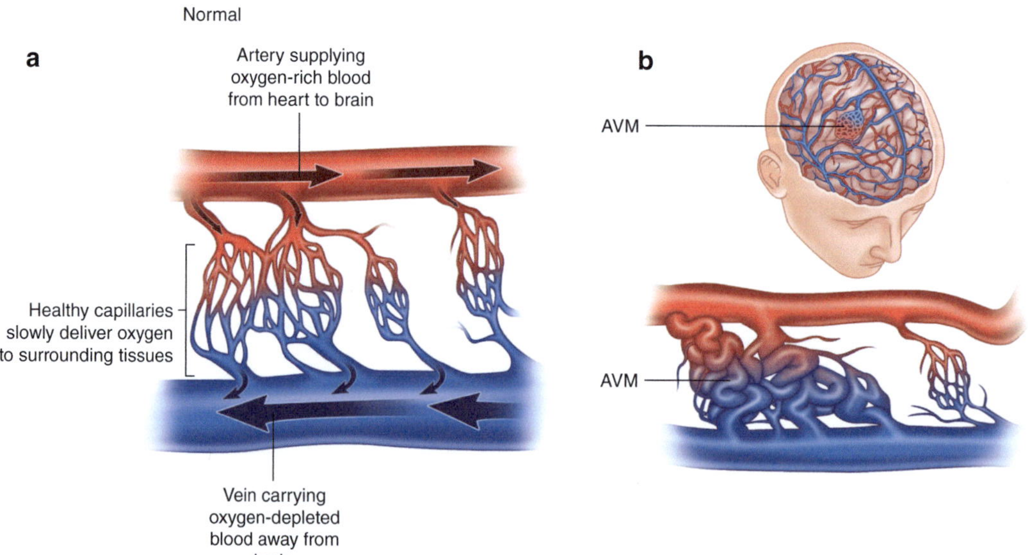

Fig. 9.1 (a) Normal vascular anatomy demonstrating capillary beds connecting high pressure arteries with low pressure veins. Hydrostatic pressure is gradually reduced across capillaries. (b) An AVM represents a tangle of blood vessels that results in direct, high-flow connections between arteries and veins without intervening capillary beds. As a result, veins are subjected to abnormally high pressure

trimester, before gradually returning to baseline [14]. Unlike other organs, such as the kidney, ovaries, and uterus in which perfusion is substantially increased, cerebral blood flow is maintained relatively constant during gestation due to the cranial cavity's relative intolerance to increased volume [15]. Mild estrogen-mediated increase in cerebral blood flow and transmission of hemodynamic force has been thought to underlie the reported risk of AVM hemorrhage during pregnancy. This is supported by the occurrence of rupture during the second and third trimesters, mirroring hemodynamic changes [16, 17]. Pregnancy is also associated with the release of a number of hormones and signaling factors including inflammatory mediators, chemokines, steroids, and growth factors which may influence AVM evolution. Moreover, animal studies have demonstrated heightened angiogenic activity in AVM tissues during late pregnancy, although there were no detectable differences in key angiogenic molecules or receptors [18]. The cerebrovascular and cardiovascular changes accompanying pregnancy are discussed in detail in Chap. 5.

Epidemiology, Presentation, and Natural Course of Arteriovenous Malformations

Scope of the Problem

Cerebral vascular malformations are relatively uncommon representing 5–9% of all intracranial space-occupying lesions; however, they are an important cause of neurologic morbidity and mortality in younger adults [19]. Developmental venous anomalies are considered the most common of these vascular malformations with a reported incidence of approximately 2% based on autopsy studies. However, these, along with capillary telangiectasias, exhibit a low tendency for neurological sequelae [20]. AVMs are relatively uncommon with prevalence between 10 and 20 per 100,000 [21–23]. While AVMs do not exhibit sex predilection, their tendency to present in young

adulthood, most commonly in the third decade of life, makes them a significant concern in women of childbearing age [24].

Clinical Manifestations and Natural Course of Arteriovenous Malformations

AVMs can cause an array of neurological manifestations related to either mass effect or hemorrhage. AVMs are the most aggressive cerebrovascular lesions, with annual rupture rates reported between 2% and 4% [25]. Hemorrhage is, by far, the most common and devastating clinical manifestation of AVMs, accounting for 40–65%, followed by seizures in 18–35%, and chronic headache or focal neurological deficit in a small proportion [26–28]. Notably, hemorrhagic presentation has been shown to occur disproportionately in the youngest (<10 years) and oldest (>50) age groups, while presentation with seizures spikes between the ages of 20–29 [29]. Risk of hemorrhage increases substantially with previous hemorrhage and older age at diagnosis, in addition to morphologic features of the AVM including deep anatomic location, exclusive deep venous drainage, and associated aneurysms [25, 30].

Contrasting the predominance of ischemic stroke in the general population, hemorrhagic stroke—such as that resulting from rupture of vascular lesions—is the most common type during pregnancy [31]. In fact, the most common cause of intracerebral hemorrhage in the expectant patient is rupture of an AVM [32]. There is a body of evidence demonstrating an association between pregnancy and/or vaginal delivery and risk of aggressive behavior (i.e., growth, rupture/hemorrhage) of AVMs [27, 33–36]. One recently published report utilizing State Inpatient Databases and employing a cohort-crossover design demonstrated a greater than threefold increase in the rate of intracranial hemorrhage during pregnancy among patients with AVMs [37]. This is considered a consequence of the hemodynamic stress that evolves through pregnancy and peaks during the second stage of labor. However, there is substantial opposing evidence, including a systematic review which was not sufficient to support increased risk of AVM hemorrhage in pregnancy [17, 38]. Therefore, there is a need for enhanced, more rigorous future research, specifically through execution of a multicenter, prospective, case crossover study.

Diagnostic Considerations for Arteriovenous Malformations in the Pregnant Patient

Initial diagnosis of AVMs is typically via non-invasive imaging during workup for the presenting cause (i.e., intracranial hemorrhage, seizures, etc.). Advancements in and availability of imaging have also increased the rate of incidental diagnosis of these pathologies [28, 39]. The presence of multiple AVMs should raise suspicion of a syndromic cause [40]. Multiple AVMs occurring in association with recurrent epistaxis, and pulmonary/hepatic AVMs are indicative of HHT [2]. While most pregnancies occur normally in patients with HHT, the potential complications including heart failure, intracranial hemorrhage, pulmonary hemorrhage, and stroke (related to paradoxical emboli) make such pregnancies "high risk" [41].

Neuroradiological Features of Arteriovenous Malformations

In the pregnant patient, acquisition of the necessary data for clinical decision making must be balanced with the concern of ionizing radiation exposure to the fetus. Computed tomography (CT) relies on ionizing radiation thereby posing potential fetal risk; however, in head and neck CT the fetus is out of the range of the scan and therefore exposed to limited radiation. In the pregnant patient, CT still remains the standard for the evaluation of suspected intracranial hemorrhage with precautions taken to reduce fetal exposure (i.e., lead shielding of abdomen and pelvis) [33, 42]. Hemorrhage from an AVM typically appears as hyperdensity in an intraparenchymal or lobar distribution, however, this is not sufficient for diagnosis. Therefore, MRI is often necessary to delineate the anatomical features, particularly the "tangle of signal voids" on T2-weighted imaging [43].

Vascular imaging, including both CT and MR angiography (CTA/MRA) is critical for the diagnosis and evaluation of AVMs [44]. Definitive diagnosis and treatment planning of a cerebral AVM is often reliant on conventional digital subtraction angiography (DSA), a catheter-based modality that utilizes ionizing radiation and iodinated contrast. DSA provides the highest spatial and temporal resolution necessary to delineate features of the AVM that are critical to management decision making. In addition to the radiation exposure, risks associated with DSA include thromboembolic complications (i.e., stroke) [45]. Despite such risks, DSA remains indicated in pregnant patients with appropriate shielding and limitation of beam time. The estimated fetal radiation exposure during DSA is between 0.17 and 2.8 mGy, sufficiently lower than the accepted limit of 50 mGy. To reduce the overall radiation exposure time while acquiring the most relevant information, it is prudent for members of the cerebrovascular team contemplating treatment to perform the DSA [38, 45]. Considerations for neuroimaging in the pregnant patient are discussed in detail in Chap. 3.

Counseling and Management of Arteriovenous Malformations

Diagnosis of an AVM is frightening for anyone, but particularly for the pregnant patient or the young adult patient, hoping to become pregnant. Such a diagnosis often leaves the expectant patient questioning how to manage both her pregnancy and the lesion in sync. Decision making regarding management in these settings is highly complex and dependent on anatomic and morphologic features of the lesion itself in addition to the patient's individual clinical factors. The occurrence of rupture and hemorrhage is a key pivotal point in decision making, with a tendency toward conservative management in unruptured or clinically silent AVMs and toward invasive management in those that have ruptured or are otherwise symptomatic. The approach to management is especially complex in the pregnant patient due to the need to balance both maternal and fetal harm. Unfortunately, there is only scarce literature and no guidelines or consensus statements to inform this unique situation.

Counseling: Patients with Arteriovenous Malformation Planning to Become Pregnant and Hereditary Concerns

Historically, the purported association between pregnancy and aggressive behavior of cerebral vascular malformations, particularly AVMs, has led women with such lesions to be sterilized, counseled against pregnancy, or to even have their pregnancies terminated. In those women in whom gestation did proceed, cesarean delivery was recommended due to concern for rupture [27, 46]. However, as described above, there is a lack of consensus on whether or not pregnancy truly confers increased risk for rupture. For a woman of childbearing age with a diagnosed AVM, a critical question may be: Should I undergo treatment before becoming pregnant? The patient should be counseled appropriately on the evidence regarding the association between pregnancy and risk of hemorrhage, which at this point is conflicting and insufficient. Therefore, the decision to treat an unruptured AVM prior to pregnancy should be consistent with the characteristics of the lesion and clinical history (i.e., previous hemorrhage) [25, 30, 47]. In a woman with a high-risk lesion or one producing severe symptoms, in whom management of the malformation is indicated, it is certainly safer for treatment to occur prior to pregnancy. It is important to note that, while radiosurgery remains an attractive approach for management of AVMs, particularly in difficult to access regions of the brain, a major limitation is its failure to achieve immediate obliteration and reduction of hemorrhage risk [39, 48]. In a study of women who became pregnant during the latency period, 2 of 18 (11.1%) experienced AVM hemorrhage compared to 2.5% of nonpregnant women [49]. Based on this evidence, albeit with limited sample size, we recom-

mend women who are treated with radiosurgery to await attempts at pregnancy until confirmed obliteration of the lesion.

Syndromic malformations represent another topic of concern in patients who are pregnant or considering becoming pregnant. In women who appear to suffer from AVMs associated with a syndromic cause, screening is warranted. HHT is one of the most common syndromes associated with cerebral AVMs and is characterized by the presence of cutaneous telangiectasias in addition to pulmonary, hepatic, and cerebral AVMs. HHT is transmitted in an autosomal dominant pattern, therefore the risk to one's offspring is 50% [50]. Screening for cerebral and pulmonary AVMs is recommended in all offspring of parent's with HHT, unless the disease is excluded by genetic testing. It has also been recommended that those screened for cerebral AVMs during infancy undergo a follow-up screen after puberty due to the potential for AVMs to grow and remodel throughout childhood [51]. Women with HHT are also recommended to be screened and treated for pulmonary AVMs prior to pregnancy; asymptomatic pulmonary AVMs identified during pregnancy should not be treated until after delivery. Finally, screening of the spine with MRI in women with HHT may be necessary to rule out spinal AVMs and thus permit regional anesthesia [41].

Management of Unruptured Arteriovenous Malformations in Pregnancy

Management of unruptured AVMs is a highly contested topic, especially in the aftermath of the heavily critiqued "A Randomized Trial of Unruptured Brain Arteriovenous Malformations" (ARUBA) study published in 2014 which was terminated early due to superiority of medical management over interventional therapy [52]. The complex decision making in management of unruptured AVMs is further complicated in the setting of pregnancy, with additional concerns regarding modality for treatment and timing in relation to delivery. The currently available

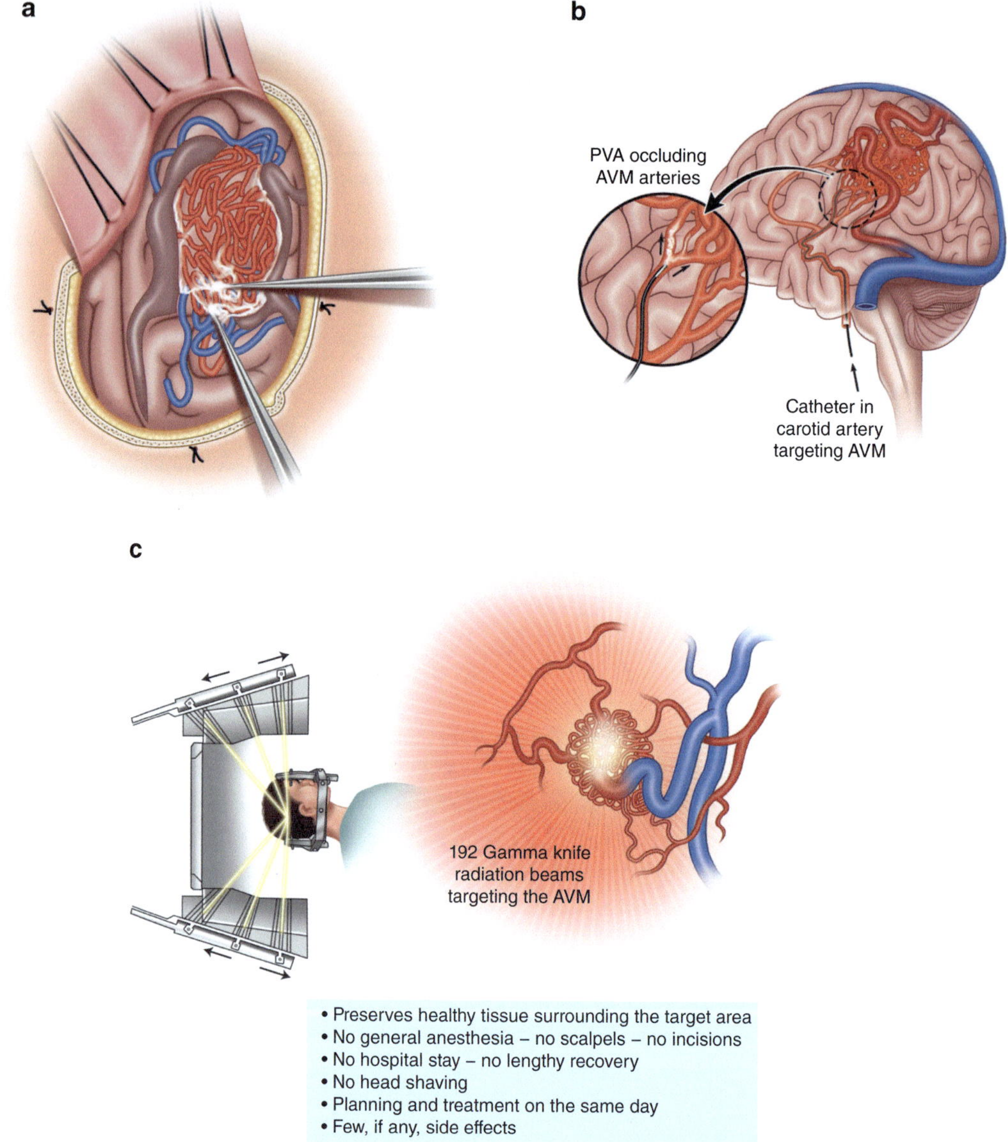

Fig. 9.2 Treatment options available for treatment of AVMs includes: (**a**) microsurgical resection, (**b**) endovascular embolization, and (**c**) radiosurgical obliteration

modalities for AVM treatment include microsurgery, neoadjuvant endovascular embolization, and radiosurgical obliteration, each with their own risk/benefit profile (Fig. 9.2). Generally, unruptured AVMs presenting in pregnancy should be approached conservatively due to their relatively low risk profile, even despite some reports of elevated rupture risk in pregnancy [38, 53]. Further supporting this, in a report of 12 patients presenting with unruptured AVM during pregnancy, all managed conservatively, one (8.3%) developed bleeding during gestation. All patients were followed to full term, with ten undergoing cesarean section and two delivering vaginally [54]. As such, intervention during pregnancy should be based on neurosurgical indications while accounting for obstetrical concerns. However, due to the paucity of data on this topic, we are unable to make specific recommendations on selection of patients for management of unruptured AVMs in pregnancy. An interdisciplinary team including a representative or representatives specialized in microsurgery, radiosurgery, and interventional procedures, as well as obstetrics/gynecology and neurocritical care should be involved in the decision making process. Guiding factors in this process should include: (1) risk of catastrophic hemorrhage, (2) maternal-fetal risk of individual therapies, and (3) stage of pregnancy. Increased risk of hemorrhage is conferred by deep venous drainage, associated nidal aneurysms, and previous rupture and these patients may warrant intervention of their unruptured AVM [25, 30]. In considering microsurgical resection, the grade of the AVM can help to predict risk of complications; for example, Spetzler-Martin grade I or II lesions have relatively low surgical risk and high probability of complete resection and obliteration [55]. Similar grading models can be applied for prediction of complications and outcomes in radiosurgery or endovascular embolization [56]. There is precedent for delay of surgery for small, low risk, ruptured AVMs until fetal maturity and delivery has occurred; this may even be extended to 2 months following delivery to permit restoration of normal cardiovascular and hemostatic factors [57, 58]. This same logic may be considered in dealing with unruptured AVMs identified during pregnancy. As with all decisions made in the clinical setting, we must strive to achieve equipoise between the true risks of the lesion and the risks associated with therapy; in the setting of unruptured AVMs in pregnancy, the risks of therapy compared to those of the lesion typically favor conservative management. In those in whom intrapartum intervention occurs, vaginal delivery in accordance with obstetric indications appears safe in patients with completely resected or obliterated AVMs [59].

Given that the most likely presentation of an *unruptured* AVM is seizures, it is of importance to briefly discuss the approach to management of seizures in pregnancy. Adequate control of seizures is critical for preservation of maternal and fetal health: seizures induce lactic acidosis, increases in uterine pressure and blood flow, and are associated with maternal and fetal hypoxia [60]. It is established that many antiepileptic drugs increase risks of congenital anomalies, such as congenital heart disease, cleft palate, neural tube defects, and finger hypoplasia. Traditional antiepileptics, such as valproate and phenobarbital, exhibit the highest risk of major malformations while newer agents, such as lamotrigine and levetiracetam, are associated with lower risk profiles [61]. Major considerations for administration of antiepileptics in the pregnant patient include supplementation of folic acid and use of monotherapy when possible for seizure control [54]. Considerations for the selection of antiepileptic agents during pregnancy are discussed in detail in Chap. 28.

Management of Ruptured Arteriovenous Malformations in Pregnancy

Ruptured AVMs resulting in intracranial hemorrhage result in substantial maternal and fetal morbidity and mortality. Emergent restoration of normal blood pressure (<140 mmHg) in hypertensive (150–220 mmHg) patients is recommended in the setting of acute intracranial hemorrhage [62]; however, it is important to balance this with maintenance of uteroplacental blood flow and utilization of safe pharmacologic agents such as labetalol, hydralazine, or nifedipine [63]. Diagnosis of the pregnant patient with intracranial hemorrhage from any cause, including AVM, should warrant consult with specialists from obstetrics/gynecology.

After initial management related to the intracranial hemorrhage, options for definitive management of the ruptured AVM include the same modalities as unruptured AVMs: microsurgical resection, endovascular embolization, radiosurgical obliteration, or a combination of the three. As in the case of unruptured AVMs, decision making in ruptured AVMs should be based on neurosurgical indications with special consideration to obstetrical concerns. After initial stabilization, the primary principle guiding management in the setting of a ruptured AVM is reducing the risk of rebleeding. It is well established that prior hemorrhage is a significant risk factor for future hemorrhage, particularly in the first year following rupture where rebleed rates spike to double that of other time points [64]. Owing to the relatively low risk of immediate rebleeding (<1% per month) from ruptured AVMs, contrasting the risk in ruptured aneurysms, delayed intervention of at least 4 weeks has been proposed to permit rehabilitation following initial hemorrhage in the general population [65]. However, it is important to note that there is evidence of increased risk of rebleeding in pregnant patients, with reported rates near 25%, compared to an annual risk of rebleeding of 7.45% in a general cohort [33, 34, 46, 57, 66]. In the pregnant patient, delayed management may be reasonable, particularly for patients in the late third trimester in whom delivery may be able to proceed prior to intervention. Delay is also supported in pregnant patients with small amounts of hemorrhage that are otherwise not at high risk for re-rupture until several weeks postpartum when maternal hemodynamics have been restored [57]. In such cases in which fetal maturity permits pre-intervention delivery, it is prudent to deliver via cesarean section [67]. If the fetus is not viable, the re-rupture risk is high, and the lesion is amenable to intervention, treatment during pregnancy is warranted [59]. Intervention during pregnancy has been reported successfully utilizing surgical [67], endovascular [68], and radiosurgical [69] means.

Each modality bears its own important risks. Microsurgical resection is substantially riskier in higher grade lesions [70]. In addition to the risk of neurological deficit associated with surgery, there is additional concern for fetal harm in the pregnant patient, particularly fetal hypoperfusion and hypoxia. Maintenance of adequate maternal hydration and hemodynamic status is critical for maintaining uterine and fetal perfusion but can be compromised in the setting of surgery via blood loss, diuresis, and even patient positioning. Diuretic agents, such as mannitol, are typically employed during microsurgical resection to minimize cerebral swelling but may cross the placenta and result fetal hypovolemia and dehydration [54]. In a small cohort of patients undergoing craniotomy for various indications, mannitol was used without complication for brain relaxation suggesting that judicious use is safe and effective in the setting of pregnancy [71]. Moreover, maternal hypotension during surgery can result in fetal hypoperfusion and hypoxia [72]. Endovascular embolization, particularly as monotherapy, does not provide total obliteration of the AVM but does allow for elimination of high-risk features such as perinidal or intranidal aneurysms which increase the re-rupture risk [73]. In addition, exposure to ionizing radiation in pregnant patients is of particular concern due to the potential fetal harm that may result. Fortunately, most reports suggest that fetal exposure during cerebral diagnostic angiography and neuroembolization is far below the safety threshold [59]. To minimize the risk of fetal harm from ionizing radiation it is critical to maintain appropriate abdominal shielding; efforts should also be made to reduce fluoroscopy time (i.e., via selective angiography of targeted vessels) and beam angling [53, 58]. Although iodinated contrast is not contraindicated in pregnancy, utilization of half strength contrast may also enhance procedural safety during embolization [53]. A major limitation of radiosurgery is the inability to achieve immediate obliteration of the AVM that would allow a patient to be freed from the risk of devastating intracranial hemorrhage. In fact, the latency of radiosurgery is typically considered to be 2 years from treatment completion; this would not warrant any protection to the pregnant patient if performed during gestation but would expose the fetus to potentially hazardous ionizing radiation [39]. We conclude, in concordance with previous groups, that radiosurgery is not an appropriate intervention to be undertaken in the pregnant patient [58].

Cavernous Malformations

Pathology and Pathogenesis of Cavernous Malformations

CMs, also known as cavernomas or cavernous angiomas, are malformations consisting of a cluster of thin-walled, dilated capillaries recognizable by their characteristic "mulberry" appearance. Histologically, the vessels, referred to as caverns, are constituted by a simple endothelial lining surrounded by a thin, fibrous adventitial layer [74]. CMs arise in two distinct forms: (1) sporadic, which are classically solitary lesions associated with a developmental venous anomaly, and (2) familial, which often presents with multiple lesions and a strong family history of neurological disease [75]. Mutations in three protein-encoding genes (*CCM1*, *CCM2*, and *CCM3*) have been identified as causative of CM and are transmitted in an autosomal dominant pattern. These proteins contribute to a larger signaling pathway that regulates angiogenesis, vessel formation, and cellular proliferation [76].

Influence of Pregnancy and Sex Hormones on Cavernous Malformation Pathogenesis

While the hemodynamic changes of pregnancy may influence pathogenesis and hemorrhage of CMs, they are low-flow lesions and generally considered to be less subject to these stresses. Consistent with this, a recently published prospective analysis of 367 deliveries demonstrated no instances of hemorrhage during this period in which acute hemodynamic stresses are expected to occur [77]. Like AVMs, CMs are influenced by circulating factors associated with pregnancy including growth factors and inflammatory mediators. Elevated levels of vascular endothelial growth factor and basic fibroblast growth factor during pregnancy are thought to underlie growth and potentiate rupture of CMs [47].

Epidemiology, Presentation, and Natural Course of Cavernous Malformations

Scope of the Problem

CMs are the second most common vascular anomaly and have a reported prevalence ranging between 0.3% and 0.5% in both autopsy and imaging studies [78–80]. Assuming a prevalence of 0.4% and an estimated 114 million births worldwide, it is expected that over half a million pregnancies will occur in women with CM [81]. Similar to AVMs, CMs tend to present during young adulthood making them a concern in women of childbearing age [82].

Clinical Manifestations and Natural Course of Cavernous Malformations

CMs rupture at an annual rate of 0.3–2.3%, making them slightly less aggressive than AVMs [30, 83]. Moreover, hemorrhagic CMs are typically less destructive due to the low flow nature of these lesions. Therefore, small hemorrhages in noneloquent tissue may be clinically silent. Any deficits related to hemorrhage are often transient and resolve within a period of days to weeks as blood is absorbed [30, 84]. Of note, there is some evidence supporting female sex as a risk factor for CM hemorrhage, although this is not conclusive [83]. The most common presentation of CM involving the cerebral hemispheres is seizures, owing to the inherent epileptogenicity of iron found at the border of the lesions [82]. Similar to AVMs, there is previous evidence suggesting that pregnancy and/or vaginal delivery confers increased risk of aggressive behavior (i.e., growth, rupture/hemorrhage) of CMs [85]. This was postulated to result from cardiovascular and hemodynamic factors as well as pregnancy-associated hormones including progesterone and growth factors [47]. However, this is refuted by more recent evidence from several large prospective and retrospective cohorts [77, 81, 86].

Diagnostic Considerations for Cavernous Malformations in the Pregnant Patient

The initial step in identification of a CM is via non-invasive imaging during the evaluation of headache, neurological deficit, or, most often, new-onset seizures. There is also an increased propensity for incidental detection with advancements and widespread availability of neuroimaging [39].

Neuroradiological Features of Cavernous Malformations

Unless the lesion is large or recently bled, CMs are typically difficult to identify on head CT. This makes MRI the gold-standard for diagnosis of CMs due to the ability to delineate key anatomic and pathologic features. Classically, CMs exhibit a reticular core with a "berry" or "popcorn" appearance that is often surrounded by a low-intensity halo [84]. In contrast to AVMs whose angioarchitecture is highlighted on angiography, the most notable radiological feature of CMs is that they are angiographically occult: that is, they do not appear on these dedicated vascular imaging studies [87].

Counseling and Management of Cavernous Malformations

Counseling: Patients with Cavernous Malformation Planning to Become Pregnant and Hereditary Concerns

Based on the most recently available and reliable data, there is no reason that the presence of a cavernous malformation should preclude a woman from considering pregnancy [77, 81, 86]. Therefore, treatment should be guided by neurosurgical considerations including anatomic location, presence of symptoms (i.e., seizures), and prior hemorrhage. When treatment is indicated, it may be prudent to intervene prior to conception to mitigate surgical or radiation risks posed to the fetus. In the setting of familial CM, which displays autosomal dominant inheritance, screening is recommended via molecular genetic testing in those in whom the familial genetic variant is isolated or otherwise via MRI of the brain and spinal cord [88].

Management of Cavernous Malformations in Pregnancy

The severity of CMs varies significantly: small hemorrhage may be clinically silent or produce transient neurological symptoms, while hemorrhage of brainstem CMs can be acutely debilitating and life-threatening. The clinical data regarding management of CMs in pregnancy is particularly limited. A treatment strategy has been proposed by Yamada et al. in which asymptomatic and mildly symptomatic lesions are managed conservatively, while those with severe or progressive symptoms are surgically resected. Certain risk factors, such as previous hemorrhage or family history may warrant intervention in a lesion that would otherwise be approached conservatively [47]. A review of 16 cases of CM identified during pregnancy determined that neurosurgical intervention is seldom necessary [89]. When surgical management is necessary, it is recommended to occur after delivery so long as there is no substantial threat to maternal or fetal wellbeing [47]. However, in cases where maternal-fetal life is compromised, such as catastrophic hemorrhage, treatment preceding delivery can be accomplished without obstetric complication [89, 90]. Historic concerns regarding CM hemorrhage in association with maternal hemodynamic changes during labor have led to a tendency for patients with asymptomatic and symptomatic lesions to undergo cesarean delivery. However, a more recent study found that vaginal delivery occurred without hemorrhagic complication in 149 of 168 pregnancies in 64 female patients with CMs [81]. Therefore, choice of delivery method should be dictated by obstetrical considerations, rather than concern for hemorrhage.

Conclusion

Management of cerebral vascular malformations is especially complicated in the context of pregnancy and requires multidisciplinary collaboration between the patient, family, obstetricians, and neurologists/neurosurgeons. While there is some evidence supporting pregnancy as a risk factor for aggressive behavior of vascular malformations (i.e., rupture, hemorrhage, progression), we do not find the evidence sufficient to definitively confirm such a relationship. For women with vascular lesions seeking counseling on becoming pregnant, we conclude that those at high risk should be treated prior to attempts at pregnancy. Women diagnosed with an unruptured or asymptomatic/mildly symptomatic lesions during pregnancy should be managed based on neurosurgical indications in consult with a team of interdisciplinary and multimodal experts; intervention is typically not warranted. Women diagnosed with a hemorrhagic lesions during pregnancy should be managed in an effort to reduce maternal and fetal morbidity and mortality; interventions taken should be in such a way as to reduce risk of fetal harm. Vaginal delivery generally appears safe in unruptured or resected/obliterated AVMs and CMs, while cesarean delivery is likely the safest approach to delivery in women with ruptured AVMs.

References

1. Flemming KD, Robert D, Brown J. 401: Epidemiology and natural history of intracranial Vascular Malformations. In: Winn HR, editor. Youmans & Winn neurological surgery. Philadelphia, PA: Elsevier; 2017.
2. Gavin CG, Kitchen ND. 400: Pathobiology of true arteriovenous malformations. In: Winn HR, editor. Youmans & Winn neurological surgery. 7th ed. Philadelphia, PA: Elsevier; 2017.
3. Nikolaev SI, Vetiska S, Bonilla X, Boudreau E, Jauhiainen S, Rezai Jahromi B, et al. Somatic activating KRAS mutations in arteriovenous malformations of the brain. N Engl J Med. 2018;378(3):250–61.
4. Al-Olabi L, Polubothu S, Dowsett K, Andrews KA, Stadnik P, Joseph AP, et al. Mosaic RAS/MAPK variants cause sporadic vascular malformations which respond to targeted therapy. J Clin Invest. 2018;128(4):1496–508.
5. Pawlikowska L, Tran MN, Achrol AS, Ha C, Burchard E, Choudhry S, et al. Polymorphisms in transforming growth factor-beta-related genes ALK1 and ENG are associated with sporadic brain arteriovenous malformations. Stroke. 2005;36(10):2278–80.
6. Ge M, Du C, Li Z, Liu Y, Xu S, Zhang L, et al. Association of ACVRL1 genetic polymorphisms with arteriovenous malformations: a case-control study and meta-analysis. World Neurosurg. 2017;108:690–7.
7. Pawlikowska L, Tran MN, Achrol AS, McCulloch CE, Ha C, Lind DL, et al. Polymorphisms in genes involved in inflammatory and angiogenic pathways and the risk of hemorrhagic presentation of brain arteriovenous malformations. Stroke. 2004;35(10):2294–300.
8. van Beijnum J, van der Worp HB, Schippers HM, van Nieuwenhuizen O, Kappelle LJ, Rinkel GJ, et al. Familial occurrence of brain arteriovenous malformations: a systematic review. J Neurol Neurosurg Psychiatry. 2007;78(11):1213–7.
9. van Beijnum J, van der Worp HB, Algra A, Vandertop WP, van den Berg R, Brouwer PA, et al. Prevalence of brain arteriovenous malformations in first-degree relatives of patients with a brain arteriovenous malformation. Stroke. 2014;45(11):3231–5.
10. Santos R, Aguilar-Salinas P, Entwistle JJ, Aldana PR, Beier AD, Hanel RA. De novo arteriovenous malformation in a pediatric patient: case report and review of the literature. World Neurosurg. 2018;111:341–5.
11. Lv X, Wang G. Review of de novo cerebral arteriovenous malformation: haemorrhage risk, treatment approaches and outcomes. Neuroradiol J. 2018;31(3):224–9.
12. Barbosa Do Prado L, Han C, Oh SP, Su H. Recent advances in basic research for brain arteriovenous malformation. Int J Mol Sci. 2019;20(21):5324.
13. So JM, Holman RE. Wyburn-Mason syndrome. Treasure Island, FL: StatPearls; 2020.
14. Sanghavi M, Rutherford JD. Cardiovascular physiology of pregnancy. Circulation. 2014;130(12):1003–8.
15. Johnson AC, Cipolla MJ. The cerebral circulation during pregnancy: adapting to preserve normalcy. Physiology (Bethesda). 2015;30(2):139–47.
16. Krause DN, Duckles SP, Pelligrino DA. Influence of sex steroid hormones on cerebrovascular function. J Appl Physiol. 2006;101(4):1252–61.
17. Liu XJ, Wang S, Zhao YL, Teo M, Guo P, Zhang D, et al. Risk of cerebral arteriovenous malformation rupture during pregnancy and puerperium. Neurology. 2014;82(20):1798–803.
18. Ceylan D, Tatarli N, Avsar T, Arslanhan A, Bozkurt SU, Bagci P, et al. In vivo effect of pregnancy on angiogenesis potential of arteriovenous malformation tissue samples: an experimental study. J Neurosurg Sci. 2017;61(2):151–6.
19. Jellinger K. Vascular malformations of the central nervous system: a morphological overview. Neurosurg Rev. 1986;9(3):177–216.

20. Aoki R, Srivatanakul K. Developmental venous anomaly: benign or not benign. Neurol Med Chir (Tokyo). 2016;56(9):534–43.

21. NORD. Arteriovenous malformation: national organization for rare diseases; 2019. https://rarediseases.org/rare-diseases/arteriovenous-malformation/.

22. Kim T, Kwon OK, Bang JS, Lee H, Kim JE, Kang HS, et al. Epidemiology of ruptured brain arteriovenous malformation: a National Cohort Study in Korea. J Neurosurg. 2018:1–6.

23. Mohr JP, Kejda-Scharler J, Pile-Spellman J. Diagnosis and treatment of arteriovenous malformations. Curr Neurol Neurosci Rep. 2013;13(2):324.

24. Hofmeister C, Stapf C, Hartmann A, Sciacca RR, Mansmann U, terBrugge K, et al. Demographic, morphological, and clinical characteristics of 1289 patients with brain arteriovenous malformation. Stroke. 2000;31(6):1307–10.

25. Kim H, Al-Shahi Salman R, McCulloch CE, Stapf C, Young WL, Coinvestigators M. Untreated brain arteriovenous malformation: patient-level meta-analysis of hemorrhage predictors. Neurology. 2014;83(7):590–7.

26. Shaligram SS, Winkler E, Cooke D, Su H. Risk factors for hemorrhage of brain arteriovenous malformation. CNS Neurosci Ther. 2019;25(10):1085–95.

27. Al-Shahi R, Warlow C. A systematic review of the frequency and prognosis of arteriovenous malformations of the brain in adults. Brain. 2001;124(Pt 10):1900–26.

28. Laakso A, Hernesniemi J. Arteriovenous malformations: epidemiology and clinical presentation. Neurosurg Clin N Am. 2012;23(1):1–6.

29. Stapf C, Khaw AV, Sciacca RR, Hofmeister C, Schumacher HC, Pile-Spellman J, et al. Effect of age on clinical and morphological characteristics in patients with brain arteriovenous malformation. Stroke. 2003;34(11):2664–9.

30. Gross BA, Du R. Natural history of cerebral arteriovenous malformations: a meta-analysis. J Neurosurg. 2013;118(2):437–43.

31. Camargo EC, Feske SK, Singhal AB. Stroke in pregnancy: an update. Neurol Clin. 2019;37(1):131–48.

32. Fairhall JM, Stoodley MA. Intracranial haemorrhage in pregnancy. Obstet Med. 2009;2(4):142–8.

33. Porras JL, Yang W, Philadelphia E, Law J, Garzon-Muvdi T, Caplan JM, et al. Hemorrhage risk of brain arteriovenous malformations during pregnancy and puerperium in a North American Cohort. Stroke. 2017;48(6):1507–13.

34. Gross BA, Du R. Hemorrhage from arteriovenous malformations during pregnancy. Neurosurgery. 2012;71(2):349–55; discussion 55–6.

35. van Beijnum J, Wilkinson T, Whitaker HJ, van der Bom JG, Algra A, Vandertop WP, et al. Relative risk of hemorrhage during pregnancy in patients with brain arteriovenous malformations. Int J Stroke. 2017;12(7):741–7.

36. Zhu D, Zhao P, Lv N, Li Q, Fang Y, Li Z, et al. Rupture risk of cerebral arteriovenous malformations during pregnancy and puerperium: a single-center experience and pooled data analysis. World Neurosurg. 2018;111:e308–e15.

37. Lee S, Kim Y, Navi BB, Abdelkhaleq R, Salazar-Marioni S, Blackburn SL, et al. Risk of intracranial hemorrhage associated with pregnancy in women with cerebral arteriovenous malformations. J Neurointerv Surg. 2021;13(8):707–10.

38. Davidoff CL, Lo Presti A, Rogers JM, Simons M, Assaad NNA, Stoodley MA, et al. Risk of first hemorrhage of brain arteriovenous malformations during pregnancy: a systematic review of the literature. Neurosurgery. 2019;85(5):E806–E14.

39. Flemming KD, Lanzino G. Management of unruptured intracranial aneurysms and cerebrovascular malformations. Continuum. 2017;23(1, Cerebrovascular Disease):181–210.

40. Willinsky RA, Lasjaunias P, Terbrugge K, Burrows P. Multiple cerebral arteriovenous malformations (AVMs). Review of our experience from 203 patients with cerebral vascular lesions. Neuroradiology. 1990;32(3):207–10.

41. Bari O, Cohen PR. Hereditary hemorrhagic telangiectasia and pregnancy: potential adverse events and pregnancy outcomes. Int J Women's Health. 2017;9:373–8.

42. Kanekar S, Bennett S. Imaging of neurologic conditions in pregnant patients. Radiographics. 2016;36(7):2102–22.

43. Tranvinh E, Heit JJ, Hacein-Bey L, Provenzale J, Wintermark M. Contemporary imaging of cerebral arteriovenous malformations. AJR Am J Roentgenol. 2017;208(6):1320–30.

44. Josephson CB, White PM, Krishan A, Al-Shahi Salman R. Computed tomography angiography or magnetic resonance angiography for detection of intracranial vascular malformations in patients with intracerebral haemorrhage. Cochrane Database Syst Rev. 2014;9:CD009372.

45. Derdeyn CP, Zipfel GJ, Albuquerque FC, Cooke DL, Feldmann E, Sheehan JP, et al. Management of brain arteriovenous malformations: a scientific statement for healthcare professionals from the American Heart Association/American Stroke Association. Stroke. 2017;48(8):e200–e24.

46. Robinson JL, Hall CS, Sedzimir CB. Arteriovenous malformations, aneurysms, and pregnancy. J Neurosurg. 1974;41(1):63–70.

47. Yamada S, Nakase H, Nakagawa I, Nishimura F, Motoyama Y, Park YS. Cavernous malformations in pregnancy. Neurol Med Chir (Tokyo). 2013;53(8):555–60.

48. Pollock BE, Garces YI, Stafford SL, Foote RL, Schomberg PJ, Link MJ. Stereotactic radiosurgery for cavernous malformations. J Neurosurg. 2000;93(6):987–91.

49. Tonetti D, Kano H, Bowden G, Flickinger JC, Lunsford LD. Hemorrhage during pregnancy in the latency interval after stereotactic radiosurgery

for arteriovenous malformations. J Neurosurg. 2014;121(Suppl):226–31.

50. Nishida T, Faughnan ME, Krings T, Chakinala M, Gossage JR, Young WL, et al. Brain arteriovenous malformations associated with hereditary hemorrhagic telangiectasia: gene-phenotype correlations. Am J Med Genet A. 2012;158A(11):2829–34.

51. McDonald J, Pyeritz RE. Hereditary hemorrhagic telangiectasia. In: Adam MP, Ardinger HH, Pagon RA, Wallace SE, Bean LJH, Stephens K, et al., editors. GeneReviews®. Seattle, WA: University of Washington; 1993.

52. Mohr JP, Parides MK, Stapf C, Moquete E, Moy CS, Overbey JR, et al. Medical management with or without interventional therapy for unruptured brain arteriovenous malformations (ARUBA): a multicentre, non-blinded, randomised trial. Lancet. 2014;383(9917):614–21.

53. Jermakowicz WJ, Tomycz LD, Ghiassi M, Singer RJ. Use of endovascular embolization to treat a ruptured arteriovenous malformation in a pregnant woman: a case report. J Med Case Rep. 2012;6:113.

54. Lv X, Liu P, Li Y. Pre-existing, incidental and hemorrhagic AVMs in pregnancy and postpartum: gestational age, morbidity and mortality, management and risk to the fetus. Interv Neuroradiol. 2016;22(2):206–11.

55. Solomon RA, Connolly ES Jr. Arteriovenous malformations of the brain. N Engl J Med. 2017;376(19):1859–66.

56. Tayebi Meybodi A, Lawton MT. Modern radiosurgical and endovascular classification schemes for brain arteriovenous malformations. Neurosurg Rev. 2018;43:49.

57. Sadasivan B, Malik GM, Lee C, Ausman JI. Vascular malformations and pregnancy. Surg Neurol. 1990;33(5):305–13.

58. Agarwal N, Guerra JC, Gala NB, Agarwal P, Zouzias A, Gandhi CD, et al. Current treatment options for cerebral arteriovenous malformations in pregnancy: a review of the literature. World Neurosurg. 2014;81(1):83–90.

59. Lv X, Li Y. The clinical characteristics and treatment of cerebral AVM in pregnancy. Neuroradiol J. 2015;28(4):385–8.

60. Beach RL, Kaplan PW. Seizures in pregnancy: diagnosis and management. Int Rev Neurobiol. 2008;83:259–71.

61. Hernandez-Diaz S, Smith CR, Shen A, Mittendorf R, Hauser WA, Yerby M, et al. Comparative safety of antiepileptic drugs during pregnancy. Neurology. 2012;78(21):1692–9.

62. Hemphill JC III, Greenberg SM, Anderson CS, Becker K, Bendok BR, Cushman M, et al. Guidelines for the management of spontaneous intracerebral hemorrhage: a guideline for healthcare professionals from the American Heart Association/American Stroke Association. Stroke. 2015;46(7):2032–60.

63. Bernstein PS, Martin JN Jr, Barton JR, Shields LE, Druzin ML, Scavone BM, et al. Consensus bundle on severe hypertension during pregnancy and the postpartum period. J Midwif Womens Health. 2017;62(4):493–501.

64. Gross BA, Du R. Rate of re-bleeding of arteriovenous malformations in the first year after rupture. J Clin Neurosci. 2012;19(8):1087–8.

65. Beecher JS, Lyon K, Ban VS, Vance A, McDougall CM, Whitworth LA, et al. Delayed treatment of ruptured brain AVMs: is it ok to wait? J Neurosurg. 2018;128(4):999–1005.

66. Pollock BE, Flickinger JC, Lunsford LD, Maitz A, Kondziolka D. Factors associated with successful arteriovenous malformation radiosurgery. Neurosurgery. 1998;42(6):1239–44; discussion 44–7.

67. Trivedi RA, Kirkpatrick PJ. Arteriovenous malformations of the cerebral circulation that rupture in pregnancy. J Obstet Gynaecol. 2003;23(5):484–9.

68. Salvati A, Ferrari C, Chiumarulo L, Medicamento N, Dicuonzo F, De Blasi R. Endovascular treatment of brain arteriovenous malformations ruptured during pregnancy--a report of two cases. J Neurol Sci. 2011;308(1–2):158–61.

69. Nagayama K, Kurita H, Tonari A, Takayama M, Shiokawa Y. Radiosurgery for cerebral arteriovenous malformation during pregnancy: a case report focusing on fetal exposure to radiation. Asian J Neurosurg. 2010;5(2):73–7.

70. Bervini D, Morgan MK, Ritson EA, Heller G. Surgery for unruptured arteriovenous malformations of the brain is better than conservative management for selected cases: a prospective cohort study. J Neurosurg. 2014;121(4):878–90.

71. Kazemi P, Villar G, Flexman AM. Anesthetic management of neurosurgical procedures during pregnancy: a case series. J Neurosurg Anesthesiol. 2014;26(3):234–40.

72. Krywko DM, King KC. Aortocaval compression syndrome. Treasure Island, FL: StatPearls; 2020.

73. van Rooij WJ, Sluzewski M, Beute GN. Brain AVM embolization with Onyx. AJNR Am J Neuroradiol. 2007;28(1):172–7; discussion 8.

74. Bokhari MR, Al-Dhahir MA. Cavernous brain angiomas. Treasure Island, FL: StatPearls; 2020.

75. Petersen TA, Morrison LA, Schrader RM, Hart BL. Familial versus sporadic cavernous malformations: differences in developmental venous anomaly association and lesion phenotype. AJNR Am J Neuroradiol. 2010;31(2):377–82.

76. Zafar A, Quadri SA, Farooqui M, Ikram A, Robinson M, Hart BL, et al. Familial cerebral cavernous malformations. Stroke. 2019;50(5):1294–301.

77. Joseph NK, Kumar S, Brown RD Jr, Lanzino G, Flemming KD. Influence of pregnancy on hemorrhage risk in women with cerebral and spinal cavernous malformations. Stroke. 2021;52(2):434–41.

78. Otten P, Pizzolato GP, Rilliet B, Berney J. [131 cases of cavernous angioma (cavernomas) of the CNS, discovered by retrospective analysis of

24,535 autopsies]. Neurochirurgie. 1989;35(2):82–3, 128–31.

79. Del Curling O Jr, Kelly DL Jr, Elster AD, Craven TE. An analysis of the natural history of cavernous angiomas. J Neurosurg. 1991;75(5):702–8.

80. Robinson JR, Awad IA, Little JR. Natural history of the cavernous angioma. J Neurosurg. 1991;75(5):709–14.

81. Kalani MY, Zabramski JM. Risk for symptomatic hemorrhage of cerebral cavernous malformations during pregnancy. J Neurosurg. 2013;118(1):50–5.

82. Gross BA, Lin N, Du R, Day AL. The natural history of intracranial cavernous malformations. Neurosurg Focus. 2011;30(6):E24.

83. Gross BA, Du R. Hemorrhage from cerebral cavernous malformations: a systematic pooled analysis. J Neurosurg. 2017;126(4):1079–87.

84. Zabramski JM, Kalani MYS. 409: Natural history of cavernous malformations. In: Winn HR, editor. Youmans & Winn Neurological Surgery. Philadelphia, PA: Elsevier; 2017.

85. Safavi-Abbasi S, Feiz-Erfan I, Spetzler RF, Kim L, Dogan S, Porter RW, et al. Hemorrhage of cavernous malformations during pregnancy and in the peripartum period: causal or coincidence? Case report and review of the literature. Neurosurg Focus. 2006;21(1):e12.

86. Witiw CD, Abou-Hamden A, Kulkarni AV, Silvaggio JA, Schneider C, Wallace MC. Cerebral cavernous malformations and pregnancy: hemorrhage risk and influence on obstetrical management. Neurosurgery. 2012;71(3):626–30; discussion 31.

87. Zyck S, Gould GC. Cavernous venous malformation. Treasure Island, FL: StatPearls; 2020.

88. Morrison L, Akers A. Cerebral cavernous malformation, familial. In: Adam MP, Ardinger HH, Pagon RA, Wallace SE, Bean LJH, Stephens K, et al., editors. GeneReviews®. Seattle, WA: University of Washington; 1993.

89. Simonazzi G, Curti A, Rapacchia G, Gabrielli S, Pilu G, Rizzo N, et al. Symptomatic cerebral cavernomas in pregnancy: a series of 6 cases and review of the literature. J Matern Fetal Neonatal Med. 2014;27(3):261–4.

90. Flemming KD, Goodman BP, Meyer FB. Successful brainstem cavernous malformation resection after repeated hemorrhages during pregnancy. Surg Neurol. 2003;60(6):545–7; discussion 7–8.

Pregnancy and Moyamoya

Arjun V. Pendharkar, Sohun S. Awsare,
and Gary K. Steinberg

Introduction

Moyamoya disease (MMD) is characterized by progressive stenosis and occlusion of the proximal intracranial circulation with concomitant proliferation and enlargement of fragile collateral perforating arteries termed "moyamoya vessels." These collaterals give rise to the characteristic angiographic "puff of smoke" signature for which the disease is named. Disease progression, namely the continued stenosis of the intracranial circulation and development of the fragile collateral network, are graded according to the Suzuki staging system (Fig. 10.1). MMD patients most commonly present with transient ischemic attacks (TIA), ischemic stroke, or intracranial hemorrhage (intraparenchymal, intraventricular, and subarachnoid). The primary modality of treatment is neurosurgical—involving cerebral revascularization via direct or indirect bypass providing extracranial blood flow to the intracranial circulation. Numerous non-randomized studies have demonstrated the efficacy of cerebrovascular bypass in reducing future ischemic and hemorrhagic stroke risk compared to historical controls [1–7]. Furthermore, a prospective randomized controlled trial showed the benefit of

surgical revascularization in reducing hemorrhagic and ischemic strokes [8].

MMD is an overall rare clinical entity with an incidence of 0.54/100,000. However, because MMD carries a 2:1 female:male predilection and a peak incidence during reproductive years, the management of MMD and pregnancy is a common cerebrovascular clinical scenario. Pregnancy is characterized by multiple physiological changes including alterations in systemic vascular resistance, blood pressure, volume status, and hematologic parameters—all of which can affect the tenuous cerebrovascular perfusion in an MMD patient.

When considering the current body of literature regarding MMD and pregnancy, it is useful to stratify the evidence into outcomes concerning patients before or after bypass surgery. Furthermore, MMD may differ significantly in different ethnic subgroups. For example, multiple demographic studies have reported adult Caucasian patients tend to present with ischemia whereas adult Asian MMD patients overwhelmingly present with hemorrhage [9]. Therefore, the studies summarized below must be interpreted in that context.

A. V. Pendharkar · S. S. Awsare · G. K. Steinberg (✉)
Stanford University School of Medicine,
Stanford, CA, USA
e-mail: arjun.v.pendharkar@kp.org;
ssa55@cornell.edu; gsteinberg@stanford.edu

© The Author(s), under exclusive license to Springer Nature Switzerland AG 2023
G. Gupta et al. (eds.), *Neurological Disorders in Pregnancy*,
https://doi.org/10.1007/978-3-031-36490-7_10

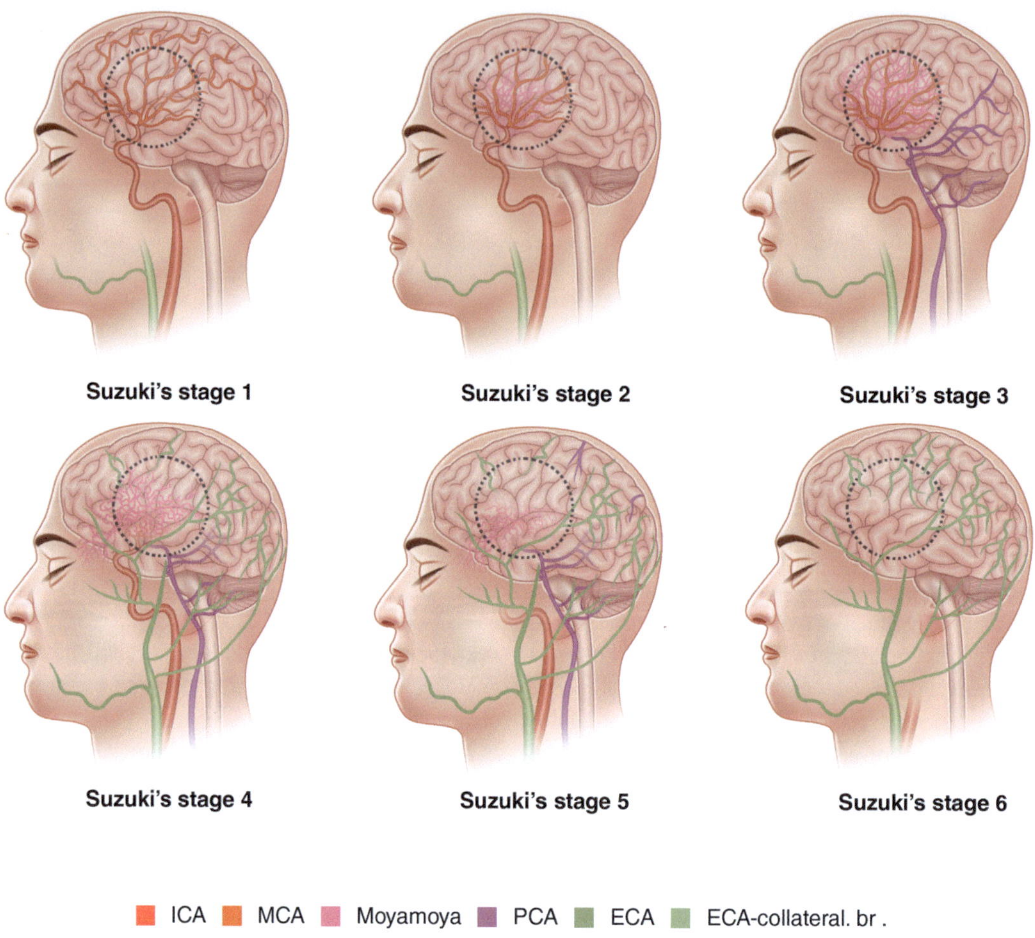

Fig. 10.1 Graphic demonstrating the angiographic staging of Moyamoya disease according to Suzuki and Takaku

Pregnancy in Untreated MMD Patients

Takahashi and colleagues conducted a retrospective survey of MMD patients in Japan. The 99 patients who accounted for 202 deliveries were previously unaware of their diagnosis of MMD at childbirth and were only later diagnosed. The clinical diagnosis for the 99 women included 32 (32.3%) with ischemic MMD and 26 (26.3%) with hemorrhagic MMD. Of the 202 deliveries, 183 (90.6%) were vaginal deliveries. This group of individuals had four instances (2%) of cerebral events during delivery and puerperium. There was one event of syncope during delivery and one event of syncope during puerperium. This cohort did not experience any adverse events dur-

ing pregnancy. Finally, in this cohort there were two instances of TIA during puerperium. Of the 99 women, 58 of them (58.6%) required bypass surgery after childbirth [10].

Two additional literature reviews have described a higher stroke risk in pregnant MMD patients not having undergone bypass. In the first literature review, Inayama and colleagues found 66 reports that included a total of 443 pregnancies. Within this search, 54 (12.1%) cases of pregnancy related stroke were determined. There were 44 (9.9%) intracranial hemorrhages and 10 (2.2%) cerebral infarctions. The antepartum period showed the highest incidence of intracranial hemorrhages with 39 instances (88.6%) while the postpartum period had three cases (6.8%) followed by the intrapartum period ($n = 2$; 4.5%). The review noted that no patient with previously diagnosed MMD developed a stroke during delivery. There were 34 instances (77.3%) of intracranial hemorrhage in patients with newly diagnosed MMD. The review also reported eight hemorrhage case deaths, of which seven (87.5%) had undiagnosed MMD at the time of the stroke. In the ten cerebral infarction cases, nine (90%) were previously undiagnosed MMD patients [11]. In the other literature review, Maragkos reported a similar event rate. Maragkos and colleagues classified the patients into three categories. The first group included patients with known MMD diagnosed before pregnancy. In this group, the 96 patients accounted for 101 pregnancies. In these pregnancies, new hypertension was observed in 16.3% and pregnancy toxemia in 11.1%. For these pregnancies, 11.4% presented with ischemic or hemorrhagic cerebrovascular events. There were no residual neurological deficits in 95.2% of the reported cases. While two (4.7%) showed mild residual deficits, no patient had severe residual neurological deficits. The second group consisted of individuals who were diagnosed with MMD during pregnancy. There were 20 studies contributing 23 cases. Pregnancy induced hypertension occurred in four cases (17.4%), toxemia in three cases (13%) and neurologic events in six cases (26%). MMD presented with an ischemic event in 34.7% of the patients and 69.5% presented as hemorrhagic [12].

Finally, in a robust pooled analysis of previously reported cases, Fluss and colleagues reviewed 12 articles that totaled 270 pregnancies after excluding patients who were diagnosed during or after delivery. In the follow-up of these patients there were 22 neurologic events recorded (9.8%). Twelve of the events were transient ischemic attacks and three events were seizures. In this cohort, there were six hemorrhagic strokes and one ischemic stroke, yielding a stroke risk of 3.1%. The remainder of the cohort had favorable neurological outcomes. These neurologic events included 15 instances during the pregnancy and seven instances in the postpartum period [13].

Indeed, the current body of evidence is limited by small sample size and retrospective nature of examination, but there is clearly an elevated risk of adverse cerebrovascular events in the untreated pregnant MMD patient.

Pregnancy in Treated MMD Patients

The elevated stroke risk during pregnancy may be due to impaired cerebral vascular reserve (CVR). In two separate reviews, both Lee's group and Park's group found diminished CVR as observed on SPECT in MMD patients is associated with development of cerebrovascular events during pregnancy. Lee and colleagues reviewed the electronic medical records of patients and included 23 patients responsible for 27 pregnancies. Ischemia was observed in 19 pregnancies (70.3%). In this cohort 23 had bilateral MMD (85.2%) while unilateral MMD was observed in four pregnancies (14.8%). There was a cerebrovascular event in 12 of the pregnancies (44.4%). Of the cerebrovascular events, 11 instances were TIA. In addition, this study explored the association between CVE and CVR on Stress SPECT. The authors found 35 hemispheres experienced a decrease or defect in perfusion on initial basal SPECT. Furthermore, 30 hemispheres showed a decreased CVR on initial stress SPECT. Within this cohort, there were 16 hemispheres that had revascularization surgery and within this group there was a decreased CVR on stress SPECT before surgery [14].

Lee's group and Park's group separately reported that diminished CVR as observed on SPECT in MMD patients is associated with development of cerebrovascular events during pregnancy [14, 15]. Since it improves cerebrovascular reserve, bypass may be protective. In a single center series, Inayama and colleagues report no adverse neurological events in 30 pregnancies in 20 women with MMD. All but five of the patients had already undergone bypass [11]. Similarly, Acker and colleagues report on a European cohort of treated MMD patients with no adverse cerebrovascular events during or after pregnancy. Acker's group reviewed 31 patients resulting in 60 pregnancies. Within this group there were two subgroups: patients with pregnancies prior to diagnosis and patients with pregnancies after diagnosis. In the first group, 25 women were responsible for 50 pregnancies. In 92% of the women, a stroke or TIA represented the onset symptom. There was a cerebral ischemic event in 8% of the patients. In the second group, there were six patients who accounted for ten pregnancies. The patients all underwent a bilateral revascularization operation prior to their pregnancy. No cerebral ischemic events occurred in these patients in the perinatal period [16]. Park's group similarly noted this difference in his retrospective chart review of 26 pregnancies and deliveries among 21 patients. The patients were divided into two groups: Group 1 was defined as those diagnosed with MMD during pregnancy and puerperium and Group 2 were those diagnosed with MMD before pregnancy. In the first group, of three patients with three pregnancies, there was one case of a pregnancy related complication (severe pre-eclampsia) and two of the three patients had motor TIAs. One of the patients had an acute cerebral infarction just before delivery and another had an acute cerebral infarction during puerperium. In these individuals, baseline SPECT and ACZ-SPECT revealed severely reduced regional CVR in more than one vascular territory in all the patients. The second group consisted of 20 patients with 23 pregnancies. Fifteen of these patients underwent more than one revascularization surgery and five patients did not undergo surgical revascularization before pregnancy. Neurologic deterioration occurred in only four cases of pregnancy, delivery and puerperium consisting of worsening TIAs. Within this group, there were statistically significant differ-

ences between those with versus without neurologic decline. In 19 deliveries without deterioration, the frequency of TIAs was less than 10 per month while in the seven deliveries with deterioration, five had more than ten TIA events per month. Additionally, there was a significant difference in the percentage of severely reduced rCVR in those without versus with neurologic deterioration (10.5% vs. 100%) [15].

MMD Treatment During Pregnancy

Although anecdotal, there is precedent for treating MMD during pregnancy. Fehnel and colleagues report the case of a 26-year-old patient at 12 weeks gestation who presented with progressive symptomatic MMD in the context of concurrent PHACES (Posterior fossa anomalies, Hemangioma, Arterial anomalies, Cardiac anomalies, Eye anomalies, and Sternal cleft and supraumbilical raphe) syndrome. She underwent uncomplicated indirect bypass (Fig. 10.2) with one self-limiting post-operative TIA and delivered at full term in an uncomplicated pregnancy without any further neurological events. At 6-year follow-up, there were no new strokes or neurological deficits, and angiography demonstrated successful revascularization [17].

At our institution, the senior author (GKS) performed uncomplicated bilateral direct bypasses (Fig. 10.3) in a 25-year-old patient at 10 weeks gestation. The patient experienced mild self-limiting post-operative TIA and went on to an uncomplicated full-term delivery. The patient subsequently completed two additional pregnancies without issue.

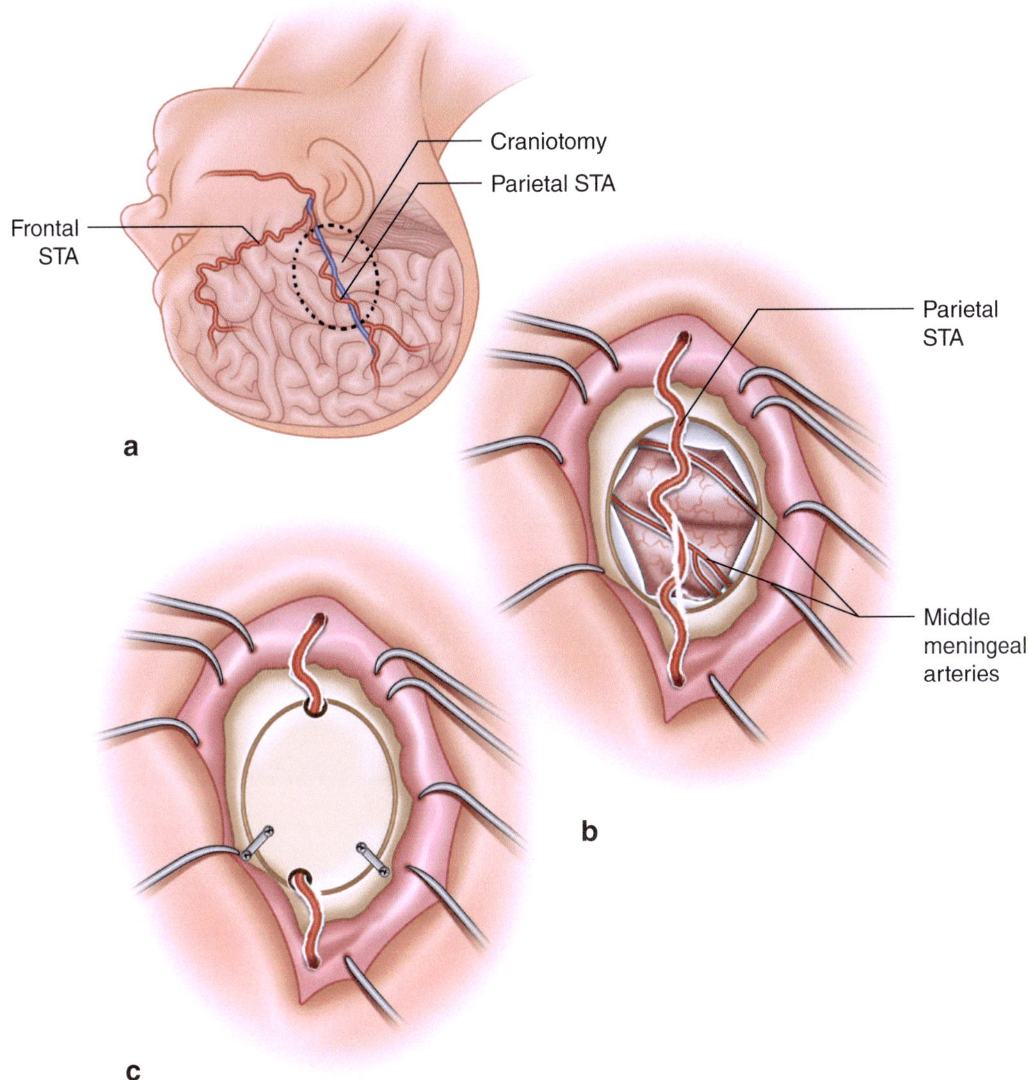

Fig. 10.2 Illustration of indirect bypass for Moyamoya disease via encephaloduroarteriosynangiosis (EDAS). (**a**) Craniotomy performed in the area of the parietal STA. (**b**) STA and vascular cuff placed over cortical surface. (**c**) Cranial flap is drilled to accommodate STA and secured with plates and screws

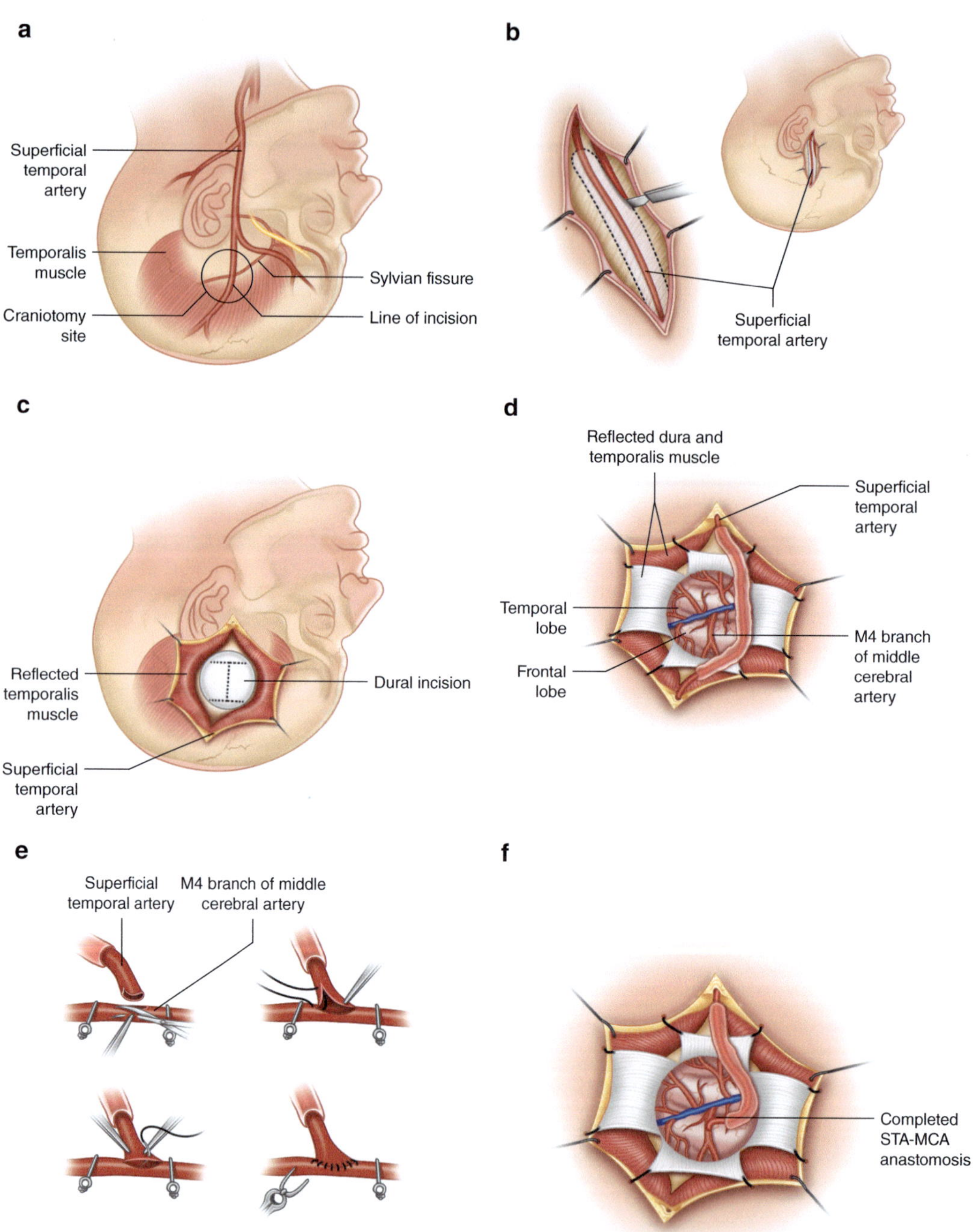

Fig. 10.3 Illustration of direct bypass for Moyamoya disease. (**a**) Identification of the superficial temporal artery (STA) and incision in proximity. (**b**) Microsurgical dissection of STA and vascular cuff. (**c**) Incision of the temporal muscle and dura. (**d**) Reflection of dura to provide wide exposure over the Sylvian fissure. An M4 branch of the middle cerebral artery is identified. (**e**) End-to-side anastomosis between distal STA and M4 branch. (**f**) Completion of anastomosis and close apposition of STA and vascular cuff to permit collateral formation

Mode of Delivery

Due to the physiological changes in pregnancy, there is a theoretical benefit to cesarean section; it may provide better control of blood pressure, as well as avoiding Valsalva and transient intracranial pressure increases during vaginal birth. In contrast, there may be a detrimental effect from anesthesia and surgical blood loss from cesarean section. Indeed, there is an increase in prevalence of cesarean sections in pregnant MMD patients in the literature, indicating that many centers recommend this as a preferred delivery method [10, 11]. However, Maragkos and colleagues conducted a systematic review and demonstrated no superiority in mode of delivery [12].

Stanford University Medical Center Experience

We have recently reported the outcomes of 59 pregnancies in 56 MMD patients occurring after cerebral revascularization at our institution (Table 10.1). In this cohort of post-bypass

Table 10.1 Stanford series (GKS)

Pre-bypass pregnancy (12)		Post-bypass pregnancy (59)
3 (25%)	Perinatal TIA Total	5 (8%)
2 (17%)	MRI confirmed Stroke	0
1 (8%)	Stroke w/Residual Deficit	0
0	Hemorrhagic Stroke	0
2 (17%)	Preeclampsia	7 (12%)
1 (8%)	Eclampsia	0
1 (8%)	Cesarean Delivery	28 (46%)

MMD patients, there were five TIAs (8%) occurring during pregnancy or within 30 days of delivery but no MRI-confirmed strokes. The 8% TIA rate is similar to reported TIA rates in non-pregnant post-bypass MMD patients. At 1-year follow-up post-delivery, no patients had any residual neurological deficits nor any MRI-confirmed strokes. Furthermore, no patients experienced a hemorrhagic stroke. When examining obstetric outcomes, there were no second or third trimester miscarriages, however, there was an elevated rate of pre-eclampsia, possibly due to an association between MMD and hypertension. There was no statistical difference in mode of delivery and rates of TIA. Interestingly, when compared to a smaller cohort of pre-bypass pregnant MMD patients, post-bypass pregnancy was an independent factor ($p = 0.0061$) for preventing perinatal stroke or TIA, suggesting bypass may be protective.

Taken together, our protocol at Stanford University Medical Center includes a preference for multidisciplinary coordinated care with the patient's obstetrician. We do recommend bypass in women with symptomatic MMD prior to conception. We recommend maintaining low-dose aspirin and careful monitoring of blood pressure during pregnancy and delivery. Regarding blood pressure, we favor permissive hypertension and weigh the risk-benefit ratio against a trend towards elevated rates of pre-eclampsia. We have no preference for vaginal or cesarean delivery. Cerebral bypass during pregnancy is reserved for symptomatic patients refractory to blood pressure augmentation. These recommendations are summarized in Fig. 10.4.

Stanford Series (GKS)

Pre-Bypass Pregnancy (12)		Post-Bypass Pregnancy (59)
3 (25%)	Perinatal TIA Total	5 (8%)
2 (17%)	MRI confirmed Stroke	0
1(8%)	Stroke w/Residual Deficit	0
0	Hemorrhagic Stroke	0
2 (17%)	Preeclampsia	7 (12%)
1(8%)	Eclampsia	0
1 (8%)	Cesarean Delivery	28 (46%)

Fig. 10.4 Summary of the Stanford Protocol for the approach to management of Moyamoya disease in women of reproductive age

Conclusions

MMD affects women in the age of fertility, and thus the pregnant patient with MMD is a common clinical scenario. Patients with untreated MMD undergoing pregnancy have a significant risk of post-partum neurological events. The data are somewhat limited, but suggest that bypass may be protective against pregnancy related strokes and TIAs due to improved cerebrovascular reserve. Careful monitoring of blood pressure, including not overtreating hypertension, is critical. There are no data to support the benefits of cesarean section compared to vaginal delivery. With closely coordinated care between neurosurgery and obstetrics, pregnant MMD patients can safely deliver without any long-lasting neurological sequelae.

References

1. Wouters A, Smets I, Van den Noortgate W, Steinberg GK, Lemmens R. Cerebrovascular events after surgery versus conservative therapy for moyamoya disease: a meta-analysis. Acta Neurol Belg. 2019;119:305–13.
2. Guzman R, Lee M, Achrol A, Bell-Stephens T, Kelly M, Do HM, et al. Clinical outcome after 450 revascularization procedures for moyamoya disease: clinical article. J Neurosurg. 2009;111(5):927–35.
3. Scott RM, Smith JL, Robertson RL, Madsen JR, Soriano SG, Rockoff MA. Long-term outcome in children with moyamoya syndrome after cranial revascularization by pial synangiosis. J Neurosurg. 2004;100(2 Suppl):142–9.
4. Houkin K, Kamiyama H, Abe H, Takahashi A, Kuroda S. Surgical therapy for adult moyamoya disease: can surgical revascularization prevent the recurrence of intracerebral hemorrhage? Stroke. 1996;27(8):1342–6. https://www.ahajournals.org/doi/10.1161/01.STR.27.8.1342.
5. Hallemeier CL, Rich KM, Grubb RL, Chicoine MR, Moran CJ, Cross DWT, et al. Clinical features and outcome in North American adults with moyamoya phenomenon. Stroke. 2006;37(6):1490–6.
6. Abhinav K, Furtado SV, Nielsen TH, Iyer A, Gooderham PA, Teo M, et al. Functional outcomes after revascularization procedures in patients with hemorrhagic moyamoya disease. Neurosurgery. 2020;86(2):257–65.
7. Derdeyn CP. Moyamoya disease and moyamoya syndrome. N Engl J Med. 2009;361(1):97–8.
8. Miyamoto S, Yoshimoto T, Hashimoto N, Okada Y, Tsuji I, Tominaga T, et al. Effects of extracranial-intracranial bypass for patients with hemorrhagic moyamoya disease: results of the Japan adult moyamoya trial. Stroke. 2014;45(5):1415–21.
9. Chiu D, Shedden P, Bratina P, Grotta JC. Clinical features of moyamoya disease in the United States. Stroke. 1998;29(7):1347–51. https://doi.org/10.1161/01.str.29.7.1347. PMID: 9660385.
10. Takahashi JC, Ikeda T, Iihara K, Miyamoto S. Pregnancy and delivery in Moyamoya disease: results of a nationwide survey in Japan. Neurol Med Chir. 2012;52:304.
11. Inayama Y, Kondoh E, Chigusa Y, Io S, Funaki T, Matsumura N, et al. Moyamoya disease in pregnancy: a 20-year single-center experience and literature review. World Neurosurg. 2019;122:684–691.e2.
12. Maragkos GA, Ascanio LC, Chida K, Boone MD, Ogilvy CS, Thomas AJ, et al. Moyamoya disease in pregnancy: a systematic review. Acta Neurochir. 2018;160:1711–9.

13. Fluss R, Ligas BA, Chan AW, Ellis JA, Ortiz RA, Langer DJ, et al. Moyamoya-related stroke risk during pregnancy: an evidence-based reappraisal. World Neurosurg. 2019;129:e582–5.

14. Lee SU, Chung YS, Oh CW, Kwon OK, Bang JS, Hwang G, et al. Cerebrovascular events during pregnancy and puerperium resulting from preexisting Moyamoya disease: determining the risk of ischemic events based on hemodynamic status assessment using brain perfusion single-photon emission computed tomography. World Neurosurg. 2016;90:66–75.

15. Park W, Ahn JS, Chung J, Chung Y, Lee S, Park JC, et al. Neurologic deterioration in patients with moyamoya disease during pregnancy, delivery, and puerperium. World Neurosurg. 2018;111:e7–17.

16. Acker G, Czabanka M, Schmiedek P, Vajkoczy P. Pregnancy and delivery in moyamoya vasculopathy: experience of a single European institution. Neurosurg Rev. 2018;41(2):615–9.

17. Fehnel KP, McClain CD, Smith ER. Indirect bypass for maternal symptomatic moyamoya in the first trimester of pregnancy: case report. J Neurosurg Pediatr. 2020;25(2):138–43.

Cerebral Venous Sinus Thrombosis in Pregnancy

11

Hai Sun

Introduction

Cerebral venous sinus thrombosis (CVST) is a rare but serious cerebrovascular disorder. The presence of a thrombus in one or more of the cerebral sinuses clinically defines the condition [1]. When accounting for all causes of stroke, CVST represents 0.5% of all etiologies [2]. Historically, the incidence of CVST was underestimated due to the clinical symptoms mimicking several other similar conditions and the reports documenting CVST were mostly based on autopsy series [2]. Today, the incidence of CVST in adults is estimated to be three to four cases per million while the incidence rises to seven cases per million in children and neonates [2]. A female predilection of CVST (i.e., women represent 75% of adult cases) has been attributed to multiple risk factors associated with this population [2]. CVST in the setting of pregnancy or puerperium is rare and this is reflected in its limited presence in the literature. However, available literature does suggest that CVST is more commonly clustered in these patients and must be addressed promptly. Advances in noninvasive diagnostic imaging methodologies allow for early detection and diagnosis of CVST thus facilitating timely intervention and improved outcomes. Additionally, ongoing clinical trials continue to advance our understanding of the condition and help clinicians act promptly to this often-elusive diagnosis.

Pathophysiology and Anatomy

The cerebral venous system is an extensive network of interconnected veins that drain both the deep and superficial circulation of the brain, ultimately emptying through the internal jugular vein (Fig. 11.1). CVST primarily affects the larger venous sinuses. The largest multicenter CVST clinical study, International Study on Cerebral and Dural Sinus Thrombosis (ISCVT), identified the anatomic location of the most commonly involved sinuses. The superior sagittal sinus (SSS) was most often affected (62%) followed by the transverse sinus (41–44%), the straight sinus (18%), and the cavernous sinus (1%) [3]. Multiple sinuses can be affected in up to 30% of cases with the SSS and the transverse sinus being the most common sites [3].

The ISCVT study also found that pregnancy is a risk factor for development of CVST. Many physiologic changes occur during pregnancy, including increase in prothrombotic proteins of the coagulation cascade, and a decrease in antithrombotic proteins, such as protein S. These abnormalities are thought to last several weeks into the post-partum period. Additionally, during

H. Sun (✉)
Department of Neurosurgery, Rutgers Robert Wood Johnson Medical School, New Brunswick, NJ, USA
e-mail: hs925@rwjms.rutgers.edu

© The Author(s), under exclusive license to Springer Nature Switzerland AG 2023
G. Gupta et al. (eds.), *Neurological Disorders in Pregnancy*,
https://doi.org/10.1007/978-3-031-36490-7_11

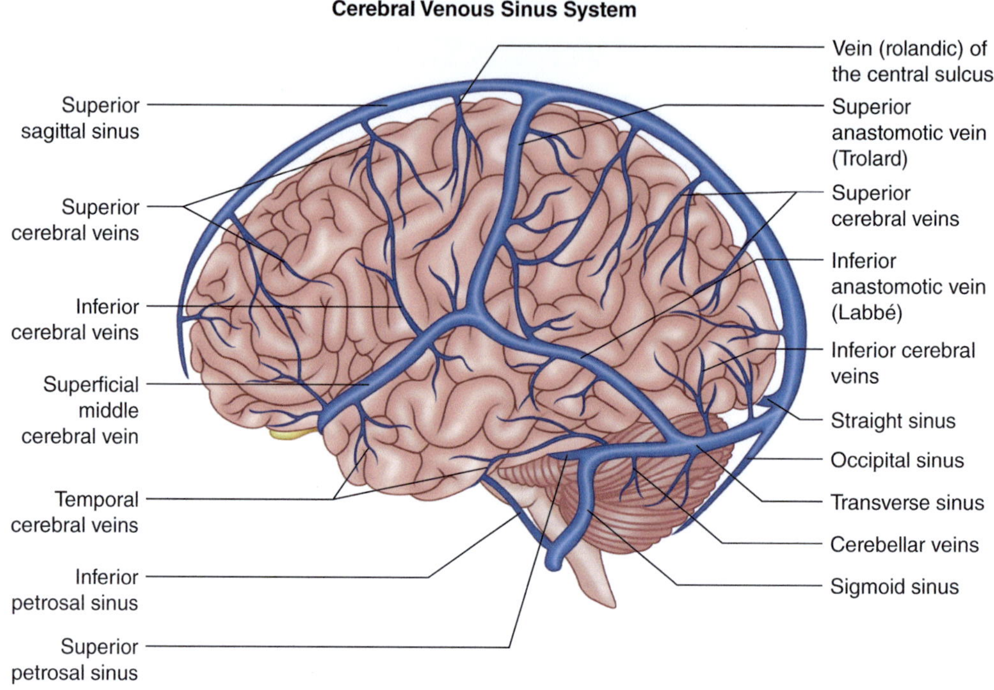

Fig. 11.1 Lateral view of cerebral veins and venous sinuses

delivery dehydration and blood loss increase blood viscosity which contributes to thrombus formation. Pregnancy-related hypertensive diseases such as pre-eclampsia, eclampsia, and HELLP (hemolysis, elevated liver enzymes, and low platelets) further contribute to a prothrombotic milieu [4]. In general, pregnancy and puerperium are associated with an increased risk of venous thrombotic events, such as deep venous thromboses (DVT) and pulmonary embolism (PE). While it has been suggested that CVST can be related to non-cerebral VTE, the ISCVT trial failed to identify a statistically significant correlation. This lack of correlation suggests that systemic and cerebral venous thrombosis may represent distinct pathophysiologic processes [3].

The pathophysiology leading to the development of CVST can be summarized by two theories, which may be separately or concomitantly implicated [2]. Regardless of which theory prevails, the outcome of CVST is the same: the lack of venous outflow causes buildup of blood proximally which ultimately leads to increased pressure in the cerebral venous system (venous hypertension) and potential devastating consequences including ICU elevations, venous infarcts, and intracranial hemorrhages [2].

Edema and CSF Obstruction Theories

The first theory of CVST pathogenesis purports that the thrombosis of the cerebral veins along with the blood–brain barrier (BBB) disruption results in the development of both vasogenic and cytotoxic edema; both of which have been demonstrated on MR imaging studies. The vasogenic edema is thought to be a direct result of the increase venous pressure and volume that induces widespread BBB disruption. Cytotoxic edema is a consequence of the decreased cerebral blood flow and perfusion which results in failure of the Na/K ATPase pump and impaired ionic hemostasis. The second theory suggests a direct thrombosis of the major cerebral venous sinuses. The thrombus causes increased pressure in the venous system which impedes the normal CSF flow patterns from the subarachnoid space to the venous circulation via the arachnoid granulations. Impaired absorption leads to the development of intracranial hypertension. Likely, these happen concomitantly.

Risk Factors and Clinical Presentation

Risk Factors

The risk factors for CVST are extensive and have been quoted to include more than 100 different underlying pathologic causes [5]. Just like other thrombosing pathologies, the Virchow triad (hematologic stasis, vascular endothelial damage, and a hypercoagulable state) is central to the development and likelihood of CVST. Broadly, the different etiological categories include hematologic, prothrombotic states (both acquired and genetic), drugs, infections, mechanical causes, autoimmunity, malignancy, and other.

The previously mentioned ISCVT study further elucidated common risk factors and epidemiology. Multifactorial causes are identified in 44% of cases while 15% of the reported cases have no underlying cause [3]. The most frequently identified causes include genetic and acquired prothrombotic states, pregnancy and puerperium, and infections. In the general population women experience more than three times the incidence of CVST than men. Young women are at particular risk given potential exposure to oral contraceptives as well as pregnancy. More generally, the reported incidence of non-cerebral venous thromboembolism (VTE) in pregnancy is approximately 13 per 1000 women [6]. Temporally, CVST risk is markedly increased during the last trimester of pregnancy and the immediate post-partum period. In a retrospective study of 113 patients with CVST, 59% presented during pregnancy or puerperium. The presence of CVST in pregnancy can be further influenced by infection, cesarean or instrumented delivery, advanced maternal age, excessive vomiting, and hyperhomocysteinemia. CVST accounts for 30–60% of all pregnancy-related strokes [6]. A pregnant woman who as suffered a previous CVST is 80 times more likely to suffer an additional episode of CVST compared to a member of the general population according to some studies [6].

Finally, of the genetic or acquired prothrombotic states, antithrombin III, protein C, and protein S deficiencies are among the most common predisposing conditions. Factor V Leiden and prothrombin (20210) mutations are less common causes. The knowledge of these prothrombotic states warrant guideline specific interventions addressed later in management.

Clinical Presentation

The diagnosis of CVST in pregnancy can be difficult given its commonly missed or overlapping symptomatology. Moreover, the clinical presentation is highly variable and can often delay a swift diagnosis. The ISCVT study revealed a median delay from the onset of symptoms to diagnosis was 7 days.

The clinical entity of CVST can be grouped into four broad symptomatologic classes.

1. *Isolated Intracranial Hypertension.* This clinical presentation includes headache with or without vomiting, papilledema, visual disturbances, and possible sixth nerve palsy. In general headache can occur in up to 89% of patients with CVST, however, this symptom has no localizing significance and provides no clue to the diagnosing physician [7]. This headache can be dull or present in an acute thunderclap fashion like subarachnoid hemorrhage. Most commonly, the headaches associated with CVST are described as dull, non-localizing, and aggravated by ICP elevating maneuvers. Papilledema may be seen in slowly developing CVST.
2. *Focal neurologic deficit and/or epilepsy.* Hemiparesis or mono-paresis are the most frequent focal neurologic signs. Depending on the specific focal symptomatology, one can infer the sinus that is thrombosed. Involvement of the SSS has a higher probability of causing bilateral motor or sensory deficits. Acute

aphasia can pinpoint a possible thrombosis in the left transverse sinus. Cognitive and neuropsychological deficits can be seen in straight sinus CVST. Seizures, either focal or generalized, are observed in 40% of patients, and CVST associated with intraparenchymal hemorrhage has an increased frequency of epileptic episodes [2].

3. *Encephalopathy.* Alterations in levels of consciousness, obtundation, coma, and multifocal signs are associated with parenchymal lesions, deep venous occlusion, and extensive sinus thrombosis.

4. *Cavernous Sinus Involvement.* This is the least common but portends the worst prognosis. It is characterized by oculomotor dysfunction, facial pain, trigeminal paresthesia, proptosis, and chemosis.

The most prevalent signs and symptoms from a pooled systematic review of CSVT in pregnancy and puerperium included headache (74%), seizure (50%), motor weakness (38%), coma or obtundation (45%), visual disturbances (24%), nausea (17%), and vomiting (23%) [8].

Diagnostics and Imaging Characteristics

Computed Tomography (CT)

Non-contrasted computed tomography (CT) may demonstrate hyperdense thrombus in a thrombosed dural sinus or vein, and is useful in identifying associated intracranial pathology (e.g., hemorrhage). Many times, thrombosed cortical veins appear as linear hyperdensities (Fig. 11.2). In some cases, hemorrhage is seen in the area associated with venous thrombosis. The most notable finding on CT scan (especially contrast enhanced CT) is the "delta sign"—this radiographic phenomenon is caused by a relatively hypodense occluded sinus contrasted against hyperdense venous collaterals and meningeal coverings [9]. The "cord sign" (denoted by thrombosed cortical or deep vein), and the

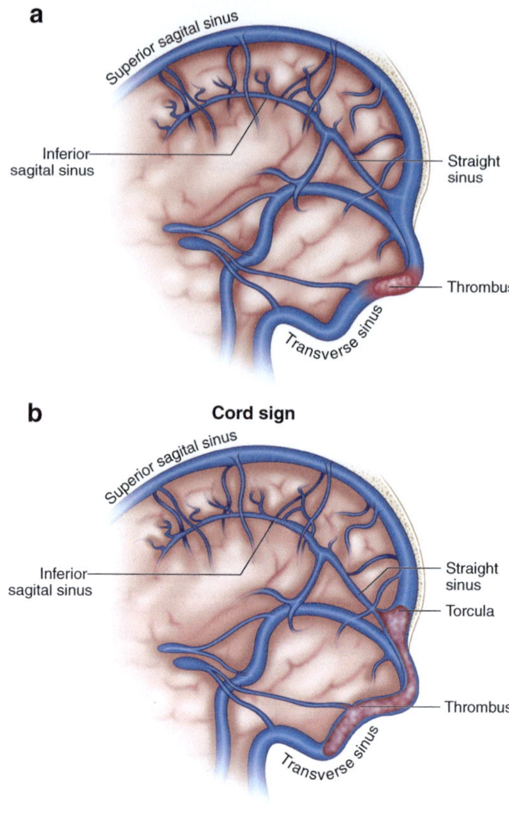

Fig. 11.2 Pathophysiological correlates of cord and attenuated vein signs. (**a**) Cord sign is observed as hyperattenuation on non-contrast CT or hyperintensity on MR imaging. This sign localizes to thrombus within a specific area of the sinus. (**b**) Attenuated vein sign is observed as delta or empty delta signs on non-contrast and contrast-enhanced CT, respectively. These represent evolution of the thrombus into the deeper venous system

"dense triangle sign" (direct visualization of the clot inside the vein) are also present in approximately 1/3 of patients [10] (Fig. 11.3). Unfortunately, routine CT is prone to false positive venous thrombus identification, the so-called pseudo-delta sign, which can be secondary to subarachnoid hemorrhage (SAH) or subdural hematoma (SDH). Additionally, the radiation associated with CT scan is an important consideration in the pregnant patient due to potential teratogenicity. For these reasons, other more sensitive imaging modalities are the mainstay of imaging detection.

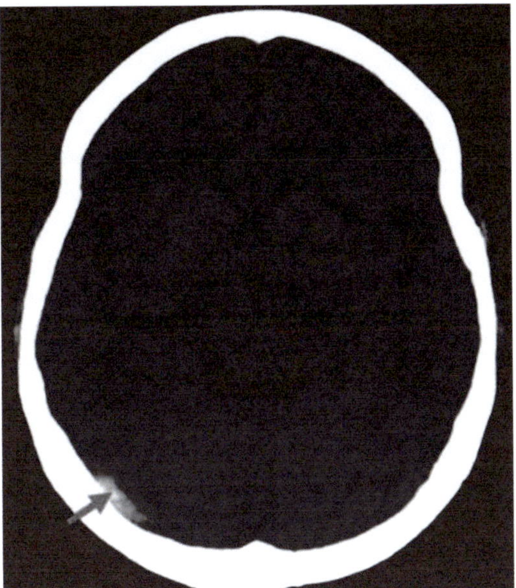

Fig. 11.3 Noncontrast computed tomography head scan showing spontaneous hyperdensity of the right transverse sinus (Saposnik et al.)

Magnetic Resonance Imaging (MRI)

Magnetic resonance imaging (MRI) and magnetic resonance venography (MRV) are the usual imaging modalities for diagnosis of CVST. Understanding the varied appearance of sinus thrombosis on MRI is critical to its usefulness as a diagnostic tool. Acute thrombosis appears isointense on T1 weighted-imaging (WI) subacute thrombus appears hyperintense on T1WI and hypointense on T2WI (Figs. 11.4 and 11.5). On gradient-refocused sequencing, thrombosis appears as a flow void. Additionally, time of flight (TOF) sequences allow MR to detect venous thromboses with high sensitivity. MRI also has the added benefit of detecting the size and extent of venous infarctions that often accompany CVST. In most cases, these sequences obviate the need for traditional angiographic imaging; however, even MR imaging has some limitations if the pathology is expressed as a partial occlu-

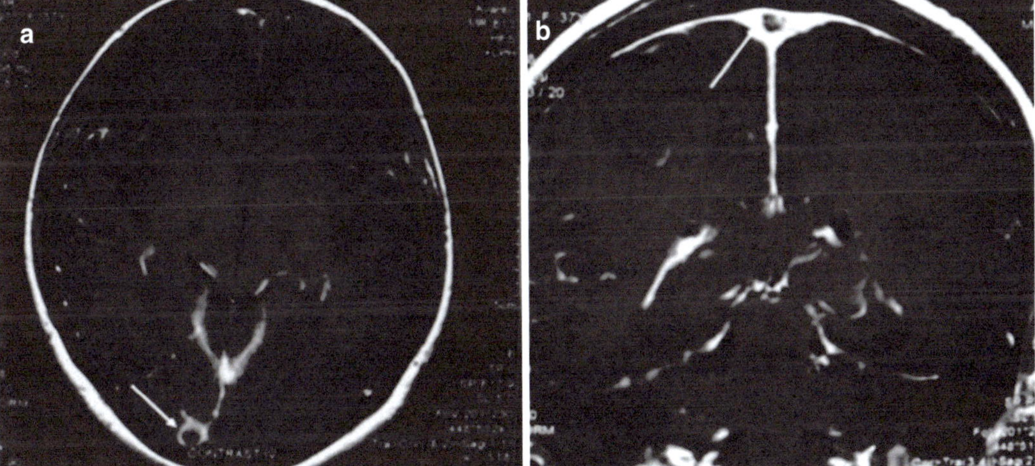

Fig. 11.4 Axial (**a**) and coronal (**b**) T1 weighted MR images after contrast administration showing a filling defect in the SSS (arrow) suggestive of sinus thrombosis (empty delta sign) (Filippidis et al.)

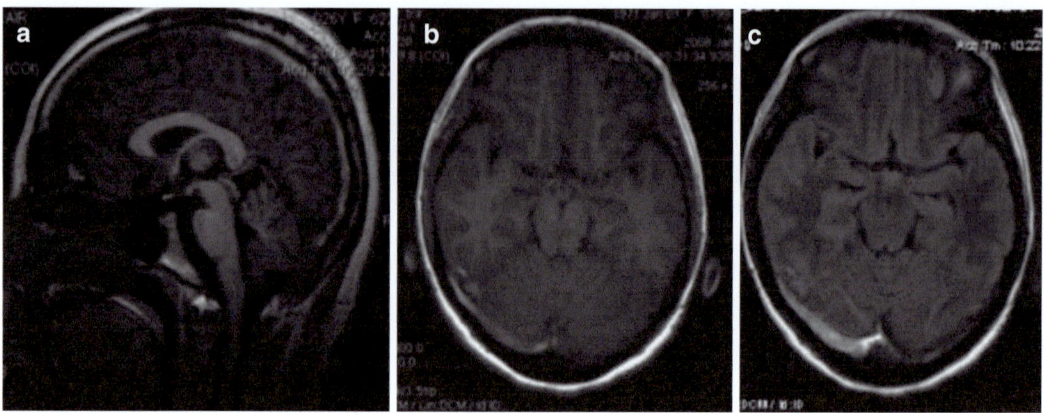

Fig. 11.5 Sagittal (**a**) and axial (**b, c**) T1-weighted MR images obtained in a 26-year-old pregnant female showing a hyperintense right transverse sinus and SSS, indicative of sinus thrombosis (Filippidis et al.)

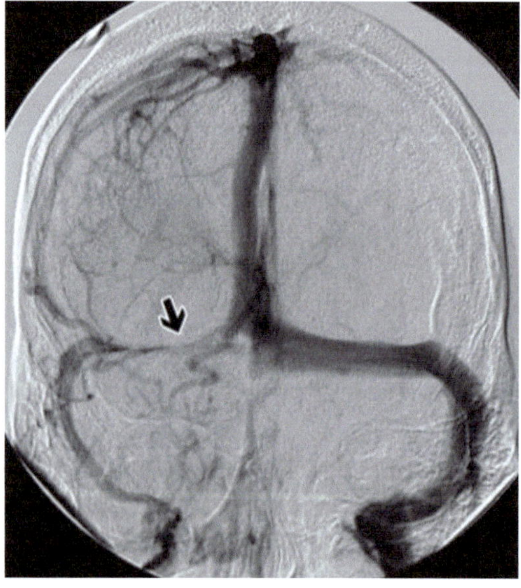

Fig. 11.6 Angiogram showing contrast in the last venous phase with an area of flow deficit in the left transverse sinus (arrow) consistent with thrombosis (Bentley et al.)

greater threat to the fetus due to ionizing radiation. A thrombosed sinus appears as an empty vessel, not filling normally with contrast, surrounded by engorged venous channels (Fig. 11.6). Thrombosed cortical veins adjacent to the main occlusion have a characteristic "hanging in space" appearance. Other times, the mark of thrombosis can be detected by abnormal dilation of collateral vessels. Although extremely sensitive in detecting CVST, there are limitations to obtaining traditional angiograms [e.g., cost, available clinicians with said expertise, dangers of contrast administration (especially in pregnancy), and time]. For these reasons, magnetic resonance imaging (MRI) has become the typical diagnostic imaging modality.

Treatment and Outcomes

Treatment

Broadly speaking to VTE in pregnancy, the current recommendations are to start heparin-based anticoagulation to prevent sequelae from a thrombus with the risks of anticoagulation needing to be considered on an individual basis [11]. Similarly, the goals of treatment for CVST are to recanalize the sinus, prevent thrombus propagation, and prevent pulmonary embolism. These goals are largely achieved by the initiation of heparin infusion, or weight-based low-molecular weight heparin (LMWH). Throughout the obstetrical and gyneco-

sion or, a normal anatomic variant, e.g., hypoplastic sinus [10]. Being non-reliant on ionizing radiation, MR-based imaging modalities have the added benefit of being safe during pregnancy.

Cerebral Angiography

While digital subtraction angiography (DSA) is much more sensitive at detecting a true venous occlusion than noninvasive techniques, it poses a logical literature, and even in the ISCVT trial, there are no guidelines put forth in regard to treatment for CVST. The ISCVT does, however, mention that over 80% of the patients enrolled in the study were treated with anticoagulants [3]. It is important to note that heparin administration is not contraindicated, even in patients with associated intracerebral hemorrhage. Currently, clinical trials are underway to determine if thrombolytic therapy has a role in reducing morbidity and mortality associated with CVST; as of yet, no such benefit has been shown [10]. For patients with transient risk factors, anticoagulation use should continue for 3–6 months; whereas patients with idiopathic CVST should remain on anticoagulation for 6–12 months; and patients with severe thrombophilia or combined permanent risk factors should remain on lifelong anticoagulation. Naturally, symptomatic treatment should be provided for seizures, cerebral edema, and hypertension to ensure the best clinical outcome. Even patients with cerebral edema requiring decompressive craniectomy have been shown to have good functional outcomes [4, 10]. Regarding specific medications traditionally used to treat cerebral edema and intracranial hemorrhage in the non-pregnant patient; levetiracetam and lamotrigine are safe antiepileptics in pregnancy as are intravenous labetalol and hydralazine for blood pressure control. There is no controlled data in human pregnancy for the use of mannitol.

Additionally, the aforementioned prothrombotic diagnoses warrant the use of anticoagulation during and after pregnancy given the increased risk of VTE. According to the American College of Obstetricians and Gynecologists Practice Bulletin on Thromboembolism in Pregnancy if a pregnant women has any of the aforementioned acquired or genetic diagnoses then prophylactic anticoagulation with heparin-based products is indicated [11].

Outcomes and Future Pregnancy

In the largest prospective observational study to date of all patients with CVST, 79% of patients recovered completely. The rate of death in the acute period was 5.6%. Prognosticators of poor outcome included: age >37 years, mental status disorders, coma, deep vein thrombosis (DVT), ICH on radiographic imaging, CNS malignancy, or infection [10]. Associated complications included: further venous thrombotic events (intra- and extracranial), seizure, headache, vision loss, and cognitive deprecation.

Patients with CVST should not become pregnant while on anticoagulation. However, after treatment is complete, data shows that despite having a higher risk of CVST recurrence, pregnancy is typically safe in women who have previous CVST. Approximately 62% of women who become pregnant post-CVST had uneventful pregnancies. However, women who had CVST were 80 times the general population to have a recurrence in a future pregnancy, and 16 times more likely to develop non-cerebral venous thromboembolism during pregnancy [6, 10].

Summary

CVST in pregnancy is a rare entity but it can have devastating sequelae. Astute clinical awareness and prompt radiographic diagnosis allow for earlier interventions. A basic understanding of the cerebral venous anatomy and pathophysiology of CVST guides the treatment paradigm. Currently, the treatment algorithm supports the initiation of heparin infusion, or weight-based low-molecular weight heparin (LMWH) with close clinic monitoring and a multidisciplinary effort across specialties. If treated appropriately patients have good outcomes and can have successful pregnancies in the future.

References

1. Nakase H. Introduction: venous brain circulation disorders. Neurosurg Focus. 2009;27(5):E1.
2. Filippidis A, Kapsalaki E, Patramani G, Fountas K. Cerebral venous sinus thrombosis: a review of the demographics, pathophysiology, current diagnosis, and treatment. Neurosurg Focus. 2009;27(5):E3.
3. Ferro JM, Canhão P, Stam J, Bousser MG, Barinagarrementeria F. Prognosis of cerebral vein and

dural sinus thrombosis: results of the international study on cerebral vein and dural sinus thrombosis (ISCVT). Stroke. 2004;35(3):664–70.

4. Liang Z-W, Wan-LiGao, Feng L-M. Clinical characteristics and prognosis of cerebral venous thrombosis in Chinese women during pregnancy and puerperium. Sci Rep. 2017;7:43866.

5. Saposnik G, Barinagarrementeria F, Brown R, Bushnell C, Cucchiara B, Cushman M, deVerber G, Ferro J, Tsai F. Diagnosis and management of cerebral venous thrombosis: a statement for healthcare professionals from the American Heart Association/American Stroke Association. Stroke. 2011;42(2011):1158–92.

6. Sousa D, Canhao P, Ferro J. Safety of pregnancy after cerebral venous thrombosis: a systematic review (2016). Stroke. 2016;47:713–8.

7. Bentley JN, Figueroa R, Vender J. From presentation to follow up: diagnosis and treatment of cerebral venous thrombosis. Neurosurg Focus. 2009;27(5):E4.

8. Kashkoush A, Ma H, Agarwal N, Panczykowski D, Tonetti D, Weiner G, Ares W, Kenmuir C, Jadhav A, Jovin T, Jankowitz B, Gross B. Cerebral venous sinus thrombosis in pregnancy and puerperium: a pooled systematic review. J Clin Neurosci. 2017;39(2017):9–15.

9. Osborne A. Diagnostic neuroradiology: a text/atlas. St. Louis: Mosby; 1993.

10. Ferro JM, Canhão P. Cerebral venous sinus thrombosis: update on diagnosis and management. Curr Cardiol Rep. 2014;16(9):523.

11. American College of Obstetricians and Gynecologists' Committee on Practice Bulletins—Obstetrics. ACOG Practice Bulletin No. 196: thromboembolism in pregnancy. Obstet Gynecol. 2018;132:e1–17.

Neurology of Preeclampsia and Eclampsia

Hannah J. Roeder and Eliza C. Miller

Introduction

Preeclampsia, a hypertensive disorder unique to human pregnancy, is among the most common of adverse pregnancy outcomes, complicating approximately 2–8% of pregnancies [1]. In its more severe manifestations, such as HELLP (hemolysis, elevated liver enzymes, low platelets) syndrome and eclampsia (preeclampsia complicated by generalized seizures), preeclampsia remains a major cause of maternal mortality both in the USA and worldwide. Hypertensive disorders account for approximately 7% of maternal deaths in the USA and 14% globally [2, 3]. Neurological complications figure prominently among the causes of maternal morbidity and mortality in women with preeclampsia, with intracerebral hemorrhage being a leading cause of death in this population [4, 5]. Thus, both neurologists and obstetricians must be familiar with the neurological manifestations of preeclampsia. In this chapter, we review the pathophysiology of preeclampsia–eclampsia (PEE) as it relates to the nervous system, as well as the prevention, diagnosis, and treatment of neurological complications in women with PEE.

History and Definitions of Preeclampsia–Eclampsia

PEE is a complex, heterogeneous disorder, and historically considerable controversy regarding its definition and classification existed. However, neurological complications have consistently been recognized as a key feature. A preeclampsia-like syndrome with neurological features was described by the ancient Greeks in the Coan Prognosis (approximately 400 BCE; often attributed to Hippocrates but likely a composite of earlier physician writers): "In pregnancy, the onset of drowsy headaches with heaviness is bad; such cases are perhaps liable to some sort of fits at the same time" [6]. However, as obstetrics was generally the purview of midwives, and not male physicians, PEE remained largely ignored by the Western medical literature until the seventeenth century, when the renowned obstetrician Francois Mauriceau described several important aspects of the syndrome, including the high morbidity of its neurological complications: "The mortal danger to mother and fetus is greater when the mother does not recover consciousness between convulsions" [7]. The term *eclampsia*, meaning "to shine/burst forth" was not introduced until the

H. J. Roeder
Department of Neurology, Carver College of Medicine, University of Iowa, Iowa City, IA, USA

E. C. Miller (✉)
Division of Stroke and Cerebrovascular Disease, Department of Neurology, Columbia University Vagelos College of Physicians and Surgeons, New York, NY, USA
e-mail: ecm2137@cumc.columbia.edu

G. Gupta et al. (eds.), *Neurological Disorders in Pregnancy*,
https://doi.org/10.1007/978-3-031-36490-7_12

eighteenth century, by the French obstetrician Boissier de Sauvages, who is first credited with differentiating eclampsia from epilepsy [8]. A prodromal syndrome which included neurological features was not recognized until a century later in 1843, when Dr. Robert Johns of the Dublin Lying-In Hospital noted that the combination of edema and "headache, weight, or giddiness in the head, ringing in the ears, [or] a temporary loss of vision" should raise alarm bells for the attending obstetrician [9]. Interestingly, he goes on to point out that "in most, if not all the cases which I state as having occurred under my own observation, these very premonitory symptoms had been present before labour, and I argue, that had they attracted the requisite attention at that period, the subsequent convulsions might have been avoided" [9]. Thus, the concept that early recognition of high-risk neurological features might prevent later maternal complications is far from new but remains highly relevant to contemporary medical practice.

In the late nineteenth and early twentieth century, prodromal features such as hypertension and proteinuria preceding eclamptic convulsions came to be known as *toxemia* or *toxemia of pregnancy*, reflecting initial prevailing theories that the syndrome was caused by a toxic or inflammatory state induced by the pregnancy. Definitions of this prodromal syndrome have since evolved, and continue to be debated and refined to this day (Table 12.1). By the 1970s, the term *toxemia* had fallen out of favor and the more modern terminology of *preeclampsia* and *hypertensive disorders of pregnancy* was adopted [8]. Hypertension and proteinuria were considered to be defining and necessary features for the diagnosis. However, in 1992, Douglas and Redman conducted an exhaustive clinical review of every case of eclampsia in the United Kingdom and found that 38% of cases were "unheralded" by hypertension or proteinuria [13]. Interestingly, their study found, in the week prior to presentation with eclampsia, headache was seen in 50% of women and visual disturbances in 19%. They concluded that while the incidence of eclampsia preceded by classic "preeclampsia" had declined, "atypical" cases remained difficult to predict, and recommended that screening and diagnostic tests consider "features other than hypertension and proteinuria" [13]. Nevertheless, despite being common and well characterized, neurological symptoms were not incorporated as a defining characteristic of preeclampsia until 2013 [14].

Currently accepted definitions of PEE are summarized in Table 12.1. Of note, the American College of Obstetricians and Gynecologists (ACOG) and the International Society for the Study of Hypertension in Pregnancy (ISSHP) have slightly different criteria for the diagnosis. Neurologists should particularly note that while both ACOG and ISSHP consider severe headaches or visual symptoms to be preeclampsia-defining, ISSHP includes additional neurological findings such as clonus, stroke, altered mental status, or eclampsia as preeclampsia-defining features. In addition, while the ACOG continues to differentiate neurological symptoms as one of several "severe features," ISSHP notes that while "distinctions between early and late onset, and mild and severe pre-eclampsia, may be useful for research purposes ... for clinical purposes, the condition should be considered as one that is at any time capable of being severe and life-threatening for mother and baby" [10, 11].

Table 12.1 ACOG and ISSHP definitions of preeclampsia–eclampsia [10, 11]

	ACOG (2019 revision)	ISSHP (2018 revision)
Preeclampsia		
New onset, persistent hypertension at or after 20 weeks pregnancy in a woman with previously normal blood pressure	• SBP of 140 mmHg or more or DBP of 90 mmHg or more on two occasions at least 4 h apart after 20 weeks of gestation in a woman with a previously normal BP	• SBP ≥140 and/or DBP ≥90 mmHg; BP should be repeated to confirm true hypertension
and	• SBP of 160 mmHg or more or DBP of 110 mmHg or more[a,b]	• If BP is severe (SBP ≥160 and/or DBP ≥110 mmHg) then BP should be confirmed within 15 min
	[Severe hypertension can be confirmed within a short interval (minutes) to facilitate timely antihypertensive therapy]	• If less severe BP, repeated readings should be taken over a few hours
		• Use liquid crystal sphygmomanometer or if unavailable, validated and appropriately calibrated automated device
Proteinuria	• 300 mg or more per 24-h urine collection (or this amount extrapolated from a timed collection) or	• 24-h urinary protein ≥300 mg per day or
	• Protein/creatinine ratio of 0.3 mg/dL or more or	• Protein/creatinine ratio ≥ 30 mg/mmol (0.3 mg/mg) or
	• Dipstick reading of 2+ (used only if other quantitative methods not available)	• When neither 24 h nor protein/creatinine ratio measures, dipstick testing showing values greater than 1 g/L, i.e., 2+
OR	New onset of any of the following:	• Acute kidney injury (creatinine ≥90 µmol/L; 1 mg/dL)
In absence of proteinuria	• Thrombocytopenia: Platelet count less than 100,000 × 10^9/L[a]	• Liver involvement (elevated transaminases, e.g., ALT or AST > 40 IU/L) with or without right upper quadrant or epigastric abdominal pain)
	• Renal insufficiency: Serum creatinine concentrations greater than 1.1 mg/dL or a doubling of the serum creatinine concentration in the absence of other renal disease[a]	• Hematological complications (thrombocytopenia—Platelet)
	• Impaired liver function: Elevated blood concentrations of liver transaminases to twice normal concentration[a]	• Count below 150,000/µL, DIC, hemolysis)
	• Pulmonary edema[a]	• Uteroplacental dysfunction (fetal growth restriction, abnormal umbilical artery Doppler wave form analysis, or stillbirth)[c]
	• **New-onset headache unresponsive to medication and not accounted for by alternative diagnoses, or visual symptoms**[a]	• **Neurological complications (eclampsia, altered mental status, blindness, stroke, clonus, severe headaches, persistent visual scotomata)**

(continued)

Table 12.1 (continued)

	ACOG (2019 revision)	ISSHP (2018 revision)
Preeclampsia variants		
Preeclampsia superimposed on chronic hypertension	• Preeclampsia in a woman diagnosed with chronic essential hypertension; diagnosis of exclusion [12]	• New onset proteinuria or other maternal organ dysfunction in a woman with a diagnosis of chronic essential hypertension
	• New onset thrombocytopenia, elevated liver transaminases, sudden development of symptoms suggestive of preeclampsia, or elevated uric acid levels suggest superimposed preeclampsia	• Rises in blood pressure are insufficient to diagnose superimposed preeclampsia • Fetal growth restriction is insufficient to diagnose superimposed preeclampsia
HELLP syndrome	• LDH elevated to 600 IU/L or more • AST and ALT elevated more than twice the upper limit of normal • Platelet count less than $100,000 \times 10^9/L$	• ISSHP does not define this as a separate condition and considers this condition to be part of the preeclampsia spectrum
Eclampsia[d]	• New-onset tonic-clonic, focal, or multifocal seizures in absence of other causative conditions (e.g., epilepsy, cerebral ischemia, intracranial hemorrhage, drug use)	• ISSHP does not define this as a separate condition and considers it among the neurological complications of preeclampsia

ACOG American College of Obstetricians and Gynecologists, *ISSHP* International Society for the Study of Hypertension in Pregnancy, *SBP* systolic blood pressure, *DBP* diastolic blood pressure, *BP* blood pressure, *ALT* alanine aminotransferase, *AST* aspartate aminotransferase, *LDH* lactate dehydrogenase, *DIC* disseminated intravascular coagulation
Bold draws attention to the neurological features of preeclampsia/eclampsia
[a] Severe feature by ACOG definition
[b] Women with gestational hypertension who present with severe-range blood pressures should be managed with the same approach as for women with severe preeclampsia, regardless of other features
[c] ISSHP includes fetal growth restriction and other placental manifestations as preeclampsia-defining features
[d] ACOG notes that women may not exhibit other signs of preeclampsia (e.g., hypertension, proteinuria) before presenting with seizures

Epidemiology of Preeclampsia–Eclampsia and Its Neurological Complications

PEE affects between 2 and 8% of all pregnancies [1]. In certain populations, the incidence is far higher; up to 50% of women with chronic hypertension develop superimposed preeclampsia, and the risk may be even higher in women with pre-existing organ dysfunction [12]. A recent Mayo Clinic study using medical-record linkage data from the Rochester Epidemiology Project (Olmsted County, Rochester, MN) took the novel approach of quantifying preeclampsia incidence on a "per-woman" rather than "per-pregnancy" basis, and found that this effectively doubled pre-eclampsia incidence from 3.3 cases per 100 pregnancies to 7.5 cases per 100 women (95% confidence interval [95%CI], 6.3–8.8) [15]. The rate is likely to be far higher in higher-risk populations [16]. Eclampsia is far less common today in high-income countries but remains a major cause of maternal death in women in low- and middle-income countries (LMICs): a recent analysis of a cluster-randomized trial in LMICs found that rates of eclampsia ranged from 19.6 to as high as 142 cases per 10,000 deliveries; overall, 6.9% of women with eclampsia died [17].

Neurological complications are common in preeclampsia and present, by definition, in all eclampsia cases. In addition to seizures, headaches, and visual symptoms, neurological complications of PEE include ischemic and hemorrhagic stroke, posterior reversible encephalopathy syndrome (PRES), reversible cerebral vasoconstriction syndrome (RCVS), peripheral neuropathy, encephalopathy, and sleep dysfunction.

Pathophysiology of Preeclampsia–Eclampsia: The "Disease of Theories"

The pathophysiology of PEE is complex and multifactorial and remains incompletely understood and hotly debated, earning it the moniker *the disease of theories* [18]. However, most authors agree that placental dysfunction is a primary disturbance [19]. Early in pregnancy, fetal trophoblast cells migrate along maternal spiral arteries in the endometrium and induce vascular remodeling, resulting in a low-resistance, high-flow state which promotes delivery of oxygen and nutrients from the maternal circulation to the placenta. The remodeling process requires complex immunological and angiogenic two-way signaling between the trophoblast and the maternal endothelium [20]. Failure of remodeling results in the so-called decidual vasculopathy, with maternal spiral arteries remaining in a high-resistance state, which leads to reduced uterine perfusion, placental ischemia, and placental release of cytokines and angiogenic factors, with a cascade of downstream vascular and inflammatory effects [21].

Vascular pathology is likely both a cause and a result of PEE. Endothelial dysfunction throughout the maternal vasculature is a key feature of PEE, including impaired nitric oxide and prostacyclin production, vascular oxidative stress, increased vasoconstrictive activity by thromboxane A2 and endothelin-1, and increased sensitivity to the vasoconstrictive effects of angiotension II [22–26]. An excess of soluble FMS-like tyrosine kinase-1 (sFlt-1), a placentally-produced anti-angiogenic factor which binds to both vascular endothelial growth factor (VEGF) and the VEGF homolog, placental growth factor (PlGF), has been shown to predict PEE in women, and animal studies support a causal role for sFlt-1 [27, 28]. Another anti-angiogenic protein, soluble endoglin (sEng), appears to combine with sFlt-1 to cause many of the severe systemic features of PEE [29]. Studies in preeclampsia rat models have also demonstrated impairment in vascular smooth muscle function [24]. Women with preeclampsia have impaired flow-mediated dilation during pregnancy and for 3 years afterwards, implicating vascular dysfunction in both the pathogenesis and long-term vascular consequences of preeclampsia [30]. Some authors propose that PEE is a maternal cardiovascular disorder, meaning a failure of the maternal vasculature to adapt to the physiological challenge of pregnancy, rather than a primary placental disorder [31].

Inflammation and immunological mechanisms also appear to play critical roles in PEE. While pregnancy has traditionally been thought of as a state of immune tolerance, recent work suggests that *immunomodulated* may better describe the complex state whereby the maternal host tolerates the allogeneic fetus [32]. Once nicknamed *the disease of primiparity*, PEE has long been noted to occur more frequently in the first pregnancy; some evidence shows an association between *primipaternity* or partner change and PEE risk, suggesting immune mechanisms [33]. Both normal pregnancy and PEE are associated with an inflammatory response, which is intensified in PEE in response to oxidative stress. Signs of inflammation such as increased C-reactive protein, platelet, and complement activation, and elevated pro-inflammatory cytokines all occur in normal pregnancy and to a greater extent in PEE. Thus, some authors have proposed that normal pregnancy and PEE exist on an inflammatory continuum, with PEE developing when inflammatory mechanisms exceed the limits of maternal compensatory capacity [34]. Increased shedding of microvesicles from the stressed placenta into the maternal circulation is seen in PEE, resulting in a cascade of proinflammatory effects, mediated in part by the recognition of danger-associated molecular patterns (DAMPs) or alarmins by the maternal inflammasome [35, 36].

Lastly, as a heterogeneous disorder, the genetics of PEE are complex. Both the maternal and fetal genome, together with their interactions, must be considered [37]. The disorder clusters in families, with a nearly three-fold higher risk in women with a family history of the disease [38]. However, the inheritance is likely polygenic and highly influenced by environmental factors [39].

Genome-wide association studies recently identified a significant susceptibility locus in the fetal genome near the FLT1 gene which encodes FMS-tyrosine kinase 1, which is biologically plausible given the known involvement of sFlt-1 and related proteins in the pathogenesis of PEE [40].

Preeclampsia–Eclampsia and the Maternal Nervous System

As described later in this chapter, PEE is associated with multiple neurological complications, including seizures, cerebral infarction, arteriopathies, intracerebral hemorrhage, encephalopathy, and peripheral neuropathies. The mechanisms by which PEE causes these complications are an underexplored area of neuroscience. However, studies have demonstrated important effects of PEE on the blood–brain barrier, the cerebral endothelium, vascular smooth muscle, and autonomic activity.

In rat models of healthy pregnancy, the cerebral vasculature adapted to the increased volume as well as increased circulating vasoconstrictors late in gestation, and autoregulation was even improved [41–43]. In contrast, plasma from preeclamptic women caused increased blood–brain barrier permeability [44]. A study in a different rat model of preeclampsia demonstrated impaired cerebral autoregulation and increased blood–brain barrier permeability in placental ischemic rats, compared to controls, an effect subsequently shown to be mediated by inflammatory cytokines [45, 46]. Studies in other animal models of PEE also support the hypothesis that PEE causes blood–brain barrier leakage and impairment of cerebral autoregulation [44, 47–49]. In clinical studies, women with PEE have shown impaired cerebral autoregulation as well as impaired cerebral vasoreactivity in response to CO_2 inhalation [50, 51]. In a neuropathological study of women who died of eclampsia, researchers found perivascular microhemorrhages and microinfarcts as well as arteriolar vasculopathy [52]. These and related effects may in part explain why intracerebral hemorrhage may occur in preeclamptic women at blood pressures that are not necessarily in the severe range [53].

Seizures are a defining feature of eclampsia. In a rat model, preeclamptic rats have been shown to have decreased seizure threshold and increased inflammatory cytokines compared to controls; the effect was inhibited by pretreatment with magnesium [54, 55]. The susceptibility of the maternal brain to seizures may be further increased by blood–brain barrier dysfunction, exposing the brain to circulating proinflammatory factors [56].

Autonomic nervous system dysfunction is also a pathophysiologic feature of PEE. In uncomplicated pregnancy, vasomotor sympathetic activity increases, but in women with hypertensive disorders of pregnancy, sympathetic activity increases to an even greater degree and parasympathetic activity decreases [57–59]. In healthy pregnancies, estrogenic effects may blunt the effect of increased sympathetic activity on vascular resistance [60]. A systematic review including 26 studies found 93.6% of women with preeclampsia demonstrated dysautonomia as assessed by cardiovascular reflex tests, heart rate variability, cardiac baroreflex gain, muscle sympathetic nerve activity, or biomarkers of sympathetic activity [61]. The atypical autonomic response in preeclampsia is also associated with a decrease in spontaneous fetal heart rate accelerations in late pregnancy, a measure of fetal well-being [58]. The sympathetic overactivity of preeclampsia normalizes after delivery [57, 62].

Maternal Neurological Complications of Preeclampsia/ Eclampsia

Seizures

The occurrence of one or more seizures superimposed on preeclampsia defines the onset of eclampsia [10]. Eclampsia is a dangerous complication of pregnancy, with high associated maternal and fetal morbidity and mortality [10]. In general, the semiology of eclamptic seizures is generalized tonic-clonic convulsions. [63] Focal seizures have been described as presentations of atypical eclampsia but should be a red flag prompting further investigation for a structural brain abnormality [64]. Electroencephalogram (EEG) abnormalities can be seen in both preeclampsia and eclampsia. One study of preeclamptic patients found that half of the EEGs were abnormal, with generalized slowing being most common [65]. In three studies that performed EEG analysis in patients with severe preeclampsia and/or eclampsia, abnormalities were seen between 70% and 80% of the time, including instances of generalized slowing, focal slowing, epileptiform discharges, seizures, alpha coma, and electrocerebral silence [65–67].

Prompt treatment of eclamptic seizures is critical. As with other medical emergencies, management of eclampsia begins with ensuring adequate maternal circulation, airway, and breathing and promptly initiating (or continuing) fetal monitoring. The patient should be placed on her side with close monitoring of vitals and oral suctioning as necessary. Magnesium is used for both treatment and prevention of eclampsia. As early as 1925, the use of magnesium sulfate to treat eclampsia was reported in the literature with a case series of 17 patients [68]. For perspective, the article also mentions *eliminative measures* (including phlebotomy, stomach lavage, castor oil, and colonic flushing with glucose and soda), which were other contemporary measures for treatment of eclampsia. The author Lazard proposed that "the sedative action of magnesium sulphate on nerve cells" was the mechanism of seizure control [68]. Even now, no single mechanism is known to be responsible for seizure control, but several are proposed. Magnesium deficiency reduces neuronal membrane surface charge and increases neuronal hyperexcitability, which supplementation corrects [69]. Magnesium acts as a central N-methyl-D-aspartate antagonist and has been shown to control NMDA-induced seizures in rats [70]. Magnesium may limit cerebral edema formation via its action on cerebral aquaporin expression, reducing seizure occurrence [71]. Magnesium acts as a smooth muscle calcium antagonist causing arterial relaxation both systemically and cerebrally, although its effect on preventing seizures via decreasing systemic blood pressure and/or inhibiting cerebral vasospasm is unknown [72]. In the general population, hypomagnesemia is known to precipitate seizures [73]. Many decades after Lazard's observations, the 1995 Eclampsia Trial Collaborative Group helped solidify magnesium as the treatment of choice for eclampsia, demonstrating its superiority to both phenytoin and diazepam in reducing recurrent eclamptic seizures [74]. Additionally, magnesium was associated with lower maternal and perinatal morbidity than phenytoin [74]. Other trials have also shown the superiority of magnesium to phenytoin and diazepam in treating eclamptic seizures [75–77]. Due to the success of magnesium in treating seizures from eclampsia, prior to the development of the current armamentarium of anti-epileptic drugs available today, magnesium was used as a treatment for seizures of all etiologies in pregnant and non-pregnant patients. This is no longer the case; however, of note, recent literature suggests there may be a potential role for magnesium in the treatment of drug-resistant seizures in the population at large [78].

The preferred magnesium regimen in the USA is a 4–6 g intravenous loading dose over 20–30 min, followed by a maintenance rate of 1–2 g/h [10]. Magnesium infusion requires close laboratory monitoring of magnesium levels and clinical monitoring of reflexes, urinary output, and respiratory status. Hypermagnesemia toxicity first presents as areflexia around 9 mg/dL with higher levels having the risk of respiratory depression (12 mg/dL) and eventually cardiac arrest (30 mg/dL) [10]. In one of the EEG studies mentioned previously, seizures persisted for two patients at serum magnesium levels of 9.6 and 11 mg/dL—both above the standard therapeutic goal for eclampsia [65]. No good data exist to guide management of magnesium-refractory eclamptic convulsions; however, it is certainly reasonable to dose benzodiazepines and consider loading a long-acting anti-epileptic drug for recurrent seizures following an adequate magnesium trial, particularly in the post-partum setting when there is no potential fetal risk, or when red flags exist to suggest possible alternative etiology of seizures.

The MAGPIE randomized controlled trial of over 10,000 women with preeclampsia admitted to hospitals in 33 countries found that magnesium lowered the risk of eclampsia by 58% (95%CI, 40–71%), such that 11 per 1000 fewer women developed eclampsia [79].

Expedient delivery of infant and placenta following the onset of eclampsia is also key to decreasing maternal and perinatal mortality. In one early study, maternal mortality was 7% with delivery within 2 h but skyrocketed to 42% with delivery beyond 24 h, and in another early study, perinatal mortality was 14% with delivery within 6 h but soared to 62% when delivery occurred between 12 and 24 h after eclampsia onset [80, 81]. Delivery may also be necessary to prevent eclampsia; the American College of Obstetricians and Gynecologists (ACOG) recommends delivery for women >37 weeks with preeclampsia, and >34 weeks with preeclampsia with severe features and in other clinical situations where the benefit outweighs the risk of preterm delivery [10].

A classic study of eclampsia found that EEG abnormalities can resolve with lowering blood pressure to a normal range, and experience from hypertensive encephalopathy and PRES in the general population support this notion [82]. However, the role of anti-hypertensives in the acute management of eclampsia remains unclear.

Regarding timing, seizures may occur antepartum, intrapartum, or postpartum. Postpartum eclamptic seizures typically occur within 48 h of delivery. Later onset of eclampsia has rarely been reported; however, such cases warrant further investigation for other seizure precipitants [83].

The obstetrician and neurologist should always consider a wide differential for seizures occurring during pregnancy and postpartum, including pre-existing epilepsy, vascular insults, space-occupying lesions, autoimmune disorders, central nervous system infections, metabolic abnormalities, and substance use/withdrawal [63]. Considerations related to seizures and epilepsy in pregnancy are detailed in Chap. 28.

Headaches

Headaches are common during pregnancy, and causes range from benign to life-threatening. Migraines are more common in women and the prevalence peaks during the childbearing years [84]. For most women, preexisting migraines improve or remit during pregnancy but for a minority, headaches can worsen or even start during pregnancy [85]. Most studies suggest that migraineurs are more like to develop preeclampsia; in one meta-analysis, 8 out of 10 studies found a positive association between migraine history and either preeclampsia or gestational hypertension [86]. One case-control study of women with preeclampsia versus controls with an uncomplicated pregnancy found an OR 4.95 (95%CI 2.47–9.92) of those with preeclampsia having a headache history [87]. Catamenial migraines with onset at menarche were most associated with preeclampsia, and women with severe preeclampsia were even more likely to have a headache history [87]. The presence of aura has not consistently been shown to affect the risk of preeclampsia in pregnant migraineurs [86]. The mechanism of the relationship between migraines and preeclampsia is unknown but possibilities include vascular reactivity, endothelial damage, platelet hyper-aggregation, and magnesium deficiency [88–93]. Notably, both migraines and preeclampsia are risk factors for ischemic stroke in women. In addition to being used for prevention and treatment of eclampsia, magnesium may be used as both a preventive and abortive medication for migraines [94–96].

Development of a new headache semiology during pregnancy may signal the onset of preeclampsia. The International Classification of Headache Disorders describes a headache attributed to PEE as a "Headache, usually bilateral and pulsating, occurring in women during pregnancy or the immediate puerperium with pre-eclampsia or eclampsia. It remits after resolution of the pre-eclampsia or eclampsia." [97] Migraines and other primary headaches must be differentiated from secondary causes of headache during pregnancy and the puerperium; differential diagnoses to be considered in addition to PEE include cerebrovascular disorders (ischemic and hemorrhagic stroke, cerebral venous thrombosis, RCVS, PRES, arterial dissection), idiopathic intracranial hypertension, space-occupying lesions, systemic or central nervous system infection, post-dural puncture headache, and pituitary apoplexy. The approach to evaluation and management of headaches during pregnancy is described in Chap. 27.

Cerebrovascular Disease

Vascular dysfunction is central to the pathophysiology of preeclampsia and eclampsia. The maternal cerebral vasculature is highly susceptible to adverse events, which may manifest as hemorrhagic stroke, ischemic stroke, RCVS, and PRES.

Ischemic and Hemorrhagic Stroke

Hypertensive disorders of pregnancy, including PEE, are well-established risk factors for maternal stroke [98–100]. Maternal stroke (stroke occurring during pregnancy, delivery, or postpartum period) occurs in an estimated 30 out of 100,000 deliveries [101]. Stroke is the most common cause of serious long-term disability following pregnancy and is the seventh leading cause of death among pregnant women in the USA [102–104]. Analysis of the Nationwide Inpatient Sample from 2000 to 2001 showed that PEE is associated with a four-fold increase (OR 4.4, 95%CI 3.6–5.4) of stroke during pregnancy [105]. Among women with preeclampsia, cerebrovascular disease is a leading cause of maternal mortality, with intracerebral hemorrhage accounting for most of the deaths [4]. In an analysis of New York State Department of Health inpatient data, among 200 strokes occurring in women with preeclampsia, the risk of stroke was greater with severe preeclampsia or eclampsia, co-existing prothrombotic states or coagulopathies, infections, and chronic hypertension [106]. Almost half of the strokes were hemorrhagic and more than 10% of the women with preeclampsia-associated stroke died during the admission for stroke [106]. In a Taiwanese population, the relative risk of stroke for women with PEE was great-

est in the third trimester and the first 3 days postpartum (with hemorrhagic strokes slightly more common than ischemic strokes) but the elevated risk for both types of strokes persisted throughout the 12-month postpartum period studied [107].

The diagnosis and management of suspected stroke in women with preeclampsia requires an interdisciplinary team, involving stroke neurologists, obstetricians, radiologists, pharmacists, anesthesiologists, critical care physicians, the patient and family, and others, depending on the clinical scenario. Sudden onset focal neurological deficits in women with preeclampsia should prompt all clinicians to consider a diagnosis of stroke and act promptly [108]. Evaluation begins with ensuring adequate circulation, airway, and breathing and measuring vital signs, including blood pressure. The team should check a fingerstick glucose level and send basic bloodwork. The clinician should obtain a brief history to establish the last known well and to identify exclusion criteria for thrombolytics, and perform a focused exam to obtain a National Institutes of Health Stroke Scale score. Specific to preeclampsia-associated stroke, antenatal and intrapartum women require fetal monitoring and administration of magnesium sulfate.

Hemorrhagic and ischemic stroke are indistinguishable by history and exam alone; therefore, neuroimaging is required (Fig. 12.1). Non-contrast computed tomography (CT) head (and CT angiogram of the head and neck if concern for a large vessel occlusion) should be obtained without delay to evaluate for hemorrhage and to assess for early ischemic signs. The fetal radiation exposure from a CT head is minimal and has not been shown to increase pregnancy or fetal complications [109, 110]. Use of abdominal/pelvic shielding, minimizing scans, and discussion with patient and family are encouraged. If immediately available, magnetic resonance imaging (MRI) is an acceptable alternative.

If CT head demonstrates a hemorrhagic stroke (intracerebral and/or subarachnoid hemorrhage), the patient should be monitored in an intensive care setting with neurology and obstetric involvement. Initial management should focus on con-

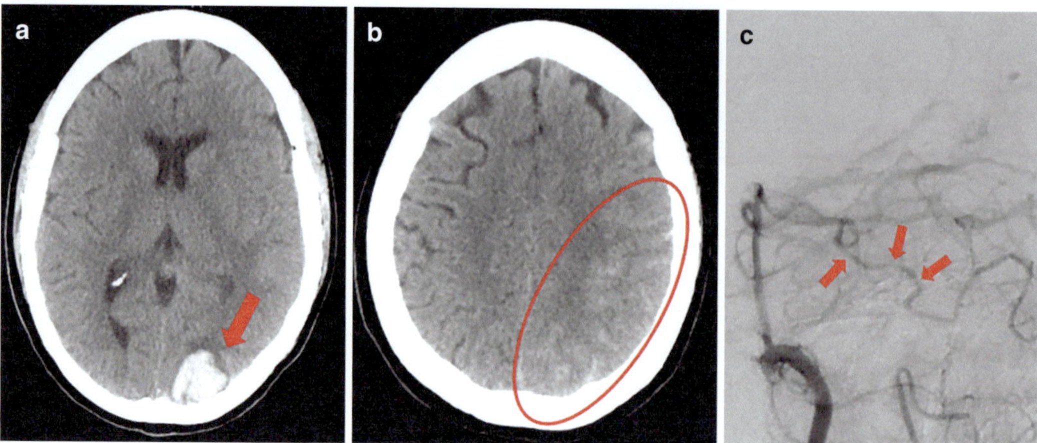

Fig. 12.1 A 40-year-old woman with history of migraines developed hypertension and severe headache a week after giving birth to her first child. Her postpartum course had been complicated by an infection requiring re-admission and intravenous antibiotics. She was treated for preeclampsia with magnesium, and symptoms improved. Shortly before planned discharge she developed recurrent headache, hypertension, and a visual field deficit. Head CT without contrast showed acute left occipital intracerebral (**a**) and subarachnoid (**b**) hemorrhage. Cerebral angiogram (**c**) showed multifocal vasoconstriction suggestive of reversible cerebral vasoconstriction syndrome. Vasospasm was confirmed with transcranial Doppler and resolved over the next few weeks

trolling blood pressure and correcting coagulopathies to avoid hemorrhage expansion. Additional imaging and evaluation may be required to identify the underlying mechanism (such as vascular malformation, venous sinus thrombosis, hypertension), and interventions to prevent recurrent hemorrhage pursued as indicated [108].

If acute onset focal neurological findings are present and brain CT is normal or shows early ischemic changes, intravenous thrombolysis and/or mechanical thrombectomy may be considered. Pregnancy is an exclusion criterion in nearly all acute ischemic stroke management trials for both thrombolysis and thrombectomy. The American Stroke Association 2018 Guidelines for management of acute ischemic stroke state "IV alteplase administration may be considered in pregnancy when the anticipated benefits of treating moderate or severe stroke outweigh the anticipated increased risks of uterine bleeding" and additionally states, "The safety and efficacy of IV alteplase in the early postpartum period (<14 days after delivery) have not been well established" [111]. A growing body of literature, mostly case reports and series, suggests thrombolysis may be beneficial in selected clinical scenarios for stroke in pregnant and postpartum women; however, a risk-benefit analysis with multidisciplinary input and patient and family counseling is recommended [112]. Pregnancy is not a reason to delay or avoid mechanical thrombectomy when clinically indicated given the high morbidity and mortality associated with proximal large vessel occlusions [108]. Steps can be taken to minimize fetal contrast and radiation exposure.

Mode and timing of delivery should also be an intradisciplinary decision considering stroke type and mechanism, maternal condition, gestational age, fetal condition and positioning, obstetric history, and patient and family preferences. Stroke is not a contraindication to vaginal birth in all scenarios, but steps may need to be taken to reduce Valsalva maneuvers and minimize intracranial pressure elevation, and Cesarean section may be preferable for women at high risk of recurrent intracranial hemorrhage [108].

Post-stroke care for women with preeclampsia should consider secondary stroke prevention (which will vary based on stroke type, mechanism, and co-morbidities), chronic management of stroke risk factors (such as hypertension, diabetes), appropriate rehabilitation care, screening and treatment of post-stroke/postpartum depression, and counseling regarding stroke risk in future pregnancies [108]. Ischemic and hemorrhagic stroke are discussed in detail in Chaps. 6 and 7, respectively.

Posterior Reversible Encephalopathy Syndrome

PRES is a neurological condition characterized by encephalopathy, headaches, seizures, cortical blindness, and/or other focal neurological signs [113]. The association between PRES and eclampsia was suggested in the first published description o11f PRES in 1996, which included 15 patients, 3 of whom had eclampsia [113]. In the general population, hypertension, autoimmune disorders, and some immunosuppressant medications are common risk factors. In pregnancy, the disorder is closely associated with PEE [114]. Similar to eclampsia, the underlying pathophysiology of PRES includes disordered cerebral autoregulation, endothelial dysfunction, and cerebral ischemia from vasospasm [115, 116]. Imaging in PRES classically demonstrates reversible vasogenic edema in bilateral occipital and parietal lobes (Fig. 12.2); however, other brain regions may also be susceptible, and the lesions and neurological deficits are not always reversible [117].

One retrospective single center study at the University of Mississippi Medical Center found imaging findings suggestive of PRES to be nearly universal in the setting of eclampsia; 46 of 47 patients with eclampsia who had neuro-imaging showed evidence of PRES and the single patient without evidence of PRES was subsequently determined to have an underlying seizure disorder [118]. In another single center case series in Japan of women with preeclampsia/eclampsia with neurological symptoms, 12 of 13 (92%) patients with eclampsia and 5 of 26 (19%) patients with preeclampsia showed evidence of PRES on MRI [119]. In two other single center case series, around half of women with eclampsia who underwent an MRI showed evidence of PRES in both studies [67, 120]. Important limitations of the retrospective reviews include bias in the selection of patients with eclampsia undergoing neuroimaging and lack of blinding, particularly of radiologists, to the clinical scenario. Nevertheless, the high prevalence of imaging characteristics of PRES among women with eclampsia has led some to coin eclampsia as *obstetric PRES* [121]. In the University of Mississippi case series, presenting PRES symptoms other than seizure included headache (87.2%), AMS (51.1%), visual disturbances (34%), nausea/vomiting (19.1%), and systolic

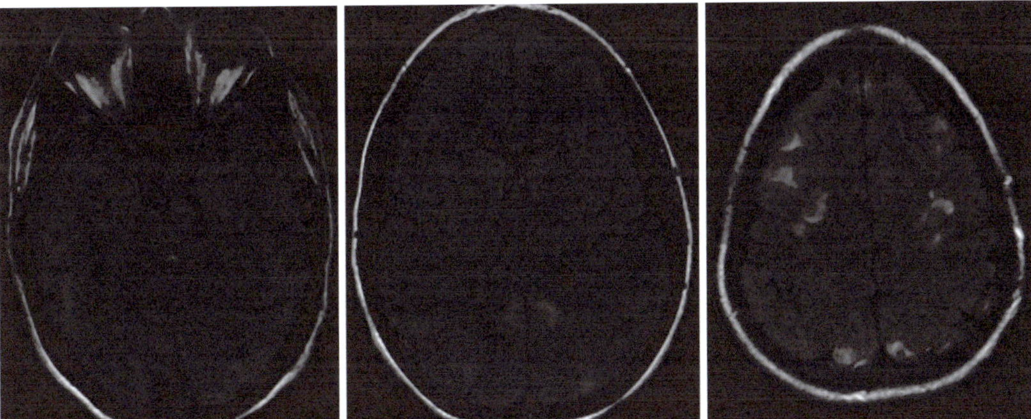

Fig. 12.2 A 30-year-old woman developed severe, progressive headache after delivering full term twins. Her pregnancy had been uncomplicated. She presented to the emergency department on postpartum day 8 with generalized seizures. MRI revealed patchy vasogenic edema consistent with the posterior reversible encephalopathy syndrome (PRES). She was treated for eclampsia with magnesium and antihypertensives. Follow-up MRI showed complete resolution of PRES related changes

blood pressure > 160 mmHg (47%) [118]. While the clinical features in PRES are similar in the pregnant and non-pregnant population, higher rates of headache and lower rates of altered mental status are described in obstetric PRES [122].

In the general population, treatment of PRES includes antihypertensives, antiepileptics, and cessation of precipitant medications as indicated. While ACOG guidelines recommend women with preeclampsia be treated with antihypertensive therapy for sustained systolic blood pressure $\geq$ 160 mmHg or diastolic blood pressure $\geq$ 110 mmHg, in preeclampsia complicated by PRES, stricter blood pressure control may be indicated [10]. In a review of eclampsia-associated PRES cases, just under half had severe systolic hypertension (SBP > 160); normalization of blood pressure to maintain cerebral and utero-placental perfusion and limit propagation of cerebral edema is the goal [118]. The choice of antihypertensive agent should consider both acuity of onset, fetal effects (prior to delivery), and maternal co-morbidities; intravenous labetalol, calcium channel blockers, or hydralazine may be used safely in pregnancy to acutely lower blood pressure [123]. Oral labetalol and calcium channel blockers may be used to maintain the desired blood pressure goal [10]. Nitroprusside should be avoided due to risk of cyanide toxicity in the mother and fetus and risk of worsening cerebral edema. Magnesium levels should be maintained in the high normal range; one study found hypomagnesemia occurred more frequently in eclampsia with PRES-related changes on MRI than in eclampsia where MRI did not demonstrate PRES [124, 125].

PRES associated with PEE may have better outcomes than in the general population [121]. The difference may be due to younger age and fewer co-morbidities among pregnant women with PRES compared to the general population with PRES [126].

Reversible Cerebral Vasoconstriction Syndrome

RCVS is a neurological disorder characterized by multi-focal cerebral vasospasm, which may lead to ischemic stroke, hemorrhagic stroke, subarachnoid hemorrhage (often cortical), and seizure. Recurrent thunderclap headaches are a pathognomonic clinical feature, and focal neurological deficits may occur when arterial vasospasm leads to hypo-perfused and/or ischemic territory [127]. Migraines, many drugs (particularly vasoactive substances), and preeclampsia are significant risk factors. Postpartum cerebral angiopathy, sometimes known by the eponym Call–Fleming Syndrome, represents a subset of RCVS, occurring most often within 1 week of delivery [128, 129]. Postpartum angiopathy is more common in women with preeclampsia and other hypertensive disorders of pregnancy [130].

Multi-focal segmental vasoconstriction on vessel imaging (CTA, MRA, conventional angiogram) is diagnostic but may be missed due to its transience. Transcranial dopplers are a preferred non-invasive neuroimaging tool to assess arterial velocity and can be used in the initial diagnosis and subsequent monitoring of RCVS [131]. Abnormalities on TCD velocities often persist following headache resolution but significantly improve or resolve over a few months [132].

Therapeutic management of RCVS is not well-established. Calcium channel blockers (both verapamil and nimodipine) are often used clinically with data that they prevent recurrent thunderclap headaches and improve TCD velocities but without strong evidence that they improve overall outcomes [133]. Long-acting verapamil may be the preferable agent [133]. Steroids were previously used to treat RCVS, but data suggests glucocorticoid therapy may lead to worse outcomes and should be avoided [134, 135]. In cases of severe cerebral vasospasm, local intra-arterial administration of calcium antagonists may be considered [136, 137]. RCVS and its postpartum variant, postpartum angiopathy, are discussed in detail in Chaps. 13 and 14.

Encephalopathy and Coma

In addition to seizures, coma superimposed on preeclampsia is another neurological manifestation defining eclampsia and portends a poor prognosis. Among women with eclampsia admitted to the intensive care unit, a low Glasgow Coma Scale score predicts mortality [138]. The workup and initial management of altered mental status and coma during pregnancy are discussed in Chap. 16.

Peripheral Neuropathy

Pregnant women are at risk for developing several neuropathies. For example, peripartum mononeuropathies involving the femoral, lateral femoral cutaneous, peroneal, and sciatic nerve may occur from stretch and/or compression during labor and delivery [139, 140]. Carpal tunnel syndrome (CTS), a median neuropathy occurring at the wrist, has increased incidence during pregnancy; however, a review at the Mayo Clinic found no correlation between pregnancy-related CTS and preeclampsia [141]. In contrast, Bell palsy, an idiopathic facial nerve palsy, may be a warning sign for preeclampsia. Bell palsy occurs more often in women of reproductive age compared to men and more commonly in pregnancy (particularly the third trimester and puerperium); proposed mechanisms include hypertension, gestational edema, viral infections, and hypercoagulability. The condition is even more frequently encountered with preeclampsia; two retrospective reviews (one from Canada and one in the USA) found preeclampsia was at least several-fold more prevalent among pregnant and postpartum women who developed Bell palsy compared to the general preeclampsia prevalence [142, 143]. In addition to cranial nerve (CN) VII palsy, case reports describe the onset of CN II (nonarteritic anterior ischemic optic neuropathy), III (pupil-sparing oculomotor), VI (abducens), and XII (hypoglossal) palsies associated with preeclampsia [144–148]. While the etiology is unknown, microvascular ischemic injury akin to a diabetic third nerve palsy may be responsible. Peripheral neuropathies affecting patients during pregnancy are described in Chap. 24.

Sleep Dysfunction

Preeclampsia may also be associated with sleep-disordered breathing and sleep architecture changes [149–151]. This phenomenon is discussed in detail in Chap. 29.

Offspring Neurological Complications Due to Maternal Preeclampsia/Eclampsia

The infant survival rate following maternal preeclampsia has vastly improved over the last several decades; however, offspring exposed to preeclampsia in utero remain at risk for systemic and neurological complications [152]. Preeclampsia is characterized by placental insufficiency and restricted oxygen supply. Abnormal umbilical artery velocimetry in women with preeclampsia may predict adverse perinatal outcomes [153]. In particular, early onset and severe preeclampsia are associated with unfavorable perinatal outcomes related to premature delivery and fetal growth restriction [154, 155].

Preeclampsia negatively affects the long-term vascular health of offspring. Hypertensive disorders of pregnancy impact vascular and renal development in offspring and make them more susceptible to hypertension, beginning in childhood and early adulthood [156–158]. One Finnish study utilizing data from the Helsinki Birth Cohort Study found an increased risk of stroke in the adult offspring of pregnancies complicated by preeclampsia (HR 1.9, 95%CI 1.2–3.0) [159]. Maternal preeclampsia and offspring vascular health are linked by genetic risk factors and often shared familial (non-genetic) exposures, but in utero exposure to preeclampsia may have direct effects on vascular, cardiac, renal, and immunologic development [160]. Supporting this hypothesis, data show siblings born from uncomplicated pregnancies do not share the same vascular abnormalities as their siblings born from pregnancies complicated by preeclampsia [161].

Offspring of preeclamptic pregnancies may have lower cognitive function and poorer mental health. A 2016 systematic review of the effects of hypertensive disorders of pregnancies on offspring health identified eight studies evaluating cognitive function, and all found evidence that hypertensive disorders of pregnancy, especially preeclampsia, negatively affect offspring intellectual abilities [162]. One study, using data from the Helsinki Birth Cohort Study, also found an elevated risk for severe mental disorders among adult offspring exposed to maternal preeclampsia [163]. A Norwegian prospective cohort study found increased risk of attention deficit hyperactivity disorder (adjusted OR 1.18, 95%CI 1.05–1.33) and autism spectrum disorder (adjusted OR 1.29, 95%CI 1.08–1.54) among children exposed to preeclampsia in utero [164].

Maternal preeclampsia may also affect an offspring's risk of developing epilepsy. One Danish study found an increased risk of epilepsy in childhood and young adulthood for offspring born at full-term to mothers with preeclampsia but no effect of maternal preeclampsia among pre-term infants. The effect size for full-term offspring was greater with preeclampsia with severe features [165]. Another retrospective cohort study using Medicaid data in South Carolina also found that maternal preeclampsia increased risk of childhood epilepsy among offspring (OR = 1.46, 95%CI 1.17–1.82) after controlling for potential confounders. In subgroup analysis, the effect again was only observed for full-term infants and not preterm infants compared to controls [166]. The effect modification seen with preterm status in both studies suggests that other preterm etiologies may be equal or greater risk factors for childhood epilepsy than preeclampsia. A Norwegian prospective cohort study also found increased risk of epilepsy in children born at term who were exposed to maternal preeclampsia (adjusted OR 1.50, 95%CI 1.05–1.33) [164]. Studies on the effect of maternal preeclampsia on other neurological conditions, including cerebral palsy and child behavior, have shown mixed results [162].

Long-Term Maternal Neurological Sequelae of Preeclampsia/Eclampsia

In the years and decades following a pregnancy complicated by preeclampsia, women are at an increased risk of many systemic chronic diseases, including neurological ones. Women with a history of preeclampsia have now been recognized to have a higher risk of vascular disease later in life. One meta-analysis of three case-control and four cohort studies calculated an OR of 1.76 (95%CI 1.43–2.21) for women with the history of preeclampsia developing ischemic stroke prior to old age [167]. The association was even greater with early-onset, severe, and recurrent preeclampsia. Preeclampsia may simply unmask preexisting subclinical risk factors and a predisposition towards vascular disease; however, it is unknown if preeclampsia may also have a causal role in developing vascular disease later in life.

An analysis of data from the California Teachers Study demonstrated that women with a history of hypertensive disorders of pregnancy who used aspirin did not have a higher risk of stroke before the age of 60 years old compared to controls (adjusted HR 0.8, 95%CI 0.4–1.7), whereas aspirin non-users had a higher risk (adjusted HR1.5, 95%CI 1.0–2.1) [168]. The same effect was not seen with statins. However, no prospective trials have evaluated aspirin use for primary stroke prevention after preeclampsia. History of preeclampsia remains an underappreciated sex-specific risk factor for vascular disease, and women with a history of preeclampsia should minimize other modifiable vascular risk factors (smoking cessation, physical activity, blood pressure management, etc.) to decrease stroke risk.

Cognitive dysfunction may persist following preeclampsia. One small study performing neuropsychiatric testing several months postpartum found significantly lower auditory-verbal memory performance in women with severe preeclampsia versus controls with an uncomplicated pregnancy [169]. A Dutch study of neurocogni-

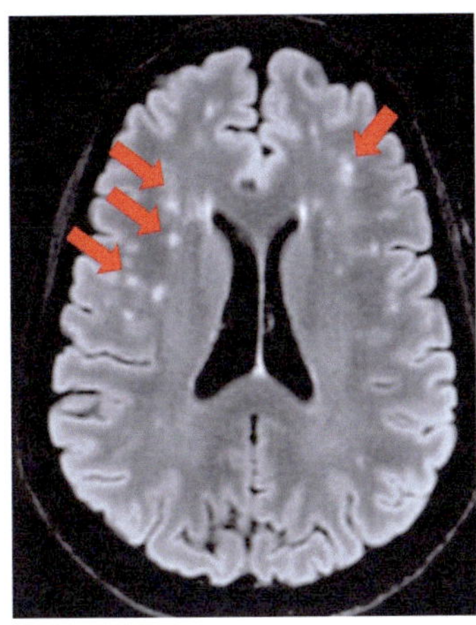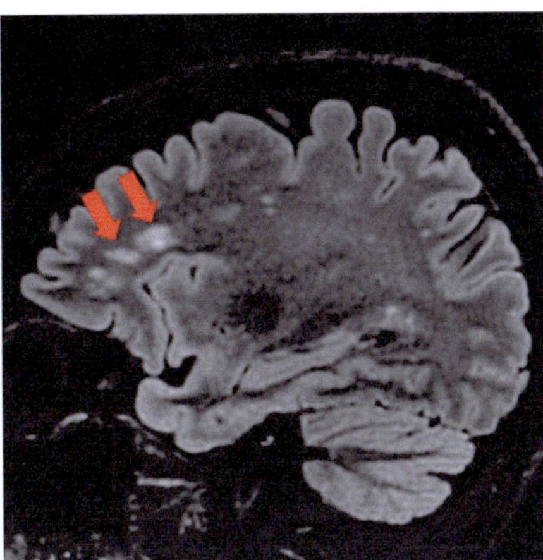

Fig. 12.3 A 49-year-old woman presented to her neurologist for evaluation of cognitive complaints. She reported a history of early onset preeclampsia in her first pregnancy at age 30. She subsequently developed chronic hypertension which was well controlled on medication. MRI showed patchy subcortical white matter hyperintensities suggestive of cerebral small vessel disease

tive functioning conducted several years postpartum found women with a history of preeclampsia or eclampsia scored worse on a subjective questionnaire of cognitive assessment and slightly worse on visuomotor functions but did not differ on other objective measures of cognitive impairment; however, they scored worse on anxiety and depression scales, which the authors hypothesized may account for differences in subjective cognitive assessment [170]. A study of cognitive function several decades following pregnancy conducted at the Mayo Clinic found that postmenopausal women with a history of preeclampsia were at greater risk than controls of cognitive impairment, particularly in executive dysfunction and verbal list impairment, which is consistent with expected cognitive effects of vascular disease (Fig. 12.3) [171].

The Neuro-Obstetrics Team and Preeclampsia–Eclampsia

Preeclampsia and eclampsia are life-threatening complications of pregnancy which can have profoundly damaging effects on the maternal and fetal nervous system. Neurological features are prominent and, in some cases, disease-defining.

Neurologists, obstetricians, family practitioners, obstetric anesthesiologists, and other clinicians who care for pregnant and postpartum women should be aware of the neurological features and complications of PEE, and have a low threshold to obtain additional diagnostic testing and involve the neurologist in clinical assessment and decision-making. Shared decision-making strategies should be employed, including the patient and her family, when caring for women with neurological complications of PEE. In addition, neurologists should obtain relevant obstetrical history and consider the long-term maternal consequences of PEE when assessing cerebrovascular and cognitive risk in women.

References

1. Duley L. The global impact of pre-eclampsia and eclampsia. Semin Perinatol. 2009;33(3):130–7.
2. CDC (Centers for Disease Control and Prevention). Pregnancy mortality surveillance system; 2020. cdc.gov/reproductivehealth/maternality-mortality/pregnancy-mortality-surveillance-system.html.
3. Say L, et al. Global causes of maternal death: a WHO systematic analysis. Lancet Glob Health. 2014;2(6):e323–33.
4. Foo L, Bewley S, Rudd A. Maternal death from stroke: a thirty year national retrospective review. Eur J Obstet Gynecol Reprod Biol. 2013;171(2):266–70.

5. Katsuragi S, et al. Analysis of preventability of stroke-related maternal death from the nationwide registration system of maternal deaths in Japan. J Matern Fetal Neonatal Med. 2018;31(16):2097–104.

6. Chesley L. Chapter 1 - Introduction, history, controversies, and definitions. In: Taylor RN, Roberts JM, Cunningham G, Lindheimer M, editors. Chesley's hypertensive disorders in pregnancy. 4th ed. London: Academic; 2015. p. 1–24.

7. Mauriceau F. Traité des maladies des femmes grosses et de celles qui sont accouchées, Vol. 1. p. 1740. Par la Compagnie des libraires.

8. Bell MJ. A historical overview of preeclampsia-eclampsia. J Obstet Gynecol Neonatal Nurs. 2010;39(5):510–8.

9. Johns R. Observations on puerperal convulsions. Dublin J Med Sci. 1843;24(1):101–15.

10. ACOG (American College of Obstetricians and Gynecologistis). Preeclampsia. ACOG Practice Bulletin No. 202. American College of Obstetricians and Gynecologists. Obstet Gynecol. 2019;133(1):e1–e25.

11. Brown MA, et al. Hypertensive disorders of pregnancy: ISSHP classification, diagnosis, and management recommendations for international practice. Hypertension. 2018;72(1):24–43.

12. ACOG (American College of Obstetricians and Gynecologists). ACOG Practice Bulletin No. 203: chronic hypertension in pregnancy. Obstet Gynecol. 2019;133(1):e26–50.

13. Douglas K, Redman C. Eclampsia in the United Kingdom. BMJ. 1994;309(6966):1395–400.

14. Roberts JM, et al. Hypertension in pregnancy: executive summary. Obstet Gynecol. 2013;122(5):1122–31.

15. Garovic VD, et al. Incidence and long-term outcomes of hypertensive disorders of pregnancy. J Am Coll Cardiol. 2020;75(18):2323–34.

16. Abalos E, et al. Global and regional estimates of preeclampsia and eclampsia: a systematic review. Eur J Obstet Gynecol Reprod Biol. 2013;170(1):1–7.

17. Vousden N, et al. Incidence of eclampsia and related complications across 10 low-and middle-resource geographical regions: secondary analysis of a cluster randomised controlled trial. PLoS Med. 2019;16(3):e1002775.

18. Pipkin FB, Rubin P. Pre-eclampsia—the 'disease of theories'. Br Med Bull. 1994;50(2):381–96.

19. Mol BWJ, et al. Pre-eclampsia. Lancet. 2016;387(10022):999–1011.

20. Brosens I, et al. The "great obstetrical syndromes" are associated with disorders of deep placentation. Am J Obstet Gynecol. 2011;204(3):193–201.

21. Parks WT. Placental hypoxia: the lesions of maternal malperfusion. Semin Perinatol. 2015;39:9.

22. Krupp J, et al. The loss of sustained Ca2+ signaling underlies suppressed endothelial nitric oxide production in preeclamptic pregnancies: implications for new therapy. Am J Phys Heart Circ Phys. 2013;305(7):H969–79.

23. Downing I, Shepherd G, Lewis P. Reduced prostacyclin production in pre-eclampsia. Lancet. 1980;316(8208):1374.

24. Goulopoulou S. Maternal vascular physiology in preeclampsia. Hypertension. 2017;70(6):1066–73.

25. Ali SM, Khalil RA. Genetic, immune and vasoactive factors in the vascular dysfunction associated with hypertension in pregnancy. Expert Opin Ther Targets. 2015;19(11):1495–515.

26. Cunningham MW Jr, et al. Agonistic autoantibodies to the angiotensin II type 1 receptor enhance angiotensin II–induced renal vascular sensitivity and reduce renal function during pregnancy. Hypertension. 2016;68(5):1308–13.

27. Levine RJ, et al. Circulating angiogenic factors and the risk of preeclampsia. N Engl J Med. 2004;350(7):672–83.

28. Powe CE, Levine RJ, Karumanchi SA. Preeclampsia, a disease of the maternal endothelium: the role of antiangiogenic factors and implications for later cardiovascular disease. Circulation. 2011;123(24):2856–69.

29. Venkatesha S, et al. Soluble endoglin contributes to the pathogenesis of preeclampsia. Nat Med. 2006;12(6):642–9.

30. Weissgerber TL, et al. Impaired flow-mediated dilation before, during, and after preeclampsia: a systematic review and meta-analysis. Hypertension. 2016;67(2):415–23.

31. Kalafat E, Thilaganathan B. Cardiovascular origins of preeclampsia. Curr Opin Obstet Gynecol. 2017;29(6):383–9.

32. Erlebacher A. Mechanisms of T cell tolerance towards the allogeneic fetus. Nat Rev Immunol. 2013;13(1):23–33.

33. Luo ZC, et al. The effects and mechanisms of primiparity on the risk of pre-eclampsia: a systematic review. Paediatr Perinat Epidemiol. 2007;21(Suppl 1):36–45.

34. Redman CW, Sargent IL, Taylor RN. Immunology of normal pregnancy and preeclampsia. In: Chesley's hypertensive disorders in pregnancy. Amsterdamv: Elsevier; 2015. p. 161–79.

35. Brien ME, et al. Alarmins at the maternal-fetal interface: involvement of inflammation in placental dysfunction and pregnancy complications (1). Can J Physiol Pharmacol. 2019;97(3):206–12.

36. Gomez-Lopez N, et al. Inflammasomes: their role in normal and complicated pregnancies. J Immunol. 2019;203(11):2757–69.

37. Gray KJ, Saxena R, Karumanchi SA. Genetic predisposition to preeclampsia is conferred by fetal DNA variants near FLT1, a gene involved in the regulation of angiogenesis. Am J Obstet Gynecol. 2018;218(2):211–8.

38. Duckitt K, Harrington D. Risk factors for preeclampsia at antenatal booking: systematic review of controlled studies. BMJ. 2005;330(7491):565.

39. Fong FM, et al. Maternal genotype and severe preeclampsia: a HuGE review. Am J Epidemiol. 2014;180(4):335–45.
40. McGinnis R, et al. Variants in the fetal genome near FLT1 are associated with risk of preeclampsia. Nat Genet. 2017;49(8):1255–60.
41. Amburgey OA, et al. Resistance artery adaptation to pregnancy counteracts the vasoconstricting influence of plasma from normal pregnant women. Reprod Sci. 2010;17(1):29–39.
42. Cipolla MJ, Bishop N, Chan S-L. Effect of pregnancy on autoregulation of cerebral blood flow in anterior versus posterior cerebrum. Hypertension. 2012;60(3):705–11.
43. Cipolla MJ, Sweet JG, Chan S-L. Cerebral vascular adaptation to pregnancy and its role in the neurological complications of eclampsia. J Appl Physiol. 2011;110(2):329–39.
44. Amburgey OA, et al. Plasma from preeclamptic women increases blood-brain barrier permeability: role of vascular endothelial growth factor signaling. Hypertension. 2010;56(5):1003–8.
45. Warrington JP, et al. Placental ischemia-induced increases in brain water content and cerebrovascular permeability: role of TNF-α. Am J Phys Regul Integr Comp Phys. 2015;309(11):R1425–31.
46. Warrington JP, et al. Placental ischemia in pregnant rats impairs cerebral blood flow autoregulation and increases blood-brain barrier permeability. Physiol Rep. 2014;2(8):e12134.
47. Clayton AM, et al. Postpartum increases in cerebral edema and inflammation in response to placental ischemia during pregnancy. Brain Behav Immun. 2018;70:376–89.
48. Wallace K, et al. Hypertension, anxiety, and blood-brain barrier permeability are increased in postpartum severe preeclampsia/hemolysis, elevated liver enzymes, and low platelet count syndrome rats. Hypertension. 2018;72(4):946–54.
49. Johnson AC, Cipolla MJ. Impaired function of cerebral parenchymal arterioles in experimental preeclampsia. Microvasc Res. 2018;119:64–72.
50. Riskin-Mashiah S, et al. Cerebrovascular reactivity in normal pregnancy and preeclampsia. Obstet Gynecol. 2001;98(5 Pt 1):827–32.
51. van Veen TR, et al. Cerebral autoregulation in normal pregnancy and preeclampsia. Obstet Gynecol. 2013;122(5):1064–9.
52. Richards A, Graham D, Bullock R. Clinicopathological study of neurological complications due to hypertensive disorders of pregnancy. J Neurol Neurosurg Psychiatry. 1988;51(3):416–21.
53. Martin JN, et al. Stroke and severe preeclampsia and eclampsia: a paradigm shift focusing on systolic blood pressure. Obstet Gynecol. 2005;105(2):246–54.
54. Huang Q, et al. Decreased seizure threshold in an eclampsia-like model induced in pregnant rats with lipopolysaccharide and pentylenetetrazol treatments. PLoS One. 2014;9(2):e89333.
55. Johnson AC, et al. The contribution of normal pregnancy to eclampsia. PLoS One. 2015;10(7):e0133953.
56. Johnson AC, et al. Inhibition of blood-brain barrier efflux transporters promotes seizure in pregnant rats: role of circulating factors. Brain Behav Immun. 2018;67:13–23.
57. Fischer T, et al. Pregnancy-induced sympathetic overactivity: a precursor of preeclampsia. Eur J Clin Investig. 2004;34(6):443–8.
58. Swansburg ML, et al. Maternal cardiac autonomic function and fetal heart rate in preeclamptic compared to normotensive pregnancies. Can J Cardiovasc Nurs. 2005;15(3):42–52.
59. Reyes LM, et al. Sympathetic neurovascular regulation during pregnancy: a longitudinal case series study. Exp Physiol. 2018;103(3):318–23.
60. Meyer MC, Cummings K, Osol G. Estrogen replacement attenuates resistance artery adrenergic sensitivity via endothelial vasodilators. Am J Phys Heart Circ Phys. 1997;272(5):H2264–70.
61. Yousif D, et al. Autonomic dysfunction in preeclampsia: a systematic review. Front Neurol. 2019;10:816.
62. Schobel HP, et al. Preeclampsia—a state of sympathetic overactivity. N Engl J Med. 1996;335(20):1480–5.
63. Thomas SV. Diagnostic Challenges with Seizures in Pregnancy. In: Epilepsy in Women, Eds. Cynthia L. Harden MD, Sanjeev V. Thomas MD, DM, Torbjörn Tomson MD, PhD. 2013;pp 75–90. https://doi.org/10.1002/9781118531037.ch7 Copyright John Wiley & Sons, Ltd.
64. Agrawal PKB, et al. Complex partial seizure with postictal aggression as a presentation of atypical eclampsia: a case report. J Karnali Acad Health Sci. 2018;1(3):45–8.
65. Sibai BM, et al. Effect of magnesium sulfate on electroencephalographic findings in preeclampsia-eclampsia. Obstet Gynecol. 1984;64(2):261–6.
66. Thomas SV, Somanathan N, Radhakumari R. Interictal EEG changes in eclampsia. Electroencephalogr Clin Neurophysiol. 1995;94(4):271–5.
67. Paolini S, et al. S21. EEG features in preeclampsia and eclampsia. Clin Neurophysiol. 2018;129:e150.
68. Lazard E. A preliminary report on the intravenous use of magnesium sulphate in puerperal eclampsia. Am J Obstet Gynecol. 1925;9(2):178–88.
69. Isaev D, et al. Surface charge impact in low-magnesium model of seizure in rat hippocampus. J Neurophysiol. 2012;107(1):417–23.
70. Cotton DB, et al. Central anticonvulsant effects of magnesium sulfate on N-methyl-D-aspartate-induced seizures. Am J Obstet Gynecol. 1993;168(3):974–8.
71. Ghabriel M, Thomas A, Vink R. Magnesium restores altered aquaporin-4 immunoreactivity following traumatic brain injury to a pre-injury state. In: Brain edema XIII. New York: Springer; 2006. p. 402–6.

72. Euser AG, Cipolla MJ. Resistance artery vasodilation to magnesium sulfate during pregnancy and the postpartum state. Am J Phys Heart Circ Phys. 2005;288(4):H1521–5.

73. Nuytten D, et al. Magnesium deficiency as a cause of acute intractable seizures. J Neurol. 1991;238(5):262–4.

74. Eclampsia Trial Group. Which anticonvulsant for women with eclampsia? Evidence from the collaborative eclampsia trial. Lancet. 1995;345(8963):1455–63.

75. Duley L, Henderson-Smart DJ, Chou D. Magnesium sulphate versus phenytoin for eclampsia. Cochrane Database Syst Rev. 2010;10:CD000128.

76. Duley L, et al. Magnesium sulphate versus diazepam for eclampsia. Cochrane Database Syst Rev. 2010;12:CD000127.

77. Lucas MJ, Leveno KJ, Cunningham FG. A comparison of magnesium sulfate with phenytoin for the prevention of eclampsia. N Engl J Med. 1995;333(4):201–5.

78. Abdelmalik PA, Politzer N, Carlen PL. Magnesium as an effective adjunct therapy for drug resistant seizures. Can J Neurol Sci. 2012;39(3):323–7.

79. Altman D, et al. Magpie Trial Collaboration Group. Do women with pre-eclampsia, and their babies, benefit from magnesium sulphate? The Magpie Trial: a randomised placebo-controlled trial. Lancet. 2002;359(9321):1877–90.

80. Menon MK. The evolution of the treatment of eclampsia. BJOG Int J Obstet Gynaecol. 1961;68(3):417–26.

81. López-Llera M. Eclampsia 1963–1966: evaluation of the treatment of 107 cases. BJOG Int J Obstet Gynaecol. 1967;74(3):379–84.

82. Jost H. Electroencephalographic records in relation to blood pressure changes in eclampsia. Am J Med Sci. 1948;216(1):57–63.

83. Chames MC, et al. Late postpartum eclampsia: a preventable disease? Am J Obstet Gynecol. 2002;186(6):1174–7.

84. Lipton RB, et al. Prevalence and burden of migraine in the United States: data from the American migraine study II. Headache. 2001;41(7):646–57.

85. Ertresvåg J, et al. Headache and transient focal neurological symptoms during pregnancy, a prospective cohort. Acta Neurol Scand. 2005;111(4):233–7.

86. Adeney KL, Williams MA. Migraine headaches and preeclampsia: an epidemiologic review. Headache. 2006;46(5):794–803.

87. Facchinetti F, et al. The relationship between headache and preeclampsia: a case–control study. Eur J Obstet Gynecol Reprod Biol. 2005;121(2):143–8.

88. Mauskop A, Altura BT, Altura BM. Serum ionized magnesium levels and serum ionized calcium/ionized magnesium ratios in women with menstrual migraine. Headache. 2002;42(4):242–8.

89. Whigham KA, et al. Abnormal platelet function in pre-eclampsia. Br J Obstet Gynaecol. 1978;85(1):28–32.

90. Hanington E, et al. Migraine: a platelet disorder. Lancet. 1981;2(8249):720–3.

91. Kisters K, et al. Plasma and membrane Ca2+ and Mg2+ concentrations in normal pregnancy and in preeclampsia. Gynecol Obstet Investig. 1998;46(3):158–63.

92. Hayashi M, et al. Characterization of five marker levels of the hemostatic system and endothelial status in normotensive pregnancy and preeclampsia. Eur J Haematol. 2002;69(5–6):297–302.

93. Yilmaz Avci A, et al. Migraine and subclinical atherosclerosis: endothelial dysfunction biomarkers and carotid intima-media thickness: a case-control study. Neurol Sci. 2019;40(4):703–11.

94. Mauskop A, et al. Intravenous magnesium sulphate relieves migraine attacks in patients with low serum ionized magnesium levels: a pilot study. Clin Sci. 1995;89(6):633–6.

95. Peikert A, Wilimzig C, Köhne-Volland R. Prophylaxis of migraine with oral magnesium: results from a prospective, multi-center, placebo-controlled and double-blind randomized study. Cephalalgia. 1996;16(4):257–63.

96. Demirkaya Ş, et al. Efficacy of intravenous magnesium sulfate in the treatment of acute migraine attacks. Headache. 2001;41(2):171–7.

97. Headache Classification Committee of the International Headache Society (IHS) The International Classification of Headache Disorders, 3rd edition. Cephalalgia. 2018;38(1):1–211. https://doi.org/10.1177/0333102417738202. PMID: 29368949.

98. Liu S, et al. Stroke and cerebrovascular disease in pregnancy: incidence, temporal trends, and risk factors. Stroke. 2019;50(1):13–20.

99. Scott CA, et al. Incidence, risk factors, management, and outcomes of stroke in pregnancy. Obstet Gynecol. 2012;120(2 Part 1):318–24.

100. Sharshar T, Lamy C, Mas J. Incidence and causes of strokes associated with pregnancy and puerperium: a study in public hospitals of Ile de France. Stroke. 1995;26(6):930–6.

101. Swartz RH, et al. The incidence of pregnancy-related stroke: a systematic review and meta-analysis. Int J Stroke. 2017;12(7):687–97.

102. Sells CM, Feske SK. Stroke in pregnancy. Semin Neurol. 2017;37:669.

103. Treadwell S, Thanvi B, Robinson T. Stroke in pregnancy and the puerperium. Postgrad Med J. 2008;84(991):238–45.

104. Creanga AA, et al. Pregnancy-related mortality in the United States, 2011–2013. Obstet Gynecol. 2017;130(2):366.

105. James AH, et al. Incidence and risk factors for stroke in pregnancy and the puerperium. Obstet Gynecol. 2005;106(3):509–16.

106. Miller EC, et al. Risk factors for pregnancy-associated stroke in women with preeclampsia. Stroke. 2017;48(7):1752–9.

107. Tang C-H, et al. Preeclampsia-eclampsia and the risk of stroke among peripartum in Taiwan. Stroke. 2009;40(4):1162–8.
108. Ladhani NNN, et al. Canadian stroke best practice consensus statement: acute stroke management during pregnancy. Int J Stroke. 2018;13(7):743–58.
109. Tremblay E, et al. Quality initiatives: guidelines for use of medical imaging during pregnancy and lactation. Radiographics. 2012;32(3):897–911.
110. Committee opinion No. 723: guidelines for diagnostic imaging during pregnancy and lactation. Obstet Gynecol, 2017. 130(4): p. e210.
111. Powers WJ, et al. Guidelines for the early management of patients with acute ischemic stroke: a guideline for healthcare professionals from the American Heart Association/American Stroke Association. Stroke. 2018;49(3):e46–99.
112. Sousa Gomes M, Guimarães M, Montenegro N. Thrombolysis in pregnancy: a literature review. J Matern Fetal Neonatal Med. 2019;32(14):2418–28.
113. Hinchey J, et al. A reversible posterior leukoencephalopathy syndrome. N Engl J Med. 1996;334(8):494–500.
114. Staykov D, Schwab S. Posterior reversible encephalopathy syndrome. J Intensive Care Med. 2012;27(1):11–24.
115. Marra A, et al. Posterior reversible encephalopathy syndrome: the endothelial hypotheses. Med Hypotheses. 2014;82(5):619–22.
116. Granata G, et al. Posterior reversible encephalopathy syndrome—insight into pathogenesis, clinical variants and treatment approaches. Autoimmun Rev. 2015;14(9):830–6.
117. Bartynski W. Posterior reversible encephalopathy syndrome, part 1: fundamental imaging and clinical features. Am J Neuroradiol. 2008;29(6):1036–42.
118. Brewer J, et al. Posterior reversible encephalopathy syndrome in 46 of 47 patients with eclampsia. Am J Obstet Gynecol. 2013;208(6):468.e1–6.
119. Mayama M, et al. Incidence of posterior reversible encephalopathy syndrome in eclamptic and patients with preeclampsia with neurologic symptoms. Am J Obstet Gynecol. 2016;215(2):239.e1–5.
120. Camara-Lemarroy CR, et al. Posterior reversible leukoencephalopathy syndrome (PRES) associated with severe eclampsia: clinical and biochemical features. Pregnancy Hypertens. 2017;7:44–9.
121. Postma IR, et al. Long-term consequences of the posterior reversible encephalopathy syndrome in eclampsia and preeclampsia: a review of the obstetric and nonobstetric literature. Obstet Gynecol Surv. 2014;69(5):287–300.
122. Liman T, et al. Clinical and radiological differences in posterior reversible encephalopathy syndrome between patients with preeclampsia-eclampsia and other predisposing diseases. Eur J Neurol. 2012;19(7):935–43.
123. Duley L, Meher S, Jones L. Drugs for treatment of very high blood pressure during pregnancy. Cochrane Database Syst Rev. 2013;7:CD001449.
124. Chardain A, et al. Posterior reversible encephalopathy syndrome (PRES) and hypomagnesemia: a frequent association? Rev Neurol. 2016;172(6–7):384–8.
125. Fang X, et al. Posterior reversible encephalopathy syndrome in preeclampsia and eclampsia: the role of hypomagnesemia. Seizure. 2020;76:12.
126. Roth C, Ferbert A. Posterior reversible encephalopathy syndrome: is there a difference between pregnant and non-pregnant patients? Eur Neurol. 2009;62(3):142–8.
127. Chen S-P, et al. Reversible cerebral vasoconstriction syndrome: current and future perspectives. Expert Rev Neurother. 2011;11(9):1265–76.
128. Call G, et al. Reversible cerebral segmental vasoconstriction. Stroke. 1988;19(9):1159–70.
129. Konstantinopoulos PA, et al. Postpartum cerebral angiopathy: an important diagnostic consideration in the postpartum period. Am J Obstet Gynecol. 2004;191(1):375–7.
130. Fugate JE, et al. Variable presentations of postpartum angiopathy. Stroke. 2012;43(3):670–6.
131. Levin JH, et al. Transcranial Doppler ultrasonography as a non-invasive tool for diagnosis and monitoring of reversible cerebral vasoconstriction syndrome. R I Med J. 2016;99(9):38.
132. Chen SP, et al. Transcranial color doppler study for reversible cerebral vasoconstriction syndromes. Ann Neurol. 2008;63(6):751–7.
133. Marsh EB, Ziai WC, Llinas RH. The need for a rational approach to vasoconstrictive syndromes: transcranial doppler and calcium channel blockade in reversible cerebral vasoconstriction syndrome. Case Rep Neurol. 2016;8(2):161–71.
134. Singhal AB, et al. Reversible cerebral vasoconstriction syndromes: analysis of 139 cases. Arch Neurol. 2011;68(8):1005–12.
135. Singhal AB, Topcuoglu MA. Glucocorticoid-associated worsening in reversible cerebral vasoconstriction syndrome. Neurology. 2017;88(3):228–36.
136. French KF, et al. Repetitive use of intra-arterial verapamil in the treatment of reversible cerebral vasoconstriction syndrome. J Clin Neurosci. 2012;19(1):174–6.
137. Elstner M, et al. Reversible cerebral vasoconstriction syndrome: a complicated clinical course treated with intra-arterial application of nimodipine. Cephalalgia. 2009;29(6):677–82.
138. Bhagwanjee S, et al. Intensive care unit morbidity and mortality from eclampsia: an evaluation of the Acute Physiology and Chronic Health Evaluation II score and the Glasgow Coma Scale score. Crit Care Med. 2000;28(1):120–4.
139. Hakim MA, Katirji MB. Femoral mononeuropathy induced by the lithotomy position: a report of 5 cases with a review of literature. Muscle Nerve. 1993;16(9):891–5.
140. Massey EW, Stolp KA. Peripheral neuropathy in pregnancy. Phys Med Rehabil Clin N Am. 2008;19(1):149–62.

141. Stolp-Smith KA, Pascoe MK, Ogburn PL Jr. Carpal tunnel syndrome in pregnancy: frequency, severity, and prognosis. Arch Phys Med Rehabil. 1998;79(10):1285–7.

142. Shmorgun D, Chan WS, Ray J. Association between Bell's palsy in pregnancy and pre-eclampsia. QJM. 2002;95(6):359–62.

143. Falco NA, Eriksson E. Idiopathic facial palsy in pregnancy and the puerperium. Surg Gynecol Obstet. 1989;169(4):337–40.

144. Giridhar P, Freedman K. Nonarteritic anterior ischemic optic neuropathy in a 35-year-old post-partum woman with recent preeclampsia. JAMA Ophthalmol. 2013;131(4):542–4.

145. Bonebrake RG, et al. Severe preeclampsia pre-senting as third nerve palsy. Am J Perinatol. 2004;21(3):153–5.

146. Thurtell MJ, et al. Isolated sixth cranial nerve palsy in preeclampsia. J Neuroophthalmol. 2006;26(4):296–8.

147. Barry-Kinsella C, et al. Sixth nerve palsy: an unusual manifestation of preeclampsia. Obstet Gynecol. 1994;83(5 Pt 2):849–51.

148. Femia G, Parratt JD, Halmagyi GM. Isolated reversible hypoglossal nerve palsy as the initial manifestation of pre-eclampsia. J Clin Neurosci. 2012;19(4):602–3.

149. Facco FL, et al. Preeclampsia and sleep-disordered breathing: a case-control study. Pregnancy Hypertens. 2013;3(2):133–9.

150. Yinon D, et al. Pre-eclampsia is associated with sleep-disordered breathing and endothelial dysfunc-tion. Eur Respir J. 2006;27(2):328–33.

151. Edwards N, et al. Pre-eclampsia is associated with marked alterations in sleep architecture. Sleep. 2000;23(5):619–25.

152. Basso O, et al. Trends in fetal and infant survival following preeclampsia. JAMA. 2006;296(11):1357–62.

153. Yoon BH, Lee CM, Kim SW. An abnormal umbilical artery waveform: a strong and indepen-dent predictor of adverse perinatal outcome in patients with preeclampsia. Am J Obstet Gynecol. 1994;171(3):713–21.

154. Buchbinder A, et al. Adverse perinatal outcomes are significantly higher in severe gestational hyper-tension than in mild preeclampsia. Am J Obstet Gynecol. 2002;186(1):66–71.

155. Stubert J, et al. Clinical differences between early- and late-onset severe preeclampsia and analysis of predictors for perinatal outcome. J Perinat Med. 2014;42(5):617–27.

156. Seidman DS, et al. Pre-eclampsia and offspring's blood pressure, cognitive ability and physical devel-opment at 17-years-of-age. Br J Obstet Gynaecol. 1991;98(10):1009–14.

157. Tenhola S, et al. Maternal preeclampsia predicts elevated blood pressure in 12-year-old children: evaluation by ambulatory blood pressure monitor-ing. Pediatr Res. 2006;59(2):320–4.

158. Vatten LJ, et al. Intrauterine exposure to preeclamp-sia and adolescent blood pressure, body size, and age at menarche in female offspring. Obstet Gynecol. 2003;101(3):529–33.

159. Kajantie E, et al. Pre-eclampsia is associated with increased risk of stroke in the adult off-spring: the Helsinki birth cohort study. Stroke. 2009;40(4):1176–80.

160. Davis EF, et al. Pre-eclampsia and offspring cardio-vascular health: mechanistic insights from experi-mental studies. Clin Sci (Lond). 2012;123(2):53–72.

161. Jayet PY, et al. Pulmonary and systemic vascular dysfunction in young offspring of mothers with pre-eclampsia. Circulation. 2010;122(5):488–94.

162. Pinheiro TV, et al. Hypertensive disorders dur-ing pregnancy and health outcomes in the off-spring: a systematic review. J Dev Orig Health Dis. 2016;7(4):391–407.

163. Tuovinen S, et al. Maternal hypertensive pregnancy disorders and cognitive functioning of the off-spring: a systematic review. J Am Soc Hypertens. 2014;8(11):832–47.e1.

164. Sun BZ, et al. Association of Preeclampsia in term births with neurodevelopmental disorders in off-spring. JAMA Psychiatry. 2020;77:823.

165. Wu CS, et al. Preeclampsia and risk for epilepsy in offspring. Pediatrics. 2008;122(5):1072–8.

166. Mann JR, McDermott S. Maternal pre-eclampsia is associated with childhood epilepsy in South Carolina children insured by Medicaid. Epilepsy Behav. 2011;20(3):506–11.

167. Brown MC, et al. Cardiovascular disease risk in women with pre-eclampsia: systematic review and meta-analysis. Eur J Epidemiol. 2013;28(1):1–19.

168. Miller EC, et al. Aspirin reduces long-term stroke risk in women with prior hypertensive disorders of pregnancy. Neurology. 2019;92(4):e305–16.

169. Brussé I, et al. Impaired maternal cognitive func-tioning after pregnancies complicated by severe pre-eclampsia: a pilot case-control study. Acta Obstet Gynecol Scand. 2008;87(4):408–12.

170. Postma IR, et al. Neurocognitive functioning follow-ing preeclampsia and eclampsia: a long-term follow-up study. Am J Obstet Gynecol. 2014;211(1):37. e1–9.

171. Fields JA, et al. Preeclampsia and cognitive impairment later in life. Am J Obstet Gynecol. 2017;217(1):74.e1–74.e11.

Reversible Vasoconstrictive Syndrome in Pregnancy

Walter Wallace Valesky, Susan W. Law, and Daniel Rosenbaum

Introduction

Historically, reversible cerebral vasoconstriction syndrome (RCVS) has had multiple terminologies and has generally been considered to be a benign condition. In recent years, focus on this condition has brought increased attention to an association with intracranial hemorrhages. This has led to a need to address, evaluate, and diagnose this condition earlier in its course. RCVS comprises a collection of symptoms including headaches and the requirement of radiographic features that show segmental, multi-focal vasoconstriction of the cerebral arteries. Additionally, these cerebrovascular imaging findings have to resolve within 12 weeks of presentation to satisfy the diagnostic criteria [1].

Known clinical presentations include thunderclap headaches, nausea, focal neurological changes, seizures, and migrainous features associated with headache. Therefore, the use of a diagnostic cerebral angiogram such as computed tomography angiography (CTA), magnetic resonance angiography (MRA), or catheter angiography is necessary to confirm the diagnosis of RCVS. There is a multitude of potential etiologies/triggers as well as multiple prior names for this syndrome including migrainous vasospasm, migrainous angiitis [2, 3], benign angiopathy of the central nervous system [4, 5], CNS pseudovasculitis [6], Call–Fleming syndrome [7], postpartum angiopathy [8], and drug-induced cerebral arteritis [9, 10]. The focus of this chapter will be on RCVS in pregnancy. Postpartum angiopathy, generally considered a subtype of RCVS, will be discussed in detail in Chap. 29.

Epidemiology

The incidence of RCVS remains unclear. Part of this lack of clarity stems from the difficulty of obtaining a prompt and accurate diagnosis. RCVS tends to affect patients who are between the ages of 20–50 years with an 80–90% predilection for females [11–17]. One study suggests that RCVS in men tend to affect those who are younger than their female counterparts by at least a decade in age [11]. It is unclear if race plays a role in RCVS, with varying reports in the few studies for which race is reported. However, it does appear that black patients are underreported in these studies [13, 17–19].

W. W. Valesky (✉) · D. Rosenbaum
Department of Neurology, Downstate Health Sciences University, Brooklyn, NY, USA
e-mail: walter.valesky@downstate.edu;
daniel.rosenbaum@downstate.edu

S. W. Law
Department of Neurology, Downstate Health Sciences University, Brooklyn, NY, USA

Department of Neurology, Kings County Hospital Center, Brooklyn, NY, USA

G. Gupta et al. (eds.), *Neurological Disorders in Pregnancy*,
https://doi.org/10.1007/978-3-031-36490-7_13

The incidence of RCVS during and following pregnancy is not known, this is in part due to the poor clarity in its nomenclature. Whereas pregnancy related RCVS has only been described in a handful of case reports [19–24], postpartum angiopathy or postpartum RCVS appears to be a much more commonly reported entity [19, 25–27] accounting for 9% of all patients with RCVS [11, 17]. It is seen in association with eclampsia and posterior reversible encephalopathy syndrome (PRES).

Pathophysiology

It is currently believed that RCVS arises from transient dysregulation of cerebral vascular tone. Whether this dysregulation is the end result of separate unrelated events culminating in a common, predictable presentation, or the result of one or more unknown isolated factors is yet to be determined. But at this time both a genetic predisposition and precipitant factors (triggers) have been hypothesized to play a role in the pathophysiology of RCVS (Fig. 13.1).

A genetic predisposition toward vascular tone dysregulation is supported by Chen et al. in their studies on brain-derived neurotropic factor (BDNF) in RCVS. This group demonstrated increased "vasoconstriction scores" in patients with RCVS who had the nucleotide polymorphism valine/methionine (val/met) genotype as opposed to those possessing the val/val or met/met genotype in codon 66 of the BDNF gene. Although the RCVS patients did not differ at baseline in their genotypes from controls without RCVS, the increased severity of RCVS in those patients point toward a genetic predisposition [28].

Multiple precipitants have been postulated to pose a role in the development of RCVS. Sympathomimetic overactivity is supported by several authors demonstrating an association with vasoconstrictive substances, serotonergic substances, pheochromocytoma, and other exposures leading to a sympathomimetic surge in patients diagnosed with RCVS [10, 11, 15–17].

Endothelial dysfunction has also been suggested as an etiology of RCVS. This is considered due to the vascular endothelial role in autoregulation. To maintain this role the endothelium must regulate vasoconstriction (thromboxane-A2 and endothelin) and vasodilation (endothelium-derived relaxing factor and nitric oxide) via various cell messengers. It is believed that injury to the endothelial lining creates an imbalance in these factors leading to dysregulation. This theory gains further support due to the overlapping features and association of RCVS with PRES, eclampsia, and migraine [29].

Oxidative stress and hormonal factors have also been proposed as etiologies of RCVS. 8-isoprostaglandin F2-alpha, which is a marker of oxidative stress and a vasoconstrictor, was shown to corelate with disease severity in patients with RCVS [30]. The association of RCVS in the postpartum period suggests a relationship with pre-eclampsia/eclampsia and therefore hormonal involvement. Hypertension is a component of both diseases, and levels of placental growth factors, sFlt-1 and TGF-beta1, known to be elevated in eclampsia, have been demonstrated in patients with RCVS in the postpartum period [31, 32].

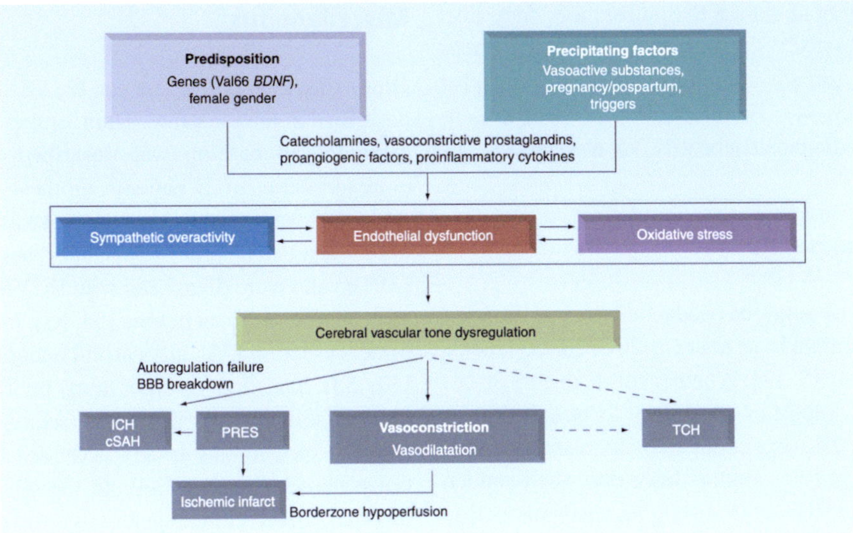

Fig. 13.1 Proposed pathophysiology of RCVS. *cSAH* cortical subarachnoid hemorrhage, *ICH* intracerebral hemorrhage, *PRES* posterior reversible encephalopathy syndrome, *TCH* thunderclap headache. (From Chen S-P, Fuh J-L, Wang S-J. Reversible cerebral vasoconstriction syndrome: current and future perspectives. *Expert Rev Neurother*. 2011;11(9):1265–1276)

Risk Factors and Precipitants

Vasoactive and Serotonergic Substances

Altered cerebrovascular tone is considered to be one of the most predominantly reported etiologies [11, 17, 31, 33–36]. This dysregulation may be idiopathic or be due to a known vasoactive or serotonergic substance. In one French study of 67 patients with RCVS, it was determined that 60% of the patients had used various vasoactive substances prior to the onset of symptoms [11]. In the aforementioned French study, cannabis, selective-serotonin reuptake inhibitors (SSRIs), nasal decongestants, and cocaine accounted for the predominance of vasoactive substance exposure in patients with RCVS. However, this distribution is not uniform with cannabis and cocaine affecting men to a greater degree, and women showing more exposure to SSRIs and decongestants in those with RCVS. Other common serotonergic substances have been reported as triggering agents for RCVS, these include methylergometrine [37], sumatriptans [38, 39], dihydroergotamines [40], and serotonin–norepinephrine reuptake inhibitors [41]. There are reports of RCVS being associated with serotonin syndrome but causality has not been established at this time [42]. Cigarette smoking (with nicotine as a vasoactive substance) also appears to be a well-investigated risk factor for RCVS but its exact role is unclear. Multiple studies categorize as many as 20–60% of patients as current smokers [11, 12, 16].

Endogenous vasoactive substances may also precipitate RCVS. Consistent with this, pheochromocytoma is commonly cited as a cause for RCVS [43, 44]. Therefore, it is prudent to consider this diagnosis when RCVS is suspected.

Migraine Headache

A history of migraine headache has been reported in the literature in as many as 20–40% of patients [11, 12, 14, 15, 17]. Whether this is due to shared pathophysiology or secondary to treatments for migraine (i.e., ergotamine/triptan medications) is not known. Prior authors have described sudden onset headaches with reversible vasoconstriction in patients with a history of migraines as "migraine angiitis" or "arterial stenosis in migraine" [2, 3]. It is likely that these case series described what would be now known as RCVS.

Endothelial dysfunction may be a common link between migraine and RCVS. Circulating endothelial progenitor cells, which function in maintenance and regeneration of the endothelial wall, are decreased in those with migraines and with RCVS [45–47]. Furthermore, eclampsia and migraines may show shared pathophysiology in the form of circulating by-products of endothelial breakdown [48–50]. Approximately 10% or more of patients with RCVS are in the post-partum state [11, 12, 17].

Cervical Artery Dissection

Mawet et al. reported on a series of patients with concomitant RCVS and cervical artery dissection [51]. Vertebral artery dissections accounted for 83% of those affected which contrasts with the normal carotid artery predominance of spontaneous cervical artery dissections. The authors point out that it is unclear which disorder preceded the other; that is, whether RCVS created upstream pressure inducing cervical artery dissection or the dissection released vasoactive substances triggering vasoconstriction. Regardless, cervical artery dissection should be included in the differential when evaluating these patients.

Miscellaneous

Other risk factors/triggers for RCVS have been described in the literature. Thunderclap headache attributed to bathing was described by Wang et al. in a series of 21 patients. Of these, 62% had multiple, segmental arterial vasoconstriction noted on magnetic resonance angiography (MRA) and were diagnosed with RCVS [52, 53]. Other causes such as trauma [54, 55], intracranial tumor resection [56], and carotid endarterectomy [57, 58] have led to what may be RCVS. In another series it was noted that seemingly mild triggers such as day-to-day activities and emotions were believed to initiate the onset of this disorder. Defecation, anger, cough, sexual activities, singing, loud speaking, sniffing, and yoga were all thought to trigger thunderclap headache with MRA confirmed vasoconstriction consistent with RCVS [59] and in one series, sexual intercourse was the precipitant in 24% of cases [60].

Pregnancy-Related Risk Factors

In the postpartum period RCVS typically presents within the first 2 weeks after delivery [11, 18, 19, 31]. It is this correlation with the postpartum state for which it is postulated that both pro-angiogenic and antiangiogenic factors may have some contribution to the development of RCVS. Some investigators have evaluated the effect of eclampsia on cerebral arterial blood flow and demonstrated that both small vessel vasoconstriction [61] and medium to large caliber vessel vasospasm [62] may be a consequence of eclampsia. Multiple authors have proposed a similar pathophysiology between postpartum angiopathy and eclampsia due to their overlapping clinical, laboratory, and radiological features [63–65].

Although the pathophysiology of RCVS remains unknown, the high prevalence of postpartum patients supports a theory of hormonal involvement. In one cohort of pregnant and postpartum women diagnosed with ischemic stroke, transient ischemic attack, cerebral venous thrombosis, or non-aneurysmal subarachnoid hemorrhage (SAH), 73% occurred in the postpartum period. Of these postpartum events, RCVS accounted for over one-third [19]. The same investigators also evaluated hemorrhagic stroke in females of childbearing age. In postpartum patients with hemorrhagic stroke, 83% were due to RCVS [18]. However, in comparison to the total number of postpartum patients, the prevalence of RCVS is extremely low and may be underdiagnosed. To illustrate, one Italian hospital reported only one case of "mild" RCVS after 900 uncomplicated deliveries for a rate of 0.11% [66]. Therefore, in approaching the evaluation of the postpartum patient with either ischemic stroke or intracranial hemorrhage, an evaluation for RCVS must be considered by the treating clinician to prevent it from being missed.

Sympathomimetic and serotonergic medications are also commonly administered in the postpartum period. Many case reports and case series of postpartum patients fail to document the absence or presence of vasoactive medications in patients with RCVS, even though these are known precipitants [20, 46, 63, 65–67]. In these reports, it is the postpartum state that is believed to be the cause of RCVS. In other case reports, where a vasoactive substance is clearly noted (e.g., bromocriptine, methylergometrine, methylergonovine), it is reported that the vasoactive substance was the trigger [9, 68]. This observation only highlights our current limited understanding of the mechanisms involved and the need for more research.

Clinical Features

Thunderclap headache is the hallmark symptom of RCVS. The headache is described as reaching maximal severity within 1 min, mimicking that of a ruptured intracranial aneurysm, and with a duration of 3–5 h. It is usually bilateral with posterior onset, occurring with associated symptoms such as nausea (47–57%), vomiting (29–40%), photophobia (24–34%), vertigo (11%), and pho-

nophobia. As stated previously, various triggers may elicit the thunderclap headache associated with RCVS, but this is not always the case as one in five will have the onset of headache at rest with no obvious precipitant [11]. In contrast with the headache of SAH, 78–100% of patients with RCVS will have recurrent thunderclap headaches, usually lasting over a period of 1–3 weeks [11, 17, 59, 60, 68].

Although the absence of headache has been noted in the literature [20], it would be a rare presentation of RCVS. In patients with history of migraine or other chronic headache, the thunderclap headaches associated with RCVS were noted to be different in character from the individual's prior headaches [11]. Additionally, all patients presenting with associated neck pain should warrant an evaluation for cervical artery dissection as there appears to be an association between these two diagnoses [51].

Focal neurologic deficits are also seen as a presenting sign of RCVS in up to 48% of patients reported [11, 14, 17, 60]. In one series of 67 patients presenting from a headache clinic, nearly a quarter had focal neurologic deficits at presentation. Of these new deficits, over half were transient, abating within 4 h. Visual symptoms seem to be most frequently seen, followed by unilateral sensory symptoms, aphasia, and hemiparesis; the majority of these deficits mimicked a transient ischemic attack with others mimicking a migraine [11]. Deficits that persist, such as hemiplegia, aphasia, hemianopia, and cortical blindness suggest a stroke and should be evaluated appropriately [34]. Seizures at onset occur in 1–17% [11, 14, 17].

While only 7–24% of patients have a history of chronic hypertension prior to the presentation of RCVS [11, 14], as many as 55% of patients have hypertension when presenting for evaluation of headache [16]. Chen et al. noted a mean presenting systolic blood pressure of 156 ± 30 mmHg [14]. Whether this elevation is due to a blood pressure surge as part of the headache itself, because of the pain, or an associated disorder has yet to be determined [34] (Fig. 13.2).

	Chen et al[7] (n=77)	Ducros et al[8] (n=89)	Singhal et al[9] (n=139)
Recruitment	Prospective, from a headache clinic	Prospective, from a single institution with an emergency headache centre and a stroke unit	Retrospective, from an internal medicine department and a stroke unit
Duration	2002–09	2004–08	1993–2009
Mean age (range)	47·7 years (10–76)	43·2 years (19–70)	42·5 years (13–69)
Sex distribution (men:women)	1:8·6	1:2·2	1:4·3
History of migraine	17%	27%	..*
History of hypertension	25%	11%	..
Any precipitant for syndrome	8%	62%	..
Post partum†	1%	13%	11%
Vasoactive substances	3%	52%	42%
Headaches at onset	100%	100%	95%
Recurrent thunderclap	100%	91%	78%
Any trigger for headaches	80%	75%	..
Focal neurological deficit	8%	25%	43%
Seizures	1%	4%	17%
Blood pressure surge	46%	34%	Some‡
Initial CT or MRI normal	..	80%	55%
Any abnormal CT or MRI	12%	37%	81%
Subarachnoid haemorrhage	0%∫	30%	34%
Intracerebral haemorrhage	0%∫	12%	20%
Cerebral infarction	8%	6%	39%
Posterior reversible encephalopathy syndrome	9%	8%	38%
CSF analysis available	18%	88%	82%
Protein concentration >60 mg/dL	0%	12%	16%
5–10 white blood cells per µL	..	17%	12%
>10 white blood cells per µL	0%	8%	3%
Death	0%	0%	2%
Persistent focal neurological deficit from stroke at follow-up	3%	6%	20%

*40% of patients had a history of headaches. †Percentages refer to female patients only. ‡No specific data were reported. ∫Haemorrhage was an exclusion criterion in this series.

Table: Large case series of reversible cerebral vasoconstriction syndrome

Fig. 13.2 Comparison of three large cohorts of RCVS. (From Ducros A. Reversible cerebral vasoconstriction syndrome. *Lancet Neurol.* 2012;11(10):906–917)

Laboratory Investigations

Generally, serum laboratory tests are noncontributory in RCVS. If inflammatory markers such as C-reactive protein and erythrocyte sedimentation rate are tested, these markers may show mild elevation [7, 69] but whether this indicates an inflammatory state from RCVS or is related to any causative state or agent preceding the symptoms of RCVS is unknown. In cases of confirmed RCVS that have undergone leptomeningeal or cerebral arterial wall biopsy, none have demonstrated inflammation on pathology sectioning [2, 4, 5, 7, 17, 32].

Common tests for cerebral angiitis such as rheumatoid factor, antinuclear antibodies, antineutrophil cytoplasmic antibodies, and tests for lyme disease are usually negative in patients with RCVS. If pheochromocytoma is the suspected precipitant, evaluation in the form of plasma or urine adrenaline, noradrenaline, metanephrine, or normetanephrine should be considered [43, 44]. Urine toxicology screens should be obtained as substances such as marijuana, amphetamines, and cocaine may trigger RCVS [34].

Cerebrospinal fluid (CSF) is commonly obtained in the evaluation of a patient presenting with a thunderclap headache. Prior to definitive diagnosis of RCVS, it is recommended that lumbar puncture (LP) be performed to exclude subarachnoid hemorrhage [70]. In patients with RCVS the CSF has been reported to be mildly abnormal in more than half of those undergoing LP. One series showed up to 97% of patients will have a CSF white blood cell count (WBC) of less than 10 WBC/μL [17, 71] with another showing a mean of 12 WBC/μL [11]. CSF protein may be normal to slightly elevated [11, 17], and CSF red blood cell count (RBC) showed a mean of 1560 RBC/μl in one series [11]. Ducros et al. recommends repeating the lumbar puncture after a few weeks to exclude chronic meningitis if the lymphocyte reaction is greater than 10 WBC/μL [34, 71]. It has also been proposed that the clinician may forgo the LP depending on the presentation. Chen et al. state that in the scenario of a patient presenting after multiple thunderclap headaches, with no neck stiffness, and with a magnetic resonance angiography (MRA) consistent with RCVS, the clinician may consider deferring the LP due to poor diagnostic yield [15]. However, this approach should be considered only when the pretest probability of CSF infection or aneurysmal subarachnoid hemorrhage is so low that the LP confers a greater chance of demonstrating a false negative result than a true positive.

Radiographic Studies and Diagnoses

While the classic findings of RCVS show segmental narrowing and dilatation commonly referred to as a "string of beads" or "beading" pattern on angiography [33], conventional angiography or MRA may initially appear normal despite diffuse vasoconstriction on subsequent imaging. Of initial computed tomography (CT) scans, nearly 90% showed no abnormalities [11]. When evaluating both magnetic resonance imaging (MRI) and CT of the brain collectively, the initial scans still showed no abnormalities in up to 55% of patients [17]. When cerebrovascular disease is seen on MRI, it is usually in the form of subarachnoid hemorrhage, intracerebral or intraparenchymal hemorrhage (ICH), cerebral infarction or reversible brain edema.

Subarachnoid Hemorrhage

RCVS-related SAH is the most commonly reported RCVS-related hemorrhage and must be distinguished from aneurysmal SAH. SAH has been observed in 22–34% of patients later diagnosed with RCVS [11, 17]. RCVS-related SAH has a particular proclivity for the puerperium. In another series of women age 18–45 with hemorrhagic stroke ($n = 130$), over 50% of those who were pregnant or postpartum (10 out of 19) were diagnosed with RCVS [18].

Radiographically, RCVS-related SAH is often small and localized to the convexity, being either unilateral or bilateral and confined to superficial cerebral sulci. It may be seen as a hyperintense signal on fluid-attenuated inversion recovery (FLAIR) MRI and as hypointense signal on T2-weighted MRI [31, 34]. Typically, RCVS-related SAH is seen early in the course of disease, within the first week [12] (Fig. 13.3).

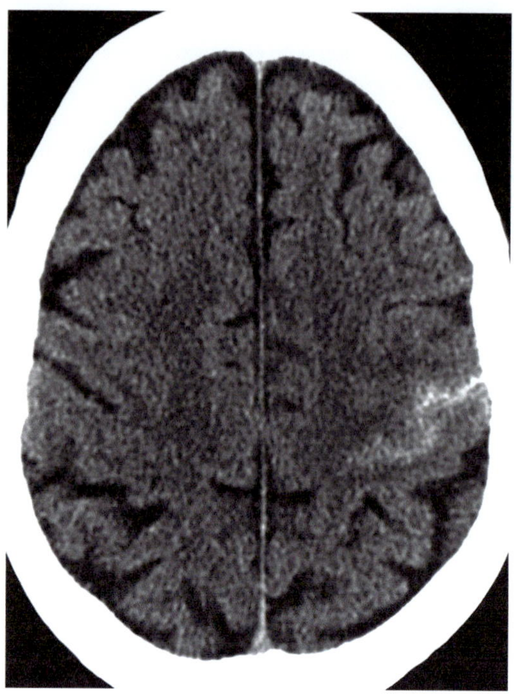

Fig. 13.3 Convexity subarachnoid hemorrhage. (From Chandra RV, Leslie-Mazwi TM, Oh D, Mehta B, Yoo AJ. Extracranial internal carotid artery stenosis as a cause of cortical subarachnoid hemorrhage. *AJNR Am J Neuroradiol*. 2011;32(3):E51–52)

Muehlschlegel et al. evaluated 38 patients with SAH related to RCVS in a retrospective analysis. They were predominantly women and substantially younger by over a decade than those with SAH not related to RCVS. Additionally, those with RCVS were noted to have medical histories consistent with chronic headache, depression or anxiety, and illicit drug or alcohol use. These patients also presented with less severe Hunt and Hess grades at presentation than did those with SAH not related to RCVS. Finally, as in prior series, all patients had subarachnoid blood located in the hemispheric convexities as opposed to blood in the sylvian fissure or basal cisterns as is commonly seen with aneurysmal SAH [72].

Intracerebral Hemorrhage

The subtleties of diagnosing SAH are usually not a factor with ICH as these disorders are usually visualized on non-contrast head CT and MRI with ease. Like RCVS-related SAH they develop early in the course of RCVS, typically diagnosed within the first week. They are typically lobar rather than deep (involving the basal ganglia) and are more likely to be isolated rather than involving multiple areas. They are seen in 12–28% of all patients presenting with RCVS [12, 16, 18].

Ischemic Stroke

Cerebral infarction is seen later in the disease process than RCVS-related SAH or ICH. Stroke usually presents in the second week, is bilateral and symmetric, with a pattern of watershed infarction. These watershed infarcts are most commonly noted between the middle cerebral artery and the posterior cerebral artery circulation and seem to spare the circulation of the anterior cerebral artery [14]. One large retrospective series demonstrated infarction in 39% of patients presenting with RCVS [17].

Cerebral infarction may be considered the most feared complications of RCVS as it leads to an increased probability of poor outcome after resolution of this syndrome with a significant odds ratio of 11 (95% CI 2.53–47.91) [16]. This is in contrast to most patients, who generally recover well after RCVS with modified Rankin score (mRs) of 0–1 reported in 78% at 2–4 months after discharge [17]. In a prior series, the duration of focal neurological deficits lasting greater than 24 h identified those patients with either ischemic stroke or intracerebral hemorrhage [11].

In pregnant patients with ischemic stroke, nearly three-quarters of patients presented in the postpartum period. And the most common mechanism of stroke in these women was RCVS, presenting in more than one-third of cases. Additionally, both preeclampsia and migraines were found to be associated with pregnancy associated stroke [19].

Cerebral Edema

Reversible cerebral edema similar to that seen in PRES can be seen in 9–38% of patients. On MRI this will be seen as a hyperintense signal on T2 FLAIR imaging most commonly in the occipital lobes and posterior parietal lobes but may also include the frontal and temporal lobes. As 85% or more of patients with PRES have been noted to have a multifocal reversible vasoconstriction and up to 35% of RCVS patients have reversible cerebral edema, a common pathogenesis has been alluded to such as altered cerebral vascular tone and endothelial dysfunction [34, 73, 74].

Angiography

Conventional catheter-based angiography is the gold standard for diagnosis of RCVS [33], but this method of evaluation is invasive and not conducive to repeated follow-up examinations. In one series it was noted that 9% of patients had a transient new neurological deficit or thunderclap headache within 1 h of completion of four-vessel angiography [11]. However, in this same series MRA missed multifocal arterial constriction in over 10% of cases that were seen on conventional angiography. Other authors report benefits of utilizing conventional angiography in cases of suspected RCVS presenting with atypical presentation (e.g., insidious headache) or a likely alternative diagnosis [73]. Additionally, these authors recommend the approach that one may preemptively attempt to make the diagnosis of RCVS utilizing the reversibility of vasoconstriction after intra-arterial vasodilator administration [75–79].

In contrast to this approach, Chen et al. have reported the utility of MRA in assessment of RCVS as a non-inferior tool in comparison to conventional angiography [14, 15]. If the decision is made to rely entirely on noninvasive testing in diagnosing RCVS, the clinician should have high suspicion for RCVS and low suspicion for alternative diagnoses with imaging showing no signs of cortical SAH or ischemic stroke [71]. However, it is likely that the decision to utilize conventional angiography in the diagnosis of RCVS will be determined on an individual basis.

On both MRA and conventional angiography the characteristic finding is that of segmental narrowing and dilation (a "string of beads" or "sausage on a string" pattern) of one or more of the cerebral arteries [7, 11, 17, 26, 33, 80] (Figs. 13.4, 13.5, and

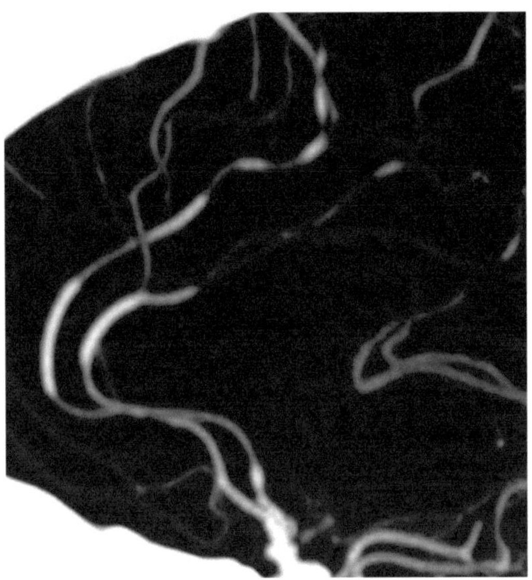

Fig. 13.4 Sagittal head CTA showing 'sausage on a string' pattern of RCVS. (From Singhal AB, Hajj-Ali RA, Topcuoglu MA, et al. Reversible cerebral vasoconstriction syndromes: analysis of 139 cases. *Arch Neurol.* 2011;68(8):1005–1012)

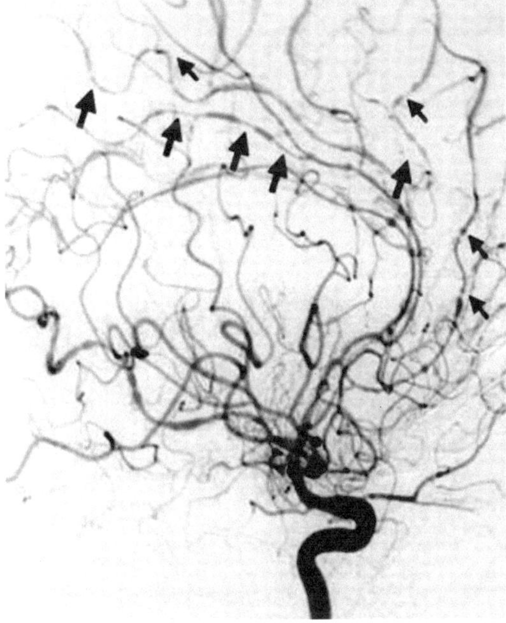

Fig. 13.5 Conventional angiography showing 'beading'. (From Hajj-Ali RA, Calabrese L. Primary angiitis of the Central Nervous System. Cleveland Clinic Center for Continuing Education. Epub July 2015. http://www.clevelandclinicmeded.com/medicalpubs/diseasemanagement/rheumatology/angiitis-of-central-nervous-system/)

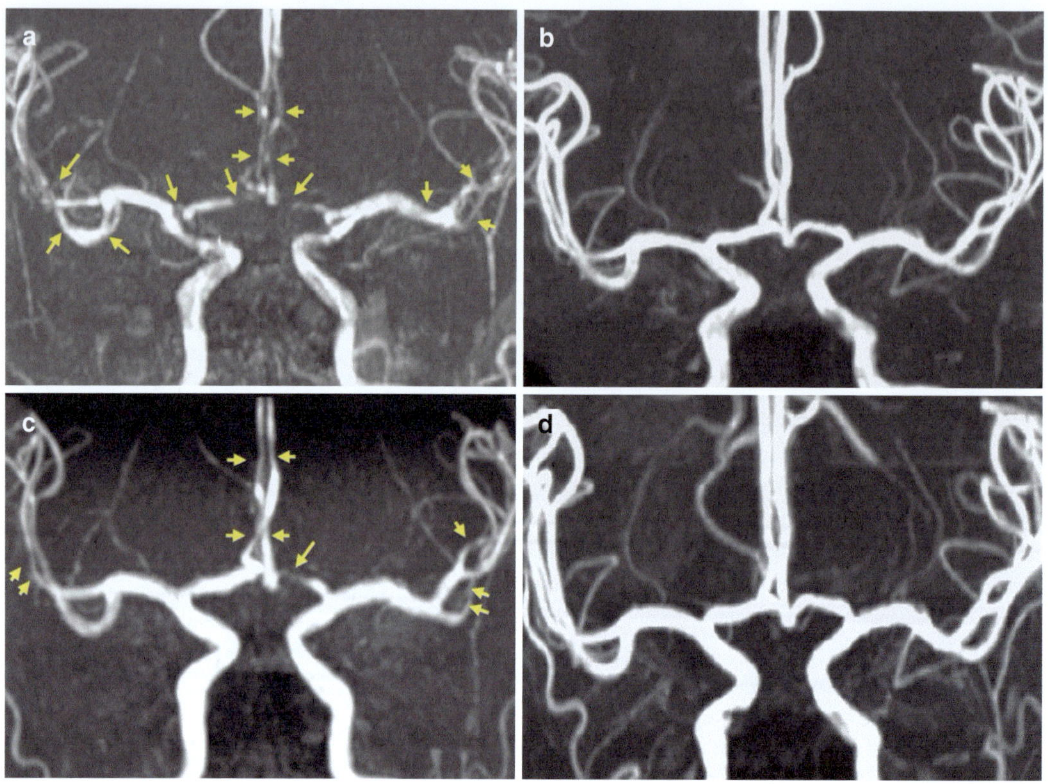

Fig. 13.6 MRA showing reversibility of vasoconstriction. (**a**) First episode of RCVS with resolution of vasoconstriction (**b**). (**c**) Recurrence of vasoconstriction on same patient followed by resolution of vasoconstriction of 13.6). second occurrence (**d**). (From Chen S-P, Fuh J-L, Lirng J-F, Wang Y-F, Wang S-J. Recurrence of reversible cerebral vasoconstriction syndrome: a long-term follow-up study. *Neurology*. 2015;84(15):1552–1558)

13.6). It is important to note that this pattern of cerebral vasoconstriction may not be noted for a week after onset of symptoms, with day 16 showing the highest number of arterial segments involved according to a Taiwanese sample of 77 patients [14]. Therefore, frequently a pattern of obtaining a repeat MRA after several days to 1 week becomes necessary if cerebral vasoconstriction is not noted and RCVS is suspected [31, 34, 36, 71, 81].

RCVS is a disease affecting the large- and medium-caliber cerebral arteries of the anterior and posterior circulation [33, 34]. It commonly involves the intracerebral arteries but has been rarely shown to involve the external carotid vessels [82]. It has been suggested that the poor association between clinical findings and radiographic evidence of vasoconstriction may be due to the involvement of small distal vessels, later demonstrating "beading" in the larger vessels [11, 34]. As these vessels are of insufficient caliber to be visualized on conventional angiography or MRA, it has been postulated that segmental vasodilation of these small, radiographically invisible vessels may be the pathophysiology of thunderclap headaches in an "initial stage" of RCVS.

Small vessel rupture causing hemorrhage may account for the RCVS-related SAH and ICH in these patients accounting for their appearance in only the first few days. Following this, a "second stage" comprising vasoconstriction of major cerebral arteries may be visualized utilizing current non-invasive radiographic imaging or conventional angiography. It would be this period of diffuse vasoconstriction accounting for not only the radiographic features, but also ischemic infarcts in the second week [12].

Transcranial Doppler

Recent strategies have implemented the usage of transcranial doppler (TCD) in the evaluation of vasospasm in patients with RCVS [83–85]. Chen et al. showed a significant difference in flow velocities of the middle cerebral artery (MCA) in patients with RCVS compared to age-matched controls. Additionally, the authors demonstrated that MCA velocities of >120 cm/s combined with a Lindegaard index >3 (ratio of the velocity of the MCA and the ipsilateral extracranial internal carotid artery), identified RCVS patients at risk of ischemic stroke and PRES [14, 83]. Other authors have attempted to utilize TCD to evaluate efficacy of treatments directed at alleviating vasospasm in the symptomatic patient. Furthermore, these same authors used TCD to evaluate treatment failures among multiple pharmacologic therapeutics directed towards symptoms and vasospasm [85].

Treatment

To our knowledge, there have been no randomized control trials evaluating treatment strategies for RCVS. The management is currently guided by observational studies and expert opinion. Importantly, inclusion of RCVS in the differential diagnosis in the patient presenting with symptoms of thunderclap headache is the first step in treatment as it is still not widely known among non-neurologists. As such, thunderclap headaches with no alternative etiology and meeting the clinical characteristics of RCVS but failing to show the radiographic features should be considered for treatment in the same manner of those showing cerebral vasoconstriction.

As most cases of RCVS are secondary to a precipitant etiology [4, 11, 17, 34, 86], it is important that a thorough history as to the etiology of RCVS is undertaken to prevent worsening severity and prolongation of symptoms. This includes removal of all vasoactive medications (i.e., decongestants, bromocriptine/ methylergometrine during pregnancy), serotonergic medications (i.e., antimigraine agents such as sumatriptan, SNRI antidepressants), or recreational drugs such as marijuana or cocaine. Additionally, an evaluation for intrinsic disease such as pheochromocytoma or cervical artery dissection should be considered depending on relevant symptoms and treatment initiated if deemed to be the causative agent. In consideration that many cases of RCVS may be exacerbated by valsalva or sexual activity [60], rest, and avoidance of sexual intercourse may be considered for a period of time deemed relevant by the clinician. Accordingly, one author also utilizes benzodiazepines to alleviate anxiety and blunt any sympathetic response that could worsen RCVS [34].

Additionally, patients who suffer from ischemic stroke, ICH, or RCVS-related SAH should be managed according to specific guidelines where applicable [70, 87, 88]. Specifically, this should apply to blood pressure management in patients with sequela of RCVS where guidelines recommend reduction of systolic blood pressure in patients with SAH to below 160 mmHg and have not found harm with lowering blood pressure to 140 mmHg with ICH. Hypotension and hypovolemia should be treated in the same manner as acute ischemic stroke to maintain perfusion and avoid organ dysfunction. This view is reflected in that of expert opinion by multiple authors as areas of vasoconstriction may reduce perfusion leading to acute ischemic stroke and its avoidance may prevent sequela of worsened ischemia and edema [14, 33–35, 89]. Antiepileptic drugs should be initiated for seizures but should be discontinued if no further seizures persist [31, 34, 35].

Calcium channel blockers, such as nimodipine, verapamil, and nicardipine, have emerged as a treatment option in RCVS based on anecdote and expert opinion. Of these options nimodipine is frequently selected due to its ability to cross the blood–brain barrier, selective affinity for cerebral arteries, and inhibitory neurohormonal effects on serotonin, catecholamine, and histamine [90]. Typical dosing consists of 30–60 mg oral nimodipine every 4 h. In the setting of worsening vasoconstriction, worsening symptoms, PRES or ischemic stroke, other authors have initiated intravenous nimodipine 0.5–2 mg/h utilizing a central venous catheter with frequent blood pressure monitoring every 2–4 h [5, 15, 23, 52, 65, 74, 91–94]. Several authors cited improvement in symptoms after initiation of nimodipine including cessation of headache or improvement in vasoconstriction in as many as 84% of patients [52, 59]. Furthermore, Cho et al. reported improvement in time to resolution of symptoms with earlier initiation of nimodipine in an observational study comprised of 82 patients. Other authors have administered intraarterial nimodipine as both a treatment option and a diagnostic test [63, 65, 79, 90, 95]. Marsh et al. described a novel approach in utilizing TCD velocities to assess treatment effect and reported improvement in seven patients with verapamil after other calcium channel blockers had failed [85].

Other treatments have been utilized for RCVS. Although previous authors have shown utilization of glucocorticoids as treatment for vasoconstrictive disease [4], it is currently thought that administration of glucocorticoids is associated with worse outcomes [17, 89, 96]. Intravenous magnesium has been used as an adjuvant medication with calcium channel blockers in cases of refractory symptoms [59, 85–97]. Epoprostenol in a dose of 1 ng/kg/min via a central venous catheter has also been used in refractory cases of progressive of RCVS [98]. Finally, in cases of progressive cerebral edema and potential herniation at least one case of decompressive craniectomy in RCVS has been reported in the literature secondary to ICH [40]. This may be considered in patients with clinical deterioration in addition to osmotic therapy such as mannitol and hypertonic saline as per guidelines [99] (Fig. 13.7).

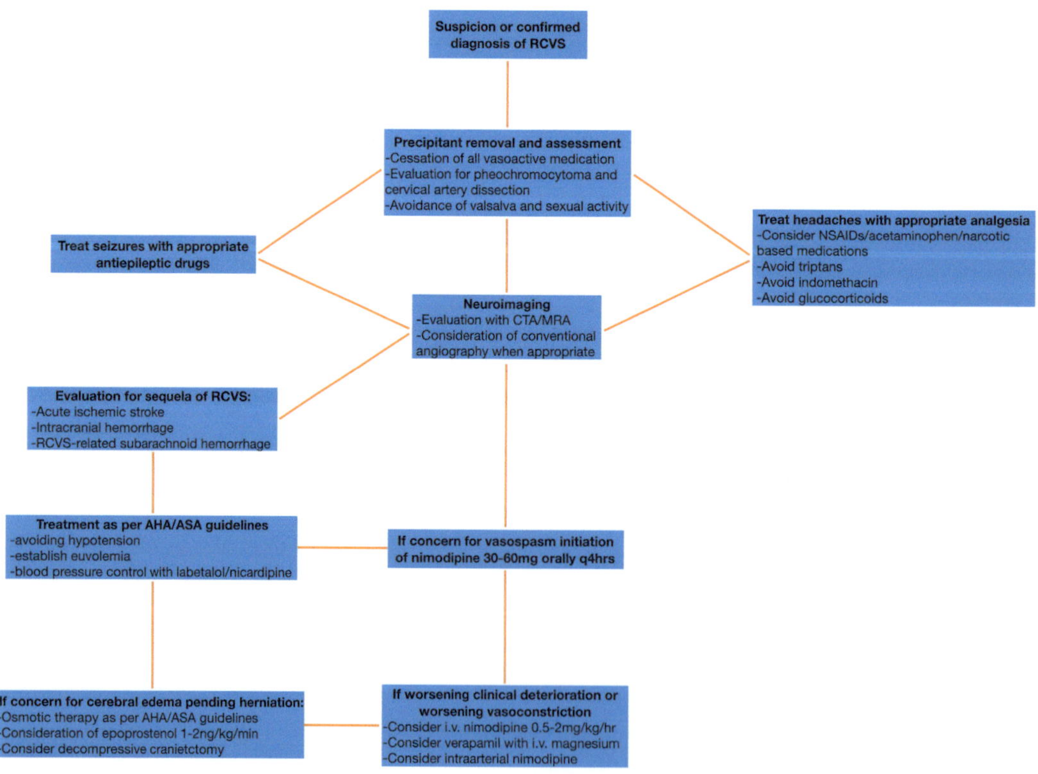

Fig. 13.7 RCVS treatment flow chart

Prognosis/Sequela

Mortality is low in patients with RCVS with rates of 1–5% cited [89] with deaths typically as a result of cerebral edema following progressive vasoconstriction [17, 25]. As the mortality rates are low it is currently unknown as to what risk factors are associated with fatal outcomes. Clinical worsening of RCVS has been evaluated in multiple studies. Katz et al. reported clinical worsening (defined by new focal neurological deficits or new onset of seizures) in one-third of their sample. Of those that worsened, 55% suffered temporary deficits that resolved within hours to days and 40% suffered permanent deficits. In their cohort, the only clinical characteristic/risk factor or radiographic finding associated with clinical worsening was ischemic stroke [16]. Following this, Singhal and Topcuoglu evaluated predictors of clinical and radiographic worsening in patients with RCVS. The predictors with the highest correlation (defined by p values) were focal neurological deficits, cerebral infarcts on baseline or final imaging, glucocorticoid usage, and treatment with intraarterial vasodilators [96]. Of note, postpartum state or pregnancy was not associated with clinical worsening.

Long-term outcomes of RCVS were reported by John et al. in a follow-up study of 45 patients (91% women) over a median of 78 months. This group noted that most headaches resolved at 3 weeks, but 53% of patients had continued headache at follow up throughout the study period. In most of these patients (43%) the impact of these headaches on daily life was minimal, but 14% described their headaches as having both a severe impact on life and being disabling. Not surprisingly, in over half of patients with persistent headaches a history of migraines was reported, and the authors postulated that one reason for this could be the subsequent elimination of antimigraine vasoconstrictive medication such as triptans after resolution of RCVS. This is an area requiring more investigation to understand the long-term consequences of RCVS [13].

The concept of recurrent RCVS is challenging the notion that this is a monophasic disease. Chen et al. reported 5% of previously diagnosed patients with RCVS returning with a diagnosis of recurrent RCVS. These patients were typically women (89%) of middle age (median age of 50 years old) and occurred at median of 35 months. The headaches associated with recurrent RCVS were similar to those from the initial diagnosis of RCVS being bilateral, severe, and sudden onset and it was found in their cohort that sexual activity as a trigger for first bout of RCVS was a predictor for recurrent RCVS [100]. While postpartum patients were not shown to be at risk for recurrence, there has been a report of recurrence of RCVS after subsequent pregnancies in a 39-year-old female [101].

Conclusions

RCVS should be considered in the evaluation of any pregnant patient with a thunderclap headache. It is a significant cause of ischemic stroke and intracranial hemorrhage in the postpartum period and should be considered in any of these conditions in the pregnant patient. There are many risk factors for RCVS such as vasoactive medications, migraine headaches, and pre-eclampsia. While RCVS is uncommon in overall pregnancies, occurring in 0.1%, approximately 10% of cases of RCVS occur in the postpartum period.

Any patient presenting with RCVS should undergo imaging with MRI/MRA of the brain including conventional angiogram in most cases. If initial imaging is not consistent with RCVS it is recommended to repeat imaging in several days to 1 week as findings on imaging can be delayed as much as 2 weeks from initial symptoms. While there are no proven therapies, treatment typically consists of a calcium channel blocker to prevent vasoconstriction. Glucocorticoids should be avoided as no inflammatory component has been identified and are risk factors for worsening. Complications such as ischemic stroke, intracranial hemorrhage, and cerebral edema should be managed as per guidelines.

Most patients have a very good prognosis but as many as 1–5% will have a fatal outcome.

Ischemic stroke is a risk factor for long-term sequela due to persistent neurologic deficits. If headaches persist beyond the acute course of RCVS, their effect on daily activities is usually minimal. Recurrent RCVS is a developing concept that has been noted in as many as 5% of patients but as the pathophysiology of RCVS is still unclear so are the risk factors for recurrence.

References

1. Headache Classification Committee of the International Headache Society (IHS) The International Classification of Headache Disorders, 3rd edition. Cephalalgia. 2018;38(1):1–211.
2. Jackson M, Lennox G, Jaspan T, Jefferson D. Migraine angiitis precipitated by sex headache and leading to watershed infarction. Cephalalgia. 1993;13(6):427–30.
3. Solomon S, Lipton RB, Harris PY. Arterial stenosis in migraine: spasm or arteriopathy? Headache. 1990;30(2):52–61.
4. Hajj-Ali RA, Furlan A, Abou-Chebel A, Calabrese LH. Benign angiopathy of the central nervous system: cohort of 16 patients with clinical course and long-term follow up. Arthritis Rheum. 2002;47(6):662–9.
5. Moskowitz SI, Calabrese LH, Weil RJ. Benign angiopathy of the central nervous system presenting with intracerebral hemorrhage. Surg Neurol. 2007;67(5):522–7; discussion 527–8.
6. Razavi M, Bendixen B, Maley JE, et al. CNS pseudovasculitis in a patient with pheochromocytoma. Neurology. 1999;52(5):1088–90.
7. Call GK, Fleming MC, Sealfon S, Levine H, Kistler JP, Fisher CM. Reversible cerebral segmental vasoconstriction. Stroke. 1988;19(9):1159–70.
8. Bogousslavsky J, Despland PA, Regli F, Dubuis PY. Postpartum cerebral angiopathy: reversible vasoconstriction assessed by transcranial Doppler ultrasounds. Eur Neurol. 1989;29(2):102–5.
9. Henry PY, Larre P, Aupy M, Lafforgue JL, Orgogozo JM. Reversible cerebral arteriopathy associated with the administration of ergot derivatives. Cephalalgia. 1984;4(3):171–8.
10. Raroque HG, Tesfa G, Purdy P. Postpartum cerebral angiopathy. Is there a role for sympathomimetic drugs? Stroke. 1993;24(12):2108–10.
11. Ducros A, Boukobza M, Porcher R, Sarov M, Valade D, Bousser M-G. The clinical and radiological spectrum of reversible cerebral vasoconstriction syndrome. A prospective series of 67 patients. Brain. 2007;130(Pt 12):3091–101.
12. Ducros A, Fiedler U, Porcher R, Boukobza M, Stapf C, Bousser M-G. Hemorrhagic manifestations of reversible cerebral vasoconstriction syndrome: frequency, features, and risk factors. Stroke. 2010;41(11):2505–11.
13. John S, Singhal AB, Calabrese L, et al. Long-term outcomes after reversible cerebral vasoconstriction syndrome. Cephalalgia. 2016;36(4):387–94.
14. Chen S-P, Fuh J-L, Wang S-J, et al. Magnetic resonance angiography in reversible cerebral vasoconstriction syndromes. Ann Neurol. 2010;67(5):648–56.
15. Chen S-P, Fuh J-L, Wang S-J. Reversible cerebral vasoconstriction syndrome: an under-recognized clinical emergency. Ther Adv Neurol Disord. 2010;3(3):161–71.
16. Katz BS, Fugate JE, Ameriso SF, et al. Clinical worsening in reversible cerebral vasoconstriction syndrome. JAMA Neurol. 2014;71(1):68–73.
17. Singhal AB, Hajj-Ali RA, Topcuoglu MA, et al. Reversible cerebral vasoconstriction syndromes: analysis of 139 cases. Arch Neurol. 2011;68(8):1005–12.
18. Miller EC, Sundheim KM, Willey JZ, Boehme AK, Agalliu D, Marshall RS. The impact of pregnancy on hemorrhagic stroke in young women. Cerebrovasc Dis. 2018;46(1–2):10–5.
19. Miller EC, Yaghi S, Boehme AK, Willey JZ, Elkind MSV, Marshall RS. Mechanisms and outcomes of stroke during pregnancy and the postpartum period: a cross-sectional study. Neurol Clin Pract. 2016;6(1):29–39.
20. Kasuya C, Suzuki M, Koda Y, et al. A headache-free reversible cerebral vasoconstriction syndrome (RCVS) with symptomatic brain stem ischemia at late pregnancy as a rare manifestation of RCVS resolved with termination of pregnancy by semi-urgent cesarean section. Oxf Med Case Reports. 2018;2018(12):101.
21. Yamauchi Y, Kaname U, Takeda T, et al. Reversible cerebral vasoconstriction syndrome associated with pregnancy. Oral presentation 19-21 May 2016. Torino, Italy. Abstract. Eur J Obstet Gynecol Reprod Biol. 2016;206:e191.
22. Fukuta T. Reversible cerebral vasoconstriction syndrome associated with pregnancy in peripartum period. Pregnancy Hypertens. 2018;13(1):S77.
23. Descamps R, Envain F, Kuchcinski G, Clouqueur E, Henon H, Gonzalez-Estevez M. Cesarean section under general anesthesia for antepartum reversible cerebral vasoconstriction syndrome: a case report. J Obstet Gynaecol Res. 2019;45(12):2461–5.
24. Tanaka K, Matsushima M, Matsuzawa Y, et al. Antepartum reversible cerebral vasoconstriction syndrome with pre-eclampsia and reversible posterior leukoencephalopathy. J Obstet Gynaecol Res. 2015;41(11):1843–7.
25. Fugate JE, Wijdicks EFM, Parisi JE, et al. Fulminant postpartum cerebral vasoconstriction syndrome. Arch Neurol. 2012;69(1):111–7.

26. Singhal AB, Bernstein RA. Postpartum angiopathy and other cerebral vasoconstriction syndromes. Neurocrit Care. 2005;3(1):91–7.
27. Singhal AB. Postpartum angiopathy with reversible posterior leukoencephalopathy. Arch Neurol. 2004;61(3):411–6.
28. Chen S-P, Fuh J-L, Wang S-J, Tsai S-J, Hong C-J, Yang AC. Brain-derived neurotrophic factor gene Val66Met polymorphism modulates reversible cerebral vasoconstriction syndromes. PLoS One. 2011;6(3):e18024.
29. Bartynski WS. Posterior reversible encephalopathy syndrome, part 1: fundamental imaging and clinical features. AJNR Am J Neuroradiol. 2008;29(6):1036–42.
30. Chen S-P, Chung Y-T, Liu T-Y, Wang Y-F, Fuh J-L, Wang S-J. Oxidative stress and increased formation of vasoconstricting F2-isoprostanes in patients with reversible cerebral vasoconstriction syndrome. Free Radic Biol Med. 2013;61:243–8.
31. Miller TR, Shivashankar R, Mossa-Basha M, Gandhi D. Reversible cerebral vasoconstriction syndrome, part 1: epidemiology, pathogenesis, and clinical course. AJNR Am J Neuroradiol. 2015;36(8):1392–9.
32. Stary JM, Wang BH, Moon S-J, Wang H. Dramatic intracerebral hemorrhagic presentations of reversible cerebral vasoconstriction syndrome: three cases and a literature review. Case Rep Neurol Med. 2014;2014:782028.
33. Calabrese LH, Dodick DW, Schwedt TJ, Singhal AB. Narrative review: reversible cerebral vasoconstriction syndromes. Ann Intern Med. 2007;146(1):34–44.
34. Ducros A. Reversible cerebral vasoconstriction syndrome. Lancet Neurol. 2012;11(10):906–17.
35. Calic Z, Cappelen-Smith C, Zagami AS. Reversible cerebral vasoconstriction syndrome. Intern Med J. 2015;45(6):599–608.
36. Sattar A, Manousakis G, Jensen MB. Systematic review of reversible cerebral vasoconstriction syndrome. Expert Rev Cardiovasc Ther. 2010;8(10):1417–21.
37. Ishibashi T, Ishibashi S, Uchida T, Nakazawa K, Makita K. Reversible cerebral vasoconstriction syndrome with limb myoclonus following intravenous administration of methylergometrine. J Anesth. 2011;25(3):405–8.
38. Kato Y, Hayashi T, Mizuno S, et al. Triptan-induced reversible cerebral vasoconstriction syndrome: two case reports with a literature review. Intern Med. 2016;55(23):3525–8.
39. Ba F, Giuliani F, Camicioli R, Saqqur M. A reversible cerebral vasoconstriction syndrome. BMJ Case Rep. 2012;2012:bcr0920114841.
40. Mullaguri N, Battineni A, George P, Newey CR. Decompression hemicraniectomy for refractory intracranial hypertension in reversible cerebral vasoconstriction syndrome. J Neurosci Rural Pract. 2019;10(2):355–9.
41. Davies G, Wilson H, Wilhelm T, Bowler J. The reversible cerebral vasoconstriction syndrome in association with venlafaxine and methenamine. BMJ Case Rep. 2013;2013:bcr2013009701.
42. John S, Donnelly M, Uchino K. Catastrophic reversible cerebral vasoconstriction syndrome associated with serotonin syndrome. Headache. 2013;53(9):1482–7.
43. Armstrong FS, Hayes GJ. Segmental cerebral arterial constriction associated with pheochromocytoma: report of a case with arteriograms. J Neurosurg. 1961;18:843–6.
44. Anderson NE, Chung K, Willoughby E, Croxson MS. Neurological manifestations of phaeochromocytomas and secretory paragangliomas: a reappraisal. J Neurol Neurosurg Psychiatry. 2013;84(4):452–7.
45. Rodríguez-Osorio X, Sobrino T, Brea D, Martínez F, Castillo J, Leira R. Endothelial progenitor cells: a new key for endothelial dysfunction in migraine. Neurology. 2012;79(5):474–9.
46. Lee ST, Chu K, Jung KH, et al. Decreased number and function of endothelial progenitor cells in patients with migraine. Neurology. 2008;70:1510–7.
47. Chen S-P, Wang Y-F, Huang P-H, Chi C-W, Fuh J-L, Wang S-J. Reduced circulating endothelial progenitor cells in reversible cerebral vasoconstriction syndrome. J Headache Pain. 2014;15:82.
48. Liman TG, Bachelier-Walenta K, Neeb L, et al. Circulating endothelial microparticles in female migraineurs with aura. Cephalalgia. 2015;35(2):88–94.
49. Salem M, Kamal S, El Sherbiny W, Abdel Aal AA. Flow cytometric assessment of endothelial and platelet microparticles in preeclampsia and their relation to disease severity and Doppler parameters. Hematology. 2015;20(3):154–9.
50. Mawet J, Debette S, Bousser M-G, Ducros A. The link between migraine, reversible cerebral vasoconstriction syndrome and cervical artery dissection. Headache. 2016;56(4):645–56.
51. Mawet J, Boukobza M, Franc J, et al. Reversible cerebral vasoconstriction syndrome and cervical artery dissection in 20 patients. Neurology. 2013;81(9):821–4.
52. Wang S-J, Fuh J-L, Wu Z-A, Chen S-P, Lirng J-F. Bath-related thunderclap headache: a study of 21 consecutive patients. Cephalalgia. 2008;28(5):524–30.
53. Silva-Néto RP. A review of 50 cases of bath-related headache: clinical features and possible diagnostic criteria. Arq Neuropsiquiatr. 2018;76(5):346–51.
54. Wilkins RH, Odom GL. Intracranial arterial spasm associated with craniocerebral trauma. J Neurosurg. 1970;32:626–33.
55. Suwanwela C, Suwanwela N. Intracranial arterial narrowing and spasm in acute head injury. J Neurosurg. 1972;36:314–23.
56. Hyde-Rowan MD, Roessmann U, Brodkey JS. Vasospasm following transsphenoidal tumor

removal associated with the arterial changes of oral contraception. Surg Neurol. 1983;20:120–4.

57. Lopez-Valdes E, Chang HM, Pessin MS, Caplan LR. Cerebral vasoconstriction after carotid surgery. Neurology. 1997;49:303–4.

58. Schaafsma A, Veen L, Vos JP. Three cases of hyperperfusion syndrome identified by daily transcranial Doppler investigation after carotid surgery. Eur J Vasc Endovasc Surg. 2002;23:17–22.

59. Chen S-P, Fuh J-L, Lirng J-F, Chang F-C, Wang S-J. Recurrent primary thunderclap headache and benign CNS angiopathy: spectra of the same disorder? Neurology. 2006;67(12):2164–9.

60. Valença MM, Andrade-Valença LPA, Bordini CA, Speciali JG. Thunderclap headache attributed to reversible cerebral vasoconstriction: view and review. J Headache Pain. 2008;9(5):277–88.

61. Hansen WF, Burnham SJ, Svendsen TO, et al. Transcranial Doppler findings of cerebral vasospasm in pre-eclampsia. J Matern Fetal Med. 1996;5:194–200.

62. Trommer BL, Homer D, Mikhael MA. Cerebral vasospasm and eclampsia. Stroke. 1988;19(3):326–9.

63. Fletcher JJ, Kramer AH, Bleck TP, Solenski NJ. Overlapping features of eclampsia and postpartum angiopathy. Neurocrit Care. 2009;11(2):199–209.

64. Donaldson JO. Eclampsia and postpartum cerebral angiopathy. J Neurol Sci. 2000;178(1):1.

65. Singhal AB, Kimberly WT, Schaefer PW, Hedley-Whyte ET. Case records of the Massachusetts General Hospital. Case 8-2009. A 36-year-old woman with headache, hypertension, and seizure 2 weeks postpartum. N Engl J Med. 2009;360(11):1126–37.

66. Anzola GP, Brighenti R, Cobelli M, et al. Reversible cerebral vasoconstriction syndrome in puerperium: a prospective study. J Neurol Sci. 2017;375:130–6.

67. Albano B, Del Sette M, Roccatagliata L, Gandolfo C, Primavera A. Cortical subarachnoid hemorrhage associated with reversible cerebral vasoconstriction syndrome after elective triplet cesarean delivery. Neurol Sci. 2011;32(3):497–501.

68. Kulig K, Moore LL, Kirk M, Smith D, Stallworth J, Rumack B. Bromocriptine-associated headache: possible life-threatening sympathomimetic interaction. Obstet Gynecol. 1991;78:941–3.

69. Singhal AB, Caviness VS, Begleiter AF, Mark EJ, Rordorf G, Koroshetz WJ. Cerebral vasoconstriction and stroke after use of serotonergic drugs. Neurology. 2002;58(1):130–3.

70. Connolly ES, Rabinstein AA, Carhuapoma JR, et al. Guidelines for the management of aneurysmal subarachnoid hemorrhage: a guideline for healthcare professionals from the American Heart Association/American Stroke Association. Stroke. 2012;43(6):1711–37.

71. Ducros A, Bousser MG. Reversible cerebral vasoconstriction syndrome. Pract Neurol. 2009;9:256–67.

72. Muehlschlegel S, Kursun O, Topcuoglu MA, Fok J, Singhal AB. Differentiating reversible cerebral vasoconstriction syndrome with subarachnoid hemorrhage from other causes of subarachnoid hemorrhage. JAMA Neurol. 2013;70(10):1254–60.

73. Miller TR, Shivashankar R, Mossa-Basha M, Gandhi D. Reversible cerebral vasoconstriction syndrome, part 2: diagnostic work-up, imaging evaluation, and differential diagnosis. AJNR Am J Neuroradiol. 2015;36(9):1580–8.

74. Pop A, Carbonnel M, Wang A, Josserand J, Auliac SC, Ayoubi J-M. Posterior reversible encephalopathy syndrome associated with reversible cerebral vasoconstriction syndrome in a patient presenting with postpartum eclampsia: a case report. J Gynecol Obstet Hum Reprod. 2019;48(6):431–4.

75. Ioannidis I, Nasis N, Agianniotaki A, Katsouda E, Andreou A. Reversible cerebral vasoconstriction syndrome: treatment with multiple sessions of intra-arterial nimodipine and angioplasty. Interv Neuroradiol. 2012;18(3):297–302.

76. French KF, Hoesch RE, Allred J, et al. Repetitive use of intra-arterial verapamil in the treatment of reversible cerebral vasoconstriction syndrome. J Clin Neurosci. 2012;19(1):174–6.

77. Farid H, Tatum JK, Wong C, et al. Reversible cerebral vasoconstriction syndrome syndrome; treatment with combined intra-arterial verapamil infusion and intracranial angioplasty. AJNR Am J Neuroradiol. 2011;32(10):E184–7.

78. Elstner M, Linn J, Müller-Schunk S, Straube A. Reversible cerebral vasoconstriction syndrome: a complicated clinical course treated with intra-arterial application of nimodipine. Cephalalgia. 2009;29(6):677–82.

79. Linn J, Fesl G, Ottomeyer C, et al. Intra-arterial application of nimodipine in reversible cerebral vasoconstriction syndrome: a diagnostic tool in select cases? Cephalalgia. 2011;31(10):1074–81.

80. Skliut M, Jamieson DG. Imaging of headache in pregnancy. Curr Pain Headache Rep. 2016;20(10):56.

81. Ghia D, Cuganesan R, Cappelen-Smith C. Delayed angiographic changes in postpartum cerebral angiopathy. J Clin Neurosci. 2011;18(3):435–6.

82. Melki E, Denier C, Théaudin-Saliou M, Sachet M, Ducreux D, Saliou G. External carotid artery branches involvement in reversible cerebral vasoconstriction syndrome. J Neurol Sci. 2012;313(1–2):46–7.

83. Chen S-P, Fuh J-L, Chang F-C, Lirng J-F, Shia B-C, Wang S-J. Transcranial color doppler study for reversible cerebral vasoconstriction syndromes. Ann Neurol. 2008;63(6):751–7.

84. Levin JH, Benavides J, Caddick C, et al. Transcranial Doppler ultrasonography as a non-invasive tool for diagnosis and monitoring of reversible cerebral vasoconstriction syndrome. R I Med J. 2016;99(9):38–41.

85. Marsh EB, Ziai WC, Llinas RH. The need for a rational approach to vasoconstrictive syndromes: tran-

scranial Doppler and calcium channel blockade in reversible cerebral vasoconstriction syndrome. Case Rep Neurol. 2016;8(2):161–71.

86. Topcuoglu MA, Singhal AB. Hemorrhagic reversible cerebral vasoconstriction syndrome: features and mechanisms. Stroke. 2016;47(7):1742–7.

87. Hemphill JC, Greenberg SM, Anderson CS, et al. Guidelines for the management of spontaneous intracerebral hemorrhage: a guideline for healthcare professionals from the American Heart Association/American Stroke Association. Stroke. 2015;46(7):2032–60.

88. Powers WJ, Rabinstein AA, Ackerson T, et al. Guidelines for the early management of patients with acute ischemic stroke: 2019 update to the 2018 guidelines for the early management of acute ischemic stroke: a guideline for healthcare professionals from the American Heart Association/American Stroke Association. Stroke. 2019;50(12):e344–418.

89. Valencia-Mendoza M, Ramírez-Rodríguez N, Vargas-Avila N, et al. Fatal reversible cerebral vasoconstriction syndrome: a systematic review of case series and case reports. J Clin Neurosci. 2019;70:183–8.

90. Cho S, Lee MJ, Chung C-S. Effect of nimodipine treatment on the clinical course of reversible cerebral vasoconstriction syndrome. Front Neurol. 2019;10:644.

91. Slivka A, Philbrook B. Clinical and angiographic features of thunderclap headache. Headache. 1995;35(1):1–6.

92. Cheng Y-C, Kuo K-H, Lai T-H. A common cause of sudden and thunderclap headaches: reversible cerebral vasoconstriction syndrome. J Headache Pain. 2014;15:13.

93. Zuber M, Touzé E, Domigo V, Trystram D, Lamy C, Mas J-L. Reversible cerebral angiopathy: efficacy of nimodipine. J Neurol. 2006;253(12):1585–8.

94. Cossu G, Daniel RT, Hottinger AF, Maduri R, Messerer M. Malignant PRES and RCVS after brain surgery in the early postpartum period. Clin Neurol Neurosurg. 2019;185:105489.

95. Klein M, Fesl G, Pfister H-W, et al. Intra-arterial nimodipine in progressive postpartum cerebral angiopathy. Cephalalgia. 2009;29(2):279–82.

96. Singhal AB, Topcuoglu MA. Glucocorticoid-associated worsening in reversible cerebral vasoconstriction syndrome. Neurology. 2017;88(3):228–36.

97. Mijalski C, Dakay K, Miller-Patterson C, Saad A, Silver B, Khan M. Magnesium for treatment of reversible cerebral vasoconstriction syndrome: case series. Neurohospitalist. 2016;6(3):111–3.

98. Thydén AL, Muhamad AA, Jacobsen A, Kondziella D. Intravenous epoprostenol for treatment-refractory reversible cerebral vasoconstriction syndrome (RCVS). J Neurol Sci. 2016;364:56–8.

99. Wijdicks EFM, Sheth KN, Carter BS, et al. Recommendations for the management of cerebral and cerebellar infarction with swelling: a statement for healthcare professionals from the American Heart Association/American Stroke Association. Stroke. 2014;45(4):1222–38.

100. Chen S-P, Fuh J-L, Lirng J-F, Wang Y-F, Wang S-J. Recurrence of reversible cerebral vasoconstriction syndrome: a long-term follow-up study. Neurology. 2015;84(15):1552–8.

101. Ursell MR, Marras CL, Farb R, Rowed DW, Black SE, Perry JR. Recurrent intracranial hemorrhage due to postpartum cerebral angiopathy: implications for management. Stroke. 1998;29(9):1995–8.

Post-Partum Cerebral Angiopathy

14

Pouya Entezami, Nicholas C. Field,
and Emad Nourollah-Zadeh

Introduction

Post-partum cerebral angiography (PPA) is a combined clinical and radiographic diagnosis that affects women within the first 6 weeks of the postpartum period. It is classically described as recurrent, sudden-onset thunderclap headaches, which are severe in nature along with radiographic evidence of segmental vasoconstriction in at least two different intracranial arteries, typically resolving within 3 months from onset. Aside from headaches, PPA can result in a wide range of focal neurological deficits.

Angiopathy of this nature, during the postpartum period, is generally accepted to be a subset of Reversible Cerebral Vasoconstriction Syndrome (RCVS), which is discussed more generally in Chap. 23. Since the 1980s, multiple papers have described various types of cerebral vasoconstriction syndromes, which were named based on association with triggers or associated conditions. These include disorders such as migraine angiitis, drug-induced angiitis, and post-partum angiopathy, representing vasocon-striction in the setting of migraine, drugs, and pregnancy, respectively.

In 1988, a series of 19 cases (including two postpartum patients) was published by Call and Fleming, outlining the clinical and radiographic appearances of cerebral vasoconstriction syndromes [1]. Call-Fleming syndrome has also been used to refer to RCVS in the literature and there are various subtypes (Table 14.1). Although multiple terminologies and associated subtypes exist [1–11], the term RCVS is used in general to simplify the clinical evaluation and research endeavors for this disorder [12–14]. Patients have similar presentations and clinical courses, regardless of the associated subtype. For this chapter, the terms RCVS and PPA are used interchangeably, though we will highlight some of the points more specific for the postpartum period.

Table 14.1 List of other terms used to describe Reversible Cerebral Vasoconstriction Syndrome, including variants

Acute benign angiopathy of the central nervous system
Call-Fleming syndrome
Central nervous system pseudovasculitis
Drug-induced cerebral arteritis
Isolated benign cerebral vasculitis
Migraine angiitis
Migranous vasospasm
Primary thunderclap headache
Post-partum cerebral angiopathy
Thunderclap headache-associated vasospasm

P. Entezami · N. C. Field
Department of Neurosurgery, Albany Medical Center,
Albany, NY, USA

E. Nourollah-Zadeh (✉)
Department of Neurology, Robert Wood Johnson
University Hospital, New Brunswick, NJ, USA
e-mail: en231@rwjms.rutgers.edu

© The Author(s), under exclusive license to Springer Nature Switzerland AG 2023
G. Gupta et al. (eds.), *Neurological Disorders in Pregnancy*,
https://doi.org/10.1007/978-3-031-36490-7_14

Currently, RCVS disorders represent the clinical manifestations associated with multifocal narrowing of the cerebral arteries. While the clinical course may include severe headaches and focal neurological deficits, the ultimate clinical outcome is generally benign. However, some patients may suffer permanent strokes, resulting in severe disability or even death.

PPA is usually associated with high blood pressure (similar to pre-eclampsia/eclampisa), however, it can also develop in the absence of hypertension. About 8–39% of these patients also have posterior reversible encephalopathy syndrome (PRES) [15].

Pathophysiology

The pathophysiology of these disorders remains uncertain, but several hypotheses have been proposed. RCVS may occur due to spontaneous or provoked dysregulation of the cerebral vascular tone via serotonergic pathways and sympathetic overactivity [16]. There is a strong association between RCVS, pre-eclampsia/eclampsia, and PRES. [17, 18] This frequent correlation highlights the potential for shared pathophysiology, namely that endothelial dysfunction is part of the process in both disorders.

Hypoperfusion in this patient cohort is caused by cerebral vasoconstriction, which is secondary to endothelial dysfunction, which can occasionally cause ischemic stroke (typically in watershed areas). Furthermore, vasogenic edema and breakdown of the blood–brain barrier can also occur accounting for the additional symptoms in patients with RCVS. This irritation of the leptomeninges stimulates the trigeminal nerve (cranial nerve V) afferents, resulting in severe headaches. Reperfusion injuries affecting smaller arteries may explain the finding of subarachnoid hemorrhage (SAH) in many patients with RCVS.

Pregnancy, in particular, causes several physiologic and hormonal changes that predispose patients to RCVS. These physiologic adaptations allow for maternal circulation to meet the increased metabolic demand during normal pregnancy [19, 20]. These compensatory mechanisms include increased plasma volume, hemodilutional anemia, decreased systemic peripheral vascular resistance, and increased heart rate and cardiac output (up to 45% increase by the second trimester and peak during labor and birth).

Furthermore, pregnancy hormones have been reported to promote changes in cerebral vasculature. Although large cerebral arteries remain structurally unaffected, the parenchymal arterioles undergo outward hypotrophic remodeling during pregnancy [21]. In other words, the arterioles develop a larger inner lumen and thinner outer wall. Moreover, cerebral capillary density increases during the pregnancy. In addition to structural remodeling, the blood–brain barrier (BBB) becomes more permeable via production of VEGF, matrix metalloproteinases, etc.

However, these normal compensatory changes during pregnancy can also be risk factors for cerebrovascular complications (such as in PPA) during special settings such as acute hypertension, ingestion of exogenous vasoactive drugs, etc. In other words, adaptations such as increased plasma volume, BBB permeability, inflammation, capillary proliferation, and remodeling of cerebral arterioles in the gestational and postpartum states increase the susceptibility to cerebral dysautoregulation, leading to microhemorrhage, regional vasogenic edema, increased inflammation, vasoconstriction, and subsequently ischemic stroke. Indeed, there has been reports of increased infiltration of inflammatory cells in cerebral arterioles and capillaries, and perivascular spaces in patients with PPA [22, 23].

Additional variations in normal physiology during the post-partum period includes a hypercoagulable state with a 4–10 times increased risk of thrombosis during pregnancy and puerperium compared to general population [24]. During the post-partum period, this can greatly increase the risk of complications secondary to hypoperfusion and changes in arterial circulation, as seen in PPA.

Epidmiology

The exact incidence of PPA and RCVS are unknown as there is a paucity of reports in the literature, partly due to heterogeneity of diagnostic criteria and the most often benign clinical course. In a French study from 2010, the incidence of RCVS was estimated to be about 0.26% of the population with only about 10% of cases occurring during the post-partum period [25]. Rates appear to be similar in other countries as well, including China [26]. While rare, PPA can be an etiology of hemorrhagic or ischemic strokes and neurological impairment in the post-partum period. Even outside the post-partum period, adult RCVS predominantly affects women, with a female-to-male ratio as high as 10:1 in some series.

Since the most severe complication of PPA is stroke, it is helpful to discuss the statistics of strokes in post-partum due to any etiology [27–30]. The rate of strokes overall (hemorrhagic or ischemic) during pregnancy is significantly increased (30 cases per 100,000 people) as compared to the general population of the same age cohort (10 per 100,000). Ischemic strokes in particular are more common than hemorrhagic ones (19.9 and 12.2 per 100,000, respectively). The stroke rate following birth in the post-partum period is roughly 14.7 per 100,000 [27]. The first 6 weeks during this post-partum period confer the highest risk [31].

The most common etiologies associated with hemorrhagic strokes are aneurysms, arteriovenous malformation, HELLP (hemolysis, elevated liver enzymes, low platelet count) syndrome, pre-eclampsia/eclampsia, and coagulopathy. The most common etiologies associated with ischemic strokes are cardioembolic, coagulopathy, and pre-eclampsia/eclampsia [18, 27]. Ischemic and hemorrhagic stroke are discussed in detail in Chaps. 6 and 7.

Clinical Findings

As with any neurological disorder, judicious and comprehensive history taking along with a thorough physical examination can quickly narrow the differential diagnosis when evaluating the post-partum patient with neurological symptoms. Sudden onset, severe headaches—commonly referred to as "thunderclap headaches"—are the most common symptom of PPA. These recurrent headaches occur in 90% of affected patients and can recur for up to 2 weeks [14, 16, 17]. Less than 10% of patients will not display these persistent headaches, but the absence of a presenting headache is exceptionally rare.

The initial headache can be similar in description to that of ruptured cerebral aneurysms, but recurrent thunderclap headaches over several days is pathognomonic for RCVS [32]. Patients frequently suffer from a migraine-like symptoms (e.g., nausea, vomiting, phonophobia, and photophobia). Other symptoms include focal neurological deficits (50%), visual field deficits (44%), encephalopathy (33%), and seizures (28%) [33].

There is a higher incidence in patients who are taking selective serotonin reuptake inhibitor (SSRIs), serotonin–norepinephrine reuptake inhibitors (SNRIs), α-sympathomimetics (e.g., pseudoephedrine and ephedrine), triptans, and Ergot alkaloids (e.g., methergine and bromocriptine). Often times, a trigger can be identified, including physical exertion, stress, straining (including during labor), and exercise, among others.

Laboratory Investigation

Laboratory investigations—including blood counts and erythrocyte sedimentation rates—are often normal in patients with RCVS. Inflammatory markers may be elevated, but this is thought to be secondary to triggers for the disorder and not as a result of RCVS itself [16, 34].

Several diagnostic tests are generally performed during evaluation, in order to rule out other similar disorders or to screen for precipitants of RCVS. Cerebral angiitis and vasculitis are common differential diagnoses, and common markers (such as Rheumatoid factor, antinuclear and antineutrophil cytoplasmic antibodies, and tests for Lyme disease) should be evaluated. Urinary measurement of vanillylmandelic acid and 5-hydroxy indoleacetic acid may also be considered to rule out pheochromocytoma.

Serum and urine toxicology screens (e.g., cocaine, amphetamines, MDMA, LSD, cannabis) should be sent to evaluate the presence of these precipitating drugs.

Cerebrospinal fluid (CSF) evaluation is usually unremarkable, though 20% of patients can have mild protein elevation (60–100 mg/dL) or pleocytosis (white blood cell count >5), most often due to associated ischemic or hemorrhagic strokes. In patients with associated subarachnoid blood, xanthachromia and elevated red blood cell counts are seen. It is recommended that CSF be retested if the white blood cell count exceeds 10 cells/µL or the protein is higher than 80 mg/dL [16].

Radiographic Evaluation

In addition to clinical symptoms, imaging in the forms of cerebral angiography and parenchymal imaging are both indicated.

Cerebral angiography can be achieved with non-invasive means such as computed tomography (CT) or magnetic resonance (MR) angiographic studies, or alternatively through cerebral digital subtraction angiography (DSA). Not only do these studies help confirm the diagnosis of PPA if suspected, they simultaneously rule out aneurysms and other vascular malformations that can share similar presentations if ruptured.

The radiographic finding of segmental vasoconstriction or "beading" is pathognomonic for cerebral vasculitides, and in the correct setting can narrow the diagnosis to RCVS (or PPA in post-partum patients). The diagnosis of PPA requires the presence of beaded vessels in at least two cerebral arteries, though these findings can be bilateral and diffuse (Fig. 14.1). Both the anterior and posterior circulations may be involved. The differential diagnosis for arterial irregularities and stenosis include internal carotid artery disease (ICAD), cerebral vasculitis (inflammatory, infectious, or neoplastic), and fibromuscular dysplasia [35].

Cerebral DSA remains the gold standard for radiographic evaluation, with sensitivity nearing 100% when compared to CT or MR angiography [36]. Furthermore, with DSA it is possible to locally inject vasodilators both as a diagnostic and therapeutic tool [37, 38].

The obvious downside of cerebral DSA is that it is more invasive than non-catheter investigations, though the rate of complication remains low (0.06–0.3%) with diagnostic cerebral DSAs. The most common complications reported are groin hematoma, while more serious complications—namely ischemic strokes and iatrogenic dissections—are possible. The rate of contrast nephropathy seen with cerebral DSAs are similar to that associated with CTA of the head [39].

Although a cerebral DSA is the gold standard modality, CTA continues to be the most commonly obtained study due to easier accessibility in most institutions, as some centers may not have neuro-angiography capabilities. The sensitivity of CTA is about 80% in RCVS-related cerebral vasoconstriction. This is similar to the utility of MRA in this patient population.

One important downside to consider in this patient population with both CT angiography and cerebral DSAs is radiation exposure and the use of iodinated contrast. However, both studies can still be considered during pregnancy, during the post-partum period, or even in patients with renal insufficiency in emergent settings without timely access to MRI or when a higher sensitivity is desired. Collaboration with colleagues in the Obstetrics department will help make appropriate imaging decisions in pregnant patients, and efforts can be made to shield the mother and fetus from radiation in these cases.

Furthermore, MRA of the neck with fat suppression can be considered to screen for cervical artery dissections. Gadolinium contrast is generally not needed during MR studies to evaluate RCVS/PPA. However, contrast should be used if an infectious or inflammatory etiology is in the differential.

Of note, appropriately timed studies (whether CT, MR, or catheter-based) should evaluate the venous structures as well, helping to rule out cerebral venous thrombosis as a cause for the patient's symptoms.

In addition to evaluation of the cerebral vasculature, the brain parenchyma should also be

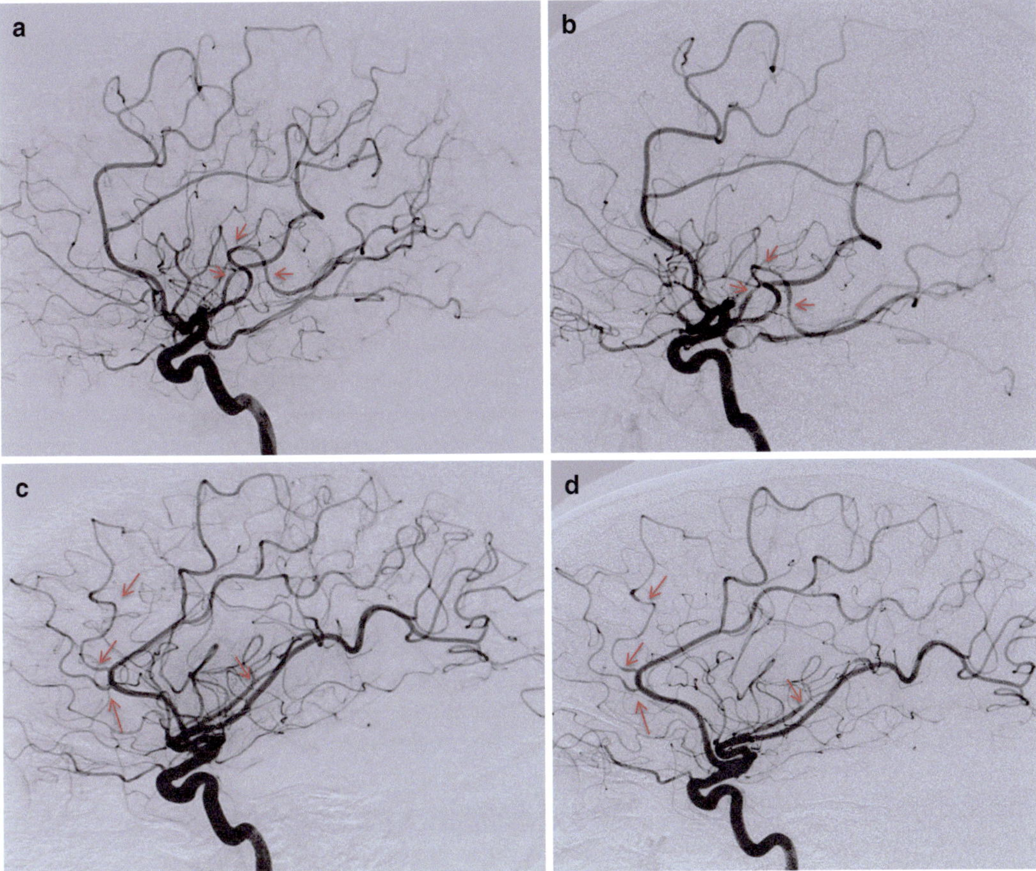

Fig. 14.1 Cerebral angiogram findings in a patient with PPA. (**a, b**) Right ICA injection on day 1 and 7, respectively. Short arrows demonstrate areas where focal, segmental beading developed on day 7 within left MCA territory. (**c, d**) Left ICA injection in the same patient on day 1 and 7, respectively. Short arrows demonstrate areas where focal, segmental beading developed on day 7 within both right MCA and right ACA territories

simultaneously imaged to assess for ischemic stroke (especially with diffusion-weighted MR), intracerebral hemorrhage (ICH), subarachnoid hemorrhage (SAH), and posterior reversible encephalopathy syndrome (PRES). Ischemic strokes often occur in the watershed territories due to aberrant perfusion, while subarachnoid hemorrhages can be seen either cortically (in the convexity sulci) or occasionally surrounding the perimesencephalon in RCVS/PPA patients.

Less common findings such as subdural hematoma (rare) and cerebral edema may be seen. Cerebral edema in the posterior parenchyma (typically occipital lobes) may herald a PRES-like syndrome, which occurs in 8–38% of all RCVS cases.

Transcranial doppler (TCD) has been investigated as an initial diagnostic tool, but its utility is limited due to its lower sensitivity when compared to the more commonly used modalities described. TCDs have a sensitivity of 42% and 67% for ACA and MCA territories, respectively. However, TCD can be a useful modality for serial trending of vasoconstriction.

Diagnostic Clinical Scores

The RCVS$_2$ Score was developed to better diagnose patients with RCVS by providing more clear guidelines (Table 14.2). RCVS$_2$ is useful in post-partum patients as well.

Table 14.2 RCVS$_2$ score

Recurrent or single thunderclap headache	
Present	5
Absent	0
Intracranial carotid artery	
Affected	−2
Not affected	0
Vasoconstrictive trigger	
Present	3
Absent	0
Sex	
Female	1
Male	0
Subarachnoid hemorrhage	
Present	1
Absent	0

A score ≥ 5 has 99% specificity and 90% sensitivity for diagnosing RCVS, while lower scores (≤2) have 100% specificity and 85% sensitivity for excluding RCVS based on the 2019 study by Rocha et al. [32] A flowchart has been made to help in diagnosing these patients (Fig. 14.1).

Other Differential Diagnoses to Consider

Several other presentations may mimic that of PPA. Some additional diagnostic considerations are discussed below.

Aneurysmal SAH is a key differential diagnosis to consider, especially given the shared thunderclap headache symptom seen in PPA. More than 30% of patients with RCVS develop SAH, however, aneurysmal SAH is a much more threatening diagnosis and should not be missed thus underscoring the importance of cerebral vascular imaging. An important radiographic finding that could potentially help differentiate between the two is the SAH pattern; in RCVS it is usually at the cortical convexity compared to the aneurysmal SAH pattern which is typically found in the basal cisterns (Fig. 14.2). Furthermore, compared to aneurysmal SAH, patients with RCVS tend to be younger, have lower Hunt-Hess and Fisher grades, higher number of affected arteries, and the presence of bilateral arterial narrowing [40].

Another diagnosis to consider is primary angiitis of the central nervous system (PACNS); which is an idiopathic multifocal inflammatory disease of the cerebral vasculature, affecting both small and medium-sized blood vessels. The PACNS typically presents with a more insidious headache as opposed to the sudden-onset/severe thunderclap headaches seen in PPA [34, 41]. Lumbar punctures are abnormal in 95% of patients, with moderate pleocytosis, elevated protein levels, and a normal glucose. These findings are similar to aseptic meningitis [42].

In a study comparing PACNS to RCVS, 70% of RCVS patients were found to have an accompanying trigger, including the use of SSRIs, SNRIs, cannabis, nasal decongestants, binge alcohol consumption, ergots, triptans, cocaine, amphetamines, nicotine patches, epinephrine, interferon-α, immunosuppressant drugs (e.g., tacrolimus, cyclosporine, cyclophosphamide), bromocriptine, indomethacin, and sulprostone usage, and notably for this chapter, post-partum state [43]. Furthermore, brain imaging is more commonly abnormal with PACN than RCVS, where imaging is abnormal in only 31% of patients. MRI of brain may show subcortical and deep white matter changes [15].

Cervical or intracranial arterial dissections may also present with headaches and focal neurological deficits and can also occur simultaneously with RCVS. One study found that 12% of patients with RCVS had an associated cervical arterial dissection. They noted that 28% of patients with this combined presentation presented in the post-partum period; thus, in patients with a high index of suspicion, vascular imaging should be extended to the neck [44].

Migraine and migraine variants are a much more common presentation of severe headaches. While some patients may have a history of migraine headaches, the sudden-onset thunderclap headaches of RCVS are usually distinct. Furthermore, RCVS is self-limited and unlikely

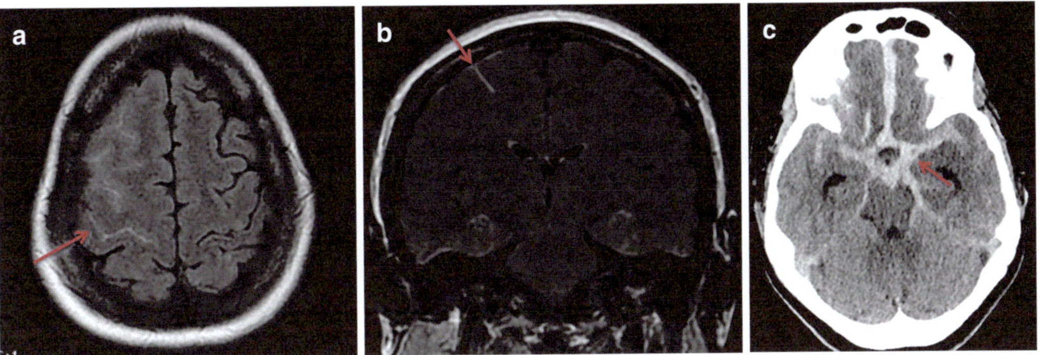

Fig. 14.2 Subarachnoid pattern in post-partum angiopathy. (**a**) Axial MRI head showing classic cortical convexity subarachnoid hemorrhage associated with PPA/RCVS. (**b**) Coronal MRI Brain showing the convexity SAH in same patient. (**c**) Axial CT head showing classic SAH pattern in basal cisterns associated with ruptured cerebral aneurysm

to recur. Incorrect diagnosis can be dangerous, as certain migraine treatments can exacerbate cerebral vasoconstriction [4].

While recurrent thunderclap headaches over several days is pathognomonic for RCVS [34], several other neurological disorders can present with severe headaches, including intracranial infections (e.g., meningitis, abscess), cerebral venous thrombosis, intracranial hypotension, and pituitary apoplexy, among others. The laboratory and imaging recommendations above will help elucidate the correct diagnosis.

Management

Currently, there is no randomized clinical trial for treatment of RCVS or PPA and management is mainly guided by expert opinion. Although the clinical course is usually benign and most patients fully recover, about one-third of patients develop transient symptoms and rarely they can have a progressive, challenging course [45]. Appropriately diagnosing PPA allows initiation of symptomatic management and supportive therapy to prevent potential neurological sequelae (Fig. 14.3).

Once the PPA diagnosis is established, it is important to stop intake of the vasoactive drug/trigger (if any). In patients with mild symptoms and no neurologic deficits, the management is mainly to treat the symptoms (i.e., pain and headache). Although in the majority of patients, clinical and angiographic resolution occur spontaneously without medical intervention, in most centers, patients with PPA are commonly started on calcium channel blockers (CCBs). Depending on symptoms, CCBs are continued for 4–12 weeks. However, this has not been extensively reviewed [46–48]. Nimodipine is the most common agent used over the first few days with dosing similar to that used in setting of aneurysmal subarachnoid hemorrhage (60 mg oral every 4 h). However, the CCB of choice after discharge is typically Verapamil, given the more affordable price and lower dosing frequency (typically 120–240 mg once daily in the sustained release formulation). In two prospective studies, Nimodipine use was associated with headache resolution in 64–83% of RCVS cases, however, it did not reduce the time course of vasoconstriction [49, 50]. Another vasodilator agent used is Magnsium sulfate, however, its utility is unknown and reported in only a few cases [51, 52].

The use of glucocorticoids in PPA is generally not recommended as it can worsen the clinical course in up to 27% of patients according to one study [53]. This underscores the importance of ruling out mimics of PPA, namely PACNS, for which glucocorticoids are the mainstay in treatment.

PPA Diagnosis- Post-partum thunder clap headache and/or neurologic deficits

ABC (Airway, Breathing, Circulation) - *Monitor O2, HR, BP, EKG)*

History (Including vasoactive drug intake)

Labs

> CBC, BMP, LFT, Calcium, Magnesium, Phosphate, Troponin, Toxicology
> *Consider: ESR, CRP and if clinically suspected vasculiteis panel*
> *Consider LP if no obvious SAH or if vasculitis/angitis/infectious etiologies in ddx*

Neurological examination

Imaging:

> MR Brain, MRA head & neck (with fat supression) if readily available
>   * Consider MR brain with contrast if PACNS in ddx
> Or
>
> CT head, CTA head & neck
>
> Other imaging modalities:
> - Cerebral angiography if dx still unclear or need to rule out dAVF, small AVM or aneurysm
> - Serial TCDs to monitor vasoconstriction
> - CT or MR venography if cerebral venous thrombosis is suspected

Fig. 14.3 Flowchart for diagnosis and initial management of post-partum angiopathy. *PACNS* primary angiitis of the central nervous system, *dAVF* dural arteriovenous fistula, *AVM* arteriovenous malformation, *SAH* subarachnoid hemorrhage

The goal of blood pressure management is to maintain appropriate cerebral perfusion pressure, thus it is imperative to avoid hypotension given the cerebral vasoconstriction in patients with PPA. Furthermore, dehydration should be avoided and patients should be volume resuscitated with a target goal of euvolemia (hypervolemia should also be avoided).

Pain and headache treatment is typically managed with a combination of acetaminophen and opioids. Of note, indomethacin and triptans should be avoided, as they are vasoactive drugs and may exacerbate the symptoms. Occasionally intravenous magnesium (2 g over 1–2 h) and oral gabapentin may provide pain relief. Patients with PPA should be instructed to avoid strenuous physical exertion and valsalva maneuver (including constipation) for a few weeks (2–4 weeks). It is also important to address constipation (a form of valsavla maneuver) since many of the patients may also be on opioids. Routine use of antiepileptic drugs (AEDs) for seizure prophylaxis should be avoided, as their use should be limited to seizure treatment. In patients with seizure, duration of AED treatment is usually about 4–12 weeks until cortical irritation is resolved. We recommend outpatient follow up with an epileptologist to determine duration of AED treatment and also to confirm its compatibility with breastfeeding. Furthermore, the use of secondary stroke prevention medications (such as antiplatelets, statins, etc.) is generally not recommended. Lastly, since PPA/RCVS recurrence is low, certain vasoactive drugs such as antidepressants can be re-introduced or started if clinically necessary.

In a subset of PPA patients with severe symptoms and neurologic deficits, it would be prudent to monitor them closely in an intensive care unit (preferably neurocritical care unit), and optimize their volume status (goal of euvolemia) and blood pressure to avoid ischemic or hemorrhagic stroke. The blood pressure should be adjusted on a case-by-case basis to maintain adequate cerebral perfusion pressure (CPP), and at the same time avoid worsening of other possible co-existing conditions such as cerebral edema or hematoma. This will depend on multiple factors including degree of vasoconstriction, neurologic examination, intracerebral hemorrhage volume (if any), severity of cerebral edema/intracranial pressure, and if there are co-existing entities such as posterior reversible encephalopathy syndrome (PRES). In patients with severe vasoconstriction, the blood pressure can be allowed up to 160–180 mmHg in an acute setting. However, as mentioned above, SBP may need to be kept lower depending on other co-existing problems. Serial TCDs may also provide important data regarding severity of vasoconstriction and help to guide medical management (Fig. 14.4).

In medically refractory vasoconstriction, endovascular treatment (either intra-arterial antispasmodic therapy and/or angioplasty) should be a consideration [23, 54–57]. Success with intra-arterial, local infusion of vasodilators such as Verapamil, Milrinone, or Nimodipine may help treat focal deficits. Large intraparenchymal hematomas causing raised intracranial pressure, though exceedingly rare with PPA, may require surgical evacuation [58].

Prognosis

Most patients with PPA do well clinically, with the vast majority (more than 90%) experiencing a full recovery within a few days or weeks. Less than 5% develop life-threatening complications such as strokes, progression of vasospasm, cerebral edema, or severe neurologic disability [59–62]. The fatality rate of RCVS is less than 1% [16, 25, 59, 61, 63, 64].

There is more concern for intractable vasoconstriction in PPA than in RCVS due to the hemodynamic and coagulability changes in post-partum females, but this has not been extensively studied. Maternal age greater than 40 years at delivery is associated with a small increased risk for hemorrhagic stroke in pregnancy and puerperium, furthering the risk in this population [65].

PPA Management

- Stop trigger/vasoactive drugs *(if any)*

- Avoid Hypotension: *BP may need to be augmented if there is severe vasoconstriction*

- Avoid Dehydration *(goal euvolemia)*

-Pain/Headache management:

    * *Acetaminophen and Opioids*
    * *May consider gabapentin and IV Magnesium*

-Vasoconstriction treatment with Calcium channel blockers
    * *Nimodipine usually while inpatient (60 mg PO q4h or 30 mg PO q2h)*
    * *Verapamil as outpatient for 4 -12 weeks (120 to 240 mg PO daily)*

-Severe and medically refractory vasoconstriction
    * *Consider endovascular treatment with intra-arterial infusion of antispasmodics or angiopalsty*

-Avoid glucocorticoids for primary treatment of PPA

-Other possible co-exisisting issues:
    * *Seizure: Limit antiepliepic use to seizure treatment. Seizure prophylaxis not indicated*
    * *PRES (if any) management*
    * *Cerebral edema and Intracerebral hemorrhage management if present.*

Fig. 14.4 Typical management of post-partum angiopathy. *PRES* posterior reversible encephalopathy syndrome

Disclosure The authors report no conflict of interest concerning the materials or methods used in this study or the findings specified in this paper.

References

1. Call GK, Fleming MC, Sealfon S, Levine H, Kistler JP, Fisher CM. Reversible cerebral segmental vasoconstriction. Stroke. 1988;19(9):1159–70.
2. Jackson M, Lennox G, Jaspan T, Jefferson D. Migraine angiitis precipitated by sex headache and leading to watershed infarction. Cephalalgia. 1993;13(6):427–30.
3. Serdaru M, Chiras J, Cujas M, Lhermitte F. Isolated benign cerebral vasculitis or migrainous vasospasm? J Neurol Neurosurg Psychiatry. 1984;47(1):73–6.
4. Singhal AB, Caviness VS, Begleiter AF, Mark EJ, Rordorf G, Koroshetz WJ. Cerebral vasoconstriction and stroke after use of serotonergic drugs. Neurology. 2002;58(1):130–3.
5. Day JW, Raskin NH. Thunderclap headache: symptom of unruptured cerebral aneurysm. Lancet. 1986;2(8518):1247–8.
6. Slivka A, Philbrook B. Clinical and angiographic features of thunderclap headache. Headache. 1995;35(1):1–6.
7. Dodick DW, Brown RD Jr, Britton JW, Huston J III. Nonaneurysmal thunderclap headache with diffuse, multifocal, segmental, and reversible vasospasm. Cephalalgia. 1999;19(2):118–23.
8. Raroque HG Jr, Tesfa G, Purdy P. Postpartum cerebral angiopathy. Is there a role for sympathomimetic drugs? Stroke. 1993;24(12):2108–10.
9. Bogousslavsky J, Despland PA, Regli F, Dubuis PY. Postpartum cerebral angiopathy: reversible vasoconstriction assessed by transcranial Doppler ultrasounds. Eur Neurol. 1989;29(2):102–5.
10. Calabrese LH, Gragg LA, Furlan AJ. Benign angiopathy: a distinct subset of angiographically defined primary angiitis of the central nervous system. J Rheumatol. 1993;20(12):2046–50.
11. Razavi M, Bendixen B, Maley JE, et al. CNS pseudovasculitis in a patient with pheochromocytoma. Neurology. 1999;52(5):1088–90.
12. Singhal AB. Cerebral vasoconstriction syndromes. Top Stroke Rehabil. 2004;11(2):1–6.
13. Calabrese LH, Dodick DW, Schwedt TJ, Singhal AB. Narrative review: reversible cerebral vasoconstriction syndromes. Ann Intern Med. 2007;146(1):34–44.
14. Frontera JA, Ahmed W. Neurocritical care complications of pregnancy and puerperum. J Crit Care. 2014;29(6):1069–81.
15. Fugate JE, Ameriso SF, Ortiz G, et al. Variable presentations of postpartum angiopathy. Stroke. 2012;43(3):670–6.
16. Ducros A. Reversible cerebral vasoconstriction syndrome. Lancet Neurol. 2012;11(10):906–17.
17. Edlow AG, Edlow BL, Edlow JA. Diagnosis of acute neurologic emergencies in pregnant and postpartum women. Emerg Med Clin North Am. 2016;34(4):943–65.
18. Razmara A, Bakhadirov K, Batra A, Feske SK. Cerebrovascular complications of pregnancy and the postpartum period. Curr Cardiol Rep. 2014;16(10):532.
19. Sanghavi M, Rutherford JD. Cardiovascular physiology of pregnancy. Circulation. 2014;130(12):1003–8.
20. Feske SK, Singhal AB. Cerebrovascular disorders complicating pregnancy. Continuum. 2014;20(1 Neurology of Pregnancy):80–99.
21. Cipolla MJ, Sweet JG, Chan SL. Cerebral vascular adaptation to pregnancy and its role in the neurological complications of eclampsia. J Appl Physiol. 2011;110(2):329–39.
22. Calado S, Vale-Santos J, Lima C, Viana-Baptista M. Postpartum cerebral angiopathy: vasospasm, vasculitis or both? Cerebrovasc Dis. 2004;18(4):340–1.
23. Samaniego EA, Dabus G, Generoso GM, Tari-Capone F, Fuentes K, Linfante I. Postpartum cerebral angiopathy treated with intra-arterial nicardipine and intravenous immunoglobulin. J Neurointerv Surg. 2013;5(3):e12.
24. Sanders BD, Davis MG, Holley SL, Phillippi JC. Pregnancy-associated stroke. J Midwifery Womens Health. 2018;63(1):23–32.
25. Ducros A, Fiedler U, Porcher R, Boukobza M, Stapf C, Bousser MG. Hemorrhagic manifestations of reversible cerebral vasoconstriction syndrome: frequency, features, and risk factors. Stroke. 2010;41(11):2505–11.
26. Liu L, Tan Q, Huang R, Hu Z. Analysis of postpartum reversible cerebral vasoconstriction syndrome in China: a case report and literature review. Medicine (Baltimore). 2019;98(45):e17170.
27. Swartz RH, Cayley ML, Foley N, et al. The incidence of pregnancy-related stroke: a systematic review and meta-analysis. Int J Stroke. 2017;12(7):687–97.
28. van Alebeek ME, de Heus R, Tuladhar AM, de Leeuw FE. Pregnancy and ischemic stroke: a practical guide to management. Curr Opin Neurol. 2018;31(1):44–51.
29. Sells CM, Feske SK. Stroke in Pregnancy. Semin Neurol. 2017;37(6):669–78.
30. Camargo EC, Feske SK, Singhal AB. Stroke in pregnancy: an update. Neurol Clin. 2019;37(1):131–48.
31. Kamel H, Navi BB, Sriram N, Hovsepian DA, Devereux RB, Elkind MS. Risk of a thrombotic event after the 6-week postpartum period. N Engl J Med. 2014;370(14):1307–15.
32. Rocha EA, Topcuoglu MA, Silva GS, Singhal AB. RCVS2 score and diagnostic approach for reversible cerebral vasoconstriction syndrome. Neurology. 2019;92(7):e639–47.
33. Martinez-Martinez M, Fuentes B, Diez-Tejedor E. Letter by Martinez-Martinez et al regarding article, "variable presentations of postpartum angiopathy". Stroke. 2012;43(6):e57; author reply e58.

34. Singhal AB, Topcuoglu MA, Fok JW, et al. Reversible cerebral vasoconstriction syndromes and primary angiitis of the central nervous system: clinical, imaging, and angiographic comparison. Ann Neurol. 2016;79(6):882–94.

35. Mukerji SS, Buchbinder BR, Singhal AB. Reversible cerebral vasoconstriction syndrome with reversible renal artery stenosis. Neurology. 2015;85(2):201–2.

36. Marder CP, Donohue MM, Weinstein JR, Fink KR. Multimodal imaging of reversible cerebral vasoconstriction syndrome: a series of 6 cases. AJNR Am J Neuroradiol. 2012;33(7):1403–10.

37. Linn J, Fesl G, Ottomeyer C, et al. Intra-arterial application of nimodipine in reversible cerebral vasoconstriction syndrome: a diagnostic tool in select cases? Cephalalgia. 2011;31(10):1074–81.

38. Bhattacharya K, Pendharkar H. Imaging of neurovascular emergencies in pregnancy and puerperium. Emerg Radiol. 2018;25(4):435–40.

39. Burton TM, Bushnell CD. Reversible cerebral vasoconstriction syndrome. Stroke. 2019;50(8):2253–8.

40. Muehlschlegel S, Kursun O, Topcuoglu MA, Fok J, Singhal AB. Differentiating reversible cerebral vasoconstriction syndrome with subarachnoid hemorrhage from other causes of subarachnoid hemorrhage. JAMA Neurol. 2013;70(10):1254–60.

41. Niu L, Wang L, Yin X, Li XF, Wang F. Role of magnetic resonance imaging in the diagnosis of primary central nervous system angiitis. Exp Ther Med. 2017;14(1):555–60.

42. Beuker C, Schmidt A, Strunk D, et al. Primary angiitis of the central nervous system: diagnosis and treatment. Ther Adv Neurol Disord. 2018;11:1756286418785071.

43. de Boysson H, Parienti JJ, Mawet J, et al. Primary angiitis of the CNS and reversible cerebral vasoconstriction syndrome: a comparative study. Neurology. 2018;91(16):e1468–78.

44. Mawet J, Boukobza M, Franc J, et al. Reversible cerebral vasoconstriction syndrome and cervical artery dissection in 20 patients. Neurology. 2013;81(9):821–4.

45. Katz BS, Fugate JE, Ameriso SF, et al. Clinical worsening in reversible cerebral vasoconstriction syndrome. JAMA Neurol. 2014;71(1):68–73.

46. Nowak DA, Rodiek SO, Henneken S, et al. Reversible segmental cerebral vasoconstriction (Call-Fleming syndrome): are calcium channel inhibitors a potential treatment option? Cephalalgia. 2003;23(3):218–22.

47. Bakhru A, Atlas RO. A case of postpartum cerebral angiitis and review of the literature. Arch Gynecol Obstet. 2011;283(3):663–8.

48. Yang L, Bai HX, Zhao X, Xiao Y, Tan L. Postpartum cerebral angiopathy presenting with non-aneurysmal subarachnoid hemorrhage and interval development of neurological deficits: a case report and review of literature. Neurol India. 2013;61(5):517–22.

49. Chen SP, Fuh JL, Lirng JF, Chang FC, Wang SJ. Recurrent primary thunderclap headache and benign CNS angiopathy: spectra of the same disorder? Neurology. 2006;67(12):2164–9.

50. Ducros A, Boukobza M, Porcher R, Sarov M, Valade D, Bousser MG. The clinical and radiological spectrum of reversible cerebral vasoconstriction syndrome. A prospective series of 67 patients. Brain. 2007;130(Pt 12):3091–101.

51. Mijalski C, Dakay K, Miller-Patterson C, Saad A, Silver B, Khan M. Magnesium for treatment of reversible cerebral vasoconstriction syndrome: case series. Neurohospitalist. 2016;6(3):111–3.

52. Chik Y, Hoesch RE, Lazaridis C, Weisman CJ, Llinas RH. A case of postpartum cerebral angiopathy with subarachnoid hemorrhage. Nat Rev Neurol. 2009;5(9):512–6.

53. Singhal AB, Topcuoglu MA. Glucocorticoid-associated worsening in reversible cerebral vasoconstriction syndrome. Neurology. 2017;88(3):228–36.

54. Bouchard M, Verreault S, Gariepy JL, Dupre N. Intra-arterial milrinone for reversible cerebral vasoconstriction syndrome. Headache. 2009;49(1):142–5.

55. Song JK, Fisher S, Seifert TD, et al. Postpartum cerebral angiopathy: atypical features and treatment with intracranial balloon angioplasty. Neuroradiology. 2004;46(12):1022–6.

56. Ringer AJ, Qureshi AI, Kim SH, Fessler RD, Guterman LR, Hopkins LN. Angioplasty for cerebral vasospasm from eclampsia. Surg Neurol. 2001;56(6):373–8; discussion 378–9.

57. Lele A, Lyon T, Pollack A, Husmann K, Reeves A. Intra-arterial nicardipine for the treatment of cerebral vasospasm in postpartum cerebral angiopathy: a case study and review of literature. Int J Neurosci. 2011;121(10):537–42.

58. Thakur JD, Chittiboina P, Khan IS, Nanda A. Unique case of postpartum cerebral angiopathy requiring surgical intervention: case report and review of literature. Neurol India. 2011;59(6):891–4.

59. Fugate JE, Wijdicks EF, Parisi JE, et al. Fulminant postpartum cerebral vasoconstriction syndrome. Arch Neurol. 2012;69(1):111–7.

60. Singhal AB, Kimberly WT, Schaefer PW, Hedley-Whyte ET. Case records of the Massachusetts General Hospital. Case 8-2009. A 36-year-old woman with headache, hypertension, and seizure 2 weeks post partum. N Engl J Med. 2009;360(11):1126–37.

61. Singhal AB, Hajj-Ali RA, Topcuoglu MA, et al. Reversible cerebral vasoconstriction syndromes: analysis of 139 cases. Arch Neurol. 2011;68(8):1005–12.

62. Hajj-Ali RA, Furlan A, Abou-Chebel A, Calabrese LH. Benign angiopathy of the central nervous system: cohort of 16 patients with clinical course and long-term followup. Arthritis Rheum. 2002;47(6):662–9.

63. Chen SP, Fuh JL, Wang SJ, et al. Magnetic resonance angiography in reversible cerebral vasoconstriction syndromes. Ann Neurol. 2010;67(5):648–56.

64. Williams TL, Lukovits TG, Harris BT, Harker RC. A fatal case of postpartum cerebral angiopathy with literature review. Arch Gynecol Obstet. 2007;275(1):67–77.

65. James AH, Bushnell CD, Jamison MG, Myers ER. Incidence and risk factors for stroke in pregnancy and the puerperium. Obstet Gynecol. 2005;106(3):509–16.

Anticoagulation for Neurovascular Disorders in Pregnancy

Patrick Bridgeman and Angela Antoniello

Introduction

Neurovascular indications for anticoagulation during pregnancy, although rare, do occur. During pregnancy and the postnatal period, women are at increased risk of acute ischemic stroke at a rate of 34 strokes per 100,000 deliveries compared to non-pregnant woman who have an incidence of 21 per 100,000 live births [1]. Pregnancy is also a risk factor for central venous thrombosis [2]. Choosing the appropriate anticoagulant treatment for pregnant patients is especially challenging. The lack of data and unclear efficacy is also reflected in the variability in practice of neurologists. In a survey sent to 384 neurologists, 88% of respondents indicated that antithrombotic therapy should be administered to pregnant patients with a history of stroke, however, differences in the agent of choice varied substantially. Aspirin was chosen by 51% of neurologists as secondary prophylaxis and 7% of respondents chose low-molecular weight heparins (LMWHs). Data regarding the use of anticoagulants for neurovascular indications in pregnancy is sparce and largely derived from observational data, including case reports and retrospective cohort studies. Throughout this chapter, data regarding use and outcomes of anticoagulation in pregnant patients with neurovascular indications will be discussed, when available. Data from other indications, such as venous thromboembolism (VTE) treatment, thrombophilia, and others, will be included to provide a picture of anticoagulant use in the pregnant patient population. Clinical considerations, including approaches to diagnosis and management, for the various neurovascular disorders are discussed in detail in other chapters of this book.

Pharmacokinetic Changes in Pregnancy

Physiologic changes in the pregnant woman result in pharmacokinetic changes that may necessitate dose adjustment, may predispose patients to increased risk of toxicity, or result in diminished efficacy or therapeutic effect. Studies evaluating pharmacokinetic parameters in pregnant patients are very limited. Drug absorption, distribution, metabolism, and excretion may be markedly different in pregnancy. Changes in regional blood flow may significantly affect absorption of enteral and intramuscular injec-

P. Bridgeman (✉)
Department of Pharmacy Practice and Administration, Ernest Mario School of Pharmacy, Piscataway, NJ, USA
e-mail: Patrick.bridgeman@pharmacy.rutgers.edu; patrick.bridgeman@rwjbh.org

A. Antoniello
Department of Pharmacy, Cooperman Barnabas Medical Center, Livingston, NJ, USA

© The Author(s), under exclusive license to Springer Nature Switzerland AG 2023
G. Gupta et al. (eds.), *Neurological Disorders in Pregnancy*,
https://doi.org/10.1007/978-3-031-36490-7_15

tions. Pregnancy-associated nausea and vomiting may also result in decreased enteral absorption.

Furthermore, the volume of distribution is increased in pregnant patients. Volume of distribution is the volume required for a drug to be evenly distributed to equal the resulting blood concentration. Many variables affect volume of distribution, including protein binding, medication lipophilicity, and patient volume status. During pregnancy, plasma volume increases by approximately 40% above baseline in part due to estrogen-mediated activation of the renin-angiotensin-aldosterone system [3]. Increases in the total fluid volume in pregnant patients lead to reduced serum concentrations compared to non-pregnant patients if the same dose is administered. Hydrophilic drugs are more likely to be affected by this change. Increases in total body fat occurring in pregnancy may decrease the volume of distribution of lipophilic medications resulting in lower serum concentrations.

Pregnant patients experience increases in glomerular filtration rate and increased renal blood flow. Increased rates of renal clearance may result in shorter half-lives of renally cleared medications. For example, enoxaparin serum concentrations are lower early and late in pregnancy. In some cases, dosage adjustments of enoxaparin may be required. Additionally, increases in hepatic blood flow may increase clearance of medications metabolized by the liver. The hepatic cytochrome P450 enzymes may increase or decrease resulting in changes in serum concentrations for medications metabolized by this pathway.

Hypoalbuminemia related to pregnancy results in reduced protein binding and increased free fraction for medications which are highly protein bound. Therefore, more active drug is available and may result in increased action of the drug. Drugs with high levels of protein binding may, therefore, require dosage adjustment [4].

Pregnancy results in several pharmacokinetic changes. Although most do not result in clinically relevant changes, providers should be aware that they may occur and be prepared to intervene if necessary. Drugs which are likely to require dose

adjustments are those that undergo increased renal clearance or those that are highly protein bound.

Food and Drug Administration Pregnancy and Lactation Labeling

For over 30 years, the United States Food and Drug Administration (FDA) has categorized fetal risk with a five-letter system (A, B, C, D and X), detailed in Table 15.1 [5]. Recently, the FDA has revised the pregnancy and lactation labeling to address concerns raised over the oversimplification of this categorization scheme as presented in drug product labeling. The current Pregnancy and Lactation Labeling Final Rule (PLLR) went into effect on June 30, 2015. For prescription drugs approved after June 30, 2015, the letter category system will no longer be utilized in the

Table 15.1 Labeling for human prescription drug and biological products

Category	Description
A	• Adequate and controlled human studies do not demonstrate fetal risk
	• Animal studies demonstrating lack of fetal risk may also be available
B	• Animal studies do not demonstrate fetal risk, but adequate and controlled human studies are lacking OR
	• Animal reproduction studies demonstrate adverse effects, but adequate and controlled human studies do not demonstrate fetal risk
C	• Animal reproduction studies demonstrate adverse effects while controlled human studies are lacking, but drug therapy benefits may outweigh risks OR
	• Adequate animal reproduction and controlled human studies are lacking
D	• Human studies or marketing data demonstrate fetal risk
	• Potential benefits of drug therapy may outweigh fetal risk
X	• Fetal harm is demonstrated by animal or human studies and/or marketing experience
	• This risk of drug therapy clearly outweighs the benefit

The above table represents pregnancy risk categories for drugs as established by the Food and Drug Administration prior to the implementation of changes per the 2015 Pregnancy and Lactation Labeling Final Rule [5]

labeling of the drug. Drugs approved prior to June 29, 2001 are not covered by the PLLR, but the pregnancy category assignments must be removed from the labeling. The changes of the PLLR will gradually be implemented for drugs approved after June 29, 2001, however, the timeline is not fully delineated. In addition to removing the pregnancy categories, other sections of the package insert or product labeling are now revised to better reflect the current information available about drug used during pregnancy. The current package insert sections "Pregnancy," "Nursing Mothers," and "Labor and Delivery" are being removed. These sections are being replaced by new section "Pregnancy," "Lactation," and "Females and Males of Reproductive Potential." Additional updates to the "Pregnancy" section include a statement regarding the existence of drug-specific pregnancy exposure registries. FDA believes this will encourage providers utilize these registries and accumulate exposure and outcome information. The pregnancy section must also contain a statement of the risk of using the drug during pregnancy, information about dosage adjustment during pregnancy, maternal adverse reactions, fetal adverse reactions, and effects on labor and delivery. For the purposes of this book chapter, the pregnancy letter categories will still be used due to provider familiarity and concurrent use with the new labeling system.

Heparin Anticoagulants

Heparin anticoagulants have been used in pregnant patients for many years. They are the first line anticoagulant for many indications in pregnancy. Utilization of UFH as a first line anticoagulant has fallen out of favor as LMWHs have several advantages over UFH, however, use of UFH may be considered in patients with renal disease or utilized near the time of delivery. There are several different LMWHs available in the United States and worldwide, including enoxaparin, dalteparin, tinzaparin, and nadroparin. LMWHs and UFH do not cross the placenta. Teratogenicity or increased rates of fetal bleeding have not been demonstrated [6]. LMWHs are renally cleared and require dosage adjustment in patients with renal dysfunction. When compared to UFH, LMWHs have a longer half-life, more predictable subcutaneous absorption, and a more predictable therapeutic effect. These characteristics make LMWHs preferable to UFH.

Beside bleeding events, other adverse reactions with heparins include allergic skin reactions, osteoporosis, and heparin-induced thrombocytopenia (HIT). Allergic skin reactions have been reported to occur with unfractionated heparin (UFH) and LMWHs. The incidence of heparin-induced skin lesions covers a wide range from 1% to 40% in pregnant patients. The etiology of the rash is a type IV delayed hypersensitivity reaction. This is different compared to HIT, which is a type I allergic reaction. In a prospective observational trial, 111 pregnant patients were evaluated for heparin-induced skin reactions. The mean onset of rash was 50.5 days. In this study, 81.8% ($n = 22$) developed a skin reaction. Nadroparin accounted for 81.8% of patients who initially developed a rash, and enoxaparin and UFH accounted for 4.5% of reactions respectively. No association between HIT and the heparin-induced rash was identified. The authors concluded skin reactions occur with high frequency in pregnant patients and the use of nadroparin should be avoided in pregnancy. The rash may resolve with switching the heparin compound administered, however, cross-reactivity has been observed and should be considered [7]. The risk of development of osteoporosis may be less with LMWHs compared to UFH. In a meta-analysis evaluating the effect of long term LMWH on bone mineral density and fracture risk in non-pregnant females, the authors concluded that LMWH may not increase fracture risk if used at therapeutic doses for 3–6 months, but that longer treatment duration may adversely affect bone mineral density [8]. Reports of osteoporosis occurring in pregnant patents have been published. Risk factors for the development of osteoporosis have not been identified yet in the pregnant population. Physicians should be aware of the possible development of osteoporosis and monitor patients accordingly. LMWHs seem to have lower rates of HIT when compared to UFH

[9]. The incidence of HIT in nonpregnant patients is approximately 3% ([10]).

The nomenclature adopted by the American College of Chest Physicians (ACCP) used to describe the categorization of dosing of LMWHs and UFH in pregnancy includes the following categories: adjusted dose UFH, prophylactic LMWH, intermediate dose LMWH, and adjusted dose LMWH [9]. Adjusted dose UFH describes when UFH is administered at 12-h intervals to achieve an aPTT within a defined therapeutic range. Prophylactic LMWH is used when describing once daily administration of at lower doses. Intermediate dose LMWH is used to describe administration of LMWH doses at 12-h intervals for prophylaxis and adjusted dose LMWH describes weight based full treatment doses (Table 15.2).

Table 15.2 Dosing strategy of UFH and LMWH

Dosing strategy	Description
UFH	
Adjusted dose	• Varying weight-based doses injected subcutaneously every 12 h to target a goal midinterval aPTT in therapeutic range
LMWH	
Prophylactic[a]	• Dalteparin 5000 units injected subcutaneously every 24 h
	• Tinzaparin 4500 units injected subcutaneously every 24 h
	• Nadroparin 2850 units injected subcutaneously every 24 h
	• Enoxaparin 40 mg injected subcutaneously every 24 h
Intermediate dose	• Dalteparin 5000 units injected subcutaneously every 12 h
	• Enoxaparin 40 mg injected subcutaneously every 12 h
Adjusted dose	• Dalteparin 200 units/kg injected subcutaneously once daily OR 100 units/kg injected subcutaneously every 12 h
	• Tinzaparin 175 units/kg injected subcutaneously once daily
	• Enoxaparin 1 mg/kg injected subcutaneously every 12 h

The above table represents various anticoagulation dosing strategies used in pregnancy as defined by the American College of Chest Physicians [9]

UFH unfractionated heparin, *LMWH* low molecular weight heparin, *aPTT* activated partial thromboplastin time

[a]Doses may be further adjusted for extremes of body weight

UFH is not teratogenic and does not result in increased risk of fetal bleeding as it does not cross the placenta [11]. A retrospective study evaluated heparin use during 100 pregnancies in 77 patients. The mean duration of heparin therapy was 17.97 weeks and all patients given heparin for treatment of VTE initially received it intravenously. There were two episodes of severe bleeding (2%), one of which was antepartum bleeding. This rate of bleeding is comparable to previously published literature on use of UFH in pregnant patients. No episodes of symptomatic fracture occurred, but bone mineral testing was not performed, therefore, changes in bone mineral density could not be evaluated. Rates of adverse fetal outcomes were similar to the general population [12].

Prolonged anticoagulant effects have been observed with the use of subcutaneous heparin. Anderson and colleagues observed pregnant patients to have a prolonged aPTT up to 28 h after discontinuation of subcutaneous heparin. The authors recommend discontinuing subcutaneous heparin 24 h prior to elective induction of labor [13].

A systematic review evaluated the safety and efficacy of LMWHs in pregnancy. A total of 2777 patients from 64 studies were included for analysis. The most common indication reported in the review was thromboprophylaxis or adverse pregnancy outcome (61 studies, 2603 pregnancies) with 15 studies (174 patients) receiving LMWH for treatment of acute VTE. In this analysis, the authors did not identify maternal deaths in the included trials. Allergic skin reactions were reported in 1.8% of patients. Enoxaparin had the lowest incidence of skin reaction compared to dalteparin or nadroparin. Across all groups, significant bleeding, usually associated with primary obstetric causes, occurred in 1.98% (1.5–2.57%). Other adverse events, such as osteoporosis and low platelet count, occurred in 3 patients and 1 patient, respectively. There were no reported cases of epidural hematoma, hemorrhagic or neurologic complications associated with epidural or spinal anesthesia identified in this review [14].

McClintok and colleagues reported the use of enoxaparin in pregnant patients with mechanical heart valves. Women were identified from a prospective database of pregnant woman and selected if the indication for anticoagulation was thomboprophylaxis in the setting of a mechanical heart valve. A total of 31 women were included in the study with a total number of 47 pregnancies. A majority of patients were treated with enoxaparin alone (72.2%) with the rest treated with a combination of enoxaparin and warfarin. Seven patients experienced a thrombotic event, and of those who experienced a thrombotic event, five were associated with enoxaparin use. Post-partum hemorrhage occurred in 12.8% ($n = 6$) of pregnancies [15].

Multiple dose formulations of enoxaparin contain benzyl alcohol as a preservative. When benzyl alcohol is administered it has been associated with neonatal death. Additionally, benzyl alcohol crosses the placenta and may be harmful to premature infants. Therefore, preservative free vials should be utilized when administered to pregnant patients [16].

Rates of post-partum hemorrhage have been evaluated in pregnant patients treated with a therapeutic dose of LMWH versus those not treated with LMWH. In a retrospective cohort study, the occurrence of post-partum hemorrhage (PPH), defined as blood loss greater than 500 mL, was 18% in the LMWH group compared with 22% in the group not treated with LMWH. The rate of severe PPH, defined as blood loss greater than 1000 mL, was not different between the two groups. The authors concluded that LMWHs were not associated with a higher incidence of PPH, however, a randomized clinical trial is required to confirm their results [17]. A subsequent meta-analysis was conducted to assess risk of PPH in patients with exposure to LMWH. The analysis included eight studies with a total of 22,162 women, and of those, 1320 were exposed to LMWH. The authors found an increased risk of PPH in the LMWH group compared to the control group (relative risk, 1.45; 1.02–2.05). However, there was no difference in the amount of blood lost or risk of transfusion at delivery [18].

Dosing recommendations for LMWH vary by indication, and dosing modifications are required in pregnancy secondary to physiologic changes

as previously described. Prophylactic doses of enoxaparin were evaluated in pregnant patients with a history of thrombophilia and recurrent pregnancy loss. The study was a multicenter prospective, open label, randomized trial where patients were assigned to receive a total daily dose of enoxaparin 40 mg or 80 mg (40 mg twice daily). A total of 180 women were enrolled in the study. There were no differences in post-partum bleeding instances, or thrombotic episodes, between the two groups. The authors concluded that both 40 mg/day or 80 mg/day regimens were well tolerated and that either dosing regimen could be used [19]. The American College of Obstetricians and Gynecologists (ACOG) recommends utilizing once daily LMWH dosing for prophylactic indications. When treatment doses are required, ACOG and ACCP guidance recommend utilizing weight adjusted dosing. Observational data evaluating once daily or twice daily weight adjusted doses have shown differences in efficacy: twice daily dosing may be preferred secondary to changes in the volume of distribution and increases in glomerular filtration rate as pregnancy progresses. Patient specific preferences should additionally be considered to ensure compliance with the prescribed regimen.

Monitoring recommendations vary depending on indication and possible need for dose increases. Routine monitoring of anti-factor Xa (anti-Xa) levels may not be required in those with normal renal function [9]. Indications to monitor anti-Xa levels in pregnant patients include recurrent thrombosis, mechanical heart valves, and high (>90 kg) or low (<50 kg) body weight [20]. If required, anti-Xa levels should be drawn 4–6 h after injection and doses adjusted to maintain an anti-Xa level of 0.6–1 units/mL for a twice daily regimen. Higher anti-Xa levels of 0.8–1.6 units/mL may be required if once daily weight adjusted regimens are utilized. Peak anti-Xa levels for patients with mechanical heart valves should be maintained between 0.8 and 1.2 units/mL.

Near the time of delivery, LMWH should be discontinued 12–24 h prior to induction of labor. Another option is to transition the patient over to intravenous UFH due to its shorter duration of action and reversibility [21].

Non-Heparin Anticoagulants

Warfarin

Warfarin crosses the placenta and is associated with adverse fetal outcomes such as fetal loss, fetal bleeding, and teratogenicity. In a systematic review evaluating the use of oral anticoagulant during pregnancy in patients with mechanical heart valves, warfarin embryopathy occurred in 6.4% of patients. The authors observed when heparin replaced warfarin for weeks 6–12 or replaced warfarin with heparin for the duration of the pregnancy, it decreased the occurrence of adverse fetal outcomes. Bleeding occurred in 2.5% of those included for analysis and most of the bleeding episodes were related to delivery. In data from the European Network of Teratology Services (ENTIS), the odds of major birth defects associated with vitamin K antagonist exposure during the first trimester was 3.86 (1.86–8.00). The most common fetal abnormalities include midfacial hypoplasia, stippled epiphyses, and central nervous system malformation. Adverse fetal outcomes related to warfarin appear to be dose-related. In a study of 52 pregnant patients with mechanical valves receiving warfarin anticoagulation, pregnancy loss occurred in 23 of 71 pregnancies. Daily doses of warfarin greater than 5 mg were significantly associated with poor pregnancy outcomes [22]. In another retrospective analysis in the same patient population comparing warfarin to a combination of heparin and warfarin, the authors found that those who required more than 5 mg daily of warfarin had significantly worse outcomes [23]. A more recent meta-analysis included 51 studies with a total of 2113 pregnancies and 1538 women. Congenital fetal anomalies occurred in 2.13% (1.34–3.33%) of live births in those who used vitamin K antagonist therapy throughout the pregnancy. Congenital fetal abnormalities occurred in 0.74% (0.19–2.33%) in those that utilized a combination of heparin and vitamin K antagonist therapy. The risk of fetal wastage in the vitamin K antagonist group was 32.53%. In the low dose subgroup, the risk of fetal wastage was 19.23%. The highest rate of fetal wastage was in the UFH group at 53.62% (41.28–65.55).

Based on this data, if warfarin must be utilized, it is ideal to maintain a daily dose of less than 5 mg/day to decrease the risk of adverse fetal outcomes. Exposure during weeks 6–12 appear to correlate with the highest risk of birth defect development. During this time period, it may be reasonable to consider an alternative anticoagulant such as a LMWH. Several guidelines recommend limiting the use of vitamin K antagonists to use in pregnant woman with mechanical heart valves only [20].

Parenteral Direct Thrombin Inhibitors

Argatroban and bivalirudin are parenteral direct thrombin inhibitors. Case reports exist on the use of argatroban during pregnancy. The first is a report of a 35-year-old female who underwent an emergency pulmonary embolectomy where argatroban was utilized as the anticoagulant during cardiopulmonary bypass. The second case report is a 26-year-old female with portal vein thrombosis who was treated with argatroban from week 33 of pregnancy through week 39. The argatroban infusion was stopped 7 h before epidural anesthesia. The patient did not experience increased blood loss and had an uneventful birth [24]. Currently there are no published reports on the use of bivalirudin in the medical literature.

Fondaparinux

Fondaparinux is a synthetic pentasaccharide that acts by binding to antithrombin and inactivates factor Xa. It has been suggested that fondaparinux may be an alternative in pregnant patients who cannot tolerate administration of heparins. With the removal of danaparoid from the United States market, fondaparinux may be the only alternative. There is data to suggest that fondaparinux may cross the placenta and exhibits measurable anti-Xa activity in umbilical blood [25]. The ACCP guidelines recommend that fondaparinux may be considered in those who cannot receive danaparoid for the treatment of HIT [9].

In a review of 65 cases where fondaparinux was used in pregnancy, no cases of major bleeding were identified. Spontaneous abortions occurred in 18 cases, preterm rupture of membranes in one case, preeclampsia in one case, and intrauterine growth retardation in two cases. The authors conclude that larger population studies are required to confirm their findings. They also state one case resulted in multiple fetal abnormalities at a rate of 1.5%, which is much higher than the general population rate of 0.16%. The authors reiterate caution interpreting these results that fondaparinux may be safe during pregnancy. They also recommend limiting its use only to patients who require management of HIT or those with severe allergic reactions to LMWH in line with recommendations from the ACCP.

Prophylactic dosing of fondaparinux is 2.5 mg daily. Treatment doses for deep vein thrombosis (DVT) or pulmonary embolism (PE) are 7.5 mg daily. When patients weigh more than 100 kg, the dose should be increased to 10 mg daily; and when they are less than 50 kg, the dose should be decreased to 5 mg daily. Fondaparinux is not recommended to be used in those with a creatinine clearance of less than 30 mL/min as it is excreted unchanged in the urine.

Direct Acting Oral Anticoagulants

Direct acting oral anticoagulants (DOACs) have become first line agents for anticoagulation for indications such as atrial fibrillation and VTE. Efficacy and safety data for DOACs in pregnancy is lacking. Medications in this class include dabigatran, rivaroxaban, apixaban, edoxaban, and betrixaban. DOACs have been shown to cross the placenta in animal models and in placental models [20]. Because placental transfer is possible, there is increased risk of teratogenicity and poor fetal outcomes. The International Society on Thrombosis and Hemostasis (ISTH) recommends avoiding the use of DOACs in pregnant women, in those women planning to become pregnant, and in

breastfeeding patients [26]. A systematic review evaluating the use of DOACs in pregnancy included a total of 357 reports and 233 unique reports. The 137 cases with pregnancy outcomes included 67 live births, 31 miscarriages, and 39 elective terminations. Abnormalities were reported in 7 cases, 3 of which may be classified as embryopathy. Until more data becomes available concerning the risk of maternal and fetal outcomes, DOACs should not be used during pregnancy. If a patient becomes pregnant while taking a DOAC it is reasonable to switch the patient to a LMWH [26].

Antiplatelets

Aspirin

Aspirin is one of the most prolific antiplatelet agents available. The use of salicin-containing willow bark for the relief of pain has been documented as far back as ancient Greece where Hippocrates recommended it for the relief of pain from childbirth. The active ingredient in willow bark was discovered in 1828 by Johann Buchner [27]. Aspirin exerts its antiplatelet effects by inhibiting the production of thromboxane A_2 within platelets. When taken orally, aspirin is rapidly absorbed in the stomach and small intestine. Ideal absorption of aspirin occurs in the stomach at a pH between 2.15 and 4.10. Absorption through the small intestine occurs at a much faster rate compared to absorption through the stomach. Aspirin crosses the placental barrier (Package insert Aspirin).

There are no controlled trials evaluating the safety and efficacy of aspirin for stroke prevention in pregnant woman. Observational data suggests that use of low-dose aspirin appears to be safe in pregnant women after the first trimester. Results of a meta-analysis conducted to evaluate the use of aspirin for the prevention preeclampsia in those with historical risk factors for development of preeclampsia included 14 clinical trials with a total 12,416 woman. Aspirin use was shown to decrease perinatal death and preeclampsia. Aspirin was also associated with a reduction in the number of spontaneous preterm births and an increase in birthweight. From a safety standpoint, the authors did not identify increased rates of antepartum bleeding or placental abruption [28]. Another study that evaluated the use of aspirin at a dose of 150 mg daily for the prevention of preeclampsia in high risk pregnancies beginning in weeks 11–14 and continued until 36 weeks did not demonstrate a difference in adverse events such as maternal bleeding between the two groups. No difference in neonatal adverse events were noted as well. However, increased utilization of maternal blood transfusion was identified in a separate trial. The U.S. Preventative Services Task Force evaluated the use of aspirin for the prevention of morbidity and mortality from preeclampsia. The authors did not find an association between short term harms and aspirin use. The authors did not identify any long term outcomes associated with low dose aspirin use, however, the data are limited [29].

For the most part, the use of low-dose aspirin in pregnancy should be limited to the second and third trimester. A majority of the data available on the use of aspirin during pregnancy is during the period of 12–28 weeks. There are exceptions where aspirin may be utilized for the prevention of early pregnancy loss. A possible link of aspirin use during the first trimester and gastroschisis has been reported. However, the dose of aspirin is not noted in this study, therefore the data may not be applicable to low-dose aspirin [30]. Another study of 1228 woman, with 615 of these patients receiving low dose aspirin preconception, did not find an increased risk of neonatal or fetal adverse events [31].

The timing of aspirin discontinuation near delivery has not been linked to maternal or fetal bleeding. The timing of low-dose aspirin discontinuation differed with variability of timing from 36 weeks through delivery. The ACOG guidelines recommend the use of low-dose aspirin for the prevention of preeclampsia in woman at high risk beginning between weeks 12 and 28. Additionally, the committee recommends that woman who were previously on aspirin for other indications prior to 12 weeks may continue to take low-dose aspirin.

Clopidogrel

Clopidogrel is an irreversible $P2Y_{12}$ inhibitor with FDA approved indications for patients with acute coronary syndrome. Clopidogrel is a prodrug that requires activation by the CYP2C19 to inhibit platelet function. Patients with genetic variations in the CYP2C19 system may experience decreased effectiveness of clopidogrel. Additionally, concomitant use with strong inhibitors of CYP2C19, such as omeprazole, decrease the effectiveness of clopidogrel. To avoid this drug interaction, administration of clopidogrel must be separated from omeprazole by 12 h or an alternative acid suppressive regimen should be utilized.

The FDA has assigned clopidogrel to pregnancy category B. Clinical trial data regarding clopidogrel use in the pregnant patient is essentially non-existent, especially for neurovascular indications. Data for other indications in pregnant patients will be discussed. Most of the data that is currently available includes those with myocardial infarction.

In the clopidogrel labeling, reproductive studies on animals have been conducted where doses of 62 and 78 times the recommended human dose were administered to rats and rabbits, respectively, and failed to demonstrate fetotoxicity. It is not known if clopidogrel or any of its metabolites cross the placenta [32].

Major adverse events associated with clopidogrel use are bleeding and thrombotic thrombocytopenic purpura. The CURE trial evaluated the use of clopidogrel in the treatment of non-ST elevation myocardial infarction in 12,562 patients. The CURE trial compared clopidogrel plus aspirin to placebo plus aspirin and determined that major bleeding occurred more frequently in the clopidogrel plus aspirin group. It is important to note that 92% of the patients in this trial received other anticoagulants. Major bleeding occurred in 3.7% in the treatment group compared with 2.7% in the placebo group ($p < 0.001$). However, the occurrence of fatal bleeding and intracranial bleeding were not statistically significantly different between the two groups. The most common type of major bleeding reported was gastrointestinal bleeding and bleeding at puncture sites. The proportion of patients that required transfusions greater than 4 units of blood was 1.2% in the treatment group. The POINT study evaluated the use of clopidogrel and aspirin vs. aspirin monotherapy initiated within 12 h for the prevention of stroke in those who experienced a high-risk TIA or minor stroke. A total of 4681 patients were enrolled in the point trial with a total follow-up time of 90 days. The primary endpoint was a composite of ischemic stroke, myocardial infarction or ischemic vascular death. The major adverse events noted in this study were major hemorrhage of 0.9% in the treatment group vs. 0.4% in the placebo group (Hazard ratio, 2.32; 95% CI, 1.10–4.87; $P = 0.02$), hemorrhagic stroke of 0.2% in the treatment group vs. 0.1% in the placebo group (Hazard ratio, 1.68; 95% CI, 0.40–7.03; $P = 0.47$) and symptomatic intracerebral hemorrhage which was not statistically different between the groups. Minor hemorrhage was statistically significantly different in the treatment group vs. the placebo group. (1.6% vs. 0.5%; Hazard ratio, 3.12; 95% CI 1.67–5.83; $P < 0.001$).

The European Society of Cardiology recommends clopidogrel can be used during pregnancy for the shortest duration possible [33]. Clopidogrel must be discontinued at least 7 days prior to any planned neuraxial anesthesia to decrease the risk of epidural hematoma. Numerous case reports have been published demonstrating the use of clopidogrel during pregnancy. A recent case report and systematic review described the use of clopidogrel for secondary stroke prophylaxis in a 33-year-old pregnant patient. The patient was being treated for secondary stroke prevention by her neurologist with clopidogrel 75 mg daily for the prior 7 years. The patient presented to the emergency department for delivery. Clopidogrel was held for 1 week prior to scheduled vaginal delivery. Labor was initiated with neuraxial anesthesia with successful delivery and minimal blood loss. No post-partum hemorrhage occurred and clopidogrel was reinstated 12 h after delivery. A systematic review published in 2014 included data for a total of 13 patients treated with clopidogrel for secondary stroke prophylaxis. Most

of the patients (10 of 13) included in this analysis did not receive clopidogrel during the first trimester of pregnancy. Fetal complications noted in the review of the patients included one fetal death, one patent foramen ovale (PFO), restrictive muscle communication, and moderate mitral insufficiency. Notably, all the patients in this review received clopidogrel for non-neurologic indications.

Ticagrelor

Ticagrelor acts on the platelet $P2Y_{12}$ ADP-receptor to reversibly inhibit platelet function. Ticagrelor may be taken with or without food and reaches a peak level of absorption in 1.5 h. It is metabolized by the CYP3A4 system to its active metabolite. Dosage adjustments are not required for hepatic or renal impairment, however, there is little experience administering ticagrelor to those with moderate hepatic impairment. The primary route of elimination is via hepatic metabolism with a mean half-life of approximately 7 h for the parent compound ticagrelor and 9 h for the active metabolite.

Ticagrelor is classified as a pregnancy category C. Doses of 20–300 mg/kg/day have been administered to evaluate reproductive effects. Doses of 300 mg/kg/day resulted in adverse outcomes such as supernumerary liver lobes and ribs, incomplete ossification of the sternebrae and displaced articulation of the pelvis. When ticagrelor was administered to rabbits, adverse outcomes occurred in offspring with a dose of 63 mg/kg/day (Package Insert Ticagrelor).

Clinical data regarding the use of ticagrelor in pregnant women is sparse and limited to case reports. One case report describes the utilization of ticagrelor in the treatment of acute myocardial infarction in a 37-year-old woman at 27 weeks of gestation. The patient had a history of hypertension and hyperlipidemia. She was admitted to the hospital for treatment of an anterior wall myocardial infarction. She was treated with aspirin, enoxaparin and ticagrelor. Due to residual thrombus during PCI, she was further treated with heparin and tirofiban. Subsequently, 12 weeks later she was admitted for an elective Cesarean section. Both aspirin and ticagrelor were discontinued

5 days prior to the procedure. The patient underwent bridging with tirofiban, which was discontinued 4 h prior to the procedure. A healthy baby was delivered, but a subtotal hysterectomy to control post-partum hemorrhage was required. The authors reported at 27 months post-delivery that no obvious adverse effects were noted in the child [34]. A second case reports the use of ticagrelor throughout the duration of pregnancy. A 37-year-old pregnant woman with Bechet's disease presented and was being treated with ticagrelor for a previous non-ST elevation myocardial infarction with ticagrelor 90 mg twice daily. The patient had additional risk factors of smoking and hypertension. Additional medications on presentation included perindopril and cyclosporine, which were discontinued. Other medications continued through pregnancy included aspirin, prednisolone, and colchicine. Ticagrelor was continued for a total of 8 months up until 7 days before planned delivery. The patient had an uneventful delivery. No significant events were noted during the post-partum period.

In summary, ticagrelor does not have enough information to recommend its use during pregnancy for either neurologic or non-neurologic indications. Moreover, data from animal studies have demonstrated adverse fetal outcomes.

Prasugrel

Prasugrel is a $P2Y_{12}$ platelet inhibitor approved by the FDA to reduce thrombotic events in those with acute coronary syndromes managed with PCI. There are no adequately controlled trials to evaluate the use of prasugrel in pregnancy for neurologic or non-neurologic indications. When administered to rabbits and rats at doses of 30 times the recommended human dose, no structural abnormalities were observed.(Effient Package insert) There is a case report of a 32-year-old African American woman being treated with prasugrel for acute coronary syndrome. The date of conception is unclear, so it could not be determined with certainty, therefore, the duration of prasugrel exposure. Prasugrel was continued up until week 38 of the pregnancy and discontinued 5 days prior to planned delivery. The patient underwent an uneventful Cesarean delivery. The patient did not experience any bleeding complications. However, utilization of prasugrel is still not recommended during pregnancy due to limited evidence [33].

Tissue Plasminogen Activator (tPA)

Alteplase (tPA) has a large molecular weight and, therefore, will most likely not cross the placenta. Alteplase was administered to rabbits during organogenesis and demonstrated to be embryocidal. When alteplase was administered at doses of 1 mg/kg to rabbits, no fetal or maternal toxicity was observed. There are no randomized controlled trials evaluating the use of alteplase in pregnancy. Observational data regarding the use of alteplase in acute ischemic stroke will be discussed below.

In data presented at the International Stroke Conference, one study utilized claims data to identify pregnant patients with acute ischemic stroke. Between 2005 and 2012, 428,564 women with stroke were identified; of those, 599 were pregnant. A total of seven pregnant patients received IV tPA. A significantly higher rate of abortive pregnancies was identified in the tPA group (28.6% vs. 4.6%). No other differences in terms of discharge disposition, length of stay or in hospital mortality were identified [35]. In another review, 18,932 pregnant stroke patients were identified, with 70 patients receiving alteplase. Of the patients that received alteplase, 55 (78.6%) were discharged home and 5 (7.1%) died [36]. In a third population study, 2603 pregnant patients were identified, with 56 (2.2%) receiving alteplase. The reported rates of intracranial hemorrhage were similar; however, mortality was higher in the tPA group. The reason for the higher mortality rate in the treatment group remains unclear.

In a study utilizing data from the American Heart Association's Stroke Registry, data from 338 pregnant or post-partum women were identified. Administration of reperfusion therapy was similar between the pregnant and post-partum group vs. the non-pregnant group (11.8% vs. 10.5%). Pregnant or post-partum women were, however, less likely to receive intravenous tPA compared to non-pregnant patients (4.4% vs. 7.9%). The authors state there was a trend toward higher rates of symptomatic intracranial hemorrhage in the pregnant and postpartum group compared to non-pregnant patients, but the difference was not statistically significant (7.5% vs. 2.6%, $P = 0.06$) for all reperfusion therapy types. In pregnant patients who received alteplase monotherapy ($n = 15$), outcomes were similar; one experienced a symptomatic intracranial hemorrhage. This study is limited by the lack of data on pregnancy outcomes [37].

A recent systematic review of the use of alteplase for acute ischemic stroke in pregnant patients included 26 articles for analysis. Of the cases that were included, 27 reported neurologic improvement and no fetal complications. Alteplase was administered in the first trimester in 13 of the reported cases. Negative outcomes in the mother, fetus or both occurred in five cases. Hemorrhagic transformation was reported in three cases [38].

Virtually all the data available to make treatment decisions on the use of alteplase in pregnancy for acute ischemic stroke is derived from case reports. Current recommendations from the American Heart Association recommend IV alteplase to be considered for pregnant patients when the anticipated benefits of treating moderate or severe stroke outweigh the risk of uterine bleeding [39].

Summary

Selecting the appropriate anticoagulant during pregnancy represents a clinical challenge, necessitating an evaluation of potential benefit and consideration for risk to baby and mother alike. LMWHs may safely be used in pregnancy if the appropriate precautions are taken. Low-dose aspirin has data supporting its use in pregnancy for prevention of preeclampsia. Data for other anticoagulant, antiplatelet and antithrombotic therapy are generally limited to case reports and few limited controlled trials.

References

1. Bushnell C, McCullough LD, Awad IA, et al, on behalf of the American Heart Association Stroke Council, Council on Cardiovascular and Stroke Nursing, Council on Clinical Cardiology, Council on Epidemiology and Prevention, and Council for High Blood Pressure Research. "Guidelines for prevention of stroke in Women"Stroke. 2014;45(5):1545–88.
2. Bousser MG, Crassard I. Cerebral venous thrombosis, pregnancy and oral contraceptives. Thromb Res. 2012;130(Suppl 1):S19–22.
3. Hytten F. Blood volume changes in normal pregnancy. Clin Haematol. 1985;14(3):601–12.
4. Loebstein R, Lalkin A, Koren G. Pharmacokinetic changes during pregnancy and their clinical relevance. Clin Pharmacokinet. 1997;33:328–43.
5. Content and format of labeling for human prescription drug and biological products; requirements for pregnancy and lactation labeling. Fed Regist. 2008;73(104):30831–68. To be codified at 21 C.F.R. §201. https://www.govinfo.gov/content/pkg/FR-2008-05-29/pdf/E8-11806.pdf.
6. Lepercq J, Conard J, Borel-Derlon A, et al. Venous thromboembolism during pregnancy: a retrospective study of enoxaparin safety in 624 pregnancies. BJOG. 2001;108(11):1134–40.
7. Schindewolf M, Gobst C, Kroll H, Recke A, Louwen F, Wolter M, et al. High incidence of heparin-induced allergic delayed-type hypersensitivity reactions in pregnancy. J Allergy Clin Immunol. 2013;132(1):131–9.
8. Gajic-Veljanoski O, Phua CW, Shah P, et al. Effects of long term low molecular wight heparin on fractures and bone mineral destiny in non pregnant adults. J Gen Intern Med. 2016;31(8):947–57.
9. Bates SM, Jaeschke R, Stevens SM, Goodacre S, Wells PS, Stevenson MD, et al. Diagnosis of DVT: antithrombotic therapy and prevention of thrombosis, 9th ed: American College of Chest Physicians evidence-based clinical practice guidelines. Chest. 2012;141:e351S–418S.
10. Warkentin TE, Levine MN, Hirsh J, et al. Heparin-induced thrombocytopenia in patients treated with low-molecular-weight heparin or unfractionated heparin. N Engl J Med. 1995;332(20):1330–5.
11. Flessa HC, Kapstrom AB, Glueck HI, Will JJ. Placental transport of heparin. Am J Obstet Gynecol. 1965;93(4):570–3.
12. Ginsberg JS, Kowalchuk G, Hirsh J, Brill-Edwards P, Burrows R. Heparin therapy during pregnancy Risks to the fetus and mother. Arch Intern Med. 1989;149(10):2233–6.
13. Anderson DR, Ginsberg JS, Burrows R, Brill-Edwards P. Subcutaneous heparin therapy during pregnancy: a need for concern at the time of delivery. Thromb Haemost. 1991;65(3):248–50.
14. Greer IA, Nelson-Piercy C. Low-molecular weight heparins for thromboprophylaxis and treatment of

venous thromboembolism in pregnancy: a systematic review of safety and efficacy. Blood. 2005;106:401.

15. McClintock C, McCowan LME, North RA. Maternal complications and pregnancy outcome in woman with mechanical prosthetic heart valves treated with enoxaparin. BJOG. 2009;116(12):1585–92.

16. Centers for Disease Control and Prevention (CDC). Neonatal deaths associated with use of benzyl alcohol-Unites States. MMWR. 1982;31(22):290–1.

17. Roshani S, Cohn DM, Stehouwer AC, Wolf H, et al. Incidence of postpartum hemorrhage in woman receiving therapeutic doses of low-molecular weight heparin: results of a retrospective cohort study. BMJ Open. 2011;1:e000257.

18. Sirico A, Saccone G, Maruotti G, et al. Low molecular weight heparin use during pregnancy and risk of post partum hemmorrhage: a systematic review and meta analysis. J Matern Fetal Neonatal Med. 2019;32(11):1893–900.

19. Brenner B, Bar J, Ellis M, et al. Effects of enoxaparin on late pregnancy complications and neonatal outcomes in woman with recurrent pregnancy loss and thrombophilia: results from the Live-Enox Study. Fertil Steril. 2005;84:770–3.

20. Scheres LJJ, Bistervels IM, Middeldorp S. Everything the clinician needs to know about evidence-based anticoagulation in pregnancy. Blood Rev. 2019;33:82–97.

21. Chan WS, Rey E, Kent NE, et al; VTE in Pregnancy Guideline Working Group; Society of Obstetricians and Gynecologists of Canada. Venous thromboembolism and antithrombotic therapy in pregnancy. J Obstet Gynaecol Can. 2014;36(6):527–53.

22. Cortufo M, DeFeo M, De Santo LS, et al. Risk of warfarin during pregnancy with mechanical valve prostheses. Obstet Gynecol. 2002;99(1):35–40.

23. Khamooshi AJ, Kashfi F, Hoseini S, Tabatabaei MB, et al. Anticoagulation for prosthetic heart valves in pregnancy. Is there an answer? Asian Cardiovasc Thorac Ann. 2007;15(6):493–6.

24. Young SK, Al-Mondhiry HK, Vaida SJ, Ambrose A, Botti JJ. Successful use of argatroban during the third trimester of pregnancy: case report and review of the literature. Pharmacotherapy. 2008;28(12):1531–6.

25. Dempfle CE. Minor tranplacental passage of fondaparinux in vivo. N Engl J Med. 2004;350:1914–5.

26. Cohen H, Arachchillage DR, Middeldorp S, Beyer-Westendorf J, Abdul-Kadir R. Management of direct oral anticoagulants in women of childbearing potential: guidance from the SSC of the ISTH. J Thromb Haemost. 2016;14(8):1673–6.

27. Desborough MJR, Keeling DM. The aspirin story-from willow to wonder drug. Br J Haematol. 2017;177(5):674–83.

28. Coomarasamy A, Honest H, Papaioannou, et al. Aspirin for the prevention of preeclampsia in woman with historical risk factors: a systematic review. Obstet Gynecol. 2003;101(6):1319–32.

29. Hendseron JT, Whitlock EP, O'Connor E, et al. Low-dose aspirin for the prevention of morbidity and mortality: a systematic review for the U.S. Preventative Services Task Force. Ann Intern Med. 2014;160:695–703.

30. Kozer E, Nikfar S, Costei A, et al. Aspirin consumption during the first trimester and congenital anomalies: a meta-analysis. Am J Obstet Gynecol. 2002;187:1623–30.

31. Ahrens KA, Silver RM, Mumford SL, et al. Complications and safety of preconception low dose aspirin among woman with prior pregnancy loss. Obstet Gynecol. 2016;127:689–98.

32. Clopidogrel prescribing information. Bridgewater: Sanofi-Aventis/Bristol-Myers Squibb Company; 2017.

33. Regitz-Zagrosek V, Roos-Hesselink J, Bauersachs J, et al., ESC Scientific Document Group. 2018 ESC guidelines for the management of cardiovascular diseases during pregnancy: the Task Force for the Management of Cardiovascular Diseases during Pregnancy of the European Society of Cardiology (ESC). Eur Heart J. 2018;39(34):3165–241.

34. Argentiero D, Savonitto S, D'Andrea P, et al. Ticagrelor and tirofiban in pregnancy and delivery: beyond labels. J Thromb Thombolysis. 2020;49:145–8.

35. Mainali S, Cool JA, Navi B, Fink M, Kamel H. Safety of stroke thrombolysis during pregnancy: a population-based analysis. Stroke. 2015;46(Suppl 1):A188.

36. Song S, Ouyang B, Knopf T, et al. Stroke outcomes and usage of IV alteplase during pregnancy in the nationwide inpatient sample 2005–2010. Stroke. 2014;45(Suppl 1):AWP321.

37. Leffert LR, Clancy CR, Bateman BT, et al. Treatment patterns and short-term outcomes in ischemic stroke in pregnancy or postpartum period. Am J Obstet Gynecol. 2016;214(6):e1–723.

38. Ryman KM, Pace WD, Smith S, Fontaine GC. Alteplase therapy for acute ischemic stroke in pregnancy: two case reports and a systematic review of the literature. Pharmacotherapy. 2019;39(7):767–74.

39. Powers WJ, Rabinstein AA, Ackerson T, et al. American Heart Association Stroke Council. 2018 Guidelines for the early management of patients with acute ischemic stroke. Stroke. 2018;49(3):e46–110.

Part III

Neurotrauma and Neurocritical Care in Pregnancy

Evaluation and Management of Altered Mental Status and Coma in the Pregnant Patient

Roger Cheng

Introduction

Altered mental status (AMS) and impaired consciousness is a frequent driver for hospital admission, and in the pregnant patient, the presence of a fetus both increases the need for urgent diagnosis and management while potentially complicating this process. Though women of child-bearing age are rarely plagued by the life-threatening neurologic disorders more commonly seen in the general population, pregnancy is associated with unique neurologic complications, and when they do occur, morbidity and mortality can be extremely high, with disorders affecting the central nervous system implicated in around 15% of cases of maternal mortality in the USA [1]. As such, rapid evaluation, diagnosis, and management of a patient presenting in a pregnant state is essential, while always considering the impact of both diagnostic tests and potential treatments on the well-being of the mother and unborn child.

Initial Approach

A basic algorithm to the initial approach to an obstetric patient presenting with coma or altered mental status is outlined schematically in Fig. 16.1.

R. Cheng (✉)
Department of Neurology, Rutgers Robert Wood
Johnson Medical School, New Brunswick, NJ, USA
e-mail: roger.cheng@rutgers.edu

History

While patients who present to the hospital with altered sensorium will be unlikely to provide useful information about their condition, establishing a basic clinical course from alternate sources of information remains crucial. In particular, the rate of onset/progression can immediately guide the clinician's diagnostic focus, with sudden onset presentations necessitating rapid workup for cerebrovascular conditions such as cerebral hemorrhage, acute ischemic stroke, or venous sinus thrombosis. Conversely, a more gradual deterioration over hours or days may prompt the clinician to undergo a more in-depth evaluation for a toxic/metabolic or infectious cause if initial findings are non-revealing. Information regarding a patient's baseline comorbidities, such as diabetes or known epilepsy, for example, may be helpful in narrowing the differential. In the pregnant patient, the obstetric course and history, as well as information regarding current and past complications of pregnancy such as preeclampsia and hypercoagulability, will further provide insight into the patient's presentation.

Physical Examination

Vital Signs

In addition to the crucial role that vital signs play in the evaluation and management of any poten-

APPROACH TO THE OBSTETRIC PATIENT WITH ALTERED CONSCIOUSNESS

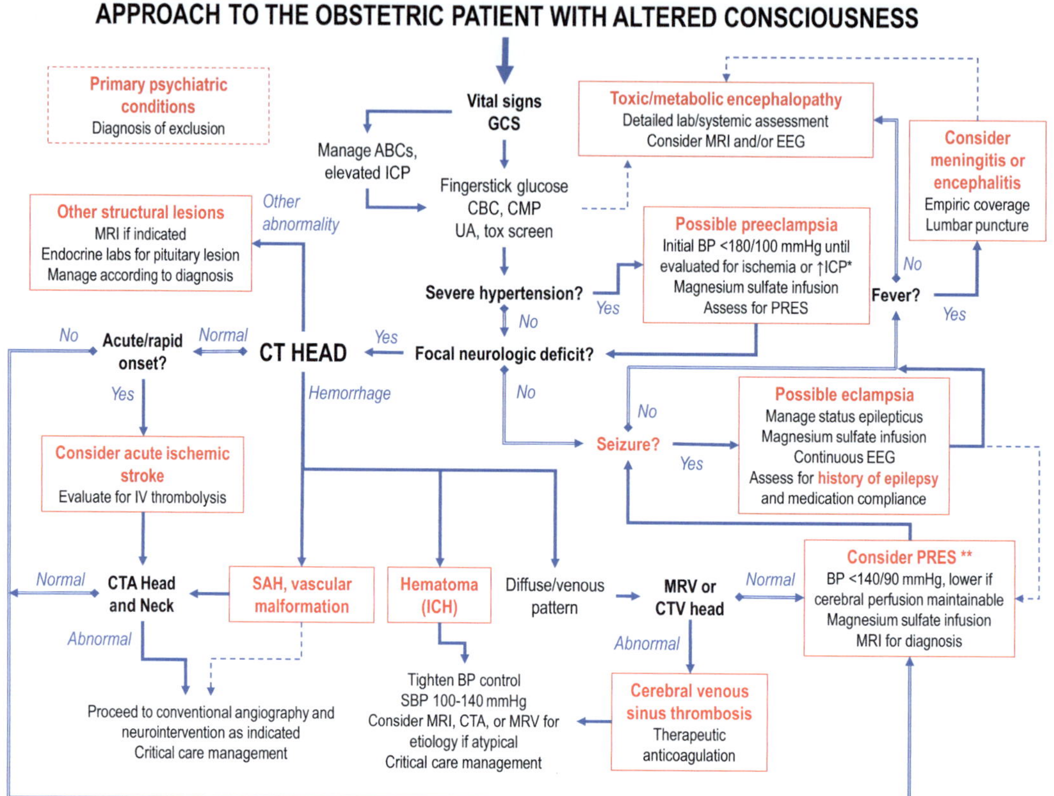

Fig. 16.1 A sample initial diagnostic algorithm for evaluation and management of a pregnant patient arriving with coma or altered mental status. *Rationale for delayed lowering of blood pressure is explained in the section on "Initial Management." **PRES can be considered a common pathway of injury in preeclampsia and eclampsia and should be presumed to exist when a severely encephalopathic patient presents with either state. *ABCs* airway, breathing, circulation, *BP* blood pressure, *CBC* complete blood count, *CMP* comprehensive metabolic panel, *CT* computed tomography, *CTA* CT angiography, *CTV* CT venography, *EEG* electroencephalography, *GCS* Glasgow Coma Scale, *ICP* intracranial pressure, *MRI* magnetic resonance imaging, *MRV* magnetic resonance venography, *PRES* posterior reversible encephalopathy syndrome, *SBP* systolic blood pressure, *UA* urinalysis

tially critically ill patient, vital sign patterns may provide some insight into the underlying diagnosis. Unstable vital signs and shock will result in alteration of consciousness regardless of underlying etiology or presence of a primary neurologic injury. Heart rate may vary with any number of normal/abnormal physiologic states as well as intoxications, however, in a patient with neurologic injury, tachycardia is frequently associated with the increased sympathetic outflow seen during cerebral hemorrhage (ICH or SAH). In combination with increased blood pressure, this may be part of a normal compensatory response to decreased cerebral perfusion (i.e., ischemia) or increased cerebral metabolic demand. However, note that there is a normal increase in heart rate seen during pregnancy as gestation progresses due to the need for increased cardiac output (CO), up to 20 bpm above baseline by 32 weeks [2]. Conversely, bradycardia when seen concomitantly with hypertension may be a sign of increased intracranial pressure (ICP). Hyper- and hypothermia may suggest underlying infection or metabolic derangement.

Neurologic Examination

Mental Status If possible, a rapid evaluation of the patient's mental status should be done on arrival, prior to treatment that may subsequently confound the clinical picture. Use of a standardized tool such as the Glasgow Coma Scale (GCS) or similar alternatives will help to quickly risk stratify, determine need for immediate interventions such as intubation, as well as help facilitate communication between members of the medical team. A systematic approach to mental status evaluation may in some cases also help to reveal coma mimics such as quadriparesis, where the patient may not be comatose at all.

Cranial Nerves Examination of brainstem reflexes may be the most reliable and specific tool for the clinician in a comatose patient. Pupillary responses are preserved even in the setting of sedation and neuromuscular blockade, and as such, may be the only available clue as to the underlying pathology. Miotic, reactive pupils may be seen in opiate intoxication or as a sign of a pontine lesion. By contrast, dilated pupils may be seen with anticholinergic toxicity. Progressive or unilateral pupillary dilation should be an immediate cue for the clinician to evaluate for and treat potential brain herniation and increased ICP. Horizontal nystagmus is common and can be the result of multiple etiologies, while vertical nystagmus is generally abnormal and indicative of brainstem dysfunction, whether structural or toxic. Dysconjugate eye position should raise concern for a structural brainstem lesion. Gaze deviation may suggest unilateral hemispheric dysfunction resulting from acute ischemia, a mass lesion, or seizure/post-ictal state, and should prompt evaluation for other signs of unilateral injury such as a facial droop (i.e., asymmetric grimace to pain) or hemiparesis.

Motor Examination While cooperation may be limited, observation and evaluation of motor response to noxious stimulus is nonetheless helpful. A patient presenting with altered sensorium but with preserved spontaneous or higher-level motor responses to stimulus (i.e., withdrawal or localization) is more likely to have a toxic/metabolic etiology that results in diffuse brain dysfunction. Conversely, there should be high suspicion for a focal, structural lesion in patients with asymmetric weakness (hemiparesis or paraparesis) or abnormal posturing. Signs of physical injury to the extremities (bruising, fractures, etc.) should prompt a careful examination for brain and spinal trauma as well.

Initial Stabilization

It goes without saying that a patient must be stabilized prior to embarking on the quest for a definitive diagnosis, and this includes neurologic stabilization in addition to airway, breathing, and circulation. If there is concern for trauma to the neuroaxis, spine precautions should be maintained. Signs of increased ICP or impending brain herniation (i.e., hypertension with bradycardia, unilaterally unresponsive pupil/CN III palsy) must trigger prompt, empiric intervention (i.e., elevation of head of bed and hyperosmolar therapy) prior to diagnostic imaging. As neurocritical care and neurosurgical interventions relevant to specific conditions are covered separately in this book, there will not be detailed discussion in this chapter. However, a few elements specific to the care of a patient presenting with coma deserve emphasis.

Airway Management

While it is often good clinical practice to secure the airway early in a patient with altered mentation and at risk of losing spontaneous airway control, it is prudent to make an extra, critical assessment of the need for intubation in the pregnant patient rather than relying on a blanket parameter such as GCS $\leq$ 8. The increased physiologic demands in pregnancy may increase the risk of potential complications from intubation and mechanical ventilation, such as precipitation of heart failure and acute respiratory distress syndrome (ARDS) [2, 3], in addition to any adverse effects of fetal exposure from the medications necessary to maintain this state. If the airway can be protected temporarily (i.e., with lateral positioning) with non-invasive delivery of oxygen, early results from initial workup may reveal rapidly reversible causes of coma (for example, opiate overdose, hypoglycemia, or a post-ictal state) that may preclude the need for intubation.

Blood Pressure Management

Severe hypertension, typically associated with eclampsia/preeclampsia, is specifically implicated in multiple pathologic processes during pregnancy which lead to neurologic injury, although hypotension can be just as detrimental. As pregnancy progresses, fetal demands on the maternal circulation with regard to need for additional cardiac output and an increased global oxygen consumption [2] means that the injured brain may be especially sensitive to systemic hemodynamic changes that result in decreased cerebral blood flow (CBF) and, therefore, oxygen delivery. This is especially true if there is increased ICP, as cerebral perfusion pressure (CPP), and by extension, CBF, is dependent on the gradient between mean arterial pressure (MAP) and ICP (CPP = MAP-ICP). In acute ischemic stroke, hypotension may likewise compromise collateral circulation to the ischemic penumbra of an affected region, potentially accelerating expansion of the infarct core and decreasing the efficacy of subsequent reperfusion procedures. This may be further compounded by the baseline hypocapnia/respiratory alkalosis seen in pregnancy [4], which may already result in cerebral vasoconstriction and affect normal compensatory autoregulation. As such, while severe hypertension should be immediately addressed, it may be prudent to slightly delay more aggressive BP lowering until structural lesions are ruled out.

Intracranial Pressure Management

Most neurocritical care interventions for ICP remain valid in a pregnant patient, however considerations must be made for her unique physiology. For example, increased circulating volume (up to 45% above baseline [2]) may necessitate increased doses of osmotic agents to achieve the same gradient for treatment of elevated ICP. In the same scenario, the previously mentioned baseline hypocapnia (PaCO$_2$ around 32 mmHg) makes hyperventilation a particularly risky intervention for both the mother as well as the fetus due to potentially decreased cerebral and uterine blood flow at even lower values [5].

Initial Studies

Laboratory

A point of care (POC) fingerstick glucose test should be obtained at the first opportunity (i.e., with vital signs and initial assessment) as hypoglycemia is a common and readily treatable cause of altered mental status. Minimum initial laboratory studies should include a complete blood count (CBC) and complete metabolic panel (CMP) covering electrolytes (including calcium), renal function tests, and liver function tests (LFTs). Patients who present febrile, or with other suspicion of infection, should have blood cultures. Urinalysis may also be helpful for an infectious workup, and while proteinuria is one of the diagnostic criteria for preeclampsia, it is notable that absence of this does not preclude the diagnosis per ACOG guidelines [6]. A urine toxicology screen may be considered in a patient presenting with unknown history and circumstances, though it should be noted that only a very small set of commonly encountered intoxicants will be detected on a rapid screen, and there are multiple hospital interventions on a critically ill patient, in particular sedatives and opiates, which may potentially confound the results. For these reasons, some advocate against its routine use [7]. Arterial/venous blood gases can be considered in cases of suspected poisonings or to guide mechanical ventilation, but for evaluation of respiratory status, there is likely already sufficient, actionable diagnostic information from other real-time monitoring sources (pulse oximetry, capnography, and exam).

Imaging

The role of imaging will vary by diagnosis/suspected diagnosis, as will be subsequently discussed. In general, a CT scan of the head will be indicated if there is suspicion for a structural lesion, along with contrast CT angiography (CTA) if a cerebrovascular disorder is suspected. While in theory, an MRI is preferable due to increased resolution of brain structures and lack of radiation exposure, the amount of time required for a usable image (minutes at best compared with seconds for a CT) during which a potentially unstable patient is inaccessible to staff and in a magnetic environment which limits use of equipment makes this an impractical option. Though it may be ultimately necessary, acute management decisions are largely made based on CT. Additional factors regarding the safety of various imaging modalities are discussed later in this chapter. In addition, neuroradiologic considerations for the pregnant patient are discussed in detail in Chap. 7.

Point of care ultrasound provides an interesting additional tool for the assessment of a comatose patient as it can be performed at bedside, however, the clinical effectiveness remains unclear. Measurement of optic nerve sheath diameter for the detection of elevated ICP has been widely reported, including specifically for use in evaluation of preeclamptic patients [8–10]. Likewise, transcranial doppler ultrasound (TCD) is a feasible method for detection of acute vascular occlusion in stroke, though this is highly dependent on a skilled operator [11]. However, the main limitation remains the inability to perform structural ultrasound imaging of the brain through the intact cranium of an adult, which still necessitates use of CT or MRI at some stage during diagnosis.

Diagnostic Process

Focusing the Differential

Despite there being several pathologic etiologies unique to pregnancy which are responsible for a large proportion of the neurologic complications, it is nonetheless helpful to approach a comatose pregnant patient in the same way as one approaches coma in any other patient. A core tenet in neurology is to not to confuse localization with an etiology, as premature focus on the latter can easily result in an anchoring bias and lead the clinician astray. As an example, one could imagine how a comatose, hypertensive pregnant patient with a normal appearing head CT could be sent down the pathway for management of preeclampsia rather than basilar stroke if

dysconjugate gaze and unilateral extensor posturing were overlooked and a CTA was not obtained. As such, while it is tempting to skip over localization and consider the myriad etiologies, it is essential to first determine whether a structural lesion can be implicated as the cause in any given presentation.

Structural causes for coma will usually be expected to also cause deficits that can be attributed to an anatomic region of the brain. Examples of this include cerebral infarction, intracranial hemorrhage, or mass lesions, which will cause specific deficits (hemiparesis, aphasia, etc.). There are metabolic processes which can cause structural lesions, however, with examples being prolonged seizures and encephalitis, or severe metabolic derangements and posterior reversible encephalopathy syndrome (PRES) which can result in cerebral edema. Conversely, there are structural causes such as obstructive hydrocephalus which may not result in a readily localizable deficit. It is important to note that for a structural lesion to result in coma, it must either involve (or progress to involve) both hemispheres of the brain or cause dysfunction at a common pathway, most commonly the reticular activating system (RAS) in the dorsal pons and midbrain. As such, particular attention should be paid to examination of brainstem reflexes. When identified, most structural lesions causing acute alteration in mental status and/or coma will require neuroimaging and emergent intervention.

If there are no clear signs of a focal deficit, or a structural cause is ruled out, processes that creating diffuse neuronal dysfunction should be considered. These will include such disparate causes as shock, hypoxia, infection/sepsis, and metabolic derangements (hypo/hyperglycemia, hyponatremia, uremia, hyperammonemia, etc.), and various intoxications. Finally, there are entities which somewhat straddle both categories, which include PRES, a disorder of autoregulation and endothelial leak associated with preeclampsia, and particularly important to consider in pregnancy, epilepsy, and psychiatric disorders. Table 16.1 illustrates some of the possible etiologies for coma and AMS in pregnancy.

Table 16.1 Causes of coma and altered mental status in pregnancy

Structural causes	Mixed/other	Toxic/metabolic causes
Ischemic stroke	Preeclampsia/eclampsia[a]	Hypo/hyperglycemia
Intracranial hemorrhage	PRES	Hypo/hypernatremia
Cerebral venous sinus thrombosis	Seizure and status epilepticus	Hypo/hyperthermia
Tumor/mass/abscess	Autoimmunity	Shock
Hydrocephalus	Quadriparesis[b]	Hypoxia
	Psychiatric[b]	Infection
		Endocrinopathy
		Renal failure
		Hepatic failure
		Intoxication and poisoning

[a] Condition unique to pregnancy
[b] Coma mimics

Structural Etiologies of Coma

Acute Ischemic Stroke

While the rate of ischemic stroke (AIS) in pregnancy is approximately three times that which is otherwise expected in this age group, it fortunately remains uncommon, estimated at around 12.2/100,000 pregnancies [12]. Multiple factors can be implicated, including the known induction of a hypercoagulable state during pregnancy increasing the risk of both embolic and thrombotic strokes, as well as increased incidence of hypertension leading to small vessel stroke. Unusual causes of stroke unique to pregnancy, such as amniotic fluid embolus, may also need to be considered. While altered consciousness may be a frequent finding in AIS, variably estimated between 4 and 38% in historical studies [13, 14], the degree of alteration reported in these studies can be hard to elucidate. For the anatomic reasons noted above (need for bi-hemispheric involvement or damage to the RAS), it is likely that some other clinical finding suggesting stroke, such as hemiparesis, will be the dominant symptom. In one study of the underlying causes of isolated AMS at presentation, only 8/127 patients had their symptoms attributable to AIS, and of these, only 2 were determined to have no other focal deficit after more detailed neurologic examination [15].

As a cause of a patient truly presenting in coma, outside of a large, completed hemispheric infarct causing surrounding cerebral edema, or extensive bilateral infarctions, basilar artery occlusion is the most likely single lesion that can be implicated. Basilar occlusions are rare, estimated at around 1% of stroke presentations [16], however due to very high morbidity and mortality if missed, the possibility must be carefully considered. Distal, "top of the basilar" occlusions are more likely to cause alterations in mental status due to involvement of the midbrain and the RAS-thalamic-cortical pathway, and motor function may actually be largely preserved aside from gaze palsies; conversely, mid-basilar infarctions affecting the pons may cause quadriparesis while leaving consciousness and vertical eye movements intact from collateral circulation from the Circle of Willis to the midbrain, resulting in "locked-in" syndrome which may initially be a coma mimic. More extensive occlusions may include combinations of all features [17]. Clinical exam should focus on examination of cranial nerves, particularly with attention to eye movements, as well as for presence of "crossed signs" of contralaterally occurring cranial nerve and limb deficits suggesting involvement of the brainstem. CT imaging of the posterior fossa is very unreliable due to surrounding bony structures, and in the acute phase, would be expected to be normal regardless. There may, however, be subtle clues such as a dense vessel sign in the basilar artery on non-contrast images. Contrast CT angiogram of the head and neck should be performed to assess for vessel patency if there is clinical suspicion. Current AHA/ASA guidelines support IV thrombolytic therapy with alteplase during pregnancy in the correct circumstances [18], and mechanical thrombectomy may also be possible (Fig. 16.2). The detail approach to evaluation and management of AIS in pregnancy is discussed in Chap. 3.

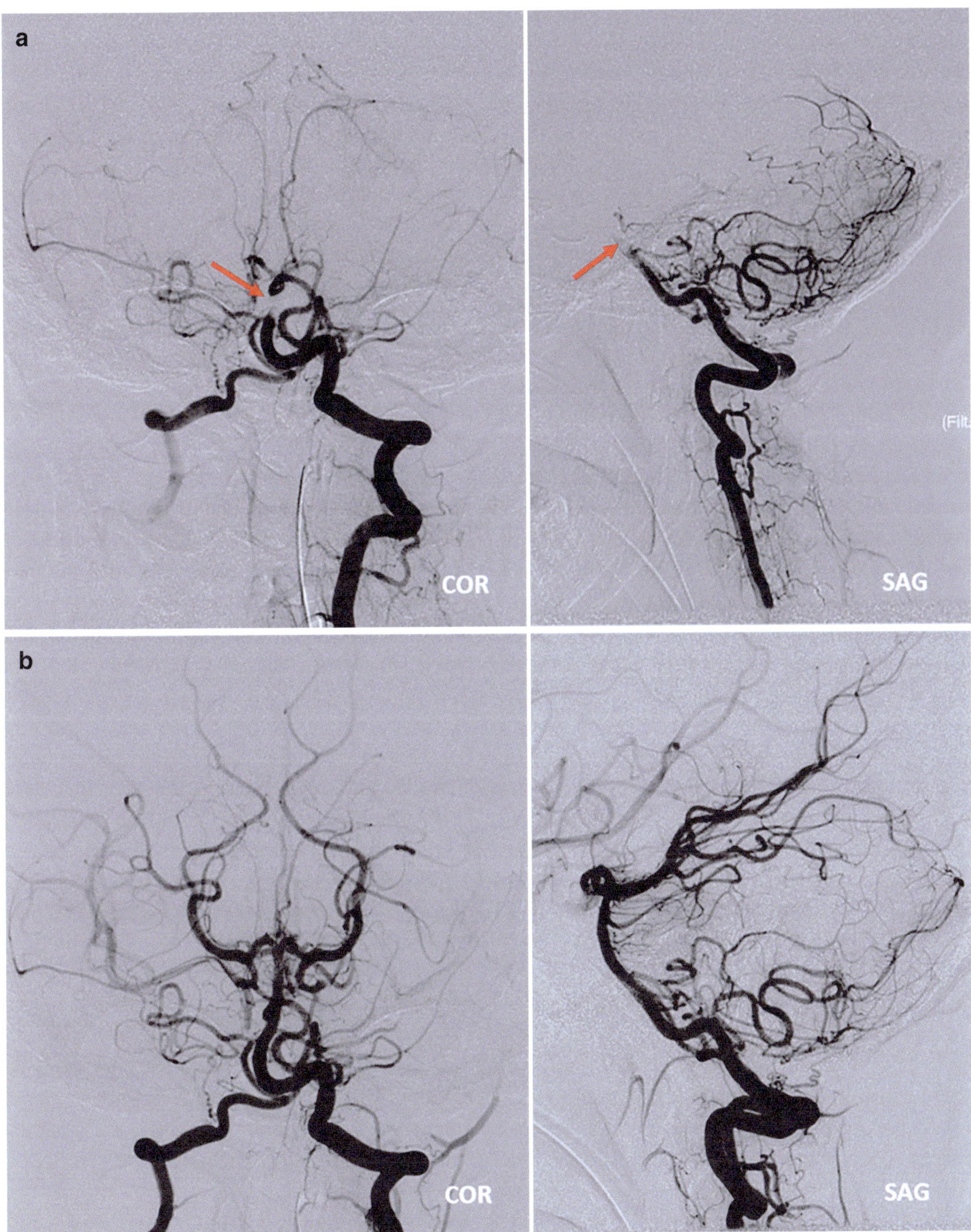

Fig. 16.2 Biplane cerebral angiographic images of a 22 year old patient presenting with distal basilar ("top-of the basilar") occlusion (**a**) and the same patient following successful mechanical thrombectomy (**b**). The initial clinical presentation was confusion, which progressed to posturing of extremities and progressive coma, triggering concern for basilar occlusion and transfer for thrombectomy. Post-reperfusion, the patient regained consciousness and was initially locked in, but subsequently regained voluntary movement in all her extremities over a period of several weeks

Cerebral Venous Sinus Thrombosis

Cerebral venous sinus thrombosis (CVST) is another thrombotic complication of pregnancy distinct from AIS, with an estimated incidence around 9.1/100,000 that is highest in the third trimester and first post-partum month [12, 19]. The pathology is the inverse of that seen in AIS, with a failure of drainage of a given brain area rather than supply, which will result in vascular congestion, cerebral edema, and hemorrhage. Seizures are also a frequent presenting symptom due to resulting cortical irritation. Extensive thrombosis or involvement of the superior sagittal sinus will affect drainage of both hemispheres, and therefore in contrast to arterial stroke, global alteration in mental status and coma may be a more common presenting sign. If there is no adequate collateral drainage, CVST may also eventually lead to increased ICP and death. Diagnosis is confirmed via imaging; non-contrast CT images may sometimes show patchy areas of vasogenic edema and/or multifocal hemorrhage in a pattern not characteristic of arterial occlusion or bleed, and occasionally, increased density of cortical vein or sinus structures can be seen. Contrast CT venography (CTV) will show the opposite, an area of non-contrast filling within the venous sinus, and non-contrast MR venography (MRV) will show absence of a flow void. Treatment is with therapeutic anticoagulation even in the presence of hemorrhage, with intravenous unfractionated heparin with transition to subcutaneous low molecular weight heparin (LMWH) through the remainder of pregnancy, and LMWH or transition to oral anticoagulants for a total treatment duration of at least 6 months [19]. Considerations pertaining to CVST in pregnancy are discussed in detail in Chap. 6.

Intracranial Hemorrhage

In comparison to cerebral ischemia, brain hemorrhages of any type can be expected to present with more profound alterations in consciousness by their nature as space occupying lesions which often occur with rapid initial expansion. Incidence of all spontaneous hemorrhages (those not due to a traumatic injury), including parenchymal (ICH), subarachnoid (SAH), and those arising from vascular malformations is likewise elevated during pregnancy, thought to be attributable to both hypertensive disorders, and possible loss of vascular compliance [20]. In addition to mass effect, blood in the subarachnoid space and ventricular system, particularly seen with SAH, may result in obstructive hydrocephalus with increased ICP and coma. Hemorrhages are readily diagnosed on non-contrast CT and an appropriate angiographic study if vascular lesion is suspected. Management includes blood pressure control, ICP management, including treatment of hydrocephalus and occasionally surgical decompression, as well as treatment of any underlying etiologies (i.e., aneurysm securement). Diagnosis and treatment of subarachnoid hemorrhage and other causes of hemorrhagic stroke are discussed in Chapters 2 and 4, respectively.

Other Structural Lesions

Most other brain lesions, such as tumors, expand slowly and are unlikely to cause acute AMS as a presenting finding. A cerebral abscess may expand more rapidly, though this is a rare occurrence and is likely to manifest other signs. However, hemorrhage into a tumor, a tumor causing transient hydrocephalus (i.e., colloid cyst), or a seizure caused by presence of an otherwise asymptomatic lesion may result in this type of clinical presentation. Of note, increased fluid retention may worsen edema caused by existing tumors, and neurohormonal changes in a pregnant patient may cause enlargement of meningiomas, vestibular schwannomas, and prolactinomas [5]. With pituitary tumors, in particular, there may be an increased risk of apoplexy, which can rarely result in coma due to compression on nearby brainstem structures. During management, careful assessment of endocrine function should be done if it occurs to avoid pregnancy complications. Finally, in a patient with existing hydrocephalus and a ventriculoperitoneal shunt, the gravid uterus during late pregnancy may obstruct shunt function, resulting in an extracranial structural cause of coma. As with all the other structural causes, appropriate imaging will be necessary for diagnosis of these conditions.

Preeclampsia, Eclampsia, and PRES

Hypertensive disorders of pregnancy are estimated to complicate 2–8% of pregnancies worldwide, and in the USA, are implicated in around 16% of maternal deaths [1, 6]. Preeclampsia is defined as new onset hypertension occurring after 20 weeks of gestation (two separate readings >140/90 mmHg, or a single occurrence >160/110 mmHg) in combination with evidence of end organ dysfunction, classically proteinuria, but now met by any thrombocytopenia, renal insufficiency, transaminitis, or new onset headache [6]. Eclampsia is diagnosed when seizures occur as the progression of this process (i.e., in the absence of other causes), however, this distinction may not be particularly important, as the underlying pathophysiology can cause significant neurologic injury even before clinical seizures are observed.

The underlying pathogenesis is complex and remains incompletely defined, however appears to be related to abnormal placentation and reduced placental perfusion. One of the effects of placental ischemia is increased placental release of antiangiogenic factors (sFLT1, sENG), which bind to and decrease circulating levels of VEGF and PIGF, growth factors necessary to maintain endothelial function. Simultaneously, other proinflammatory factors are released, as are autoantibodies to angiotensin II type 1. The end result is aberrant systemic vasoconstriction and hypertension, with leaky, impaired vascular endothelium [6, 21]. In the CNS, hypertension and vasculopathy along with coagulopathy (i.e., from thrombocytopenia or liver dysfunction) may already independently account for increased risk of cerebral hemorrhage in preeclamptic states, but the combination also results in loss of cerebral autoregulation and leaky blood–brain barrier, leading to vasogenic cerebral edema. The posterior circulation appears to be particularly vulnerable to this injury (though not exclusively so), resulting in a characteristic, symmetric, usually posterior dominant pattern of leukoencephalopathy on imaging (Fig. 16.3). These radiographic findings along

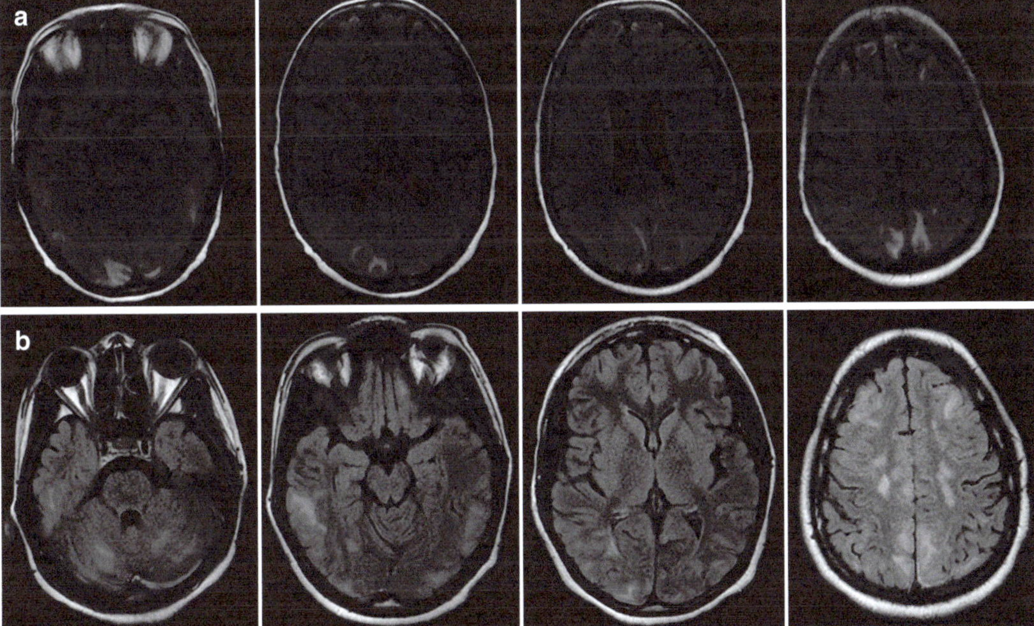

Fig. 16.3 Axial, T2 FLAIR MRI images at several levels showing a typical, posterior dominant pattern of vasogenic edema associated with PRES (sequence **a**), as well as a more diffuse, fulminant presentation involving frontal lobes and cerebellum (sequence **b**). Patient A presented clinically with acute onset encephalopathy and apparent aphasia, while patient B had persistent coma in the setting of eclampsia. Both patients recovered with appropriate management

with the resulting clinical findings of encephalopathy (up to and including coma), visual disturbance, and seizures define the posterior reversible encephalopathy syndrome (PRES) [22], which may be the common pathway of neurologic injury for most of the hypertensive disorders of pregnancy.

As it pertains to coma, severe PRES can be a sufficient causative factor, however, as aggressive blood pressure reduction is the hallmark of management, imaging to rule out a structural cause (and less importantly, to rule in PRES) is crucial. A known diagnosis of preeclampsia is insufficient, as the underlying systemic dysfunction may result in other causes of coma, for instance, ICH as previously noted, or cerebral edema as the result of hepatic failure. Both are potentially situations in which relative hypotension would result in accelerated cerebral ischemia. Once this is done, however, aggressive BP reduction to at least SBP <140 mmHg and DBP <90 mmHg should be undertaken, as despite the name, injury can frequently be irreversible and result in cell death and permanent injury. Magnesium sulfate infusion should also be initiated at this stage if a patient presents with alteration in consciousness as this is indicative of preeclampsia with severe features at high risk of progression to eclampsia [6]. If there is progression to eclampsia, magnesium should remain the first line agent for seizures, though delivery of the fetus/placenta would be indicated (and curative) at this stage, if not already considered. Pre-eclampsia, eclampsia, and PRES are described in detail in Chap. 33.

Of note, the aberrant vasoconstriction seen with preeclampsia can also occur in the brain, resulting in a vasospastic syndrome known as reversible cerebral vasoconstrictive syndrome (RCVS). This typically manifests clinically as severe, thunderclap headache, with focal deficits and encephalopathy seen in some cases. Due to appearance in the same population, this may occasionally lead to confusion with PRES, however imaging will typically be normal, or in severe cases may show small amounts of SAH or areas of edema corresponding to ischemia rather than diffuse vasogenic edema. An angiographic study will confirm the diagnosis, though CTA and MRA may not be able to adequately image the affected, distal vessels. Due to the typically mild nature, treatment is generally with oral calcium channel blockers. In rare cases, the vasoconstrictive process can progress to permanent ischemia and will warrant more aggressive intervention [5]. RCVS, more generally, and postpartum angiopathy, a specific RCVS variant, are discussed in Chapters 23 and 29, respectively.

Toxic and Metabolic Causes of Coma

Hypo- and Hyperglycemia

Hypoglycemia may easily result in AMS, and has myriad of underlying causes, but is easily detected and treated. A pregnant patient receiving adequate prenatal care is unlikely to be thiamine deficient, but repletion prior to administration of glucose must be considered in the right clinical scenario. Hyperglycemic coma in non-insulin dependent diabetics is linked to hyperosmolar state, which typically is seen with serum glucose >600 mg/dL or serum osmolality >320 mOsm/kg [23]. In type I diabetes and coma from DKA, an upper limit is more difficult to define, and specifically in pregnancy, euglycemic DKA has been reported [24]. History of type I diabetes and a lab testing establishing acidosis would be helpful. Initial management in both cases is with rehydration prior to insulin administration.

Hypo- and Hypernatremia

Mild hyponatremia (>130 mEq/L) is common in pregnancy and typically asymptomatic, however, acute worsening may occur, for instance, with vomiting and consumption of hypotonic fluids, and may easily become symptomatic [25]. Severe hyponatremia (<125 mEq/L) may lead to acute AMS, seizures, and cerebral edema. Care must be taken to correct sodium gradually if severe hyponatremia has been chronic as this may result in osmotic demyelination syndrome affecting the brainstem, which may itself result in coma and quadriparesis. Conversely, severe hypernatremia (>160 mEq/L) may also depress consciousness due to hyperosmolality but would be unlikely to occur spontaneously in a patient with intact thirst response and access to water.

Infection

While any infection may potentially cloud mental status, there should be a high level of concern for CNS infection if an, otherwise, healthy patient presents with significant AMS/coma, signs of infection such as fever but no indication of overwhelming systemic infection such as septic shock. Physical findings such as meningismus can be unreliable. There are no specific deviations from workup and empiric therapy resulting from a pregnant state only. Management of intracranial infections, including meningitis and encephalitis, is discussed in detail in Chap. 30.

Renal and Hepatic Impairment

In addition to electrolyte abnormalities, severe uremia during renal failure may contribute to depressed level of consciousness. Similarly, hepatic failure may lead independently to cerebral edema, or may be associated with hyperammonemia, which will depress mental status. Impairment of both will potentially affect clearance of medications which may confound the clinical picture. Dysfunction of these organs may occur because of preeclampsia, or independently of that process.

Endocrinopathies

Severe endocrine dysfunction in pregnancy is rare as most of these will preclude maintenance of the pregnant state, though theoretically, discontinuation of treatments during pregnancy could occur. When considering a patient presenting with significant AMS, aside from pituitary apoplexy as noted previously, Sheehan's syndrome, or postpartum pituitary infarction usually associated with hemorrhage, could result in panhypopituitarism and subsequent postpartum presentation for decreased level of consciousness from hypocortisolism (Addisonian crisis) or a severe hypothyroid state [26]. Pituitary neoplasms and their resultant endocrinopathies are discussed in detail in Chap. 12.

Intoxications and Poisonings

While there is likely lower incidence in the pregnant population compared with the overall population, intentional and accidental intoxications do occur. Usually this will be revealed by obtaining an exposure/medication history, or by observing resolution of symptoms over time with supportive care as other causes are investigated. Recognizing certain clinical toxidromes may also be helpful. As an example, recognizing the combination of pinpoint pupils, depressed respiratory drive, and decreased bowel sounds associated with opiate overdose in an unresponsive patient will prompt use of naloxone, which will be both diagnostic and therapeutic. As discussed previously, toxicology screens can be useful in the correct context, but the results must be critically evaluated against the known clinical data.

Mixed/Miscellaneous Causes of Coma

Seizures and Epilepsy

The most common cause of seizures in pregnancy overall is not eclampsia, but rather pre-existing epilepsy [27]. In a large registry study of pregnancies in mothers with epilepsy, the incidence of seizures was similar to the patients' baseline, and status epilepticus was fairly uncommon (1.8%) [28]. In patients presenting with AMS and a history of epilepsy, a post-ictal state, or non-convulsive status epilepticus (NCSE) must be considered when there is no clear explanation, and EEG may be required to rule out the possibility.

It is important to differentiate the seizures of eclampsia and that of primary epilepsy, as treatments differ. Magnesium sulfate does not generally play a role in the latter case, and seizures are treated with benzodiazepines and traditional antionvulsant agents as first line rather than for refractory control despite known teratogenic potential. It is notable, however, that patients with epilepsy can still develop eclampsia, and there may be patients who have a first seizure during pregnancy who have an alternate explanation; the presence/absence of the other signs of preeclampsia (hypertension, other organ dysfunction) will make the distinction. In particular, a presentation with status epilepticus rather than isolated seizure may suggest an alternative underlying pathology (frequently eclampsia and PRES) rather than primary epilepsy [29]. Management of epilepsy, including pre-conception planning and titration or initiation of alternative pharmacologic agents, is discussed in Chap. 8.

Autoimmune Conditions

Generally, there is a lower incidence and relapse rate of autoimmune conditions during pregnancy, often followed by a rebound/increase in the postpartum period. A well-studied example of this is seen in the reported clinical course of multiple sclerosis during pregnancy, which follows this pattern even when disease modifying therapies must be temporarily discontinued [30]. Clinical presentations are varied and can mimic infectious encephalitis or even mass lesions. Despite the rarity, this should be considered as part of the differential diagnosis. Considerations for evaluation and management of multiple sclerosis, Guillain-Barré, and myasthenia gravis during pregnancy are described in Chap. 9, 18, and 26.

Coma Mimics

Quadriparesis, resulting from pontine lesions (the previously mentioned locked-in syndrome) or occasionally high cervical spinal cord injury may resemble coma or an altered mental state on superficial examination if the presence of volitional cranial nerve mediated movements and other signs of underlying consciousness are not observed. Severe neuromuscular weakness of any cause (acute polyneuropathy, myasthenia gravis, botulism) may also present with a similar clinical picture if presented at a late stage in evolution. In all of these situations, there is often associated respiratory failure which will lead to a presentation in true coma, however after successful resuscitation and stabilization, careful neurologic examination to assess for signs of underlying consciousness should be performed. In the case of suspected spinal cord injury, a careful history and examination for signs of trauma, as well as

history of possible spinal procedures (i.e., epidural anesthesia for delivery) should trigger appropriate definitive diagnostic imaging, in this case MRI of the affected spinal segments. Neurotrauma in the pregnant patient is discussed in detail in Chap. 25.

Finally, after all other causes have been eliminated, consideration of psychogenic coma (conversion disorder, malingering), or other primary psychiatric conditions such as catatonia must be considered. This diagnosis is again established by careful neurologic examination which may provide clues to a non-structural cause for findings, or occasionally with supporting studies such as EEG which show a normal underlying brain pattern. However, these signs can frequently be deceiving or unreliable, and prior to settling on a psychogenic etiology, all other possible causes should be thoroughly explored. Mental health diseases arising during pregnancy are discussed in detail in Chap. 22.

Subsequent Management and Diagnostic Considerations

Due to the vastly disparate causes of coma, there is limited guidance possible beyond initial management and diagnosis due to very divergent treatment paths. However, there are some common considerations that exist when the diagnosis is unclear or with shared characteristics.

Management of Agitation and Delirium

Patients who present with severe encephalopathy can manifest with both hypoactive and hyperactive behaviors. In the latter case, sedation is occasionally needed to prevent inadvertent self and fetal harm, as well as harm to medical staff. In the case of pregnancy, optimal drug choice can be unclear. In general, due to the established teratogenicity of benzodiazepines, use in pregnancy should be avoided unless for indications such as status epilepticus or alcohol/GABA agonist withdrawal. Instead, the typical antipsychotics, such as haloperidol, are recommended by ACOG consensus guidelines as first line for severe agitation [31]. Dexmedetomidine may be an attractive maintenance option due to lack of respiratory depression, making it viable for use in non-intubated patients with severe agitation. After intubation, IV sedative/hypnotic agents may be unavoidable, and propofol is generally recommended, with opiates as necessary for analgesia [5, 32, 33]. Benzodiazepine infusions are less desirable in the critical care setting for all patients, and this holds true still in pregnancy.

Diagnostic Role of Electroencephalography (EEG)

When imaging and initial laboratory studies are unable to establish the diagnosis, yet AMS persists, EEG may be a useful tool to quickly exclude non-convulsive seizures/status epilepticus. While it is non-invasive and can be done at bedside, equipment and technician availability may vary widely between facilities, particularly during off hours, and placement in the emergency department or obstetric triage may be challenging due to the need to move patients around to facilitate flow. However, there are now commercially available devices involving a limited electrode montage that can be placed by staff after only minimal training and orientation. With recent literature reporting a comparable detection rate with limited montage vs. traditional EEG for status epilepticus and findings requiring immediate intervention in the hospital, this may provide for expanded access to this tool during initial workup of encephalopathy going forward [34, 35].

Diagnostic Role of Lumbar Puncture (LP)

Cerebrospinal fluid analysis may be immensely helpful for situations where CNS infection is suspected but unable to be confirmed from systemic tests such as blood cultures, or in cases of non-specific encephalitis. As exclusion of infection may prevent prolonged empiric antimicrobial exposure for the patient and fetus, pregnancy should not be a limiting factor when the test is otherwise indicated. There are no specific contraindications for LP from pregnancy itself, outside of the typical exclusions (coagulopathy, intracranial mass lesion, etc.). Positioning of the patient may be more difficult than normal, however, and anatomical landmarks may be more difficult to establish. If image guidance is necessary, use of a non-ionizing modality such as real-time ultrasound would be highly preferable due to the location of the fetus relative to the lumbar spine, with fluoroscopy reserved only for when the study is absolutely necessary.

Safety of Neuroimaging

As a general rule, pregnancy should not change the choice of imaging modality when evaluating a patient with an acute neurologic deficit, as any potential for harm to both the mother and fetus resulting from delayed diagnosis would likely outweigh any potential harm from the imaging technique. Concerns regarding ionizing radiation apply to any patient and should be considered when choosing a modality, regardless of pregnancy status. Specifically, regarding neuroimaging during pregnancy, CT studies of the head and neck result in minimal additional radiation exposure to the fetus, and when the study is otherwise indicated, use is widely accepted and established in guidelines [36, 37]. Iodinated contrast used in CT and traditional angiography has not been shown in humans to cause fetal harm during pregnancy, nor harm to an infant during breastfeeding, though screening should be done for hypothyroidism in the infant. Conversely, there is evidence that gadolinium-based MRI contrast may deposit in fetal tissue, with incompletely established physiologic effects, so careful evaluation of necessity prior to use is recommended [37]. Neuroimaging considerations during pregnancy are discussed in detail in Chap. 7.

Conclusion

The range of possible pathologies underlying coma and other states of altered mental status remains vast even in pregnancy, and the clinician must contend with a very broad differential diagnosis and potentially very divergent management pathways. Recognition of the unique physiologic states that exist during pregnancy will help guide the clinician along this process, and understanding is crucial to optimal management in this frequently medically challenging patient population.

References

1. Creanga AA, Syverson C, Seed K, Callaghan WM. Pregnancy-related mortality in the United States, 2011–2013. Obstet Gynecol. 2017;130:366–73.
2. Ouzounian JG, Elkayam U. Physiologic changes during Normal pregnancy and delivery. Cardiol Clin. 2012;30:317–29.
3. Guntupalli KK, Karnad DR, Bandi V, Hall N, Belfort M. Critical illness in pregnancy: part II: common medical conditions complicating pregnancy and puerperium. Chest. 2015;148:1333–45.
4. Lapinsky SE, Kruczynski K, Slutsky AS. Critical care in the pregnant patient. Am J Respir Crit Care Med. 1995;152:427–55.
5. Frontera JA, Ahmed W. Neurocritical care complications of pregnancy and puerperum. J Crit Care. 2014;29:1069–81.
6. ACOG Practice Bulletin No. 202: gestational hypertension and preeclampsia. Obstet Gynecol. 2019;133:e1s.
7. Traub SJ, Wijdicks EF. Initial diagnosis and management of coma. Emerg Med Clin North Am. 2016;34:777–93.
8. Dubost C, Le Gouez A, Jouffroy V, Roger-Christoph S, Benhamou D, Mercier FJ, et al. Optic nerve sheath diameter used as ultrasonographic assessment of the incidence of raised intracranial pressure in preeclampsia: a pilot study. Anesthesiology. 2012;116:1066–71.
9. Robba C, Santori G, Czosnyka M, Corradi F, Bragazzi N, Padayachy L, et al. Optic nerve sheath diameter measured sonographically as non-invasive estimator of intracranial pressure: a systematic review and meta-analysis. Intensive Care Med. 2018;44:1284–94.
10. Brzan Simenc G, Ambrozic J, Prokselj K, Tul N, Cvijic M, Mirkovic T, et al. Ocular ultrasonography for diagnosing increased intracranial pressure in patients with severe preeclampsia. Int J Obstet Anesth. 2018;36:49–55.
11. Mattioni A, Cenciarelli S, Eusebi P, Brazzelli M, Mazzoli T, Del Sette M, et al. Transcranial Doppler sonography for detecting stenosis or occlusion of intracranial arteries in people with acute ischaemic stroke. Cochrane Database Syst Rev. 2020;2:CD010722.
12. Swartz RH, Cayley ML, Foley N, Ladhani NNN, Leffert L, Bushnell C, et al. The incidence of pregnancy-related stroke: a systematic review and meta-analysis. Int J Stroke. 2017;12:687–97.
13. Li J, Wang D, Tao W, Dong W, Zhang J, Yang J, et al. Early consciousness disorder in acute ischemic stroke: incidence, risk factors and outcome. BMC Neurol. 2016;16:140.
14. Bogousslavsky J, Van Melle G, Regli F. The Lausanne Stroke Registry: analysis of 1,000 consecutive patients with first stroke. Stroke. 1988;19:1083–92.
15. Benbadis SR, Sila CA, Cristea RL. Mental status changes and stroke. J Stroke Cerebrovasc Dis. 1994;4:216–9.
16. Reinemeyer NE, Tadi P, Lui F. Basilar artery thrombosis. StatPearls. Treasure Island: StatPearls Publishing; 2020 [cited 2020 May 15]. http://www.ncbi.nlm.nih.gov/books/NBK532241/.
17. Demel SL, Broderick JP. Basilar occlusion syndromes. Neurohospitalist. 2015;5:142–50.
18. Demaerschalk BM, Kleindorfer DO, Adeoye OM, Demchuk AM, Fugate JE, Grotta JC, et al. Scientific rationale for the inclusion and exclusion criteria for intravenous alteplase in acute ischemic stroke a statement for healthcare professionals from the American Heart Association/American Stroke Association. Stroke. 2016;47:581–641.
19. Cheryl B, McCullough LD, Awad IA, Chireau MV, Fedder WN, Furie KL, et al. Guidelines for the prevention of stroke in women. Stroke. 2014;45:1545–88.
20. Camargo EC, Feske SK, Singhal AB. Stroke in pregnancy. Neurol Clin. 2019;37:131–48.
21. Phipps EA, Thadhani R, Benzing T, Karumanchi SA. Pre-eclampsia: pathogenesis, novel diagnostics and therapies. Nat Rev Nephrol. 2019;15:275–89.
22. Hinchey J, Chaves C, Appignani B, Breen J, Pao L, Wang A, et al. A reversible posterior leukoencephalopathy syndrome. N Engl J Med. 1996;334:494–500.
23. Kitabchi AE, Umpierrez GE, Murphy MB, Kreisberg RA. Hyperglycemic crises in adult patients with diabetes: a consensus statement from the American Diabetes Association. Diabetes Care. 2006;29:2739–48.
24. Munro JF, Campbell IW, McCuish AC, Duncan LJP. Euglycaemic diabetic ketoacidosis. Br Med J. 1973;2:578–80.
25. Pazhayattil GS, Rastegar A, Brewster UC. Approach to the diagnosis and treatment of hyponatremia in pregnancy. Am J Kidney Dis. 2015;65:623–7.
26. Laway BA, Mir SA. Pregnancy and pituitary disorders: challenges in diagnosis and management. Indian J Endocrinol Metab. 2013;17:996–1004.
27. Karnad DR, Guntupalli KK. Neurologic disorders in pregnancy. Crit Care Med. 2005;33:S362–71.

28. Battino D, Tomson T, Bonizzoni E, Craig J, Lindhout D, Sabers A, et al. Seizure control and treatment changes in pregnancy: observations from the EURAP epilepsy pregnancy registry. Epilepsia. 2013;54:1621–7.
29. Rajiv KR, Radhakrishnan A. Status epilepticus in pregnancy – can we frame a uniform treatment protocol? Epilepsy Behav. 2019;101:106376.
30. Vukusic S, Hutchinson M, Hours M, Moreau T, Cortinovis-Tourniaire P, Adeleine P, et al. Pregnancy and multiple sclerosis (the PRIMS study): clinical predictors of post-partum relapse. Brain J Neurol. 2004;127:1353–60.
31. ACOG Practice Bulletin No. 92: use of psychiatric medications durinsg pregnancy and lactation. Obstet Gynecol. 2008;111:1001–20.
32. Kaur M, Singh PM, Trikha A. Management of critically ill obstetric patients: a review. J Obstet Anaesth Crit Care. 2017;7:3.
33. Pacheco LD, Saade GR, Hankins GDV. Mechanical ventilation during pregnancy: sedation, analgesia, and paralysis. Clin Obstet Gynecol. 2014;57:844–50.
34. Kamousi B, Grant AM, Bachelder B, Yi J, Hajinoroozi M, Woo R. Comparing the quality of signals recorded with a rapid response EEG and conventional clinical EEG systems. Clin Neurophysiol Pract. 2019;4:69–75.
35. Westover MB, Gururangan K, Markert MS, Blond BN, Lai S, Benard S, et al. Diagnostic value of electroencephalography with ten electrodes in critically ill patients. Neurocrit Care. 2020;33:479.
36. Chansakul T, Young GS. Neuroimaging in pregnant women. Semin Neurol. 2017;37:712–23.
37. Committee on Obstetric Practice. Committee opinion no. 723: guidelines for diagnostic imaging during pregnancy and lactation. Obstet Gynecol. 2017;130:e210–6.

Management of Neurological Trauma in the Pregnant Patient

Christopher E. Talbot and Antonios Mammis

Introduction

A pregnant mother presenting with traumatic brain injury (TBI), especially in moderate to severe cases, creates unique and complex care decisions for providers. As this presentation is rare compared to the total incidence of TBI, there is an overall scarcity of studies guiding care of these patients. Additionally, appropriate care will often require consideration of both the lives of the mother and fetus. The viability and gestational age of the fetus become forefront variables in the care of the injured mother and may carry strong ethical considerations. For instance, a viable fetus may have profound effect on the care decisions made for an otherwise neurologically devastated mother. Not only does this stir a complex ethical discussion, but also a profound consideration of obstetrical care which the typical TBI provider (i.e., intensivist, neurosurgeon, etc.) is not familiar with.

In the following chapter, the authors will present prominent considerations in the care of the pregnant TBI patient and examine any existing literature. This shall be presented first as a brief review of TBI for the provider who does not encounter TBI regularly (i.e., obstetrician), followed by a review of specific TBI practices and their considerations for a pregnant patient, and finally a brief discussion addressing the ethical considerations of caring for both mother and fetus.

A Review of TBI

Traumatic brain injury may be stratified into mild, moderate, and severe categories based on the patient's presenting Glasgow Coma Scale (GCS). The GCS is a tool which measures the patient's best eye, motor, and verbal responses. The GCS has been used to stratify TBI as mild (14–15), moderate (9–13), or severe (3–8) [1]. Traditionally, mild TBI has been used synonymously with concussion and usually implies a good prognosis.

Multiple studies have shown an inverse relationship between GCS and mortality, with mortality rates reaching between 65% and 78% as GCS decreases to a minimum score of 3 [2–4]. Despite the GCS being a validated and reliable tool for communication and prognosis, characteristics of the traumatic event, healthcare response, acute clinical course, clinical exam, and radiographic exams are also imperative in guiding providers through treatment decisions and goals of care discussions. Furthermore, GCS is an inade-

C. E. Talbot
Department of Neurological Surgery, Rutgers New Jersey Medical School, Newark, NJ, USA

A. Mammis (✉)
Department of Neurological Surgery, NYU Grossman School of Medicine, New York, NY, USA
e-mail: antonios.mammis@nyulangone.org

G. Gupta et al. (eds.), *Neurological Disorders in Pregnancy*,
https://doi.org/10.1007/978-3-031-36490-7_17

quate descriptor of the patient's neurological status past the acute period.

It is important to define a few frequently used terms to describe a prolonged diminished mental status. In addition to the standard facets of the neurological exam, terminology exists to better describe the patient's states of consciousness and arousal. In severe TBI, this can be challenging and frequently terms such as "brain death" and "persistent vegetative state" are misused [5]. "Brain death" is the irreversible loss of all brainstem reflexes and persistent apnea in a comatose patient without the presence of other confounders. The concept of brain death is widely accepted by most as death of the individual. The additional demonstration of complete loss of perfusion throughout the entire brain is used by a portion of clinicians through computed tomographic angiography (CTA) or nuclear medicine perfusion (NMP) techniques [6]. "Coma" is a state of absent arousal, consciousness, and eye-opening lasting at least 1 h. Patients in a "vegetative state" are awake but unaware of self or environment. The prefix of "persistent" is added to vegetative state when this state has persisted for longer than 1 month, but this does not imply irreversibility. "Minimally conscious state" was proposed as a subgroup of patients exhibiting function higher than that of vegetative state but not consistently. Lastly, "locked-in" syndrome is a state of preserved awareness but disruption of corticospinal and corticobulbar pathways resulting in quadriplegia, severely impaired cranial nerve motor function, and aphonia or hypophonia. These functions may include intermittent command following, verbal response, or purposeful behavior. With the exception of brain death, a patient in any one of these may have the potential to recover function and move into another higher-functioning state [5, 7–10].

In many circumstances, there are additional variables or conditions which prevent the above states from being diagnosed in an individual who has suffered severe TBI. Confidence in one of the above diagnoses requires stabilization, reduction of confounding factors, and usually advanced imaging such as MRI. As such, the decision to pursue or withdraw aggressive treatment for a severe TBI patient remains difficult to navigate in many situations where prognosis is not clear. Previous wishes of patients either relayed verbally, in a written advanced directive, or not shared can also play an important role in decision making.

In 2016, the fourth edition of "Guidelines for Management of Severe Traumatic Brain Injury" was released by the Brain Trauma Foundation (New York, New York) and later published in 2017 [4]. This work reviewed 189 publications and divided systematic and evidence-based recommendations into 18 topics. Although widely accepted, adherence to these guidelines is variable and the impact of adherence on patient outcomes requires further studies [11–13].

TBI Guidelines and the Pregnant Patient

As stated previously, there is an extreme absence of data to guide care of the pregnant patient who has sustained TBI. The exact incidence of PVS or brain death post-TBI in the pregnant patient is unknown. The literature shows a large number of mothers who suffered debilitating neurological injury secondary to motor vehicle accidents; however, the exact incidence and how it compares to the general population is unknown [14, 15].

The Brain Trauma Foundation guidelines do not specify this subgroup of patients and many of the influential publications used to form these guidelines exclude pregnancy in their studies. The authors of this chapter conducted a literature review and were unable to identify any Class I or Class II evidence regarding this patient population. As such, the following discussion identifies TBI care topics as described in the Brain Trauma Foundation guidelines and possible additional considerations in the pregnant patient. These considerations have been identified either through Class III evidence, case reports, or the author's own theory or deduction based on known physiological or pathological principles in TBI or pregnancy. Topics without any additional considerations or contributing evidence in the pregnant TBI patient have been identified as such.

Treatments

Decompressive Craniectomy

The Brain Trauma Foundation offers level IIA recommendations for a large frontotemporoparietal decompressive craniectomy (DC) for reduced mortality and improved neurologic outcomes in patients with severe TBI [4]. In the author's review of the literature, there were multiple case reports of DC for pregnant patients sustaining severe TBI [16–18]. There were found to be multiple instances of DC in pregnant or post-partum patients for other etiologies of increased intracranial pressure (ICP) such as intracranial hemorrhage, arteriovenous malformation rupture, and venous sinus thrombosis [19–21]. In some cases, it may be appropriate to coordinate emergent DC with emergent cesarean section [16]. Execution of this dual-operation would likely benefit from interdisciplinary discussion and planning between obstetric, neurosurgery, anesthesia, and perioperative teams. There were no studies to change or influence this guideline in the pregnant patient.

Prophylactic Hypothermia

Hypothermia has been previously utilized in TBI treatment for reducing tissue damage through reduction of cerebral metabolic demand and reduction of ICP. However, this therapy's benefit has been weighed against the risks of coagulopathy, immunosuppression, cardiac dysrhythmia, and death. The Brain Trauma Foundation offers level IIB recommendation that early and short-term hypothermia is not recommended to improve outcomes in these patients [4]. Although hypothermia has been shown to improve neurologic outcome in cardiac arrest, pregnancy is considered a relative contraindication [22, 23]. There was no evidence to change or influence the Brain Trauma Foundation guideline on prophylactic hypothermia.

Hyperosmolar Therapy

Mannitol and hypertonic therapy are commonly administered in the context of elevated ICP for their ability to decrease brain volume and therefore ICP. In the case of mannitol, it is now known that the reduction of ICP is attributed to reduction of blood viscosity and decreased circulatory or flow resistance within circulation. In the third edition of guidelines from the Brain Trauma Foundation, mannitol was recommended for control of elevated ICP [4]. However, this recommendation was not carried forward in the fourth edition given insufficient evidence in regard to outcomes. The guidelines do recognize an increased use of hypertonic saline in the setting of refractory elevated ICP as compared to mannitol. Mannitol is assigned as a pregnancy Category C agent by the FDA, meaning animal reproduction studies have shown an adverse effect on the fetus; however, there have been no adequate human studies. Although a number of case reports utilized these therapies to reduce ICP [24], there were no studies to change or influence the Brain Trauma Foundation's recommendation on hyperosmolar therapy in the pregnant patient.

Cerebrospinal Fluid Drainage

Placement of an external ventricular drain has been routinely performed in patients with suspected intracranial pathology leading to increased ICP for its ability to both measure ICP in the closed position and provide therapeutic drainage of cerebrospinal fluid (CSF) in an open position. The use of this system in severe TBI has been a controversial topic. The Brain Trauma Foundation provides level III recommendations stating placement of EVD may be considered to lower ICP in patients with a GCS <6 during the first 12 h after injury and that continuous drainage with EVD at the level of the midbrain may be more effective at lowering ICP than intermittent drainage [4]. Although the authors found multiple case reports of EVD placement in the pregnant patient [25–28], there was no evidence to further modify or influence this guideline in the pregnant patient with severe TBI.

Ventilation Therapies

Rapid sequence intubation for airway protection is a generally accepted practice in any patient with suspected severe TBI and GCS <9 [29–32]. The use of prophylactic hyperventilation has been controversial and the Brain Trauma Foundation offers level IIB recommendation that prolonged prophylactic hyperventilation with partial pressure of carbon dioxide in arterial blood ($PaCO_2$) of 25 mmHg or less is not recommended [4]. Although low $PaCO_2$ is believed to decrease ICP through vasoconstriction and decreases in cerebral blood volume, the decreased cerebral blood flow may result in cerebral ischemia. Alternatively, increased $PaCO_2$ may result in cerebral hyperemia and increased ICP. The authors found no evidence for consideration of this guideline in the pregnant TBI patient.

Anesthetics, Analgesics, and Sedatives

These pharmacologic agents have been used in the management of TBI patients for several reasons including control of ICP, seizure prophylaxis, and patient comfort. ICP may be reduced by not only limiting elevations caused by agitation, coughing, and other Valsalva-like actions, but also through reduction of the cerebral metabolic rate. The Brain Trauma Foundation provides three level IIB guidelines: (1) administration of barbiturates to induce burst suppression as prophylaxis for reduction of ICP is not recommended, (2) high-dose barbiturate administration is recommended to control elevated ICP refractory to maximal standard medical and surgical treatment, and (3) administration of propofol for control of ICP is not recommended for improvement in outcome and may be associated with increased morbidity at high doses [4]. The authors could not find any evidence to contribute to these practices in the pregnant TBI patient. Of note, the US FDA considers barbiturates as pregnancy Category D meaning there is enough evidence showing these medications can cause fetal damage. Propofol is considered a pregnancy Category B medication, meaning it is considered safe to use if there is a clinical need. Anesthetic and analgesic considerations during pregnancy are discussed in detail in Chaps. 10 and 11, respectively.

Steroids

In neurocritical care, steroids are commonplace and used routinely to reduce vasogenic cerebral edema and therefore ICP in the context of brain tumors. Although a historical debate has surrounded their use in neurologic trauma, multiple studies have shown no benefit of steroids on outcome in severe TBI [33]. The Corticosteroid Randomization After Significant Head Injury (CRASH) trial was a multicenter randomized clinical trial which compared mortality between moderate and severe TBI patients receiving corticosteroids versus placebo [34, 35]. Steroid-allocated patients received a 2 g loading dose of methylprednisolone followed by an additional 19.2 g over 48-h continuous infusion for a total of 21.2 g [36]. This dose is equivalent to 106.0 mg hydrocortisone [37, 38]. The study was halted when there was determined to be a higher risk of death in the treatment group (21.1% vs. 17.9%) regardless of injury severity or time since injury [34]. The Brain Trauma Foundation provides level I recommendations against the use of high-dose methylprednisolone in severe TBI patients [4].

In obstetrics, antenatal corticosteroids have been shown to reduce the morbidity and mortality of hyaline membrane disease through accelerated fetal lung development and improved lung function immediately post-partum [39]. This therapy consists of either two doses of 12 mg intramuscular betamethasone or four doses 6 mg intramuscular dexamethasone. These doses each convert to 640.0 mg hydrocortisone [37, 38].

In equivalents of hydrocortisone over a 48-h period, it appears a much larger dose of steroid is administered for fetal lung maturation than was used in the CRASH trial treatment group. The agents above further differ in other properties [37] In terms of duration of action, methylprednisolone lasts between 12 and 36 h whereas dexamethasone and betamethasone are each long acting, lasting between 36 and 54 h.

Methylprednisolone is the only agent of these three that demonstrates mineralocorticoid activity. Lastly, both dexamethasone and betamethasone have anti-inflammatory potencies 30 times greater than hydrocortisone versus methylprednisolone which has a potency only 5 times greater.

Recently, multiple in vivo and clinical studies have suggested a neuroprotective role of certain sex steroid hormones such as estrogen and progesterone [40–47]. The neuroprotective mechanism of these hormones has been postulated to be a multifactorial mechanism through protection against glutamate toxicity, antioxidant action, anti-inflammatory action, improved cerebral blood flow, and possible action against apoptotic pathways [46–49]. These findings have led to a generalized belief that pregnant women, with inherent elevation of estrogen and progesterone, may demonstrate improved outcomes in TBI. Despite the above cited research, several other studies have failed to support this relationship [50–53].

Nutrition

The Brain Trauma Foundation offers level IIA recommendation to attain basal caloric replacement by the 5th day post-injury and to avoid under-nutrition past the 7th day post-injury to decrease mortality [4]. The guidelines also offer level IIB recommendations to provide transgastric jejunal feeding over nasogastric or orogastric means to reduce the incidence of ventilator-associated pneumonia [4].

Infection Prophylaxis

The Brain Trauma Foundation provides level IIA recommendations for early tracheostomy to reduce mechanical ventilation days and avoidance of providine-iodine oral care as this does not reduce ventilator-associated pneumonia and may increase risk of acute respiratory distress syndrome [4]. They provide level III evidence that antimicrobial-impregnated EVD catheters may prevent catheter-related infections [4]. The authors were unable to find any significant studies to contribute to or modify these recommendations in the pregnant patient with severe TBI. Of note, cephalosporins are considered pregnancy Category B and IV vancomycin is pregnancy Category C.

Deep Vein Thrombosis Prophylaxis

Severe TBI patients are at risk for venous thromboembolism (VTE) not only because of their lack of mobilization and potential neurological deficits causing weakness or flaccidity, but also secondary to a hypercoagulable state induced by the brain injury. Predictors of deep vein thrombosis (DVT) include age, subarachnoid hemorrhage, an Injury Severity Score >15, and extremity injury [54]. This risk has been quantified and approximated to be 3–4 times increased over a non-TBI sample [55]. The Brain Trauma Foundation provides level III recommendations for low molecular weight heparin (LMWH) or low-dose unfractionated heparin to be used in combination with mechanical prophylaxis such as serial compression devices, however initiation of pharmaceutical prophylaxis should be weighed with the risk of potential expansion of intracranial hemorrhage [4].

Pregnant women are five times more likely to develop DVT as compared to non-pregnant women and the frequency of DVT is similar throughout all three trimesters [56]. Additionally, pulmonary embolism (PE) is the leading cause of maternal death in the US and other developed nations [56–58]. Unfractionated heparin is considered pregnancy Category C by the US FDA whereas LMWH is designated as pregnancy Category B.

As identified above, both severe TBI and pregnancy are independent risk factors for DVT and VTE which may put individuals at risk for significant morbidity and mortality. The relationship of these combined risk factors in the pregnant patient who has sustained severe TBI is unknown. Without further studies, it is unknown whether these two combined risk factors produce a purely summative effect on the patient's risk for DVT or VTE. Mechanical prophylaxis should be initiated as deemed clinically safe, possibly with routine screening for DVT on admission. Pharmaceutical prophylaxis in the form of unfractionated heparin should be initiated after the benefit of such is determined to outweigh the risk of expanding intracranial hemorrhage. Considerations for the use of anticoagulation during pregnancy are discussed in Chap. 28.

Seizure Prophylaxis

Severe TBI puts patients at risk for seizures and epilepsy [4]. Clinically evident post-traumatic seizure may have an incidence of as high as 12% and perhaps even greater for subclinical seizures. Post-traumatic epilepsy is defined as recurrent seizures more than 7 days following injury.

The Brain Trauma Foundation provides two level IIA recommendations regarding seizure prophylaxis [4]. First, the prophylactic use of phenytoin or valproate is not recommended for preventing late (>7 days post-injury) post-traumatic seizure. Second, phenytoin is recommended to decrease the incidence of early (<7 days post-injury) post-traumatic seizure when the benefit is felt to outweigh the risk of such treatment.

Anti-epileptic drug (AED) use during pregnancy has for the most part been studied in the epilepsy population, and levetiracetam is believed to be a risk factor for major congenital malformations when used during pregnancy [59]. That risk increases with polytherapy and additional AEDs. Valproate use during pregnancy may increase rates of autism but typically shows better control of seizures in the pregnant epileptic population [60]. The risk of spina bifida increases with exposure to valproate, digit hypoplasia with phenytoin, oral clefts with phenobarbital, and neural tube defects with carbamazepine [61].

There are no significant studies investigating post-traumatic seizure incidence or prophylaxis in the pregnant severe TBI patient. Selection of AEDs during pregnancy is discussed in Chap. 8.

Monitoring

Intracranial Pressure

ICP monitoring has become an essential objective measure in the assessment and care of severe TBI patients. The correlation between elevated ICP and secondary brain injury has been well established, and a clinician's ability to access ICP data is crucial in guiding other therapies. The Brain Trauma Foundation provides level IIB recommendation for use of ICP monitoring in severe TBI patients to reduce in-hospital and 2-week post-injury mortality [4].

There exist many case reports of ICP monitoring devices such as EVDs in pregnant patients; however, there is no significant evidence to contribute to or alter the Brain Trauma Foundation's recommendation.

Cerebral Perfusion Pressure

In regard to cerebral perfusion pressure (CPP) monitoring in the severe TBI patient, the Brain Trauma Foundation has a level IIB recommendation for CPP monitoring to decrease 2-week mortality [4].

During in utero development, the fetus is completely dependent on the placenta, uteroplacental exchange, and uterine perfusion [62, 63]. The placental hemodynamics are poorly understood and difficult to monitor precisely in a clinical setting. There are detrimental effects of hypoperfusion of the placenta as well as maternal hypertension, however, the authors were unable to find precise parameters or guidelines in the literature. There is no significant evidence to contribute to or alter the Brain Trauma Foundation's recommendation.

Advanced Cerebral Monitoring

Advanced cerebral monitoring techniques include the assessment of blood flow and oxygenation by transcranial doppler sonography, arteriovenous oxygen content difference ($AVDO_2$) monitoring, and local tissue oxygen and carbon dioxide tension measurements.

The Brain Trauma Foundation provides a level III recommendation for use of jugular bulb monitoring of $AVDO_2$ to help guide management decisions [4]. This guideline is thought to reduce mortality and improve outcomes at 3- and 6-months post-injury.

Thresholds

Blood Pressure

The Brain Trauma Foundation provides a level III guideline to consider maintenance of SBP at $\geq$100 mmHg for patients 50–69 years old or at

≥110 mmHg or above for patients 15–49 or over 70 years old to decrease mortality and improve outcomes [4].

Agent selection is also complicated by the pregnant patient and is discussed in relation to ischemic and hemorrhagic stroke in Chaps. 3 and 4, respectively. Notably, nicardipine is considered FDA pregnancy Category C.

Intracranial Pressure

The Brain Trauma Foundation guidelines have level IIB and II recommendations for the treatment of ICP above 22 mmHg to decrease mortality and use of ICP values, clinical findings, and brain CT findings to make management decisions, respectively [4]. There are no significant studies to contribute to or modify this recommendation for the pregnant TBI patient.

Cerebral Perfusion Pressure

The Brain Trauma foundation states a level IIB recommendation for target CPP value for survival and favorable outcomes to be between 60 and 70 mmHg [4]. The guidelines further comment whether 60 or 70 mmHg is the minimum optimal CPP threshold is unclear and may depend upon the patient's autoregulatory status. They also provide a level III recommendation for avoiding aggressive attempts to maintain CPP above 70 mmHg with fluids and pressors due to the risk of adult respiratory failure. There are no significant studies to contribute to or modify this recommendation for the pregnant TBI patient. Details on the effect of pregnancy on cerebral perfusion and autoregulation are described in Chap. 20.

Advanced Cerebral Monitoring

The Brain Trauma Foundation guidelines have level III recommendation that jugular venous saturation of <50% may be a threshold to avoid in order to reduce mortality and improve outcomes [4]. There are no significant studies to contribute to or modify this recommendation for the pregnant TBI patient.

Additional Considerations

In addition to the above discussion on the Brain Trauma Foundation guidelines, the topics below were identified by the authors to be pertinent for appropriate care of the pregnant TBI patient.

Hospital Resources and Transfer of Patients

Many primary care hospitals lack neurocritical care units, trauma teams, and/or neurosurgeons accustomed to caring for severe TBI patients. In the presentation of a pregnant patient with severe TBI and possible additional injuries, availability of the above services in addition to obstetricians and neonatal intensivists comfortable with emergent and preterm delivery is preferred. A multidisciplinary approach provides the breadth of knowledge and resources necessary for this complex presentation, however, a high-level of evidence for such a recommendation to improve outcomes is non-existent [17, 64]. There is also unclear evidence that admission to larger volume hospitals result in improved care in severe TBI patients. Higher volume hospitals may be associated with lower in-hospital mortality for severe TBI patients [65, 66]. Appropriate assessment and decision making requires presence of both neurosurgical and obstetric teams for a multidisciplinary approach. Decision to transfer a patient to a higher-level care facility should be made only after considering the patient's neurological, hemodynamic, and obstetric stability as well as any possible consequences of transfer such as prolonged time to treatment and the inherent risks of patient transport.

Assessing Fetal Status and Timing of Delivery

Determining fetal status is a responsibility of the obstetrician and should be conducted as soon as possible in a pregnant patient who has sustained a trauma. Fetal monitoring is considered part of the secondary survey in a pregnant trauma patient [67, 68]. This assessment is crucial in a pregnant patient presenting with severe TBI, and signs of fetal compromise or distress should be identified with haste as they could have a considerable impact on the patient's acute clinical course. Assessment of fetal status includes patient's obstetric and gynecologic history (if available), gynecologic examination, and fetal cardiotocography [67, 68].

Emergency cesarean section is indicated with fetal distress, antepartum hemorrhage, or circumstances otherwise life-threatening to the fetus and/or mother [69]. If no emergent delivery is indicated, the gestation of the fetus may be continued safely by systemically supporting the mother to maintain a near-normal physiological state [15]. Several case reports have been published in which mothers with devastating, non-recoverable neurological injury, such as brain death, have undergone maximal treatment for the protective benefit of the fetus. In these cases, the mother was deemed to be in a stable and non-salvageable neurological state [15, 17, 70]. Whitney et al. present a case of decompressive hemicraniectomy on a severely injured pregnant mother in order to control ICP. This patient was not brain dead on presentation, surgery was an option regardless of fetal gestational age, and the fetus was of not-yet-viable gestational age [17].

Depending on the degree of neurological injury, maintenance of a normal and safe physiological state in the mother will require supportive measures and interventions. A mother who is diagnosed with brain death will require mechanical ventilation, and many severely injured patients will require nutritional support [71]. In addition, the loss of vagal tone or sympathetic storming phenomenon may result in profound hemodynamic instability with times of hypertension or hypotension [15].

Imaging Considerations

Imaging considerations for the pregnant patient range from consequences of irradiation to the fetus to comfort and safety of the patient. Routine imaging of the head and brain (CT or MRI) is usually performed with the patient in the supine position and the patient frequently is transferred from the bed to table in this position. As such, there is unlikely mechanical risk of harm with frequent CT head and angiography suite transfers of the pregnant patient.

In computed tomography (CT), fetal radiation doses for examinations of the head or chest are minimal and, therefore, do not complicate the risk-benefit analysis because the fetus is not directly imaged [72]. In CT imaging of the abdomen or pelvis, radiation dose should be considered because the fetus is likely to be directly exposed.

Magnetic resonance brain imaging (MRI brain) may be helpful in prognostication as it can help identify specific lesions associated with better or worse long-term outcomes. Gadolinium is not routinely used in the assessment of traumatic lesions. Haghbayan et al. found MRI was helpful in the identification of lesions which were difficult to discern on CT imaging such as those of the brain stem or diffuse axonal injury [73]. In that regard, MRI is useful in providing prognostic information; however, large well-controlled studies are necessary [1]. A large retrospective study by Ray et al. found there to be no increased risk of harm to the fetus associated with MRI during the first trimester. However, administration of gadolinium at any time during pregnancy was associated with an increased risk of rheumatological, inflammatory, or infiltrative skin conditions and stillbirth or neonatal death [74]. Considerations for neuroimaging in the pregnant patient are discussed in detail in Chap. 7.

Caring for Both Mother and Fetus

Pregnancy adds a potentially complicating variable to the patient who has sustained traumatic neurological injury. In addition to the paucity of evidence guiding our care, there also emerges an ethical discussion in which providers must consider the status of both the mother and fetus. This dilemma of "a body with two lives" may complicate an otherwise clear clinical course if the patient had presented without pregnancy [75].

These situations have been described many times in the literature and range in severity for both mother and fetus. In the events of brain death, devastating neurological injury without salvageable function, or otherwise grave prognosis for the mother, many clinicians will then focus care toward achieving good fetal outcome [17, 76, 77]. In some cases, mothers declared brain dead or in other vegetative state have undergone life-saving or life-preserving measures in order to maintain the fetus until viable for delivery [17].

However, in severe TBI, the mother may not present neurologically devastated or her chances for neurological recovery may be unclear. It is in these circumstances that the decision making process for neurosurgeons and other providers becomes more complex. Interests and therapies for the mother and fetus may potentially compete and require compromise at the expense of optimal treatment for either. It is in these situations that no agreed upon guidelines or recommendations exist. Major factors contributing to the care plan include the hemodynamic stability of both mother and fetus, the gestational age and history of fetus, and the neurological stability and salvageability of mother. Other factors which may influence management include the experience of a care plan which includes neurosurgery and obstetrics. If family is available, information on status and possible prognosis should be shared so the next of kin may make an informed decision. Medical, legal, and ethical considerations pertaining to neurological conditions during pregnancy are discussed in detail in Chap. 21.

With the paucity of evidence and lack of clinical trials in treating the pregnant patient who presents with TBI, it is impossible to provide substantial guidelines in this chapter. Instead, the authors have provided selected care considerations ranging from first basic obstetric considerations that the neurosurgeon may not be familiar with followed by selected guidelines in brain trauma and their possible implications in care of the pregnant patient. The reader is asked to keep in mind the lack of evidence for this small and specific population of patients and that many landmark studies which guide our care of the TBI patient excluded pregnant patients from their samples [78, 79].

Conclusion

In this chapter, the guidelines for management of severe TBI were reviewed and compared to any existing evidence for care in a pregnant TBI patient. There were minimal studies to contribute to these guidelines in a pregnant patient which is to be expected in this rare patient presentation. However, important points were made regarding the use of steroids and DVT prophylaxis. High-dose steroids are used to accelerate fetal lung maturation if a preterm delivery is expected but steroids have also been shown to have a negative effect on mortality in the TBI patient. Additionally, both pregnancy and TBI are proven risk factors for development of DVT and VTE but these have not been studied together in a multivariate model. Lastly, some considerations were discussed regarding a multidisciplinary approach, specific injuries to the mother or fetus that accompany TBI, and a brief ethical discussion regarding decisions involving both mother and fetus. It is hoped that this chapter serves as an initial reference for providers as well as a pathway toward further studies to guide care decisions.

References

1. Mena JH, Sanchez AI, Rubiano AM, Peitzman AB, Sperry JL, Gutierrez MI, Puyana JC. Effect of the modified glasgow coma scale score criteria for mild traumatic brain injury on mortality prediction: comparing classic and modified glasgow coma scale score model scores of 13. J Trauma. 2011;71:1185–93.
2. Fearnside MR, Cook RJ, Mcdougall P, Mcneil RJ. The Westmead head injury project outcome in severe head injury. A comparative analysis of pre-hospital, clinical and CT variables. Br J Neurosurg. 1993;7:267–79.
3. Chesnut RM, Chesnut RM, Marshall LF, Klauber MR, Blunt BA, Baldwin N, Eisenberg HM, Jane JA, Marmarou A, Foulkes MA. The role of secondary brain injury in determining outcome from severe head injury. J Trauma. 1993;34:216.
4. Carney N, Totten AM, O'Reilly C, et al. Guidelines for the management of severe traumatic brain injury, fourth edition. Neurosurgery. 2017;80:6–15.

5. Andrews K, Murphy L, Munday R, Littlewood C. Misdiagnosis of the vegetative state: retrospective study in a rehabilitation unit. Br Med J. 1996;313:13–6.

6. Berenguer CM, Davis FE, Howington JU. Brain death confirmation: comparison of computed tomographic angiography with nuclear medicine perfusion scan. J Trauma. 2010;68:553–8.

7. Wade DT. How often is the diagnosis of the permanent vegetative state incorrect? A review of the evidence. Eur J Neurol. 2018;25:619–25.

8. Laureys S, Owen AM, Schiff ND. Brain function in coma, vegetative state, and related disorders. Lancet Neurol. 2004;3:537–46.

9. Jennett B, Plum F. Persistent vegetative state after brain damage. A syndrome in search of a name. Lancet (London, England). 1972;1:734–7.

10. Giacino JT, Ashwal S, Childs N, et al. The minimally conscious state: definition and diagnostic criteria. Neurology. 2002;58:349–53.

11. Khormi YH, Gosadi I, Campbell S, Senthilselvan A, O'Kelly C, Zygun D. Adherence to brain trauma foundation guidelines for management of traumatic brain injury patients and its effect on outcomes: systematic review. J Neurotrauma. 2018;35:1407–18.

12. Aiolfi A, Benjamin E, Khor D, Inaba K, Lam L, Demetriades D. Brain trauma foundation guidelines for intracranial pressure monitoring: compliance and effect on outcome. World J Surg. 2017;41:1543–9.

13. Hirschi R, Rommel C, Letsinger J, Nirula R, Hawryluk GWJ. Brain trauma foundation guideline compliance: results of a multidisciplinary, international survey. World Neurosurg. 2018;116:e399–405.

14. Sim KB. Maternal persistent vegetative state with successful fetal outcome. J Korean Med Sci. 2001;16:669–72.

15. Bush MC, Nagy S, Berkowitz RL, Gaddipati S. Pregnancy in a persistent vegetative state: case report, comparison to brain death, and review of the literature. Obstet Gynecol Surv. 2003;58:738–48.

16. Dawar P, Kalra A, Agrawal D, Sharma BS. Decompressive craniectomy in term pregnancy with combined cesarean section for traumatic brain injury. Neurol India. 2013;61:423–5.

17. Whitney N, Raslan AM, Ragel BT. Decompressive craniectomy in a neurologically devastated pregnant woman to maintain fetal viability. J Neurosurg. 2012;116:487–90.

18. Neville G, Kaliaperumal C, Kaar G. "Miracle baby": an outcome of multidisciplinary approach to neurotrauma in pregnancy. BMJ Case Rep. 2012;2012:bcr2012006477. https://doi.org/10.1136/bcr-2012-006477.

19. Gioti I, Faropoulos K, Picolas C, Lambrou MA. Decompressive craniectomy in cerebral venous sinus thrombosis during pregnancy: a case report. Acta Neurochir (Wien). 2019;161:1349–52.

20. Penarrocha M, Penarrocha D, Bagan J, Penarrocha M. Post-traumatic trigeminal neuropathy. A study of 63 cases. Med Oral Patol Oral y Cir Bucal. 2012;17:e297–300.

21. MacMillan DS. Intracerebral hemorrhage with herniation in a second-trimester pregnant female. Air Med J. 2018;37:203–5.

22. Jeejeebhoy FM, Zelop CM, Lipman S, et al. Cardiac arrest in pregnancy: a scientific statement from the American Heart Association. Circulation. 2015;132:1747–73.

23. Kikuchi J, Deering S. Cardiac arrest in pregnancy. Semin Perinatol. 2018;42:33–8.

24. Jing Z, Yanping L. Middle cerebral artery thrombosis after IVF and ovarian hyperstimulation: a case report. Fertil Steril. 2011;95:2435.e13–5.

25. Reschke M, Sweeney JM, Wong N. Spinal anesthesia performed for cesarean delivery after external ventricular drain placement in a parturient with symptomatology from an intracranial mass. Int J Obstet Anesth. 2019;37:122–5.

26. Moore DM, Meela M, Kealy D, Crowley L, McMorrow R, O'Kelly B. An intrathecal catheter in a pregnant patient with idiopathic intracranial hypertension: analgesia, monitor and therapy? Int J Obstet Anesth. 2014;23:175–8.

27. Spike J. Brain death, pregnancy, and posthumous motherhood. J Clin Ethics. 1999;10:57–65.

28. Hallsworth D, Thompson J, Wilkinson D, Kerr RSC, Russell R. Intracranial pressure monitoring and caesarean section in a patient with von Hippel-Lindau disease and symptomatic cerebellar haemangioblastomas. Int J Obstet Anesth. 2015;24:73–7.

29. Davis DP, Peay J, Sise MJ, Vilke GM, Kennedy F, Eastman AB, Velky T, Hoyt DB. The impact of prehospital endotracheal intubation on outcome in moderate to severe traumatic brain injury. J Trauma. 2005;58:933–9.

30. Bernard SA, Nguyen V, Cameron P, et al. Prehospital rapid sequence intubation improves functional outcome for patients with severe traumatic brain injury: a randomized controlled trial. Ann Surg. 2010;252:959–65.

31. von Elm E, Schoettker P, Henzi I, Osterwalder J, Walder B. Pre-hospital tracheal intubation in patients with traumatic brain injury: systematic review of current evidence. Br J Anaesth. 2009;103:371–86.

32. Gaither JB, Spaite DW, Bobrow BJ, Denninghoff KR, Stolz U, Beskind DL, Meislin HW. Balancing the potential risks and benefits of out-of-hospital intubation in traumatic brain injury: the intubation/hyperventilation effect. Ann Emerg Med. 2012;60:732–6.

33. Alderson P, Roberts I. Corticosteroids in acute traumatic brain injury: systematic review of randomised controlled trials. BMJ. 1997;314:1855–9.

34. Roberts I, Yates D, Sandercock P, et al. MRC CRASH trial. Lancet. 2004;364:1321–8.

35. Edwards P, Arango M, Balica L, et al. Final results of MRC CRASH, a randomised placebo-controlled trial of intravenous corticosteroid in adults with head injury-outcomes at 6 months. Lancet (London, England). 2005;365:1957–9.

36. The CRASH trial management group, The CRASH trial collaborators. The CRASH trial protocol (corticosteroid randomisation after significant head injury) [ISRCTN74459797]. BMC Emerg Med. 2001;1:1.

37. Adrenal cortical steroids. In: Drug facts and comparisons. 5th ed. St. Louis: Facts and Comparisons, Inc.; 1997.

38. Meikle AW, Tyler FH. Potency and duration of action of glucocorticoids. Effects of hydrocortisone, prednisone and dexamethasone on human pituitary-adrenal function. Am J Med. 1977;63:200–7.

39. Bonanno C, Wapner RJ. Antenatal corticosteroids in the management of preterm birth: are we back where we started? Obstet Gynecol Clin North Am. 2012;39:47–63.

40. Roof RL, Hall ED. Estrogen-related gender difference in survival rate and cortical blood flow after impact-acceleration head injury in rats. J Neurotrauma. 2000;17:1155–69.

41. Roof RL, Hall ED. Gender differences in acute CNS trauma and stroke: neuroprotective effects of estrogen and progesterone. J Neurotrauma. 2000;17:367–88.

42. Wise PM, Dubal DB, Wilson ME, Rau SW, Böttner M. Minireview: neuroprotective effects of estrogen - new insights into mechanisms of action. Endocrinology. 2001;142:969–73.

43. Wise PM, Dubal DB, Wilson ME, Rau SW, Böttner M, Rosewell KL. Estradiol is a protective factor in the adult and aging brain: understanding of mechanisms derived from in vivo and in vitro studies. Brain Res Brain Res Rev. 2001;37:313–9.

44. Kondo Y, Suzuki K, Sakuma Y. Estrogen alleviates cognitive dysfunction following transient brain ischemia in ovariectomized gerbils. Neurosci Lett. 1997;238:45–8.

45. Chen X, Li Y, Kline AE, Dixon CE, Zafonte RD, Wagner AK. Gender and environmental effects on regional brain-derived neurotrophic factor expression after experimental traumatic brain injury. Neuroscience. 2005;135:11–7.

46. Rogers E, Wagner AK. Gender, sex steroids, and neuroprotection following traumatic brain injury. J Head Trauma Rehabil. 2006;21:279–81.

47. Amantea D, Russo R, Bagetta G, Corasaniti MT. From clinical evidence to molecular mechanisms underlying neuroprotection afforded by estrogens. Pharmacol Res. 2005;52:119–32.

48. Stein DG. Is progesterone a worthy candidate as a novel therapy for traumatic brain injury? Dialogues Clin Neurosci. 2011;13:352–9.

49. Tyagi E, Agrawal R, Ying Z, Gomez-Pinilla F. TBI and sex: crucial role of progesterone protecting the brain in an omega-3 deficient condition. Exp Neurol. 2014;253:41–51.

50. Ottochian M, Salim A, Berry C, Chan LS, Wilson MT, Margulies DR. Severe traumatic brain injury: is there a gender difference in mortality? Am J Surg. 2009;197:155–8.

51. Davis DP, Douglas DJ, Smith W, Sise MJ, Vilke GM, Holbrook TL, Kennedy F, Eastman AB, Velky T, Hoyt DB. Traumatic brain injury outcomes in pre- and post-menopausal females versus age-matched males. J Neurotrauma. 2006;23:140–8.

52. Coimbra R, Hoyt DB, Potenza BM, Fortlage D, Hollingsworth-Fridlund P. Does sexual dimorphism influence outcome of traumatic brain injury patients? The answer is no! J Trauma. 2003;54:689–700.

53. Theis V, Theiss C. Progesterone effects in the nervous system. Anat Rec. 2019;302:1276–86.

54. Ekeh AP, Dominguez KM, Markert RJ, McCarthy MC. Incidence and risk factors for deep venous thrombosis after moderate and severe brain injury. J Trauma. 2010;68:912–5.

55. Reiff DA, Haricharan RN, Bullington NM, Griffin RL, McGwin G, Rue LW. Traumatic brain injury is associated with the development of deep vein thrombosis independent of pharmacological prophylaxis. J Trauma. 2009;66:1436–40.

56. Devis P, Knuttinen MG. Deep venous thrombosis in pregnancy: incidence, pathogenesis and endovascular management. Cardiovasc Diagn Ther. 2017;7:S300–19.

57. James AH, Jamison MG, Brancazio LR, Myers ER. Venous thromboembolism during pregnancy and the postpartum period: incidence, risk factors, and mortality. Am J Obstet Gynecol. 2006;194:1311–5.

58. Simpson EL, Lawrenson RA, Nightingale AL, Farmer RDT. Venous thromboembolism in pregnancy and the puerperium: incidence and additional risk factors from a London perinatal database. Br J Obstet Gynaecol. 2001;108:56–60.

59. Mawhinney E, Craig J, Morrow J, et al. Levetiracetam in pregnancy: results from the UK and Ireland epilepsy and pregnancy registers. Neurology. 2013;80:400–5.

60. Bromley RL, Mawer G, Clayton-Smith J, Baker GA. Autism spectrum disorders following in utero exposure to antiepileptic drugs. Neurology. 2008;71:1923–4.

61. Hernández-Díaz S, Smith CR, Shen A, Mittendorf R, Hauser WA, Yerby M, Holmes LB. Comparative safety of antiepileptic drugs during pregnancy. Neurology. 2012;78:1692–9.

62. Schenone MH, Mari G, Schlabritz-Loutsevitch N, Ahokas R. Effects of selective reduced uterine perfusion pressure in pregnant rats. Placenta. 2015;36:1450–4.

63. Burton GJ, Fowden AL. The placenta: a multifaceted, transient organ. Philos Trans R Soc B Biol Sci. 2015;370(1663):20140066. https://doi.org/10.1098/rstb.2014.0066.

64. Burkle CM, Tessmer-Tuck J, Wijdicks EF. Medical, legal, and ethical challenges associated with pregnancy and catastrophic brain injury. Int J Gynecol Obstet. 2015;129:276–80.

65. Alali AS, Gomez D, McCredie V, Mainprize TG, Nathens AB. Understanding hospital volume-outcome relationship in severe traumatic brain injury. Clin Neurosurg. 2017;80:534–41.

66. Wada T, Yasunaga H, Doi K, Matsui H, Fushimi K, Kitsuta Y, Nakajima S. Relationship between hospi-

tal volume and outcomes in patients with traumatic brain injury: a retrospective observational study using a national inpatient database in Japan. Injury. 2017;48:1423–31.

67. Huls CK, Detlefs C. Trauma in pregnancy. Semin Perinatol. 2018;42:13–20.

68. Petrone P, Asensio JA. Trauma in pregnancy: assessment and treatment. Scand J Surg. 2006;95:4–10.

69. Choate JW, Lund CJ. Emergency cesarean section: an analysis of maternal and fetal results in 177 operations. Am J Obstet Gynecol. 1968;100:703–15.

70. Chiossi G, Novic K, Celebrezze JU, Thomas RL. Successful neonatal outcome in 2 cases of maternal persistent vegetative state treated in a labor and delivery suite. Am J Obstet Gynecol. 2006;195:316–22.

71. Koh ML, Lipkin EW. Nutrition support of a pregnant comatose patient via percutaneous endoscopic gastrostomy. J Parenter Enter Nutr. 1993;17:384–7.

72. Goldberg-Stein SA, Liu B, Hahn PF, Lee SI. Radiation dose management: part 2, estimating fetal radiation risk from CT during pregnancy. Am J Roentgenol. 2012;198:W352–6.

73. Haghbayan H, Boutin A, Laflamme M, Lauzier F, Shemilt M, Moore L, Zarychanski R, Douville V, Fergusson D, Turgeon AF. The prognostic value of MRI in moderate and severe traumatic brain injury. Crit Care Med. 2017;45:e1280–8.

74. Ray JG, Vermeulen MJ, Bharatha A, Montanera WJ, Park AL. Association between MRI exposure during pregnancy and fetal and childhood outcomes. J Am Med Assoc. 2016;316:952–61.

75. Kho GS, Abdullah JM. Management of severe traumatic brain injury in pregnancy: a body with two lives. Malays J Med Sci. 2018;25:151–7.

76. Lane A, Westbrook A, Grady D, O'Connor R, Counihan TJ, Marsh B, Laffey JG. Maternal brain death: medical, ethical and legal issues. Intensive Care Med. 2004;30:1484–6.

77. van Bogaert LJ, Dhai A. Ethical challenges of treating the critically ill pregnant patient. Best Pract Res Clin Obstet Gynaecol. 2008;22:983–96.

78. Kreitzer N, Lyons MS, Hart K, Lindsell CJ, Chung S, Yick A, Bonomo J. Repeat neuroimaging of mild traumatic brain-injured patients with acute traumatic intracranial hemorrhage: clinical outcomes and radiographic features. Acad Emerg Med. 2014;21:1084–91.

79. Lelubre C, Taccone FS. Transfusion strategies in patients with traumatic brain injury: which is the optimal hemoglobin target? Minerva Anestesiol. 2016;82:112–26.

Intracranial Infections in Pregnancy: Meningitis and Encephalitis

Pinki Bhatt and Susan E. Boruchoff

Introduction

Pregnant women have multiple alterations in immune function, as is necessary to maintain fetal tolerance, including:

- Increase in the level of estradiol which reduces T-lymphocyte response and cell-mediated immunity.
- Increase in B-lymphocyte response and antibody production.
- Increase in progesterone level which can suppress the maternal immune response.

As a result, pregnant women have increased susceptibility to T-cell mediated infections. However, despite the immunologic changes that characterize pregnancy, common infections are more common than opportunistic ones.

With a few specific exceptions, there is a paucity of data regarding intracranial infections that is specific to pregnant women.

This chapter will discuss both common infections and opportunistic infections predominantly seen in the pregnant population. Figure 18.1 describes a general approach to the pregnant patient with infection of the central nervous system (CNS). As with all potential CNS infections, consultation with an Infectious Diseases specialist is an important part of management.

P. Bhatt (✉)
Division of Allergy/Immunology and Infectious Disease, Department of Medicine, Rutgers Robert Wood Johnson Medical School,
New Brunswick, NJ, USA
e-mail: pb518@rwjms.rutgers.edu

S. E. Boruchoff
Division of Infectious Disease, Department of Medicine, Rutgers Robert Wood Johnson Medical School, New Brunswick, NJ, USA

Fig. 18.1 General approach to pregnant women with CNS infection

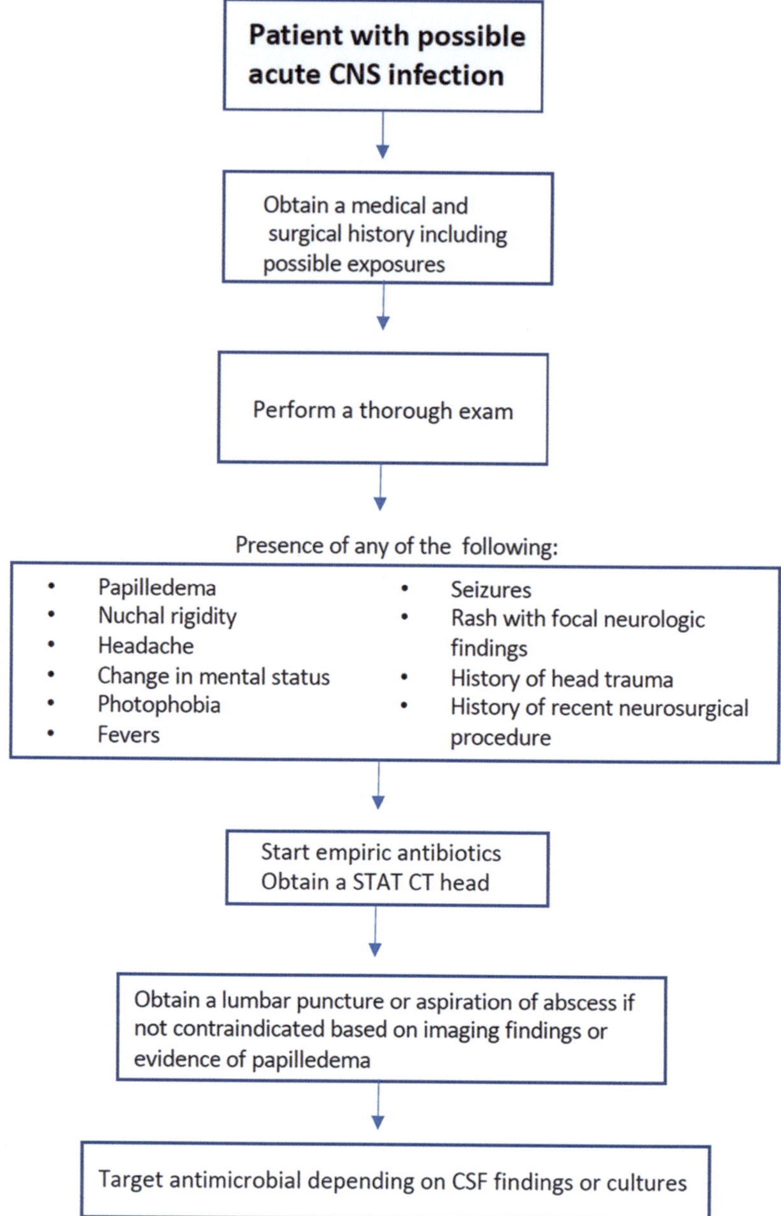

Meningitis

Meningitis, defined as inflammation of the meninges usually caused by infection, is diagnosed by the finding of elevated numbers of white blood cells (WBC) in the cerebrospinal spinal fluid (CSF). The clinical presentation may be either acute, subacute or chronic, and the rapidity of the clinical presentation may be helpful in determining the urgency of the diagnostic workup, as well as the pathogens that may be implicated and the empiric treatments to initiate while awaiting microbiologic results.

Acute meningitis is defined as the sudden onset of meningeal symptoms over the course of hours to a couple of days. Chronic meningitis is characterized as a more subacute onset of meningeal signs and symptoms along with abnormal CSF for at least 4 weeks. Common infectious causes of acute and chronic meningitis will be described below.

Bacterial Meningitis

Despite effective antibiotics, bacterial meningitis continues to cause significant morbidity and mortality world-wide. In general, pregnancy has not been associated with an increased risk of bacterial meningitis with common pathogens other than *Listeria monocytogenes.*

Etiology and Epidemiology

Following the initiation of routine immunization for infants, such as conjugate *Haemophilus influenzae* type b vaccine in 1990, 7-valent *Streptococcus pneumoniae* conjugate (pneumococcal) vaccine (PCV7) in 2000 and 13-valent pneumococcal vaccine (PCV13) in 2010, the frequency of bacterial meningitis has decreased. In addition, the peak age group for bacterial meningitis has shifted from children under the age of 5 to adults.

Pregnant patients are susceptible to most of the same organisms that affect non-pregnant adults, specifically *S. pneumoniae, N. meningitidis, L. monocytogenes,* and Enterobacteriaceae. Table 18.1 highlights the most common organisms that cause community acquired bacterial meningitis in pregnant patients [1, 2].

Since the development of the *H. influenzae* type B (Hib) vaccination the most common pathogen to cause community-acquired bacterial

Table 18.1 Most common pathogens causing community acquired bacterial meningitis in pregnant patients

Common	Less common
Streptococcus pneumoniae	*Haemophilus influenzae*
Neisseria meningitidis	*Streptococcus agalactiae* (Group B streptococcus; GBS)
Listeria monocytogenes	Group A streptococcus
	Neisseria gonorrhoeae
	Enterobacteriaceae

meningitis is *S. pneumoniae,* with a reported case fatality rate of 19–37% [3]. It is important to recognize that while the incidence of *H. influenzae* type B in the USA has decreased due to routine childhood vaccination, it is still a significant problem in developing countries largely due to vaccine expense.

N. meningitidis can cause an acute fulminant meningitis (meningococcal meningitis)—this is a medical emergency. It typically affects previously well, young adults. Due to its tendency to progress rapidly over a matter of hours, mortality can be very high if not treated quickly and appropriately. In the USA serogroups B, C, and Y each account for approximately one third of cases [4]. Outside of the USA, serogroups A and C account for large-scale epidemics and outbreaks in South America, Africa ("meningitis belt") and parts of Asia. Serogroup W is a less common cause of disease but is especially known for its largest outbreak in 2000 and 2001 associated with the Hajj in Mecca, with several cases brought back to other countries in Asia, Europe, and the USA [5]. Although *N. meningitidis* is the most frequent cause of invasive disease in adolescents, there have only been two reported cases of meningococcal meningitis during pregnancy. There are also case reports of neonatal intrauterine transmission in pregnant women positive for nasopharyngeal or cervical carriage of *N. meningitidis* [6].

L. monocytogenes accounts for 2–8% of bacterial meningitis in the USA with a mortality rate of up to 29%. The organism is typically found in dust, soil, water, sewage, or decaying matter. Outbreaks have been reported after consumption of contaminated food such as coleslaw, milk, cheese, certain meats or raw vegetables. Symptomatic listeriosis has been reported in all stages of pregnancy. Maternal illness can be mild with undifferentiated fever or a flu-like syndrome or can be asymptomatic and self-limited. Though it typically causes disease in newborns, adults over the age of 60 or immunocompromised patients, particularly those with defects in T-cell function, it has been reported to cause meningitis in patients with other predisposing conditions such as diabetes mellitus, liver disease, chronic renal disease or pregnancy [7, 8]. Of the cases of *L. monocytogenes* meningitis in pregnancy described in the literature, the average age of pregnant women was 26 years without any predisposing conditions identified. A high rate of fetal loss, still birth, invasive disease in the newborn and maternal death were reported [1]. Most of the cases of listeria meningitis have occurred in healthy pregnant women which argues that health care providers should be alert to the possibility of listeria meningitis in all pregnant women with signs and symptoms of meningitis and/or listeriosis.

Streptococcus agalactiae (group B streptococcus; GBS) can be isolated from the vaginal or rectal cultures of 15–35% of asymptomatic pregnant women. Carriage may be transient or intermittent but is frequently chronic (40%), which increases the risk of transmission from mother to infant. GBS is a common cause of meningitis in neonates and can also rarely cause meningitis in adults. Risk factors in adults include age older than 60 years, diabetes mellitus, pregnancy or the postpartum state, cardiac disease, malignancy, renal failure, hepatic failure, use of steroids or alcoholism [7]. In a meta-analysis of 141 adults with GBS meningitis, 1 was pregnant and 6 were in the post-partum state [9].

Meningitis due to Enterobacteriaceae in pregnant women has not been specifically reported.

Pathogenesis

Bacterial meningitis in pregnant and non-pregnant patients typically occurs by hematogenous spread to the CNS either by colonization of the nasopharynx with subsequent blood stream invasion, invasion of CNS due to a localized source or direct entry into CNS from a contiguous infection, trauma, neurosurgery, cerebrospinal leak or infected medical devices (CSF shunts, intracerebral pressure monitors or cochlear implants). Of the six cases of pneumococcal meningitis reported in pregnant patients in the Netherlands between 2005 and 2010, four were due to otitis [1].

Clinical Manifestations

There is nothing different or distinctive about the presentation of acute bacterial meningitis in pregnancy. The classic symptoms of acute bacterial meningitis are sudden onset of fever, change in mental status, headache, photophobia, nausea, and nuchal rigidity. Less common manifestations include seizures, aphasia, coma, cranial nerve palsy, rash, and papilledema. Concomitant infections can also be present such as sinusitis or otitis, pneumonia or endocarditis, which could provide clues to the etiology of meningitis [10]. Most patients who present with *H. influenzae* meningitis have a concurrent or underlying condition such as sinusitis, otitis media, epiglottis, pneumonia, diabetes mellitus, alcoholism, asplenia or splenectomy, head trauma with CSF leak or an immune deficiency [7]. Similarly, patients with *S. pneumoniae* meningitis often have a contiguous or distant focus of pneumococcal infection such as otitis media, sinusitis, mastoiditis, pneumonia or endocarditis. As mentioned previously, *L. monocytogenes* meningitis can have a more indolent presentation in pregnant patients with the most common findings being fever and altered mental status. However, any suspicion of meningitis should raise the question of Listeria. The presentation of CNS infection by *L. monocytogenes* may include seizures, cranial nerve deficits, and tremors which should raise the suspicion of a space-occupying lesion such as an abscess [7, 8]. *N. meningitidis* infection is often accompanied by rashes. The classic finding is a petechial rash or palpable purpura, but the presence of pustular skin lesions should also raise concern for Neisserial infection. The petechial rash is not specific to meningococcal infection as it can also be associated with other pathogens such as *Staphylococcus aureus*, rickettsial disease (Rocky Mountain Spotted Fever) or enteroviruses. Maculopapular rash or arthritis have also been described in patients with meningococcal meningitis. The classic signs of meningismus (Kernig and Brudzinski) may be helpful if present, although one study of 297 adults with suspected meningitis found them to be only 5% sensitive to indicate meningitis [11].

Diagnosis

Caution is advised before a lumbar puncture (LP) is considered in patients with possible elevated intracranial pressure with attendant risk of cerebral herniation, thrombocytopenia or a suspected

Table 18.2 Cerebrospinal fluid findings in bacterial meningitis

Cerebrospinal fluid parameter	Typical findings
Opening pressure	Elevated, 200–500 mmH$_2$O
White blood cell count	>1000/mm^3
Percentage of neutrophils	≥80%
Protein	100–500 mg/dL
Glucose	≤40 mg/dL
CSF-to-serum glucose ratio	≤0.4
Gram stain	Positive in 60–90%
Culture	Positive in 70–85%

Table 18.3 Suggested antimicrobial treatment for acute meningitis

Microorganism	Treatment
Streptococcus pneumoniae	Ceftriaxone or cefotaxime (if penicillin MIC <1.0 µg/mL); vancomycin (if penicillin MIC ≥1.0 µg/mL)
Haemophilus influenzae type b	Ceftriaxone or cefotaxime or cefepime
Listeria monocytogenes	Ampicillin or penicillin G +/− aminoglycoside
Neisseria meningitidis	Penicillin G or ampicillin; third generation cephalosporin if penicillin MIC ≥0.1 µg/mL
Streptococcus agalactiae (Group B Streptococcus)	Ampicillin or penicillin G +/− aminoglycoside
Enterobacteriaceae (*Escherichia coli*, *Klebsiella* spp.)	Ceftriaxone or cefotaxime

spinal epidural abscess. If there is a high suspicion of an intracranial mass either due to presence of papilledema or focal neurological deficit, or if the patient is immunocompromised, presents with new onset seizure or an abnormal level of consciousness, a CT of the head or an MRI of the brain should be obtained first. Otherwise, an immediate LP should be obtained if there is any suspicion for meningitis. If there is any delay in performing the LP, blood cultures should be obtained and empiric antibiotics started as quickly as possible, prior to the LP.

Table 18.2 highlights the classic CSF profile in bacterial meningitis. Virtually all cases have elevated CSF opening pressure. Other CSF findings include elevated white blood cell (WBC) >1000/µL with neutrophilic predominance (≥80%). However, in meningitis caused by *L. monocytogenes*, a predominance of lymphocytes in CSF can be seen. Typical chemistries include CSF glucose <40 mg/dL, CSF to serum glucose ratio of ≤0.4, and a protein concentration of >200 mg/dL. Gram stain is positive in 60–90% of culture positive cases. CSF cultures are usually positive unless the patient has already received antibiotics. It is important, however, to recognize that while antibiotics administered prior to obtaining CSF may render the cultures negative, they should not alter the gram stain findings. Blood cultures are often positive (50–90%) and are especially helpful if CSF cannot be obtained or if CSF cultures are negative [7, 10].

Treatment

If high suspicion for bacterial meningitis remains and no etiology is found by an LP or if an LP is delayed, empiric antibiotics should be started after obtaining blood cultures. Suggested antimicrobial treatment options for bacterial meningitis are listed in Table 18.3. Although prospective data is not available in terms of timing of antimicrobial therapy, several retrospective studies have shown that delays in the administration of antibiotics for acute bacterial meningitis increase the risk of unfavorable outcome such as mortality or residual neurological deficits by up to 30% per hour of treatment delay. Another retrospective study found a 1.5-fold increased risk of in-hospital mortality when the treatment delay exceeded 6 h [12, 13]. Adjunctive dexamethasone use in patients with pneumococcal meningitis has been shown to reduce unfavorable outcomes and mortality, but a significant difference in outcomes was not seen in patients with meningitis caused by other bacterial pathogens [14].

Prognosis

Despite prompt diagnosis and treatment, mortality can remain high in pregnant patients with acute bacterial meningitis. Risk factors for unfavorable outcome include otitis or sinusitis, absence of rash, low score on the Glasgow Coma scale on admission, tachycardia, positive blood cultures, elevated erythrocyte sedimentation rate, thrombocytopenia and a low CSF WBC count [14]. A study of 15 cases of pneumococcal meningitis in pregnant women in Nigeria between 1958 and 1962 reported three maternal deaths and seven fetal losses (abortion, stillbirth or neonatal death) with a high rate of neurologic sequelae in surviving women. As would be expected, those with the most severe impairment in consciousness at the time of admission had the worst outcomes [15]. The study's author also compared the incidence and outcome of pneumococcal meningitis in pregnant women with those caused by other organisms and concluded that the increased susceptibility for pyogenic meningitis in pregnancy was specific for this organism.

Prevention

The most common causes of bacterial meningitis during pregnancy can be prevented through routine vaccination. Vaccines are available for *S. pneumoniae, N. meningitidis,* and *H. influenzae.*

In the USA, children undergo routine childhood immunization against *H. influenzae* and thus vaccination is not necessary for adults except for those with prior or impending splenectomy. In most developing countries, national immunization programs have been established to introduce Hib vaccines to all children. However, in some countries in Africa and Asia approximately 60% of children are still unvaccinated [16].

Meningococcal vaccines are typically administered to all adolescents in the USA. The quadrivalent meningococcal conjugate vaccine against Serogroups A, C, Y, and W135 is given to all adolescents 11–12 years of age with a booster at age 16 and the serogroup B meningococcal vaccine is given to young adults 16–23 years old.

The prevention of meningitis due to *L. monocytogenes* is an important consideration for pregnant patients. As there is no vaccine, prevention involves avoiding exposure to the organism. Most cases are sporadic and due to contaminated food. Women should be counseled to avoid unpasteurized dairy foods. Pregnant women should also be vigilant about washing all utensils and surfaces that have come into contact with meat to avoid cross-contamination [8].

Non-bacterial Meningitis/ Encephalitis

Non-bacterial meningitis is also referred to as *aseptic meningitis.* Infectious causes may include viral, fungal, mycobacterial, spirochetal, and rickettsial organisms. Aseptic meningitis may also be caused by malignancy or certain medications. The presentation can be similar to that of bacterial meningitis with fever, headache, and stiff neck, but the onset is often less acute and the sensorium is often less affected. Here, we discuss the most common causes of non-bacterial meningitis.

Viral

Viral infections of the CNS can result in aseptic meningitis or encephalitis, the latter characterized by altered mental status, altered behavior, motor or sensory deficits or speech/movement abnormality. The distinction between the two can frequently be blurred as some patients can present with clinical symptoms of both ("meningoencephalitis"). Analysis of the CSF is required as an initial step to distinguish between meningitis and encephalitis and for establishment of the etiology with further testing, such as CSF polymerase chain reaction (PCR) testing for herpes simplex (HSV)-1, HSV-2 or enteroviruses depending on the clinical presentation and exposure history. Increased CSF WBC (usually less than 250/mm^3) with predominance of lymphocytes, elevated protein concentration (though less than 150 mg/dL), and normal glucose concentration are findings consistent with a viral CNS infection. Here we present the most common viral infections of the CNS. Table 18.4 includes a more comprehensive table of types of non-bacterial meningitis pathogens and suggested treatments.

1. Herpes Simplex Virus (HSV)

    The optimal method for establishing the etiologic diagnosis of HSV meningitis or encephalitis is detection of HSV-1 or-2 DNA in the CSF by polymerase chain reaction (PCR), either via a dedicated HSV PCR or as part of a multiplex assay ("meningitis panel").

Table 18.4 Suggested therapy for viral causes of meningitis/encephalitis

Pathogen	Treatment
Cytomegalovirus (CMV)	Ganciclovir or valganciclovir or foscarnet
Epstein-Barr (EBV)	No specific treatment
Herpes Simplex (HSV)	Acyclovir
Human Herpesvirus 6 (HHV6)	Ganciclovir or foscarnet or cidofovir
Human immunodeficiency virus (HIV)	Antiretroviral therapy
Influenza	Oseltamivir
JC	If applicable or possible, reduction of immunosuppression
Measles	Ribavirin
Varicella-zoster (VZV)	Acyclovir
West Nile	No specific treatment

CSF viral culture is rarely positive in the early stages of infection and use of PCR has largely replaced use of viral cultures in most laboratories. The CSF profile includes pleocytosis (predominantly lymphocytes) with normal CSF glucose.

HSV-2 generally causes viral meningitis in immunocompetent patients. The majority of patients with primary HSV-2 meningitis have genital lesions which typically precede CNS symptoms. However, the genital lesions may not be apparent or symptomatic, especially in women, so the finding of HSV-2 in the CSF of a pregnant woman—or even the diagnosis of aseptic meningitis without an alternate microbial etiology—should prompt an examination to look for genital lesions, as genital HSV in the mother has significant implications for management of the fetus and newborn. HSV meningitis is typically not associated with significant morbidity or mortality.

In contrast, HSV encephalitis is almost exclusively due to HSV-1, which is the most common cause of fatal sporadic encephalitis world-wide.

Prompt diagnosis and treatment is important for HSV encephalitis, as this can be fatal if left untreated and the prognosis for neurologic recovery is directly related to the patient's level of consciousness at time of pre-sentation. Early initiation of treatment with acyclovir leads to better outcomes, not only for the mother but the baby as well. Neurological impairments such as status epilepticus in a mother with known history of epilepsy and another case with recurrent seizure and anterograde memory loss 1 year after the infection have been reported [17–19].

2. Cytomegalovirus (CMV)

Although rare and typically seen in patients with acquired immune deficiency syndrome (AIDS), CMV encephalitis can occur in immunocompetent patients and has been associated with other neurologic sequelae. CMV infection of the CNS can present as cerebral mass lesion, transverse myelitis or polyradiculomyelitis. Clinical manifestations are not different from other infectious encephalitis. Diagnosis is made by finding CMV DNA by PCR in the CSF.

3. Measles

Measles during pregnancy is associated with increased risk of maternal and fetal complications [20, 21]. Maternal neurologic complications associated with measles include encephalitis, subacute sclerosing panencephalitis (SSPE), and acute disseminated encephalomyelitis (ADEM).

Fungal Infections

Fungal meningitis is more common in patients with compromised cellular immune function. The most common pathogenic fungi to cause meningitis are *Cryptococcus neoformans, Coccidioides immitis,* and *Histoplasma capsulatum.* Though rare in pregnancy, this should be considered in those with unexplained headaches, altered mentation, and certain risk factors or environmental exposures. The clinical presentation can be similar to bacterial meningitis. For the purpose of this chapter, other fungal organisms such as Aspergillus or zygomycetes will not be discussed.

Cryptococcus neoformans

C .neoformans, the most common cause of fungal meningitis in immunocompromised patients (especially AIDS), has been reported in pregnant women. The organism is typically found in soil and bird droppings world-wide. The CSF profile typically shows pleocytosis with a mononuclear predominance, elevated protein, and low glucose. This organism causes a basilar meningitis which may lead to block of CSF drainage, and elevated intracranial pressure can be associated with significant morbidity and mortality. A positive Cryptococcal antigen in the CSF strongly supports the diagnosis. Treatment includes Amphotericin B alone or in combination with flucytosine. There is no data regarding fetal teratogenic effects. A few cases of cryptococcal meningitis have been reported in immunocompetent and HIV-infected pregnant women with a positive mother-baby outcome and no reports of cryptococcal disease in the infant after birth [22–24].

Coccidioides immitis

Coccidioides (*C. immitis* and *C. posadasii*) are dimorphic fungi endemic in the deserts of the southwestern region of the USA, Mexico, and Central and South America. Coccidiomycosis is usually a self-limiting infection, however, the risk of disseminated disease following an asymptomatic pulmonary infection is increased in immunocompromised patients, with pregnancy as a well-recognized risk factor. If meningitis occurs during pregnancy, it can have devastating complications. Pregnant women residing in an endemic area with symptoms suggestive of the coccidioidal meningitis should be tested. Serum or CSF [1, 3]-beta-D-glucan may be elevated in patients with CSF involvement. Definitive diagnosis requires histopathologic identification, a positive culture with *Coccidioides* spp. and serologic testing. Complement fixation assay to detect coccidioidal antibodies is an important method to diagnose coccidioidal meningitis. The decision to treat depends on the stage of pregnancy and degree of illness. Pregnant women with coccidioidomycosis should be managed by infectious diseases specialists in collaboration with maternal-fetal medicine specialists. Azole antifungals are typically contraindicated, especially in the first trimester, and therefore intrathecal amphotericin B deoxycholate is used instead for treatment of coccidioidal meningitis [25].

Histoplasma capsulatum

Histoplasmosis, caused by *Histoplasma capsulatum,* is found worldwide but more common in Central America and North America (particularly in the Midwestern states such as Ohio and Mississippi River valleys). Infection may be asymptomatic or present as pulmonary disease, however, disseminated histoplasmosis should be considered in those with risk factors for the disease and presence of fever, fatigue, and weight loss with other end organ involvement. CNS involvement should be suspected if the patient has altered mental status or other neurologic abnormalities. Establishing the diagnosis of histoplasma meningitis can be difficult but if suspected, CSF (fungal culture, *Histoplasma* antigen test, anti-*histoplasma* antibody test), serum (fungal blood culture, *Histoplasma* antigen test, anti-*histoplasma* antibody test), urine *Histoplasma* antigen testing and possibly bone marrow fungal culture should be obtained [26, 27]. If suspicion remains high, diagnosis of histoplasmosis should not be excluded if CSF cultures do not yield *H. capsulatum* and a meningeal or brain biopsy may be required to make the diagnosis. Due to poor penetration of most antifungals into the CSF, treatment for *Histoplasma* meningitis can be difficult and should be managed in conjunction with an infectious disease specialist. Induction therapy with liposomal amphotericin B for 4–6 weeks is generally recommended followed by itraconazole for at least a year, or an azole anti-fungal for life if the patient is at risk for relapse [26–28]. Treatment in pregnant women can be challenging as azoles are contraindicated in the first trimester due to the risk of teratogenicity.

Mycobacterial

Primary active tuberculosis (TB) can progress into TB meningitis especially in adults with an underlying immunocompromising condition. CNS TB accounts for about 1% of tuberculosis cases and about 4% of extrapulmonary disease in the USA [29], however, prior epidemiological studies have estimated that 10% of patients with active TB can develop TB meningitis with an incidence as high as 20.6 per 1,000,000 in highly endemic countries [30, 31]. Some case reports have been published implying the rarity of its disease in the pregnant population [32–34]. Symptoms of TB meningitis, such as stiff neck, headache, and fevers, can be similar to bacterial meningitis. However, TB meningitis typically has a subacute presentation with onset of clinical presentation ranging from 1 to 3 weeks and in some cases, more than 3 weeks [35]. TB meningitis should be suspected in patients with the above clinical manifestations and risk factors such as history of prior TB infection, prior TB exposure, and travel to or past/present residence in a country with high TB burden. Work up should include radiographic imaging such as CT or MRI of the brain as well as CSF examination with opening pressure, routine CSF studies, nucleic acid amplification test (NAAT), and acid-fast bacilli (AFB) smear and culture of the CSF. The diagnosis of TB meningitis can be made in the setting of typical CSF findings for TB meningitis (lymphocytic pleocytosis, low glucose concentration, elevated protein concentration), moderately elevated opening pressure (180–300 mmH$_2$O), positive CSF AFB smear, positive NAAT, or culture positive for *M. tuberculosis*. It should be noted, however, that the number of AFB in the CSF of patients with TB meningitis is very low so AFB smears of CSF are rarely positive and a large volume of CSF must be obtained in order to increase the yield of AFB culture. Empiric treatment for TB meningitis should not be delayed due to the high complication rate and morbidity if left untreated. Treatment consists of prompt administration of anti-tuberculous therapy in conjunction with gluco-corticoids. Complications such as hydrocephalus can be seen at the time of treatment and can be managed with serial lumbar punctures with clinical monitoring, however, due to the nature of rapid neurological decompensation, surgical consultation is typically warranted. Pregnant women with TB meningitis should undergo treatment as untreated TB can pose a greater risk to both the mother and the baby than potential complications of any of the medications [36]. To maximize adherence and as recommended by World Health Organization (WHO), TB therapy should be administered as directly observed therapy with

clinical case management. We recommend referring to the WHO guidelines regarding anti-tuberculous treatment and agents. Due to the complexity of the disease, patients with TB meningitis should also be managed in conjunction with an infectious disease specialist.

Spirochetal

Syphilis

Neurosyphilis, infection of the CNS by *Treponema pallidum*, can occur at any time after initial syphilis infection. Clinical manifestations in pregnant patients are similar to non-pregnant patients, described further in Table 18.5. Diagnosis requires CSF examination, with characteristic findings of lymphocytic pleocytosis (<100 cells/μL), elevated protein concentration (<100 mg/dL), and a reactive CSF-Venereal Disease Research Laboratory (VDRL) test. Treatment includes aqueous penicillin G (18–24 million units per day, administered as three to four million units intravenous [IV] every 4 h, or 24 million units daily as a continuous infusion) for 10–14 days, or procaine penicillin (2.4 million units intramuscular [IM] once daily) plus probenecid (500 mg orally four times a day), both for 10–14 days [37].

Parasitic

Malaria, Cerebral

Pregnant women are particularly vulnerable to malaria, specifically from severe disease caused by *Plasmodium falciparum*. Cerebral malaria is the most severe neurological complication seen in patients infected with malaria. The cerebral edema and elevated intracranial pressure commonly associated with cerebral malaria contributes to the high mortality rate in *P. falciparum* malaria. Persistent neurocognitive deficits are also seen which can last for decades [38]. Symptoms include impaired consciousness, delirium, and/or seizures with the severity depending on time between onset of symptoms and initiation of therapy, parasite burden, and

Table 18.5 Clinical manifestations of neurosyphilis

	Early neurosyphilis	Late neurosyphilis
Duration	<1 year after initial infection	>1 year after initial infection up to decades after primary infection
Clinical manifestations	Symptomatic meningitis	Dementia
	Cranial neuropathies or ocular disease	Personality change
	Meningovascular stroke + meningitis	General paresis
		Tabes dorsalis
		Sensory ataxia
		Incontinence

immune response. In patients with abnormal neurological clinical presentations, the diagnosis of cerebral malaria requires the presence of *P. Falciparum* in peripheral blood smear. CSF findings can be normal in patients with cerebral malaria, however, mild pleocytosis, elevated protein, and low glucose can also be seen. Intravenous Artesunate is currently the treatment of choice for cerebral malaria in pregnancy. If suspicion is high in an immigrant or returning traveler from an endemic location, treatment should be started promptly as untreated cerebral malaria is almost universally fatal [39, 40]. Because the risk of complications and poor outcomes is so high, and because some of the prophylactic medications are not approved in pregnancy, pregnant women should be discouraged from travel to endemic areas.

Space Occupying Abscess

Intracranial space occupying abscess can occur either by a direct spread (20–60% of cases) or hematogenous spread. Though rare in pregnancy, the etiology of abscess is similar to non-pregnant patients with most arising from sinus or odontogenic sources. The most frequent organisms causing brain abscess are *Staphylococcus* and *Streptococcus* spp. See Table 18.6 for primary sources of infection and associated microorganisms [41]. MRI should be performed to detect the lesion, with tissue sampling via stereotactic CT-guided aspiration or surgery for gram stain, aerobic/anaerobic, mycobacterial, and fungal culture. Modified acid-fast stain should be per-

Table 18.6 Primary sources and associated microorganisms of common intracranial space occupying abscesses

Source of infection	Organisms
Heart (Endocarditis)	*Staphylococcus aureus*
	Viridans streptococci
Lungs	*Actinomyces* spp.
	Fusobacterium spp.
	Streptococcus spp.
Neurosurgical procedures	*Enterobacter* spp.
	Pseudomonas aeruginosa
	Staphylococcus spp.
	Streptococcus spp.
Sinusitis and dental infections	*Bacteroides* spp.
	Enterobacteriaceae
	Fusobacterium spp.
	Haemophilus spp.
	Prevotella spp.
	Staphylococcus aureus
	Streptococcus spp.
Otitis media or mastoiditis	*Actinomyces*
	Bacteroides spp.
	Enterobacteriaceae
	Nocardia spp.
	Pseudomonas aeruginosa
	Prevotella spp.
	Staphylococcus aureus
	Streptococcus spp.
Penetrating head trauma	*Clostridium* spp.
	Enterobacteriaceae
	Pseudomonas aeruginosa
	Staphylococcus spp.
	Streptococcus spp.

formed if there is high suspicion for *Nocardia* spp. [42]. Once diagnosed, immediate neurosurgical intervention is necessary to decrease morbidity and mortality, along with long-term intravenous antibiotics targeted toward the identified organism. As the most common source is odontogenic, good oral hygiene plays a pivotal role in prevention of brain abscess during pregnancy.

Conclusion

Pregnant women have enhanced susceptibility to some types of infections due to underlying alterations in immune function. Though data regarding intracranial infections specific to pregnant women is limited, this chapter highlighted a general approach to management of CNS infections in pregnant women. For optimal management of these complex infections, an Infectious Diseases specialist should be consulted early as part of a multidisciplinary approach.

References

1. Adriani KS, Brouwer MC, van der Ende A, van de Beek D. Bacterial meningitis in pregnancy: report of six cases and review of the literature. Clin Microbiol Infect. 2012;18(4):345–51.
2. Oordt-Speets AM, Bolijn R, van Hoorn RC, Bhavsar A, Kyaw MH. Global etiology of bacterial meningitis: a systematic review and meta-analysis. PLoS One. 2018;13(6):e0198772.
3. Landrum LM, Hawkins A, Goodman JR. Pneumococcal meningitis during pregnancy: a case report and review of literature. Infect Dis Obstet Gynecol. 2009;2009:63624.
4. Cohn AC, MacNeil JR, Clark TA, Ortega-Sanchez IR, Briere EZ, Meissner HC, et al. Prevention and control of meningococcal disease: recommendations of the Advisory Committee on Immunization Practices (ACIP). Morb Mortal Wkly Rep Recomm Rep. 2013;62(2):1–28.
5. Centers for Disease Control and Prevention (CDC). Serogroup W-135 meningococcal disease among travelers returning from Saudi Arabia. MMWR Morb Mortal Wkly Rep. 2000;49(16):345.
6. Kurlenda J, Kaminska-Pabich A, Grinholc M. Neonatal intrauterine infection with Neisseria meningitidis B. Clin Pediatr (Phila). 2010;49(4):388–90.
7. Bennett JE, Dolin R, Blaser MJ. Mandell, Douglas, and Bennett's principles and practice of infectious diseases: 2-volume set. Amsterdam: Elsevier Health Sciences; 2014.
8. Janakiraman V. Listeriosis in pregnancy: diagnosis, treatment, and prevention. Rev Obstet Gynecol. 2008;1(4):179.
9. van Kassel MN, van Haeringen KJ, Brouwer MC, Bijlsma MW, van de Beek D. Community-acquired group B streptococcal meningitis in adults. J Infect. 2020;80(3):255–60.
10. Bijlsma MW, Brouwer MC, Kasanmoentalib ES, Kloek AT, Lucas MJ, Tanck MW, et al. Community-acquired bacterial meningitis in adults in The Netherlands, 2006–14: a prospective cohort study. Lancet Infect Dis. 2016;16(3):339–47.
11. Thomas KE, Hasbun R, Jekel J, Quagliarello VJ. The diagnostic accuracy of Kernig's sign, Brudzinski's sign, and nuchal rigidity in adults with suspected meningitis. Clin Infect Dis. 2002;35(1):46–52.
12. Bodilsen J, Dalager-Pedersen M, Schonheyder HC, Nielsen H. Time to antibiotic therapy and outcome in bacterial meningitis: a Danish population-based cohort study. BMC Infect Dis. 2016;16:392.
13. Koster-Rasmussen R, Korshin A, Meyer CN. Antibiotic treatment delay and outcome in acute bacterial meningitis. J Infect. 2008;57(6):449–54.
14. van de Beek D, de Gans J, Spanjaard L, Weisfelt M, Reitsma J, Vermeulen M. Clinical features and prognostic factors in adults with bacterial meningitis. N Engl J Med. 2005;352:950.
15. Lucas AO. Pneumococcal meningitis in pregnancy and the puerperium. Br Med J. 1964;1(5375):92–5.
16. World Health Organization. Haemophilus influenzae type b (Hib); 2013.
17. Dupuis O, Audibert F, Fernandez H, Frydman R. Herpes simplex virus encephalitis in pregnancy. Obstet Gynecol. 1999;94(5):810–2.
18. Gunduz A, Beskardes AF, Kutlu A, Ozkara C, Karaagac N, Yeni SN. Herpes encephalitis as a cause of nonconvulsive status epilepticus. Epileptic Disord. 2006;8(1):57–60.
19. Hankey GJ, Bucens MR, Chambers JS. Herpes simplex encephalitis in third trimester of pregnancy: successful outcome for mother and child. Neurology. 1987;37(9):1534.
20. Atmar RL, Englund JA, Hammill H. Complications of measles during pregnancy. Clin Infect Dis. 1992;14(1):217–26.
21. Ogbuanu IU, Zeko S, Chu SY, Muroua C, Gerber S, De Wee R, et al. Maternal, fetal, and neonatal outcomes associated with measles during pregnancy: Namibia, 2009-2010. Clin Infect Dis. 2014;58(8):1086–92.
22. Chen C-P, Wang K-G. Cryptococcal meningitis in pregnancy. Am J Perinatol. 1996;13(01):35–6.
23. Costa ML, Souza JP, Oliveira Neto AF, Pinto ESJL. Cryptococcal meningitis in HIV negative pregnant women: case report and review of literature. Rev Inst Med Trop Sao Paulo. 2009;51(5):289–94.
24. Ngwenya S. Cryptococcal meningitis in pregnancy, the neglected diagnosis: a case report. Gynecol Obstet Res Open J. 2016;3(2):23–5

25. Goldstein EJ, Johnson RH, Einstein HE. Coccidioidal meningitis. Clin Infect Dis. 2006;42(1):103–7.
26. Bloch KC, Myint T, Raymond-Guillen L, Hage CA, Davis TE, Wright PW, et al. Improvement in diagnosis of histoplasma meningitis by combined testing for histoplasma antigen and immunoglobulin G and immunoglobulin M anti-histoplasma antibody in cerebrospinal fluid. Clin Infect Dis. 2018;66(1):89–94.
27. Wheat J, Myint T, Guo Y, Kemmer P, Hage C, Terry C, et al. Central nervous system histoplasmosis: multicenter retrospective study on clinical features, diagnostic approach and outcome of treatment. Medicine (Baltimore). 2018;97(13):e0245.
28. Wheat L, Batteiger B, Sathapatayavongs B. Histoplasma capsulatum infections of the central nervous system. A clinical review. Medicine (Baltimore). 1990;69(4):244.
29. Centers for Disease Control and Prevention. Reported tuberculosis in the United States 2018. https://www.cdc.gov/tb/statistics/reports/2018/national_data.htm.
30. Bourgi K, Fiske C, Sterling TR. Tuberculosis meningitis. Curr Infect Dis Rep. 2017;19(11):39.
31. Murthy J. Tuberculosis meningitis: the challenges. Neurol India. 2010;58(5):716–22.
32. Gasparetto EL, Tazoniero P, Neto AC. Disseminated tuberculosis in a pregnant woman presenting with numerous brain tuberculomas: case report. Arq Neuropsiquiatr. 2003;61(3B):855–8.
33. Kent SJ, Crowe SM, Yung A, Lucas CR, Mijch AM. Tuberculous meningitis: a 30-year review. Clin Infect Dis. 1993;17(6):987–94.
34. Prévost MR, Fung FK, KM. Tuberculous meningitis in pregnancy—implications for mother and fetus: case report and literature review. J Matern Fetal Med. 1999;8(6):289–94.
35. Pehlivanoglu F, Yasar K, Sengoz G. Tuberculous meningitis in adults: a review of 160 cases. Sci World J. 2012;2012:1.
36. Centers for Disease Control and Prevention. Treatment for TB disease & pregnancy. https://www.cdc.gov/tb/topic/treatment/pregnancy.htm.
37. Clement ME, Okeke NL, Hicks CB. Treatment of syphilis: a systematic review. JAMA. 2014;312(18):1905–17.
38. Idro R, Jenkins NE, Newton CRJC. Pathogenesis, clinical features, and neurological outcome of cerebral malaria. Lancet Neurol. 2005;4(12):827–40.
39. Saba N, Sultana A, Mahsud I. Outcome and complications of malaria in pregnancy. Gomal J Med Sci. 2008;6(2):26.
40. Seal SL, Mukhopadhay S, Ganguly RP. Malaria in pregnancy. J Indian Med Assoc. 2010;108(8):487–90.
41. Brook I. Microbiology and treatment of brain abscess. J Clin Neurosci. 2017;38:8–12.
42. Braun TI, Kerson LA, Eisenberg FP. Nocardial brain abscesses in a pregnant woman. Rev Infect Dis. 1991;13(4):630–2.

Part IV

Neuro-Inflammatory, Neuromuscular, and Musculoskeletal Disorders in Pregnancy

Neuroanesthesia in the Parturient

Carl L. Esser, Matthew B. Berman,
Sanjeev Sreenivasan, Gaurav Gupta,
and Christopher Fjotland

Intro

Very infrequently is the anesthesiologist faced with providing neuroanesthesia during pregnancy which makes it very challenging for even the most experienced individuals. The challenge lies in achieving the appropriate balance between protecting the mother and determining safety for the fetus [1]. Anesthetic management of patients during pregnancy is largely theoretical since there is insufficient evidence and studies to completely qualify exact methods and/or guidelines to be followed [2]. Normal physiology is altered in the parturient which adds to the complexity of management and anesthesia care [1, 2]. Ultimately, there should be avoidance of damaging drug effects for the fetus and safe delivery of anesthesia techniques [3].

Most cases that are indicated for intervention include trauma including head injury, intracranial vascular lesions, intracranial tumor, and spinal cord tumors and lesions [3]. A multi-disciplinary approach is needed for these patients including collaboration among the obstetrician, neurosurgeon, and neuroanesthetist [4]. Due to the rarity of these cases, management of obstetric patients that requires any neurological intervention requires a team approach with close communication between the neurosurgeon, obstetrician, and anesthesiologist regarding the sequence, timing, mode of delivery, and the neurosurgical intervention [4].

There are currently no standardized guidelines for the management of the pregnant patient with neurological pathology and, ultimately, the anesthetic management for that patient if she were to require an intervention [5]. One case study has shown that 7 out of 16 pregnant patients who underwent neurosurgery had no obstetric complications and delivered full term [5]. This chapter focuses on the anesthetic management for pregnant patients who require neurosurgical intervention prior to or during delivery.

C. L. Esser · M. B. Berman · S. Sreenivasan
Robert Wood Johnson Medical School, Rutgers
University, New Brunswick, NJ, USA
e-mail: cwf22@rwjms.rutgers.edu;
sa2034@rwjms.rutgers.edu

G. Gupta (✉)
Neurosurgery, Rutgers Robert Wood Johnson
Medical School, New Brunswick, NJ, USA
e-mail: guptaga@rutgers.edu

C. Fjotland
Department of Anesthesiology, Rutgers Robert Wood
Johnson Medical School, New Brunswick, NJ, USA

Neuroanesthesia and Intraoperative Management for the Pregnant Patient

Intraoperative monitoring for pregnant patients is really no different from the general population and should include all standard American Society of Anesthesiology (ASA) monitors as well as

© The Author(s), under exclusive license to Springer Nature Switzerland AG 2023
G. Gupta et al. (eds.), *Neurological Disorders in Pregnancy*,
https://doi.org/10.1007/978-3-031-36490-7_19

fetal heart rate (FHR) monitoring if the fetus is beyond 20 weeks gestation. Invasive arterial pressure monitoring is warranted with two large bore intravenous (IV) catheters. A central venous catheter may be needed depending on the nature of the procedure and the anticipated need for vasopressor use [6]. Utilization of isonatremic, isotonic, and glucose-free solutions with hourly urine output monitoring is necessary to reduce the risk of cerebral edema and hyperglycemia [7]. Optimal operative positioning is the dorsal decubitus position with trunk rotation to the left with a log roll to help prevent aortocaval compression [8].

Careful airway assessment and management planning is necessary as always with pregnant patients. Smaller than usual oral endotracheal tubes should be used for general anesthesia with all difficult airway equipment on hand including the laryngeal mask airway (LMA) in case of difficult intubation and fiberoptic laryngoscopy if necessary for awake intubation [9]. These patients are considered "full stomachs" and present a high risk for aspiration so they should be given a non-particulate antacid such as 30 mL of sodium citrate (Bicitra), an H_2 receptor antagonist such as famotidine (20 mg IV) and metoclopramide (10 mg) to help decrease the acidity and volume of gastric contents. Anesthetic induction should be a combination of rapid sequence due to increased risk of aspiration and a slow "neuro induction" to help minimize a hemodynamic response to intubation, especially in patients with elevated intracranial pressure (ICP) or an intracranial aneurysm [10]. General anesthesia can be maintained with either total IV anesthesia using propofol or a balanced IV plus volatile anesthesia. Nitrous oxide is contraindicated because it can increase ICP, impair autoregulation, expand air bubbles, increase cerebral blood flow and cerebral metabolic rate, and may contribute to (postoperative nausea and vomiting) PONV [11].

Even though pregnant patients require about a 30% reduction in MAC, research shows that a regular dose of volatile anesthetic should be used to avoid awareness [12]. Volatile anesthetics suitable for anesthesia during pregnancy include sevoflurane and isoflurane and these are appro-

priate for neuro-anesthesia as they reduce cerebral metabolic rate, have the least effect on ICP and provide a level of cerebral protection [12]. Prolonged hyperventilation is not recommended in pregnancy [13]. Normal arterial carbon dioxide tension ($PaCO_2$) is 28–32 mmHg during pregnancy owing to an increase in minute ventilation and studies have shown that hyperventilation to a $PaCO_2$ <25 mmHg is associated with adverse patient outcomes [13]. Severe hypocarbia may impair fetal oxygen delivery by shifting the maternal oxygen-hemoglobin dissociation curve to the left [13]. However, a $PaCO_2$ between 28 and 30 mmHg is usually sufficient for surgical conditions without interfering with fetal oxygenation [13, 14].

Some case studies have shown the use of a single, low dose of mannitol had no overt maternal or fetal/neonatal adverse effects either acutely or longitudinally [15]. Even though mannitol has been shown to cross the placenta and may accumulate in the fetus, a one-time dose and dosages used clinically (0.5–1 g/kg) are unlikely to cause severe fluid or electrolyte abnormalities in the fetus [15]. Furosemide is an alternative to mannitol [16]. Dexmedetomidine is another medication that has often been thought to be contraindicated in pregnancy, but again multiple case reports have shown no long-term adverse effects for parturients or fetuses [17, 18].

Hypotension needs to be aggressively treated, especially systolic blood pressure <90 mmHg to ensure adequate uteroplacental perfusion and maintain targeted cerebral perfusion pressure of 50–70 mmHg. Ephedrine was once considered the drug of choice for pregnant patients for treating hypotension, however, recent studies have shown no evidence of deleterious effects of phenylephrine on fetal wellbeing. For the reverse, labetalol is both effective for the mother to treat hypertension and safe for the fetus [19]. Intracranial pressure also should be kept below 20 mmHg and managed as needed with osmotic diuretics such as hypertonic saline, mannitol (0.25–1 g/kg) and raising the head of the bed by 15–20° [20].

If it is determined the fetus should be delivered prior to a neurosurgical procedure, regional or neuraxial anesthesia can be considered. Epidural anesthesia provides the advantage of maintaining stable blood pressure parameters and allowing neurological status assessment during surgery [12, 21]. Most studies have concluded that if the pregnancy is in the third trimester with a viable fetus, up-front delivery is the first choice to keep the risk of the maternal death not higher than in non-pregnant females undergoing such surgery [21]. Early delivery would also bypass the need for obstetric intervention if the FHR tracing becomes concerning during a neurosurgical procedure. Additionally, the delivery of the fetus before surgery eliminates concern for adverse pregnancy outcome when interventions for cerebral protection are used such as hyperventilation, induced hypertension or hypotension, or administration of mannitol [15]. The optimal time to perform surgery during pregnancy is still a matter of debate [22].

Upon emergence, the pregnant patient should be fully awake with airway reflexes intact. There also needs to be an effort to prevent coughing and straining upon emergence which could worsen ICP or an intracranial hemorrhage. Prevention may be facilitated through administration of lidocaine 75–100 mg, fentanyl 25–50 µg, or a titration of dexmedetomidine at the end of the operation [17].

should consider both the mother and child [23, 24]. If the fetus is not near term, neurosurgery can be performed without attempt of delivery with continuous FHR monitoring and readiness to deliver the baby immediately if fetal distress develops. However, if the fetus is near or at term, cesarean section follow by craniotomy may be the safest option to ensure the best maternal and fetal outcomes [23].

Modest short-term hyperventilation may be temporarily used to reduce elevated ICP or to help improve surgical exposure during craniotomy. Aggressive fluid resuscitation is encouraged even in normotensive patients as signs of hypovolemia may be masked in pregnancy due to the relative hypervolemic and hemodiluted state [25]. To prevent uterine atony after cesarean section, avoidance of high concentrations of volatile anesthetics should occur together with use of uterotonic drugs [26]. Drug infusions should be titrated with strict monitoring of arterial blood pressure and continuous FHR monitoring. Most studies say emergent cesarean section after traumatic head injury is the best option for the fetus [23]. For patients with possible cervical spine injury, fiberoptic intubation techniques may be preferable to avoid further injury [27].

The management of the pregnant patient with neurotrauma is discussed in detail in this chapter.

Trauma and Traumatic Brain Injury

Trauma actually complicates 6–7% of all pregnancies and is a leading cause of maternal death and morbidity [23]. In fact, trauma is the leading cause of non-obstetric maternal death in the USA [23]. Incidence of trauma during pregnancy is 8%, 40%, and 52% in the first, second, and third trimesters, respectively [24]. Maternal resuscitation follows the standard guidelines for trauma management. The fetus should be assessed during or immediately after maternal stabilization and it should be determined if an emergent cesarean section is warranted or not [24]. While initial stabilization of the mother should take priority, further assessment and subsequent management

Intracranial Tumors

Primary central nervous system tumors occur in about 6 in 100,000 females, but are similar in frequency in both pregnant and non-pregnant women [28]. There is much evidence and a strong correlation between pregnancy hormones and the growth of meningiomas owing to the expression of sex hormone receptors by tumor cells [29]. Sometimes treatment for these tumors can be postponed into the postpartum as long as no aggressive behavior or irreversible deficits are anticipated [29]. If necessary, non-urgent surgery should be performed during the second trimester when preterm contractions and spontaneous abortion are the least likely [29].

As with other neurosurgical procedures during pregnancy, anesthetic concerns include proper positioning, avoidance of extremes of blood pressure, possible induction of labor, and treatment of postpartum hemorrhage during anesthesia [9]. A balanced and prolonged discussion between the neurosurgeon, obstetrician, and anesthesiologist regarding the use of diuretics for brain relaxation is necessary due to purported risks during pregnancy [3].

Systemic steroids, which are a hallmark of medical management for CNS tumors, are often avoided due to the risk of causing suppression of the fetal pituitary-adrenal axis [30]. Awake brain tumor resection has its unique advantages and should be considered when indicated even in patients who are pregnant. In such cases, local anesthetic infiltration serves as the mainstay of analgesia and low infusions of either propofol, remifentanil and/or dexmedetomidine are utilized for mild sedation particularly during opening and closing. This approach may help to minimize fetal exposure to anesthetics. Ultimately, adequate preoperative preparation and counseling are necessary so that the patient understands the entire process and what to expect [31].

Considerations for evaluating and managing the pregnant patient with brain tumors and sellar lesions are described in detail in Chaps. 36 and 37.

Vascular Lesions

Intracranial hemorrhage is responsible for 5–12% of all maternal deaths, however, the overall incidence of cerebrovascular pathologies in pregnant patients is low, between 0.01% and 0.05% of all pregnancies [32]. Maternal mortality may be as high as 35–80% for aneurysmal and 28% for arteriovenous malformation (AVM)-related hemorrhages [32]. Most often, hemorrhage due to AVM or aneurysm occurs during the third trimester and the primary goal is to maintain cardiovascular stability [32]. The risk of bleeding is purportedly increased during pregnancy owing to the physiologic changes associated with pregnancy such as increased intravascular volume and cardiac output along with the effects of hormones on vessel walls [33]. Subarachnoid hemorrhage (SAH) is the most common consequence of a ruptured intracranial aneurysm or AVM [34]. SAH may be up to five times more common during pregnancy as compared with non-pregnant states and is associated with significant morbidity and mortality [32].

Hormonal changes and hemodynamic stress may cause an increase in the risk of aneurysm development and rupture during pregnancy; and these changes are mostly seen in the last 3 months of pregnancy or during the process of labor [35]. Other reported factors that may potentiate aneurysm progression during pregnancy include high levels of relaxin and increased wall tension from intraparenchymal artery hypoplasia [35].

When a pregnant patient arrives complaining of a headache, evaluation of the patient must be thorough and requires a detailed neurologic assessment. Eclampsia is one of the differential diagnoses of SAH because of similarity of presenting symptoms such as seizures and acute-onset elevated blood pressure and needs to be ruled out [32].

Neurosurgical resection offers the best treatment option for a ruptured AVM either alone or in combination with preoperative embolization. Embolization alone as the sole treatment only provides a 20% recovery rate. Surgical intervention mainly depends on the risk of rupture or rebleeding of the vascular lesions as well as the gestational age of the fetus. All marginally viable fetuses should be monitored perioperatively or even delivered prior to neurosurgery if gestational age allows [36]. If there is a high risk of rupture or re-rupture, then the patient should undergo delivery followed by immediate surgical repair [36]. It is advised that for gestational ages beyond 34 weeks, cesarean section under general anesthesia be performed followed immediately by aneurysm surgery [37]. Hypotension should be avoided due to the risk of hypoperfusion to the fetus as well as osmotic agents which can cause fetal hyperosmolarity [37]. In early pregnancy cases when an aneurysm is clipped, the pregnancy can progress until term and delivery can proceed vaginally with care taken to minimize acute maternal hypertension [37]. Endovascular treatment, most often via aneurysm coiling, represents another viable option for management of cerebral aneurysms. Notably, maternal complications were more than twice as frequent in patients who underwent clipping versus coiling for aneurysm rupture. However, there is debate as to whether surgical clipping or coil embolization provides greater long-term stability [37]. Endovascular intervention is also associated with risk of fetal irradiation due to reliance on ionizing radiation.

Anesthetic goals during AVM or aneurysm surgery are to avoid rapid swings in transmural pressure by minimizing arterial and ICP changes and cerebral perfusion pressure should be maintained to provide flow to areas of potentially abnormal autoregulation [37]. Elective cesarean section has been suggested in women with an untreated or partially treated AVM, especially if it has bled during pregnancy to try to avoid hemodynamic changes of labor which ultimately could stress the fragile vessels of the malformation [32].

The approach to the patient with ruptured and unruptured vascular lesions, including a detailed discussion of data regarding the link between pregnancy and hemorrhage, is provided in Chaps. 8 (Aneurysms) and 9 (AVMs).

References

1. Singh S, Sethi N. Neuroanesthesia and pregnancy: uncharted waters. Med J Armed Forces India. 2019;75(2):125–9. https://doi.org/10.1016/j.mjafi.2018.10.001.
2. Wang LP, Paech MJ. Neuroanesthesia for the pregnant woman. Anesth Analg. 2008;107(1):193–200. https://doi.org/10.1213/ane.0b013e31816c8888.
3. Griffiths S, Durbridge JA. Anaesthetic implications of neurological disease in pregnancy. Contin Educ Anaesth Crit Care Pain. 2011;11(5):157–61. https://doi.org/10.1093/bjaceaccp/mkr023.
4. Molina-Botello D, Rodríguez-Sanchez JR, Cuevas-García J, et al. Pregnancy and brain tumors; a systematic review of the literature. J Clin Neurosci. 2021;86:211–6. https://doi.org/10.1016/j.jocn.2021.01.048.
5. Reitman E, Flood P. Anaesthetic considerations for non-obstetric surgery during pregnancy. Br J Anaesth. 2011;107:i72–8. https://doi.org/10.1093/bja/aer343.
6. Sim JH, Lee JH, Lee CH, Ryu SA, Choi SS. Anesthetic management during cesarean delivery in a pregnant woman with ruptured cerebral arteriovenous malformation: a case report. Anesth Pain Med. 2017;12(3):220–3. https://doi.org/10.17085/apm.2017.12.3.220.
7. Vandse R, Cook M, Bergese S. Case report: perioperative management of a pregnant poly trauma patient for spine fixation surgery. F1000Res. 2015;4:171. https://doi.org/10.12688/f1000research.6659.2.
8. Xia Y, Ma X, Griffiths BB, Luo Y. Neurosurgical anesthesia for a pregnant woman with macroprolactinoma. Medicine (Baltimore). 2018;97(37):e12360. https://doi.org/10.1097/MD.0000000000012360.
9. Mushambi MC, Kinsella SM, Popat M, et al. Obstetric Anaesthetists' Association and Difficult Airway Society guidelines for the management of difficult and failed tracheal intubation in obstetrics. Anaesthesia. 2015;70(11):1286–306. https://doi.org/10.1111/anae.13260.
10. Johnston JR, Moore J, McCaughey W, et al. Use of cimetidine as an oral antacid in obstetric anesthesia. Anesth Analg. 1983;62(8):720–6.
11. Kim JH, Kim N, Lee SK, Kwon YS. Effect of pregnancy on postoperative nausea and vomiting in female patients who underwent nondelivery surgery: multicenter retrospective cohort study. Int J Environ Res Public Health. 2022;19(22):15132. https://doi.org/10.3390/ijerph192215132.
12. Upadya M, Saneesh P. Anaesthesia for non-obstetric surgery during pregnancy. Indian J Anaesth. 2016;60(4):234–41. https://doi.org/10.4103/0019-5049.179445.
13. Navot D, Donchin Y, Sadovsky E. Fetal response to voluntary maternal hyperventilation. A preliminary report. Acta Obstet Gynecol Scand. 1982;61(3):205–8. https://doi.org/10.3109/00016348209156557.
14. Huch R. Maternal hyperventilation and the fetus. J Perinat Med. 1986;14(1):3–17. https://doi.org/10.1515/jpme.1986.14.1.3.
15. Basso A, Fernández A, Althabe O, Sabini G, Piriz H, Belitzky R. Passage of mannitol from mother to amniotic fluid and fetus. Obstet Gynecol. 1977;49(5):628–31.
16. Al-Balas M, Bozzo P, Einarson A. Use of diuretics during pregnancy. Can Fam Physician. 2009;55(1):44–5.
17. Cortegiani A, Accurso G, Gregoretti C. Should we use dexmedetomidine for sedation in parturients undergoing caesarean section under spinal anaesthesia? Turk J Anaesthesiol Reanim. 2017;45(5):249–50. https://doi.org/10.5152/TJAR.2017.0457812.
18. Kitsiripant C, Kamata K, Kanamori R, Yamaguchi K, Ozaki M, Nomura M. Postoperative management with dexmedetomidine in a pregnant patient who underwent AVM nidus removal: a case report. JA Clin Rep. 2017;3:17. https://doi.org/10.1186/s40981-017-0085-6.

19. Crooks BNA, Deshpande SA, Hall C, Platt MPW, Milligan DWA. Adverse neonatal effects of maternal labetalol treatment. Arch Dis Child Fetal Neonatal Ed. 1998;79(2):F150–1. https://doi.org/10.1136/fn.79.2.F150.

20. Godoy DA, Robba C, Paiva WS, Rabinstein AA. Acute intracranial hypertension during pregnancy: special considerations and management adjustments. Neurocrit Care. 2022;36(1):302–16. https://doi.org/10.1007/s12028-021-01333-x.

21. Haggerty E, Daly J. Anaesthesia and non-obstetric surgery in pregnancy. BJA Educ. 2021;21(2):42–3. https://doi.org/10.1016/j.bjae.2020.11.002.

22. Rosen MA, Weiskopf RB. Management of anesthesia for the pregnant surgical patient. Anesthesiology. 1999;91(4):1159. https://doi.org/10.1097/00000542-199910000-00033.

23. Kho GS, Abdullah JM. Management of severe traumatic brain injury in pregnancy: a body with two lives. Malays J Med Sci MJMS. 2018;25(5):151–7. https://doi.org/10.21315/mjms2018.25.5.14.

24. Irving T, Menon R, Ciantar E. Trauma during pregnancy. BJA Educ. 2021;21(1):10–9. https://doi.org/10.1016/j.bjae.2020.08.005.

25. Crowhurst JA. Intravenous fluid administration in pregnancy: maintenance and acute hydration. Emerg Med. 1996;8(s1):63–8. https://doi.org/10.1111/j.1442-2026.1996.tb00545.x.

26. Shuhaiber S, Koren G. Occupational exposure to inhaled anesthetic. Is it a concern for pregnant women? Can Fam Physician. 2000;46:2391–2.

27. Pedaballe AR, Chhabra HS, Tandon V, Chauhan P, Verma R. Acute traumatic cervical spinal cord injury in a third-trimester pregnant female with good maternal and fetal outcome: a case report and literature review. Spinal Cord Ser Cases. 2018;4:93. https://doi.org/10.1038/s41394-018-0127-y.

28. Shiro R, Murakami K, Miyauchi M, Sanada Y, Matsumura N. Management strategies for brain tumors diagnosed during pregnancy: a case report and literature review. Medicina (Mex). 2021;57(6):613. https://doi.org/10.3390/medicina57060613.

29. Rodrigues AJ, Waldrop AR, Suharwardy S, et al. Management of brain tumors presenting in pregnancy: a case series and systematic review. Am J Obstet Gynecol MFM. 2021;3(1):100256. https://doi.org/10.1016/j.ajogmf.2020.100256.

30. Bandoli G, Palmsten K, Forbess Smith CJ, Chambers CD. A review of systemic corticosteroid use in pregnancy and the risk of select pregnancy and birth outcomes. Rheum Dis Clin N Am. 2017;43(3):489–502. https://doi.org/10.1016/j.rdc.2017.04.013.

31. Al Mashani AM, Ali A, Chatterjee N, Suri N, Das S. Awake craniotomy during pregnancy. J Neurosurg Anesthesiol. 2018;30(4):372. https://doi.org/10.1097/ANA.0000000000000424.

32. Fairhall JM, Stoodley MA. Intracranial haemorrhage in pregnancy. Obstet Med. 2009;2(4):142–8. https://doi.org/10.1258/om.2009.090030.

33. Aoyama K, Ray JG. Pregnancy and risk of intracerebral hemorrhage. JAMA Netw Open. 2020;3(4):e202844. https://doi.org/10.1001/jamanetworkopen.2020.2844.

34. Meeks JR, Bambhroliya AB, Alex KM, et al. Association of primary intracerebral hemorrhage with pregnancy and the postpartum period. JAMA Netw Open. 2020;3(4):e202769. https://doi.org/10.1001/jamanetworkopen.2020.2769.

35. Onat T, Daltaban İS, Tanın ÖŞ, Kara M. Rupture of cerebral aneurysm during pregnancy: a case report. Turk J Obstet Gynecol. 2019;16(2):136. https://doi.org/10.4274/tjod.galenos.2019.23080.

36. Lv X, Liu P, Li Y. The clinical characteristics and treatment of cerebral AVM in pregnancy. Neuroradiol J. 2015;28(3):234–7. https://doi.org/10.1177/1971400915589692.

37. Barbarite E, Hussain S, Dellarole A, Elhammady MS, Peterson E. The management of intracranial aneurysms during pregnancy: a systematic review. Turk Neurosurg. 2016;26(4):465–74. https://doi.org/10.5137/1019-5149.JTN.15773-15.0.

Analgesia and Pain Management During Pregnancy

Robert Ross and Kate Balbi

Labor Analgesia

There are three stages of labor, and in providing analgesia, it is imperative that the clinician have an understanding of what each stage entails, as well as the modulation of related pain pathways.

Pain during the first stage of labor (cervical dilation) is primarily caused by uterine contraction and changes in the both the cervix and lower uterine segment. This pain is transmitted by visceral nerve fibers that enter the spinal cord from T10 to L1. During the second stage of labor (complete cervical dilation to delivery) pain is primarily caused by distention and ischemia of the pelvic floor, perineum, and vagina. This pain is transmitted by somatic nerve fibers that enter the spinal cord from S2 to S4. The third stage of labor begins after delivery and is completed when the placenta, which separates from the uterine wall, is passed through the vaginal orifice [1].

While neuraxial anesthesia remains the most effective and most widely used form of pain relief during labor, intravenous anesthesia, inhaled anesthesia, and post-operative pain management will all be discussed.

Neuraxial

Neuraxial techniques are advantageous as they allow the parturient to remain awake without sedative side effects, while providing a predictable and sufficient analgesia for labor and delivery. The primary anesthetic goal of epidural analgesia for this patient population is to provide maximum sensory relief, with minimal motor involvement—to preserve the patient's ability to push and facilitate vaginal delivery of the newborn.

Epidural Epidural analgesia involves threading a catheter into the epidural space to allow for continuous analgesia. For labor analgesia, the catheter is usually placed from L2 to L5 and can be performed with the patient in the sitting or lateral position. To locate the epidural space, a tactile technique known as "loss of resistance" is implemented and, when performed correctly, the introducer (Tuohy needle) does not piece the dura [2].

While specific combinations vary by institution, analgesia is achieved by an epidural infusion containing both a local anesthetic and a narcotic. The synergistic effect of using dilute concentrations of local anesthetics combined with narcotics enables the clinician to maximize pain relief, with minimal effect on the patient's

R. Ross (✉) · K. Balbi
Department of Anesthesiology, Rutgers Robert Wood Johnson Medical School and University Hospital, New Brunswick, NJ, USA
e-mail: rr1095@rwjms.rutgers.edu

G. Gupta et al. (eds.), *Neurological Disorders in Pregnancy*,
https://doi.org/10.1007/978-3-031-36490-7_20

ability to actively participate in the second stage of labor.

Dilute concentrations of amide local anesthetics including bupivacaine and ropivacaine are the most commonly used, with the addition of the commonly used narcotics such as fentanyl and sufentanil. An advantage of an epidural is that the catheter can be dosed with a more potent local anesthetic, for the conversion to a cesarean section, retained placenta, post-delivery dilation and evacuation, laceration repair, or post-partum tubal ligation. An epidural catheter provides access to the epidural space; what local anesthetic combination is administered through the catheter will determine the degree of sensory and motor blockade.

Spinal While the most common indication for a spinal in the parturient is a cesarean section, spinal anesthesia can be used for vaginal delivery or a postpartum procedure such as laceration repair, retained placenta, or post-partum tubal ligation. For a vaginal delivery, a spinal can be especially helpful for pain associated with the second stage of labor and an instrumented delivery.

For a cesarean section, a hyperbaric solution of local anesthetic is typically used. This allows for a high sensory level with a short onset of action. The block can be supplemented with a narcotic to improve the quality of anesthesia, and epinephrine to prolong the duration of the block. Performing a spinal injection involves using a 24–26 gauge "pencil-point" needle to reduce the risk of a post-dural puncture headache [2].

Combined Spinal Epidural (CSE) CSE is a technique that involves both administering subarachnoid medication and then placing an epidural catheter. When compared to an epidural, advantages of a CSE include lower maternal and fetal plasma concentrations of medications, faster onset of analgesia, a denser block, and lower failure rate. When compared to a spinal, a CSE results in less hypotension, allows for the extension of the blockade with the epidural catheter and is technically easier in obese patients.

Disadvantages of a CSE include a post-dural puncture headache and the inability to test that the epidural is in the correct position until after the spinal anesthesia has worn off [2].

Contraindications to Neuraxial Anesthesia

1. Patient refusal
2. Infection at the needle insertion site
3. Significant coagulopathy
4. Hypovolemic shock
5. Increased intracranial pressure
6. Inadequate provider expertise.

Complications of Neuraxial Anesthesia

Unintentional dural puncture Unintentional dural puncture in the obstetric patient is cited at 1.5% of which approximately half will experience a post-dural puncture headache [3]. Symptomatic patients can be managed conservatively with hydration, analgesics, and caffeine. An epidural blood patch can be offered to those that fail to respond to conservative therapy.

Other side effects include pruritus, nausea, shivering, and urinary retention. Rare but serious side effects include meningitis, epidural hematoma, arachnoiditis, and nerve or spinal cord injury. Due to the systemic vessel engorgement seen in pregnant women, parturients are at a higher risk of unintentional intravascular injection. An intravascular injection of local anesthetic can lead to local anesthetic systemic toxicity that may manifest as tinnitus, seizures, or cardiac arrest [1].

Intravenous Analgesia

Opioids Although all opioids cross the placenta, they are commonly used for pain relief in the parturient. Fetal side effects of opioids include decreased fetal heart rate variability and dose-related respiratory depression. Maternal side effects include hypoventiliation, nausea, vomiting, and pruritis. The specific opioid selected is often based on local availability and provider preference as the incidence of side effects are largely dose-dependent rather than drug-dependent. Butorphanol, a synthetic opioid with agonist-antagonist properties is commonly used for labor analgesia [1].

Remifentanil Remifentanil, which undergoes rapid hydrolysis by plasma and tissue esterases, has been used for labor analgesia. Remifentanil's rapid onset and offset make it a good choice for the cyclical pain associated with uterine contractions. Although not comparable to pain relief provided by neuraxial anesthesia, patient-controlled analgesic (PCA) via remifentanil is a good alternative for those not a candidate for neuraxial approaches. When used as a PCA, 1:1 nursing and continuous pulse oximetry and capnography is strongly recommended [1].

Non-opioid Analgesia

Acetaminophen Acetaminophen, a weak inhibitor of both cyclooxygenase (COX)-1 and COX-2, is the first-line treatment for mild pain in a parturient [2].

Ketamine Ketamine, an antagonist at NMDA receptors, is a dissociated analgesic and works synergistically when administered with opioids. While not recommended for labor analgesia, ketamine's rapid onset is ideal for urgent situations such as episiotomy or induction of general anesthesia in a hemodynamically unstable patient [2].

Inhaled Anesthesia

Nitrous, when administered with 50% oxygen, is a mild analgesic and is offered at some centers for labor analgesia. It is self-administered and when not administered in conjunction with opioids, it does not cause respiratory depression,

hypoxia or loss of protective airway reflexes. Side effects include nausea, dizziness, paresthesias, and dry mouth. Although nitrous does cross the placenta, adverse effects on the fetus have not been noted [1].

Post-operative Pain

Neuraxial Anesthesia Neuraxial opioid administration is the gold standard for post-cesarean analgesia. Neuraxial opioids exert their effect on spinal cord receptors and when dosed appropriately, they do not cause respiratory depression. Although there is a higher incidence of pruritis when opioids are administered neuraxially, analgesia is superior compared to intravenous or oral opioids. Because neuraxial opioids exert their effect on spinal cord receptors, intrathecal administration is superior to opioids administered in the epidural space. Common opioids used are fentanyl, which is lipid soluble and short acting, and morphine, which has a prolonged duration of action [1].

Regional Blocks

Transversus abdominis plane (TAP) block, usually preformed under ultrasound guidance is accomplished by administering local anesthetic medication in the fascial plane between the internal oblique and transversus abdominis muscles. This block is administered bilaterally and is ideal for post-cesarean section pain in those unable to receive long-acting morphine neuraxially [2].

Conclusion

It is important for clinicians to understand the pain pathways involved in labor to adequately provide analgesia. Neuraxial anesthesia includes epidural, spinal, and CSE and are the most effective and most widely used form of analgesia during labor. Advantages of neuraxial anesthesia include providing sensory pain relief while preserving motor and mental status. Complications from neuraxial anesthesia are rare and include headache and pruritus. Alternatives to neuraxial anesthesia include intravenous medication, inhaled and regional anesthesia.

References

1. Chestnut D, Wong C, Tsen L, Ngan Kee WD, Beilin Y, Mhyre J et al. Chestnut's obstetric anesthesia: principles and practice. 5th ed. Lubbock: S L Saunders; 2014.
2. Miller RD, Eriksson LI, Fleisher LA, Wiener-Kronish JP, Cohen NH, Young WL. Miller's anesthesia. 8th ed. Lubbock: S L Saunders; 2014.
3. Choi PT, Galinski SE, Takeuchi L, Lucas S, Tamayo C, Jadad AR. PDPH is a common complication of neuraxial blockade in parturients: a meta-analysis of obstetrical studies. Can J Anaesth. 2003;50(5):460–9.

Management of Multiple Sclerosis in Pregnancy

Konstantin Balashov and Yaritza Rosario

Introduction: Multiple Sclerosis and Pregnancy

Multiple Sclerosis (MS) is a chronic inflammatory and neurodegenerative disease of the central nervous system. Although MS affects over 700,000 individuals in the USA and more than two million individuals worldwide, its etiology remains unknown. The disease progression and specific symptoms of MS are unpredictable and vary from person to person. Initially, most patients experience episodes of disease flare-up (relapses) followed by complete or partial improvement of symptoms (remission). Later stages of the disease may be associated with progressive neurological disability. While individuals of all ages are affected by MS, it is more commonly diagnosed in young adults and its prevalence is significantly increased in women compared to men. More than half of women diagnosed with MS will develop the disease during their reproductive years, making pregnancy issues a prevalent concern [1].

There are several key questions that health professionals treating MS need to be aware of when treating their female patients of childbearing age (Table 21.1).

Table 21.1 Reproductive and pregnancy-related questions in multiple sclerosis (MS)

Stage	Topic of discussion
Prior to conception	Q1. Can MS patients use contraceptive medications?
	Q2. Is it difficult to get pregnant with a diagnosis of MS?
	Q3. If needed, can MS patients use assisted reproductive technology?
	Q4. Should patients discontinue MS medications prior to pregnancy?
Pregnancy	Q5. Does MS activity change during pregnancy?
	Q6. Are pregnancy-related complications more common in MS? Is special obstetrics care required?
	Q7. Can a patient have an MRI during pregnancy?
	Q8. Is IV steroid treatment safe during pregnancy or breastfeeding?
Postpartum	Q9. Will MS disease activity increase after pregnancy?
	Q10. What is the effect of breastfeeding on MS activity?
	Q11. When should a patient restart MS medication? Can breastfeeding patients take MS medications?
	Q12. Will children of MS patients have an increased risk of developing this illness in the future?

K. Balashov (✉)
Department of Neurology, Boston Medical Center and Boston University School of Medicine, Boston, MA, USA
e-mail: balashov@bu.edu

Y. Rosario
Rutgers Robert Wood Johnson Medical School, Piscataway, NJ, USA

G. Gupta et al. (eds.), *Neurological Disorders in Pregnancy*,
https://doi.org/10.1007/978-3-031-36490-7_21

Contraception in MS

A key counseling point is to advise patients that MS does not affect fertility and therefore, effective contraception should be implemented if pregnancy is not desired. Oral contraceptive use is not associated with greater risk of MS relapses and appears to be safe for women with MS [2, 3]. Disease-modifying therapies for MS do not appear to decrease the effectiveness of hormonal contraception [3].

Pregnancy Rates in MS

MS may cause sexual dysfunction, either directly (e.g., loss of libido, erectile dysfunction, vaginal dryness, inability to achieve orgasm) or indirectly through other symptoms related to MS (e.g., bladder symptoms, fatigue, spasticity, depression) [4]. However, pregnancy rates among patients with MS are comparable to pregnancy rates in woman without MS. Based on the recent retrospective analysis of submitted administrative claims, pregnancy rates among patients with MS have increased from 7.91% to 9.47% between 2006 and 2014. At the same time, pregnancy rates for women without MS decreased from 8.83% to 7.75%. Pregnant women with MS were older by approximately 3 years (average age: 32.5 years) than pregnant women without MS [5].

The Use of Reproductive Technology in MS

The risk of MS exacerbations and increased radiological disease activity (on brain MRI) has been reported in selected case series describing patients with relapsing-remitting MS exposed to gonadotropin-releasing hormone and follicle-stimulating hormone as a part of assisted reproductive technology infertility treatment [6, 7]. The recent meta-analysis of 220 clinical cases confirmed an increased frequency of MS relapses following assisted reproductive technology [8].

The practicing clinicians shall discuss with patients the increased risks associated with reproductive technology.

MS Medications During Pregnancy in People with MS

Multiple disease-modifying treatments (DMTs) are available for patients with MS. The overall goal is to initiate DMTs early in the course of the disease. Currently, none of the DMTs are approved by the US Food and Drug Administration (FDA) for use during pregnancy. The decision whether to prescribe or not prescribe a particular DMT prior to or during pregnancy remains at the discretion of the prescriber, who will need to discuss potential benefits and risks of the drug with their patient. It is important to note that selected DMTs are strongly contraindicated during pregnancy and shall not be used. Women with MS are not discouraged from conceiving, but should be advised on the precautions surrounding the use of specific DMTs prior to conception and during pregnancy. The question then becomes which is the most appropriate DMT choice (if any) when considering pregnancy planning.

The appropriate time frame to discontinue DMTs prior to conception to avoid pregnancy-related complications is not fully understood for most therapies. In general, it would be prudent to consider the half-life of DMTs when planning discontinuing therapy prior to pregnancy. Extra vigilance is needed when prescribing DMTs that have teratogenic potential/impact nucleic acid synthesis or repair, (e.g., Teriflunomide and Cladribine). When possible, it may be best to avoid these medications for female and male MS patients who plan to conceive children. In addition, select DMTs have been associated with a risk of rebound disease activity upon discontinuation (e.g., Fingolimod and Natalizumab). Therefore, prescribers need to be aware of this risk for severe rebound relapses when discontinuing such medications for women of childbearing age who desire pregnancy or are not on reliable birth control [9].

DMTs and safety of its use prior or during pregnancy are described as follows.

Interferons and Glatiramer Acetate

Interferon beta-based drugs and Glatiramer Acetate have the longest record in terms of safety profile, although there are many other DMTs with a higher efficacy profile. There have been no well-controlled randomized studies of Interferon beta-based drugs and Glatiramer Acetate in pregnant women with MS. The approved label for Interferon beta-1b was updated in 2019 to reflect that available data, which includes prospective observational studies, have not generally indicated a drug-associated risk of major birth defects with Interferon beta-1b during pregnancy. Some neurologists suggest that it is reasonable for females who do not wish to discontinue therapy, to safely continue the use of either Interferons or Glatiramer Acetate until they have a confirmed pregnancy, at which time point they can discontinue the use of these therapies [9]. It is important to understand that if these medications are restarted in the postpartum period, their efficacy may be limited in the first several months and will not offer reduction in relapse rate during this time [4].

Dimethyl Fumarate

The safety of Dimethyl Fumarate during pregnancy has not been established. The recommendation is for women with MS to use effective contraception while on this therapy and to consider alternate therapy if pregnancy is desired [4]. The same recommendation is applicable to Diroximel Fumarate, the recently approved DMT with the mechanism of action similar to Dimethyl Fumarate.

Fingolimod

Females should be advised to use reliable contraception while on Fingolimod. This oral agent may pose an increased risk of adverse fetal outcome, therefore, the recommendation is to discontinue fingolimod 2 months prior to conception [9]. For accidental/unintended pregnancy while on Fingolimod, it is advisable to discontinue this therapy immediately after confirmed pregnancy. The same recommendation is applicable to siponimod, the recently approved DMT with the mechanism of action similar to Fingolimod.

Teriflunomide

Teriflunomide is typically not prescribed for women of childbearing age, due to the relatively high risk of teratogenicity (FDA pregnancy category X). The general recommendation is to maintain effective contraception methods while on this therapy and stop this medication prior to conception. The female patient may need to undergo rapid accelerated elimination of the drug, as Teriflunomide has a very long half-life in plasma. Once discontinued, it is advisable that she maintains effective contraception methods for over a month until the plasma concentration is 0.02 mg/L on two occasions 14 days apart [4]. If plans of pregnancy are several years in the future, the patient should stay on effective contraception for 2 additional years or undergo rapid elimination [4]. An option to bridge therapy, with either Interferon beta or Glatiramer Acetate, will prevent the patient from remaining untreated after discontinuing Teriflunomide.

It is also advisable that males with MS who plan on fathering a child avoid the use of this medication as the drug is secreted in the semen, which is in turn a potential exposure to the fetus [9].

Cladribine

Cladribine is contraindicated during pregnancy due to the risk of fetal harm, including teratogenicity and embryo-fetal related death based on animal studies with Cladribine IV. The manufacturer recommends that, in addition to hormonal contraception, a second barrier method should be implemented during treatment and for at least 4 weeks after the last dose in the treatment course. The general advice is that females should not become pregnant for a minimum of 6 months upon completion of a Cladribine dosing regimen [4].

Natalizumab

Natalizumab is often prescribed to patients with more aggressive disease. This medication is also associated with increased risk of disease rebound once it is discontinued. The average time frame in which a relapse can occur is approximately 12–16 weeks after discontinuation of Natalizumab [10]. Therefore, a female patient with MS who is considering pregnancy should be advised to discuss their treatment options with her provider and not self-discontinue therapy.

Natalizumab is not known to cross the placenta during the first trimester of pregnancy, but does so during the second and third trimester [4]. Some authors suggest, for patients with highly active MS, to consider Natalizumab treatment over a 6–8 week extended interval, with the last dose given at less than 30 weeks gestation [9]. Hematologic monitoring of the newborn will be necessary for infants exposed to Natalizumab during the pregnancy. If both the patient and prescriber decide to discontinue Natalizumab prior to conception, it is advisable that the patient continues reliable contraception until the risk of rebound relapse has passed (6–12 months) before trying to conceive [9].

Ocrelizumab

Ocrelizumab is a humanized monoclonal IgG antibody; immunoglobulins are known to cross the placenta which in turn exposes the fetus to this therapeutic agent. It has been reported that infants exposed to other anti-CD20 agents have experienced transient B cell depletion and lymphopenia [11]. Due to possible B cell depletion, infants will need to be monitored if exposed during pregnancy.

Alemtuzumab

Alemtuzumab is contraindicated during pregnancy. The general manufacturer's recommendation for Alemtuzumab is to avoid pregnancy during treatment and for a minimum of 4–6 months after therapy is discontinued for both female and male patients. For 4 years after Alemtuzumab discontinuation, patients are still at increased risk of autoimmune thyroid disease, immune thrombocytopenic purpura, Goodpasture's syndrome, and other autoimmune

disorders [12]. Due to the extended time span in which these disorders can occur it may be possible that these occur during pregnancy and may affect both mother and fetus. Therefore, it will be important for female patients to comply with monthly testing (full blood count, kidney function, thyroid function) in order to identify any abnormalities in the early phases [4].

MS Disease Activity During Pregnancy

MS is an immune-mediated disease. The maternal immune system is complex and governed by multiple factors. There are significant changes in the immune system in pregnancy that include adjustment of maternal tolerance and protection of the fetus [13]. Naturally, MS activity also changes during and after pregnancy. Relative to the preconception period, MS relapse rate decreases during pregnancy by more than 35%, especially in the last trimester [5].

Pregnancy-Related Complications in MS

The recent retrospective US administrative claim analysis suggests that the higher proportion of woman with MS than without had premature labor, infection, cardiovascular disease, anemia/ acquired coagulation disorder, acquired fetal damage and congenital fetal malformation [14]. A diagnosis of MS should not influence obstetric management, for example, whether the patient can have an epidural, or vaginal delivery vs. cesarean section. The retrospective cohort data from the British Columbia MS Clinics' database showed that MS was not significantly associated with assisted vaginal delivery or Cesarean section [15]. Extra care may be required for women with significant neurological disability. For example, significant spasticity would need to be taken into consideration when planning obstetric care [4].

The Use of MRI During Pregnancy

In general, MRI without IV contrast is not contraindicated at any time during pregnancy However, most gadolinium contrast solutions can cross the placenta and result in fetal exposure and gadolinium retention. It increases the risk of stillbirth and neonatal death. Therefore, brain MRI with IV contrast should be avoided when possible [16].

The Use of IV Steroid Treatment During Pregnancy or Breastfeeding

Methylprednisolone has pregnancy category C (use with caution if benefits outweigh risks). The recently published UK consensus on pregnancy in multiple sclerosis suggests that MS relapses can be treated with corticosteroids during pregnancy [4]. Some neurologists prefer to use intravenous immunoglobulin instead of methylprednisolone during pregnancy. A clinical trial addressing this issue would be reasonable to further investigate the safest and most effective treatment for an MS relapse during pregnancy. Furthermore, there is no indication to stop breastfeeding if methylprednisolone is required to treat a postpartum relapse [17].

MS Disease Activity After Pregnancy

Relative to the preconception period, MS relapse rate increases during puerperium by approximately 70%, and remains elevated in the postpartum year's last three quarters [5]. However, MS patients should be advised that pregnancy does not increase the risk of worsening long-term disability [4]. For example, the recent data analysis of the prospectively followed cohort of 2466 of MS patients provided evidence of protective effects of pregnancy against neurological disability accrual over the 10-year period [18].

The Effect of Breastfeeding on MS Activity

The health benefits of breastfeeding for both mother and infant have long been established [19]. There were multiple studies on the role of breastfeeding in MS. The recent meta-analysis of available publications suggests that breastfeeding is protective against postpartum relapses in MS. The probability of postpartum relapses was decreased approximately by 40% in breastfeeding compared with non-breastfeeding MS patients [20].

MS patients who are agreeable to breastfeeding should be counseled on the possible benefits of exclusive breastfeeding. It appears that exclusive breastfeeding may decrease the risk of postpartum MS relapse [9]. For those who do not wish to breastfeed counseling on DMT reinitiating is advisable.

Restarting MS Medication After Pregnancy

There is no conclusive data in regard to infant exposure to DMTs via breastmilk. The recent UK consensus on pregnancy in MS suggests that the benefits of breastfeeding while on Glatiramer Acetate and Interferon beta-based drugs outweigh any risk and should be encouraged [4]. Other authors suggest that resuming Glatiramer Acetate or Interferon beta in the postpartum period does not reduce the risk of MS relapses within the first 6 months postpartum and prefer restarting the above medications at 6–12 months postpartum [9].

Oral agents (dimethyl fumarate, fingolimod, teriflunomide, and cladribine) and alemtuzumab are contraindicated during breastfeeding due to potential harmful effects on the infants' development [4, 9]. The same authors are more open to the use of natalizumab in breastfeeding patients [4, 9]. In regard to ocrelizumab, animal data does show medication excretion into breast milk, therefore, it is advisable to avoid this therapy if planning to breastfeed [4, 9].

The Risk of MS Among Children of MS Patients

Although the etiology of MS is not known, multiple genes have been implicated in MS pathogenesis. Therefore, compared to the general population, the risk of MS among children of patients with MS is significantly increased. Based on the recent analysis of 18 family studies, the risk of MS inheritance with one affected parent was estimated at 1.45%, increasing to approximately 18% with two affected parents [21].

Conclusion

While MS is a chronic condition that can be associated with significant neurological disability, patients should be counseled that pregnancy is not a contraindication. In addition, MS does not affect fertility rates. Pregnancy counseling will need to be a simultaneous conversation when discussing MS treatment options and general prognosis. Patients and their partners will need to be educated on different factors related to disease activity associated with pregnancy. It will also be necessary to consider MS treatment modification during pregnancy. The clinician has a key role in educating the patient appropriately and alleviating any concerns surrounding MS and pregnancy.

References

1. Buraga I, Popovici RE. Multiple sclerosis and pregnancy: current considerations. ScientificWorldJournal. 2014;2014:513160, 1.
2. Bove R, Rankin K, Chua AS, Saraceno T, Sattarnezhad N, Greeke E, et al. Oral contraceptives and MS disease activity in a contemporary real-world cohort. Mult Scler. 2018;24(2):227–30.
3. Houtchens MK, Zapata LB, Curtis KM, Whiteman MK. Contraception for women with multiple sclerosis: guidance for healthcare providers. Mult Scler. 2017;23(6):757–64.
4. Dobson R, Dassan P, Roberts M, Giovannoni G, Nelson-Piercy C, Brex PA. UK consensus on pregnancy in multiple sclerosis: 'Association of British Neurologists' guidelines. Pract Neurol. 2019;19(2):106–14.
5. Houtchens MK, Edwards NC, Phillips AL. Relapses and disease-modifying drug treatment in pregnancy and live birth in US women with MS. Neurology. 2018;91(17):e1570–e8.
6. Correale J, Farez MF, Ysrraelit MC. Increase in multiple sclerosis activity after assisted reproduction technology. Ann Neurol. 2012;72(5):682–94.
7. Hellwig K, Schimrigk S, Beste C, Muller T, Gold R. Increase in relapse rate during assisted reproduction technique in patients with multiple sclerosis. Eur Neurol. 2009;61(2):65–8.
8. Bove R, Rankin K, Lin C, Zhao C, Correale J, Hellwig K, et al. Effect of assisted reproductive technology on multiple sclerosis relapses: case series and meta-analysis. Mult Scler. 2019;26:1352458519865118.
9. Langer-Gould AM. Pregnancy and family planning in multiple sclerosis. Continuum (Minneap Minn). 2019;25(3):773–92.
10. Portaccio E, Moiola L, Martinelli V, Annovazzi P, Ghezzi A, Zaffaroni M, et al. Pregnancy decision-making in women with multiple sclerosis treated with natalizumab: II: maternal risks. Neurology. 2018;90(10):e832–e9.
11. Chakravarty EF, Murray ER, Kelman A, Farmer P. Pregnancy outcomes after maternal exposure to rituximab. Blood. 2011;117(5):1499–506.
12. Coles AJ, Cohen JA, Fox EJ, Giovannoni G, Hartung HP, Havrdova E, et al. Alemtuzumab CARE-MS II 5-year follow-up: efficacy and safety findings. Neurology. 2017;89(11):1117–26.
13. Bonney EA. Immune regulation in pregnancy: a matter of perspective? Obstet Gynecol Clin N Am. 2016;43(4):679–98.
14. Houtchens MK, Edwards NC, Schneider G, Stern K, Phillips AL. Pregnancy rates and outcomes in women with and without MS in the United States. Neurology. 2018;91(17):e1559–e69.
15. van der Kop ML, Pearce MS, Dahlgren L, Synnes A, Sadovnick D, Sayao AL, et al. Neonatal and delivery outcomes in women with multiple sclerosis. Ann Neurol. 2011;70(1):41–50.
16. Ray JG, Vermeulen MJ, Bharatha A, Montanera WJ, Park AL. Association between MRI exposure during pregnancy and fetal and childhood outcomes. JAMA. 2016;316(9):952–61.
17. Boz C, Terzi M, Zengin Karahan S, Sen S, Sarac Y, Emrah MM. Safety of IV pulse methylprednisolone therapy during breastfeeding in patients with multiple sclerosis. Mult Scler. 2018;24(9):1205–11.
18. Jokubaitis VG, Spelman T, Kalincik T, Lorscheider J, Havrdova E, Horakova D, et al. Predictors of long-term disability accrual in relapse-onset multiple sclerosis. Ann Neurol. 2016;80(1):89–100.

19. Haghikia A, Hellwig K. Multiple sclerosis. In: Neurological illness in pregnancy: principles and practice; 2016. p. 142–52.
20. Krysko KM, Rutatangwa A, Graves J, Lazar A, Waubant E. Association between breastfeeding and postpartum multiple sclerosis relapses: a systematic review and meta-analysis. JAMA Neurol. 2019;77:327.
21. O'Gorman C, Lin R, Stankovich J, Broadley SA. Modelling genetic susceptibility to multiple sclerosis with family data. Neuroepidemiology. 2013;40(1):1–12.

Guillain-Barré Syndrome in Pregnancy

Shellen Arora, David Atherton, and Shan Chen

Introduction

Guillain-Barré syndrome is a type of acute or subacute demyelinating peripheral neuropathy typically presenting with sensory complaints and rapidly progressive symmetric ascending limb weakness over the course of days. It can lead to quadriparesis, respiratory failure, and autonomic dysfunction with labile blood pressure and arrhythmia in severe cases, making it potentially life threatening. Neurological examination often shows symmetric proximal and/or distal muscle weakness with normal or reduced sensation and, characteristically, hyporeflexia or areflexia. Cranial nerve deficits are seen in some patients. Guillain-Barré syndrome is due to a dysfunctional autoimmune process that targets the peripheral nervous system, most commonly the myelin sheaths of motor and sensory axons.

Guillain-Barré syndrome (GBS) can be divided into several subtypes depending on the phenotype, pathophysiology, and neurophysiological features. Acute inflammatory demyelinating polyneuropathy (AIDP) is the most common form of GBS and was the first to be recognized over a century ago. Acute motor axonal (AMAN) and acute sensorimotor axonal (AMSAN) variants have been described in the last three decades and are mediated by molecular mimicry targeting peripheral nerve motor or motor and sensory axons rather than myelin sheaths in the AIDP form. Miller-Fisher syndrome (MFS) is a rare but known form of GBS presenting with external ophthalmoplegia, gait ataxia, and absent tendon reflexes. Other rare phenotypic variants have also been described including pure sensory variant, restricted autonomic manifestations, and the pharyngeal-cervical-brachial pattern [1]. Bickerstaff brainstem encephalitis (BBE) is also considered a GBS variant which presents following varicella zoster virus or cytomegalovirus infections with drowsiness, altered mental status, cerebellar ataxia, possibly external ophthalmoplegia, brisk reflexes, and extensor plantar response rather than absent reflexes. These cases are often associated with brainstem dysfunction and T2 signal abnormalities in the brainstem and basal ganglia with little, if any, enhancement on brain MRI.

Typically, nerve conduction studies (NCS) in the AIDP form of GBS show evidence of demyelinating features with prolonged distal latencies and reduced conduction velocities, as well as conduction block or temporal dispersion in motor and sensory nerves. Sural nerve sparing is common and unique in GBS and can differentiate it from other neuropathies such as diabetic

S. Arora
West Virginia School of Osteopathic Medicine, Lewisburg, WV, USA

D. Atherton · S. Chen (✉)
Division of Neuromuscular Disorders and ALS, Rutgers, Department of Neurology, Robert Wood Johnson Medical School, New Brunswick, NJ, USA
e-mail: chens5@rwjms.rutgers.edu

neuropathy or chronic inflammatory demyelinating polyneuropathy (CIDP). Nerve conduction studies in the AMAN and AMSAN form of GBS show evidence of axonal damage with significantly reduced amplitudes accompanied by either normal or slightly reduced conduction velocities in motor and/or sensory nerves. CSF analysis commonly shows elevated protein levels with normal cell counts and can support the diagnosis of GBS. Once diagnosed, patients with GBS are treated with either intravenous immunoglobulin (IVIg) or plasmapheresis/plasma exchange (PE) along with best supportive medical management.

Guillain-Barré Syndrome in Pregnancy

Pregnant and non-pregnant patients with GBS have similar presentations involving complaints of weakness that may gradually lead to paralysis. Weakness starts in the lower extremities and ascends to the upper body, affecting respiratory and bulbar muscles in some cases. One case series identified two main groups of pregnant GBS patients with distinct clinical features, namely the AIDP and the AMANs groups [2]. This analysis of 45 pregnant women with GBS who were admitted to three medical centers in China revealed that pregnant women in the AIDP group (25 out of 45) more often present with distal limb weakness, distal paresthesia, and autonomic dysfunction, whereas pregnant women in the AMAN group (20 out of 45) more often present with limb weakness and dyspnea ($P < 0.01$). In addition, multivariate logistic regression analysis confirmed that limb weakness and limb weakness with dyspnea, in addition to preceding diarrhea, were significantly associated with the AMAN form of GBS and are thus considered predictors. It is important to note that the AMAN form is more common in Asia than in Western countries.

The occurrence of GBS during the third trimester of pregnancy is associated with increased risk of respiratory failure, suggesting the need for close monitoring during this period [3].

Postpartum flares can also commonly occur because of delayed hypersensitivity [4]. Individuals having suffered GBS in the past may also experience relapse throughout gestation, more commonly in the third trimester, and into the postpartum period.

Risk Factors of Guillain-Barré Syndrome in Pregnancy

GBS can rarely complicate pregnancy, and it is generally believed that it can increase maternal and neonatal morbidity and mortality.

Pre-existing risk factors for GBS are poorly understood and even less is known about predispositions among pregnant women. Generally, risk is thought to be conferred through both environmental triggers and genetic factors. Previously identified environmental factors include preceding infectious agents, vaccination, or surgical procedures.

Prodromal viral infection is a well-known trigger for GBS [5]. Reports of GBS during pregnancy in the literature show that the most common infectious triggers are respiratory or gastroinstenstinal virus such as Epstein-Barr virus (EBV), Campylobacter jejuni, cytomegalovirus (CMV), and, most recently, the Zika virus, and during the pandemic, the COVID-19 virus. In Salvador, Brazil, outbreaks of acute exanthematous illness (AEI), Guillain-Barré syndrome (GBS), and microcephaly were attributed to Zika virus in 2015. Notably, the Zika virus can trigger GBS in adults in addition to causing microcephaly and other congenital neurological abnormalities in neonates, making it of particular concern for pregnant women. Therefore, any women suspected of having being infected with the Zika virus must be closely monitored to prevent devastating GBS complications and potential neurodevelopmental abnormalities in the fetus [6].

As is observed in the non-pregnant patient population, *Campylobacter jejuni*, which commonly causes enteritis characterized by abdominal pain, fever, and diarrhea, can lead to post-infectious GBS in pregnant women, especially the axonal (AMAN) form. Pregnant patients with GBS might report a history of enteric disease or diarrhea occurring weeks or months prior to the neurological symptoms, making *C. jejuni* infection an easily missed trigger due to a prolonged prodromal period before the GBS symptom onset [7]. One study in India examined the prevalence of anti-Zika and anti-C. *jejuni* antibodies among patients with GBS using enzyme-linked immunosorbent assay (ELISA) and found that anti-C. *jejuni* antibodies were present in 46.6% of patients diagnosed with GBS and while anti-Zika antibodies were present in 15.5% [8]. This study confirms that both of these organisms are associated with a substantial proportion of GBS cases.

Additional non-infectious risk factors for GBS during pregnancy have also been identified through epidemiological methods. In one recent study of 228 cases of GBS among 1,108,541 women who delivered in the province of Quebec, Canada, between 1989 and 2013, the overall incidence was 1.42 per 100,000 person-years [9]. Notably, the incidence was six-to-seven fold higher for women with immune-mediated and rheumatologic disorders, three-fold higher for women who had blood transfusion, and two-fold higher for women with preeclampsia. Women with immune-related conditions that occurred early in life had the highest cumulative risk of GBS among pregnant patients excluding infectious triggers. In addition, preeclampsia was the only pregnancy-specific risk factor identified to be associated with GBS in pregnancy. Other pregnancy-specific risk factors, including placental disorders, gestational diabetes mellitus, preterm birth before 37 weeks of gestation, intrauterine growth restriction, postpartum hemorrhage, and multiple pregnancy, were not shown to predict incidence of GBS [9].

There are also rare case reports of the association of GBS with ketoacidosis in diabetic patients. In these cases, patients developed onset of neurological symptoms following control of ketoacidosis and hyperglycemia. Notably, transport of ketone bodies across the placental barrier leading to hypoxia and eventual fetal distress could be responsible for early termination or abortion in pregnant patients diagnosed with GBS that are

experiencing an episode of diabetic ketoacidosis rather than GBS itself [10]. Therefore, any signs of motor weakness or neuropathy in patients with a history of diabetes should warrant consideration for GBS [11]. Cases of GBS associated with miscarriage and abortion are extremely rare making it difficult to draw conclusions; some studies show no association [10] and others suggest these severe consequences are indeed related and can be effectively prevented or resolved with intervention [6].

The exact cause of Guillain-Barre syndrome is unknown. At the molecular level, molecular mimicry, antiganglioside antibodies and, possibly complement activation are thought to be involved in the pathogenesis of GBS [12]. Pregnant patients with GBS have been found to have an increase in humoral immunity due to an increase in IL-10 production, but an overall decrease in cellular immunity [13]. These changes might be related to the occurrence of GBS during pregnancy and the puerperium.

Diagnosis

GBS consists of a spectrum of neuropathic disorders with distinct pathogenesis and clinical presentations as discussed above [14], thus making the diagnosis quite challenging. However, accurate and timely diagnosis of GBS is critical for clinical practice, especially in the early phase of the disease course when treatment is most effective and close ICU monitoring can prevent life-threatening complications. Early diagnosis of GBS in pregnant women is more challenging and commonly delayed due to initial non-specific symptoms that can mirror changes in pregnancy. For example, one case reported a patient presenting with pain and progressive heaviness of both lower limbs in her third trimester of pregnancy without any antecedent infective episode and was thought to be due to the stress of pregnancy. On the third postpartum day, the patient developed weakness in all four limbs and electromyography (EMG), NCS, and CSF analysis confirmed the GBS diagnosis [15]. In addition, other pregnancy-specific symptoms and complications such as eclampsia, abnormal contractions with threatened abortion, fetal abnormalities, etc. may mask or mimic symptoms of GBS leading to a delayed or missed diagnosis.

The initial diagnosis of Guillain-Barré remains clinical. Acute or subacute onset and rapidly progressive weakness are red flag features of GBS. Co-existing bulbar weakness, distal numbness and tingling in fingers and/or toes, neck and/or lower back pain, autonomic dysfunction with urinary retention, constipation, volatile blood pressure and heart rate, and respiratory compromise are all signs of extensive peripheral nerve damage in which the diagnosis of GBS must be considered [16]. Neurological findings including symmetric weakness with reduced reflexes should raise a suspicion in an otherwise healthy woman. EMG/NCS is often performed during the workup of these clinical phenotypes and results consistent with demyelinating sensory and motor polyneuropathy or polyradiculoneuropathy confirm the diagnosis. Further, albuminocytologic dissociation in CSF with elevated protein content and normal mononuclear leukocyte count is strongly indicative of GBS [17]. Both CSF analysis and NCS can be quite useful in patients with atypical features of GBS, GBS mimics, or any diagnostic doubt. However, it is important to recognize that the CSF abnormalities may not be present until the second or even third week after onset of symptoms. Similarly, during the acute phase lasting from a couple of days up to 1 week after onset, EMG/NCS may remain normal.

A high index of clinical suspicion, thorough history taking, and detailed examination are critical to make the clinical diagnosis. In some cases, repeat EMG/NCS or CSF studies will be indicated to confirm. It is important to remember that there is an extensive list of diseases that are GBS mimics including toxic/metabolic/nutritional polyneuropathy, myopathy, infectious, inflammatory, neoplastic infiltration of spinal nerve roots or peripheral nerves, neuromuscular junctional disorders, and etc. which must be considered and ruled out. Misdiagnosis can be avoided by history, examination, and a combination supportive or exclusionary testing [18].

In recent years, a growing number of antiganglioside antibodies in serum or spinal fluid have been identified in patients with GBS spectrum disorders. Variable ganglioside antibodies, either alone or in combination, may be associated with the different forms of GBS. For example, anti-GQ1b, in addition to GT1a, is associated with at least 90% of cases of MFS and BBE variants; anti-GM1 and GD1a and GalNAc-GD1a are associated with AMAN; anti-GM1 and GD1a are associated with AMSAN. These serum antibodies can be measured by ELISA to the gangliosides themselves or their combinatory complexes (GM1a, GM1b, GM2, GM3, GD1a, GalNAc-GD1a, GD1b, GD2, GD3, GT1a, GT1b, GQ1b, GA1) in commercial laboratories [12].

Screening for viral infection in pregnant GBS patients carries an important role not only in supporting the diagnosis but also in intervening during the antenatal period to mitigate the risk of major neurodevelopmental sequelae, such as congenital CMV or neonatal Zika infection. For example, a report has described a case of a full-term neonate presenting with symptomatic congenital CMV infection with hepatosplenomegaly, "blueberry muffin" rash, intracranial calcifications, thrombocytopenia, and respiratory distress who was born to a mother with history of GBS during the first trimester of pregnancy. This underscores the importance of screening for CMV infection if GBS has been diagnosed in a pregnant woman [19].

Brain imaging, though not always necessary, may be important if there is altered mental status or unexplained cranial nerve involvement as can be seen in BBE.

The clinical, electrophysiological, laboratory, and radiological features should be thoroughly examined and considered together to reach an accurate diagnosis in the timeliest fashion. Early recognition will ensure that patients receive critical interventions when they are most effective and are monitored for life-threatening complications. Complicated or atypical cases with suspicion for a GBS variant warrant consultation at tertiary medical centers with neurologists and EMG experts specialized in neuromuscular disorders.

Management

Once the diagnosis of GBS is made, management of the pregnant patient generally follows the same principles as for non-pregnant individuals. Early treatment carries a favorable outcome. Methods of management for pregnant patients diagnosed with GBS include ventilatory support, IVIg, PE, adequate nutrition, infection control, pain control, physiotherapy, and psychological support [3]. Patients with GBS need multidisciplinary supportive care to prevent or to manage these diverse complications and to ensure timely transfer to the intensive care unit (ICU) when indicated.

Immunomodulation

The mainstay of management comprises administration of IVIg or PE for immunomodulation, both of which are considered generally safe for pregnant women. The effectiveness of IVIg and PE, but not corticosteroids, has been established for the treatment of GBS by multiple randomized controlled trials (RCTs) [17, 20].

PE involves the replacement of the patient's plasma with normal healthy plasma or substitute in order to remove autoreactive antibodies. Most commonly, the paradigm of five to six PE treatments every other day is recommended for GBS patients. Human albumin is a commonly used replacement fluid, while some use fresh frozen plasma. PE is typically performed through a central venous catheter; rarely peripheral venous access is used. Complications related to PE include those associated with the catheter placement procedure (e.g., vascular injury, infection), hypotension, allergic reactions, and hypocalcemia (which is the most commonly associated laboratory abnormality).

Immunoglobulin is often administered intravenously at 0.4 g/kg of body weight for five consecutive days. IVIg functions by modulating the immune reaction at the level of T cells, B cells, and macrophages, interfering with antibody production and degradation, modulating the complement cascade, and exerting effects on the cytokine network. However, the precise mechanism of action of IVIg in GBS is not yet clear [21]. IVIg has a very good safety profile, especially for long-term administration. It does, however, have some noteworthy side effects that can range from mild to severe: (1) mild infusion-rate-related reactions such as headaches, myalgia, or fever; (2) moderate but inconsequential events such as aseptic meningitis and skin rash; and (3) severe, but rare, complications, such as thromboembolic events likely due to increased plasma viscosity and renal tubular necrosis resulting in acute renal failure in some cases requiring dialysis [22]. It is generally believed that IVIg and PE have similar efficacy and benefit. However, if patients are known to have associated ganglioside IgG auto-antibodies against GM1, GM1b, or GalNAc-GD1a, IVIg may be more effective than PE and is preferred in these situations. Administration of IVIg was shown to be associated with good maternal and fetal outcomes in pregnant patients with sensory GBS in a small case study [23].

A meta-analysis comparing PE versus IVIg showed no evidence of superiority in the efficacy or safety in the management of GBS and another autoimmune neuromuscular disorder, myasthenia gravis. Additionally, no significant difference was found in terms of hospital stay length or ventilator support time [24]. However, in a retrospective cohort study of 6642 records (2637 treated with PE and 4005 treated with IVIg) from the 2002 to 2014 Nationwide Inpatient Sample, PE was found to likely be associated with poorer healthcare utilization outcomes as compared to IVIg, including prolonged hospitalization by approximately 7.5 days, greater hospitalization costs by approximately $46,000, and increased risk of in-hospital death with an odds ratio of 2.78. These effects were not changed after controlling for confounders through risk adjustment, propensity score adjustment, or matching [25]. In practice, deciding between IVIg and PE often depends on individual features of the patient and their disease course. IVIg often is initiated as the first therapy and is more likely to be completed due to its ease of timely administration. Immunoglobulin (Ig) has also been administered via the subcutaneous route as an alternative treatment option for indicated chronic autoimmune disorders, especially in patients with limited intravenous access. However, data supporting the use of subcutaneous Ig in GBS patients is lacking. In general, steroids are avoided in GBS patients, although steroid therapy is generally considered safe during pregnancy. However, steroids are not shown to hasten the recovery or improve the long-term outcome of GBS patients and may even cause worsening of weakness when used in high doses. The use of steroids is advocated by some in GBS variants where symptoms do not respond to conventional IVIg and PE therapies. For example, there were reports of successful treatment using steroids in cases of AMSAN and BBE, both of which are GBS variants [26, 27].

Unfortunately, there are no consensus statements or RCTs on the treatment strategy for severe GBS cases when patients fail to improve on IVIg or PE; this is considered treatment failure. In fact, about 25–30% of patients with GBS ultimately require artificial ventilation and approximately 20% are unable to walk after 6 months despite employing current immunotherapies. The International GBS Outcome study (IGOS) did not show better outcomes after a second IVIg course in GBS with poor prognosis, though the study was limited by its observational design, small numbers, and baseline characteristic imbalances. Moreover, about 10% of GBS patients have a secondary deterioration within the first 8 weeks after starting IVIg. In these cases of treatment-related fluctuation (TRF), repeated IVIg treatment is required [28].

Emerging biological therapeutic agents have been proposed and attempted, but are limited to single case reports or series. A recent Cochrane study analyzing RCTs that have evaluated pharmacological agents other than IVIg, PE, or steroids determined that all of the available studies were too small to demonstrate clinically important benefit or harms [29].

One emerging therapy is rituximab, a genetically engineered antibody that depletes CD20+ B cells and is FDA approved for the treatment of non-Hodgkin's lymphoma, CD20+ chronic lymphocytic leukemia, and rheumatoid arthritis. Although it carries a favorable side effect profile, the evidence of its efficacy in severe cases of dysimmune demyelinating disease was primarily restricted to CIDP with very limited data on effectiveness in GBS. Moreover, no large prospective RCTs evaluating its use in GBS are available. Eculizumab is recombinant humanized monoclonal antibody against the complement protein C5 and has been used to treat paroxysmal nocturnal hemoglobinuria (PNH), atypical hemolytic uremic syndrome (aHUS), and recently was FDA-approved to treat seropositive generalized myasthenia gravis (gMG) and AQP4+ neuromyelitis optica spectrum disorder (NMOSD). Additionally, eculizumab was found to be safe in a small phase 2 trial for use in GBS. While complement inhibition combined with IVIg treatment might improve outcome in GBS, their combined efficacy remains uncertain. Future agents targeting other immune mediators and cytokines, such as the anti-CD52 monoclonal antibody, alemtuzumab, are also on the horizon and may play a role in GBS management. As of now, however, none of these newer agents has been approved for the treatment of GBS by the FDA [30]. Moreover, little is known about the efficacy of these newer pharmacologics and immunotherapies in pregnant women with GBS.

Monitoring and Supportive Measures

GBS is a complex and rapidly evolving disorder in which patients can present with ascending limb paralysis and quickly develop other complications due to diffuse peripheral nerve damage, including respiratory compromise, cardiac arrhythmias, and autonomic dysfunction. Mild hyponatremia has been found in 7–26% of patients and severe sodium level reduction resemblant of syndrome of inappropriate antidiuretic hormone secretion (SIADH) ([Na$^+$]: 105 to 120 mEq/L) may also occur. Patients may also develop mild transient proteinuria and rarely glomerulonephritis. Serum CK level is found to be elevated in 33% of patients, often up to 4 times higher than the upper limit of normal.

Patients with GBS may have severe autonomic dysfunction; some have urinary retention and constipation, some have light-fixed pupils and excessive sweating, whereas others have cardiac dysrhythmia (10–75% patients report cardiac arrhythmia with more than 50% patients present with an abnormal EKG) or labile blood pressure. The exact mechanism is unknown and clinically difficult to predict among these distant presentations.

Reported increases in the mortality rate among pregnant GBS patients are most likely attributed to the presence of cardiac arrhythmias and/or pulmonary emboli [31]. GBS afflicted pregnant women must be closely monitored for the development of respiratory failure and autonomic dysfunction. Anti-hypertensive medications are generally to be avoided. In addition, all the immunomodulating therapies affect the immune system. Thus, patients may get infections more easily, even serious or fatal infections.

Supportive measures include venous thromboembolism prophylaxis, aggressive physical therapy, pressure ulcer prevention, enteral nutrition, pain control, management of bowel and bladder dysfunction, and respiratory support.

Subcutaneous heparin has been shown to possibly lower risk of thromboembolic events including deep vein thrombosis in intensive care patients with severe muscle weakness.

Nonsteroidal anti-inflammatory drugs (NSAIDs) may provide some pain relief but often do not provide full analgesic benefit for the patient, and should be avoided during pregnancy if possible. NSAID use in early pregnancy is associated with an increased risk of miscarriage and congenital malformation. The U.S. Food and Drug Administration (FDA) is warning that use of NSAIDs around 20 weeks or later in pregnancy may cause rare but serious kidney problems in an unborn baby. This can lead to low levels of amniotic fluid surrounding the baby and possible complications. Pain can be severe and needs to be treated sufficiently. Opioids can also be used, but it may worsen autonomic symptoms, especially constipation. Patients with GBS are encouraged to do strength exercises even during the acute paralytic phase and should continue with rehabilitation to restore mobility and function after acute hospitalization [32].

Management After Guillain-Barré Syndrome

Most GBS patients recover and are able to resume their normal activities. However, despite current treatment options, many patients have residual deficits. In addition to engaging physical and occupational therapy to help restore motor and ambulatory functions, other long-term health consequences persisting after acute hospital management must be addressed.

Chronic Neuropathic Pain, Fatigue, and Depression

Pain is a prevalent clinical feature of GBS. Patients with GBS often present with two main types of pain: aching muscle pain and neuropathic pain.

Pain often occurs during the acute paralytic phase of GBS and may persist even after muscle strength is recovered. Pain experienced in the acute phase is mostly nociceptive, caused by inflammation of nerve roots and peripheral nerves that activate the nociceptors [33]. Over time, GBS patients develop neuropathic pain as they move past the acute phase, which is described as non-nociceptive pain because it does not arise from activation of the pain receptors but arises from the degeneration and regeneration of nerves associated with chronic neuropathy [33]. Consistent with this, the chronic pain is typically described as sharp, shooting, or burning. Sensory disturbance such as numbness in distal limbs is also a common concurrent complaint. Overuse of recovering muscles or compensating muscles can also result in pain in tendons, ligaments, and joints, usually described as achiness deep in the muscles or around the joints which often resolves once muscle strength improves. Many medications can be used to reduce neuropathic pain including NSAIDs, opioids, corticosteroids, anticonvulsants, tricyclic antidepressants, and neuroleptics [34], but often high doses and combinations of different pharmacologic categories are needed. This can lead to the development of more side effects and, in general, need to be used with extreme caution in pregnant women to avoid maternal-fetal complications.

Among the analgesics indicated for post-GBS pain is gabapentin, one of the first-line treatments and perhaps the most commonly used agent in clinical practice for neuropathic pain in non-pregnant patients. It exerts its analgesic effects by binding to voltage-dependent calcium channels in the spinal cord, which reduces afferent traffic and excitation of nociceptive neurons that are responsible for hyperalgesia. The drug is also known to cross the blood–brain barrier and therefore is responsible for the modulation of central pain pathways, including decreased production of glutamate in sensory or motor nociceptive fibers [35]. In a double-blinded, placebo-controlled, cross-over study, patients with GBS experiencing either acute pain or neuropathic pain reported significantly reduced Fentanyl consumption, lower sedation scores, and fewer side effects associated with gabapentin use compared to other agents. Owing to its tolerability and relatively few side effects, gabapentin is the drug of choice for chronic neuropathic pain following GBS. However, its ability to be used in pregnant women is limited as it is considered category C due to the lack of research or well-controlled studies verifying its safety in human pregnancy.

While the symptoms of pain can occur prior to the onset of weakness and persist for at least 2 years following resolution, fatigue is more pervasive with a high prevalence during the early recovery phase and potential persistence through decades after other symptoms resolve [34]. Fatigue contributes significantly to morbidity and adversely affects the quality of life in GBS patients. Although fatigue is highly subjective, its severity can be evaluated through measurements like the Fatigue Severity Scale (FSS). Interestingly, one study demonstrated that presence of fatigue at admission (FSS ≥ 4, reported in 39% of GBS patients) was significantly associ-ated with ventilator requirement and neuropathic pain. Furthermore, the presence of fatigue at discharge (FSS ≥ 4, 12%) was associated with disability, anxiety, and extended duration of rehabilitative stay. Fatigue did not correlate with age, gender, antecedent illness, muscle weakness, depression, or sleep disturbances [36]. Despite being a pervasive problem, there are limited studies or clinical trials addressing fatigue in GBS. Generally speaking, the impact of fatigue on daily life can be improved or minimized by energy reservation strategies, which can be developed through activities like exercise. One RCT showed that high intensity relative to lower intensity exercise significantly reduced disability in patients with GBS. Overall, various types of exercise programs improve physical outcomes such as functional mobility, cardiopulmonary function, isokinetic muscle strength, and reduced fatigue in patients with GBS.

Lifestyle changes can help fatigue using energy reservation strategies very few studies on the efficacy of pharmacologic therapies to help combat post-GBS fatigue showed little benefits. Amantadine has been shown to improve fatigue in patients with multiple sclerosis but has been ineffective in GBS patients. Stimulants such as modafinil, methylphenidate, or dextroamphet-amine are also used in patients with multiple sclerosis with some benefits but none was studied in GBS patients. Of an important note, modafinil and methylphenidate are both pregnancy category C and no stimulant has been proven safe during pregnancy. Depression is also a significant problem following GBS, with approximately 1 in 15 patients (6.7%) diagnosed with GBS meeting depression criteria based on Hospital Anxiety and Depression Scale scores. In addition, depressive symptoms were found to be present at 3 months post-diagnosis, with notable relief of depression after bicycle exercise training [37]. Among 76 GBS survivors enrolled in an Australian study that evaluated long-term GBS related outcomes, 18% reported moderate to extreme depression using the Depression Anxiety Stress Scale, with higher scores among women.

Anxiety, depression, and brief episodes of reactive psychosis are more frequently reported in patients with GBS in high dependency settings or ICUs, particularly those with severe GBS experiencing quadriparesis and cranial nerve involvement or requiring ventilation [38]. Treating concurrent psychological issues, particularly depression, plays an important role in the recovery from GBS.

Prediction Models and Prognosis

GBS is a very heterogeneous disease with variable disease courses and outcomes. Several novel prediction models have been proposed and validated to provide accurate prognostic data in different phases of GBS and to help in selecting patients for individualized care.

In the emergency room, the Erasmus GBS Respiratory Insufficiency Score (EGRIS) can be used as to predict the probability of respiratory insufficiency in the first week after admission for GBS. The model uses the following parameters: severity of weakness (expressed as the MRC sum score), the number of days between onset of weakness and admission, and facial and/or bulbar weakness. If the predicted chance of developing respiratory insufficiency is high, the patient should be admitted to the ICU instead of a general ward [39].

About 25% of GBS patients require artificial ventilator support. It was shown that time from onset to admission of <7 days, inability to cough, inability to stand, inability to lift the elbows or head from the bed, and increased liver enzyme levels was predictive of increased probability of needing artificial ventilation in a French study of 722 GBS patients [40]. Another study identified similar parameters predicting the need for mechanical ventilation: time from onset to admission <7 days, muscle weakness on admission, facial and/or bulbar weakness, and IgG antibody against GQ1b [41].

Once intubated, factors that predict successful weaning from the ventilator are age < 60 years, lack of autonomic dysfunction, and vital capacity >20 mL/kg or an improvement in vital capacity of 4 mL/kg [12]. Conversely, autonomic dysfunction, advanced age, and pulmonary comorbidity are associated with a long duration of mechanical ventilation and the need for tracheostomy [42]. A high grade on the GBS Disability Scale at neurological examination at 2 weeks after admission, diarrhea preceding GBS onset, and advanced age are all predictors of poor long-term outcome [43].

Mortality from GBS varies between 3% and 7%, most commonly from respiratory insufficiency, pulmonary infection, autonomic dysfunction, and cardiac arrest. Predictors of mortality are advanced age, severe disease, increased comorbidity, pulmonary and cardiac complications, mechanical ventilation, and systemic infection. A large proportion of the deaths occur >30 days from onset, and a subsequent study has shown that the majority of patients who died were in the recovery phase [44]. Therefore, it is important to continue close monitoring and supportive care after patients are discharged from the ICU.

Most pregnant women with GBS carry a good prognosis. The majority of them recover with no residual deficits and have an uncomplicated labor and delivery following pregnancy. Poor prognostic factors among pregnant patients with GBS include marked decrease in muscular strength, need for ventilatory assistance, and reduced amplitude of evoked motor potential on EMG/NCS [4]. About 5% of patients initially diagnosed with GBS are eventually found to have chronic inflammatory demyelinating polyradiculoneuropathy (CIDP) with acute onset (A-CIDP) [28]. This subgroup of patients requires long-term immunotherapies unlike most GBS patients. There was also a case report of relapsing GBS during the immediate postpartum period following an initial GBS during the third trimester and a full recovery. Presumably, surgery and anesthesia may be triggers for relapse in association with an overall increase in pro-inflammatory cytokines in the postpartum period. The patient responded to a repeat course of IVIg [45].

In summary, Guillain-Barre syndrome (GBS) rarely complicates pregnancy, and can be associated with high maternal and perinatal morbidity if not properly identified and treated. Neurologists, intensivists, and obstetricians should work together to provide the best care of these patients.

References

1. Dimachkie MM, Barohn RJ. Guillain-Barré syndrome and variants. Neurol Clin. 2013;31(2):491–510. https://doi.org/10.1016/j.ncl.2013.01.005.
2. Gu YW, Lin J, Zhang LX, et al. Classification of pregnancy complicating Guillain-Barré syndrome. Zhonghua Yi Xue Za Zhi. 2019;99(18):1401–5. https://doi.org/10.3760/cma.j.issn.0376-2491.2019.18.009.
3. Vasudev R, Raina TR. A rare case of Guillain-Barré syndrome in pregnancy treated with plasma exchange. Asian J Transfus Sci. 2014;8(1):59–60. https://doi.org/10.4103/0973-6247.126695.
4. Bahadur A, Gupta N, Deka D, Mittal S. Successful maternal and fetal outcome of Guillain-Barré syndrome complicating pregnancy. Indian J Med Sci. 2009;63(11):517–8. https://doi.org/10.4103/0019-5359.58882.
5. Sejvar JJ, Baughman AL, Wise M, Morgan OW. Population incidence of Guillain-Barré syndrome: a systematic review and meta-analysis. Neuroepidemiology. 2011;36(2):123–33. https://doi.org/10.1159/000324710.
6. Barbi L, Coelho AVC, de LCA A, Crovella S. Prevalence of Guillain-Barré syndrome among Zika virus infected cases: a systematic review and meta-analysis. Braz J Infect Dis. 2018;22(2):137–41. https://doi.org/10.1016/j.bjid.2018.02.005.
7. Ang CW, Krogfelt K, Herbrink P, et al. Validation of an ELISA for the diagnosis of recent campylobacter infections in Guillain-Barré and reactive arthritis patients. Clin Microbiol Infect. 2007;13(9):915–22.
8. Baskar D, Amalnath D, Mandal J, Dhodapkar R, Vanathi K. Antibodies to Zika virus, campylobacter jejuni and gangliosides in Guillain-Barré syndrome: a prospective single-center study from Southern India. Neurol India. 2018;66(5):1324–31. https://doi.org/10.4103/0028-3886.241402.
9. Auger N, Quach C, Healy-Profitós J, Dinh T, Chassé M. Early predictors of Guillain-Barré syndrome in the life course of women. Int J Epidemiol. 2018;47(1):280–8. https://doi.org/10.1093/ije/dyx181.
10. Affes L, Elleuch M, Mnif F, et al. Guillain Barré syndrome and ketoacidosic decompensation of diabetes during pregnancy: about a case and review of the literature. Pan Afr Med J. 2017;26:1–6. https://doi.org/10.11604/pamj.2017.26.86.11091.
11. Akpınar ÇK, Doğru H, Balcı K. A possible Guillain-Barré syndrome associated with diabetic ketoacidosis: a case report and literature review. J Turgut Ozal Med Cent. 2016;23(1):96–9. https://doi.org/10.5455/jtomc.2015.2725.
12. van den Berg B, Walgaard C, Drenthen J, Fokke C, Jacobs BC, van Doorn PA. Guillain-Barré syndrome: pathogenesis, diagnosis, treatment and prognosis. Nat Rev Neurol. 2014;10(8):469–82. https://doi.org/10.1038/nrneurol.2014.121.
13. Prashant SV, Nakum K, Bhatia N. A relapsing case of Guillain-Barré syndrome (GBS)- with full term pregnancy. Natl J Integr Res Med. 2015;6(4):119–20.
14. Yuki N, Hartung H-P. Guillain–Barré Syndrome. N Engl J Med. 2012;366(24):2294–304. https://doi.org/10.1056/nejmra1114525.
15. Zafar MS, Naqash M, Bhat T, Malik G. Guillain-Barré syndrome in pregnancy: an unusual case. J Family Med Prim Care. 2013;2(1):90. https://doi.org/10.4103/2249-4863.109965.
16. Fernando T, Ambanwala A, Ranaweera P, Kaluarachchi A. Guillain-Barré syndrome in pregnancy: a conservatively managed case. J Family Med Prim Care. 2016;5:688–90.
17. Pradhan D, Dey S, Bhattacharyyaa P. A case of successful management of Guillain-Barré syndrome in pregnancy. JNMA J Nepal Med Assoc. 2015;53(198):134–6.
18. Levin KH. Variants and mimics of Guillain-Barré syndrome. Neurologist. 2004;10(2):61–74. https://doi.org/10.1097/01.nrl.0000117821.35196.0b.
19. Pollak-Christian E, Lee K-S. Importance of diagnostic work-up of Guillain-Barré syndrome in pregnancy. BMJ Case Rep. 2016;2016:bcr2016216826. https://doi.org/10.1136/bcr-2016-216826.
20. Dua K, Banerjee A. Guillain-Barré syndrome: a review. Br J Hosp Med (London). 2010;71(9):495–8.
21. Stangel M, Pul R. Basic principles of intravenous immunoglobulin (IVIg) treatment. J Neurol. 2006;253(S5):v18–24. https://doi.org/10.1007/s00415-006-5003-1.
22. Dalakas MC. The use of intravenous immunoglobulin in the treatment of autoimmune neuromuscular diseases: evidence-based indications and safety profile. Pharmacol Ther. 2004;102(3):177–93.
23. Matsuzawa Y, Sakakibara R, Shoda T, Kishi M, Ogawa E. Good maternal and fetal outcomes of predominantly sensory Guillain-Barré syndrome in pregnancy after intravenous immunoglobulin. Neurol Sci. 2010;31(2):201–3. https://doi.org/10.1007/s10072-009-0188-6.
24. Ortiz-Salas P, Velez-Van-Meerbeke A, Galvis-Gomez CA, JH RQ. Human immunoglobulin versus plasmapheresis in Guillain–Barré syndrome

and myasthenia gravis. J Clin Neuromuscul Dis. 2016;18(1):1–11. https://doi.org/10.1097/cnd.0000000000000119.

25. Beydoun HA, Beydoun MA, Hossain S, Zonderman AB, Eid SM. Nationwide study of therapeutic plasma exchange vs intravenous immunoglobulin in Guillain-Barré syndrome. Muscle Nerve. 2020;61(5):608–15. https://doi.org/10.1002/mus.26831.

26. Almohammedi R, Aljohani S, Bakheet M. Pulse-steroid therapy in a 37-year-old man with acute motor and sensory axonal neuropathy: a case report. Clin Case Rep. 2019;7:506. https://doi.org/10.1002/ccr3.2000.

27. Okayasu H, Yasui-Furukori N, Kadowaki T, Funakoshi K, Hirata K, Shimoda K. Bickerstaff's brainstem encephalitis suspected as functional neurologic disorders. Int Med Case Rep J. 2020;13:177–81. https://doi.org/10.2147/imcrj.s249818.

28. van Doorn PA. Diagnosis, treatment and prognosis of Guillain-Barré syndrome (GBS). Presse Med. 2013;42(6):e193. https://doi.org/10.1016/j.lpm.2013.02.328.

29. Doets AY, Hughes RA, Brassington R, Hadden RD, Pritchard J. Pharmacological treatment other than corticosteroids, intravenous immunoglobulin and plasma exchange for Guillain-Barré syndrome. Cochrane Database Syst Rev. 2020;2020:CD008630. https://doi.org/10.1002/14651858.cd008630.pub5.

30. Doets AY, Jacobs BC, van Doorn PA. Advances in management of Guillain-Barré syndrome. Curr Opin Neurol. 2018;31(5):541–50. https://doi.org/10.1097/WCO.0000000000000602.

31. Campos da Silva F, de Moraes Paula G, CV DSEA, Mendes de Almeida DS, Ubirajara Cavalcanti Guimarães R. Guillain-Barré syndrome in pregnancy: early diagnosis and treatment is essential for a favorable outcome. Gynecol Obstet Investig. 2009;67(4):236–7. https://doi.org/10.1159/000209215.

32. Walling AD, Dickson G. Guillain-Barré syndrome. Am Fam Physician. 2013;87:191–19738.

33. Ruts L, van Koningsveld R, Jacobs BC, van Doorn PA. Determination of pain and response to methylprednisolone in Guillain-Barré syndrome. J Neurol. 2007;254(10):1318–22.

34. Farmakidis C, Inan S, Milstein M, Herskovitz S. Headache and pain in Guillain-Barré syndrome. Curr Pain Headache Rep. 2015;19(8):1–7.

35. Pandey CK, Bose N, Garg G, et al. Gabapentin for the treatment of pain in Guillain-Barré syndrome: a double-blinded, placebo-controlled, crossover study. Anesth Analg. 2002;95(6):1719–23. https://doi.org/10.1097/00000539-200212000-00046.

36. Khanna M, Gupta A, Nagappa M, Taly A, Haldar P, Ranjani P. Prevalence of fatigue in Guillain-Barré syndrome in neurological rehabilitation setting. Ann Indian Acad Neurol. 2014;17(3):331. https://doi.org/10.4103/0972-2327.138521.

37. Merkies IS, Kieseier BC. Fatigue, pain, anxiety and depression in Guillain-Barré syndrome and chronic inflammatory demyelinating polyradiculoneuropathy. Eur Neurol. 2016;75(3–4):199–206. https://doi.org/10.1159/000445347.

38. Khan F, Pallant JF, Ng L, Bhasker A. Factors associated with long-term functional outcomes and psychological sequelae in Guillain–Barré syndrome. J Neurol. 2010;257(12):2024–31. https://doi.org/10.1007/s00415-010-5653-x.

39. Walgaard C, Lingsma HF, Ruts L, Drenthen J, van Koningsveld R, Garssen MJ, van Doorn PA, Steyerberg EW, Jacobs BC, Walgaard C, et al. Prediction of respiratory insufficiency in Guillain–Barré syndrome. Ann Neurol. 2010;67(6):781–7. https://doi.org/10.1002/ana.21976.

40. Sharshar T, Chevret S, Bourdain F, Raphaël JC, French Cooperative Group on Plasma Exchange in Guillain–Barré Syndrome. Early predictors of mechanical ventilation in Guillain–Barré syndrome. Crit Care Med. 2003;31(1):278–83.

41. Yamagishi Y, Kusunoki S. The prognosis and prognostic factor of Guillain-Barré syndrome. Rinsho Shinkeigaku. 2020;60(4):247–52. https://doi.org/10.5692/clinicalneurol.cn-001398.

42. Nguyen TN, Badjatia N, Malhotra A, Gibbons FK, Qureshi MM, Greenberg SA. Factors predicting extubation success in patients with Guillain–Barré syndrome. Neurocrit Care. 2006;5(3):230–4. https://doi.org/10.1385/NCC:5:3:230.

43. IGOS GBS prognosis tool. IGOS International GBS Outcome Study [online], 2014.

44. van den Berg B, Bunschoten C, van Doorn PA, Jacobs BC, van den Berg B, et al. Mortality in Guillain-Barre syndrome. Neurology. 2013;80(18):1650–4. https://doi.org/10.1212/WNL.0b013e3182904fcc.

45. Meenakshi-Sundaram S, Swaminathan K, Karthik SN, Bharathi S. Relapsing Guillain-Barre syndrome in pregnancy and postpartum. Ann Indian Acad Neurol. 2014;17:352–4.

Myasthenia Gravis in Pregnancy and Delivery

23

Megan M. Leitch

Abbreviations

AChR- Ab	Acetylcholine receptor antibody
IVIg	Intravenous immunoglobulins
MG	Myasthenia gravis
MUSK	Muscle specific tyrosine kinase

Clinical Background

Myasthenia gravis (MG) is an autoimmune disorder of the neuromuscular junction, characterized by fluctuating weakness of skeletal muscles. MG has a bimodal age of onset in men and women. The peak annual age for incidence of disease is at ages 20–24 and 70–75 for women [1]. There are two clinical forms of myasthenia: ocular and generalized. Patients with ocular MG have symptoms limited to eyelids and extraocular muscles, causing diplopia and ptosis. In generalized MG, weakness affects ocular muscles in addition to limb, bulbar, and respiratory muscles, causing fatigable limb weakness, dysphagia, dysarthria, and dyspnea. More than 50% of patients with MG present with ocular symptoms and about half of patients who present with ocular MG will remain purely ocular.

In a patient clinically suspected of having MG, additional testing should be undertaken. Serologic testing should start with searching for autoantibodies against the acetylcholine receptor (AChR-Ab). If AchR-Abs are negative, testing for muscle specific tyrosine kinase (MuSK) is recommended. If antibody testing is negative, electrodiagnostic tests including repetitive nerve stimulation or single fiber electromyography can be done to look for evidence of neuromuscular junction disease. Additionally, many patients with MG will have evidence of thymic gland pathology. Ten to fifteen percent of MG patients have thymomas and as many as 70% have thymic gland hyperplasia [1]. Thymectomy is standard of care for all patients with evidence of thymoma on chest imaging and for AchR-Ab positive patients with generalized MG [2].

A variety of medications are used in the treatment of MG. Pyridostigmine is an acetylcholinesterase inhibitor and is used as the standard first-line treatment for nearly all myasthenic patients to help control symptoms. If pyridostigmine fails to fully control a patient's symptoms, the patient is typically started on a steroid. Generally, a nonsteroidal immunosuppressant such as azathioprine, cyclosporin, mycophenolate mofetil, or methotrexate is started if there is a contraindication to steroids or if the patient needs a high dose of steroids to control their symptoms. Data from randomized control trials and expert consensus recommends using azathioprine as an initial immunosuppressant [3].

M. M. Leitch (✉)
Department of Neurology, Rutgers Robert Wood
Johnson Medical School, New Brunswick, NJ, USA
e-mail: mml196@rwjms.rutgers.edu

A myasthenic crisis is the most feared complication of MG and is defined as respiratory failure with the need for mechanical ventilation. Approximately 15–20% of patients with MG experience a crisis in their lifetime. A crisis is more likely to occur within the first 2 years of the disease but can occur at any time. In one study, 76% of crises began with worsening generalized weakness, 19% by bulbar symptoms, and 5% by worsening respiratory function [4]. Common triggers of a myasthenic crisis include respiratory infection, aspiration, post-thymectomy, emotional stress, certain medications, early pregnancy, and the postpartum period ([4]; Rowland). Plasmapheresis or intravenous immunoglobulin (IVIg) are both effective in treating a myasthenic crisis and can also be used to treat severe or refractory generalized myasthenia.

Preconception Care in Myasthenia Gravis

It is not uncommon to see pregnant women with MG, as the disease does not affect fertility and is prevalent in women of childbearing age. MG has a variable but potentially serious effect on pregnancy. In a review of the literature involving 322 pregnancies in 225 myasthenic mothers, 31% had no change in MG symptoms, 28% improved, and 41% had a clinical worsening during pregnancy [1]. Additionally, 30% had an exacerbation of their myasthenia in the postpartum period. Another study of 18 patients found 11% had improvement, 39% had clinical worsening, and 50% remained clinically stable [5]. The highest risk periods for an exacerbation of symptoms are during the first trimester and the early postpartum period. In most women, MG symptoms improve during the second and third trimester coinciding with the normal immunosuppression that occurs during later stages of pregnancy (Djelmis).

Ideally, all myasthenic patients considering pregnancy should receive preconception counseling to maximize their clinical condition and minimize the use of immunosuppressive drugs. Many myasthenic patients also suffer with autoimmune thyroid disease, so thyroid status should be checked during pregnancy planning and again when the patient becomes pregnant [6]. Pregnancy during the first year after diagnosis puts the mother at a higher risk of lift-threatening complications from the disease [7]. It is generally recommended that women wait 1–2 years after diagnosis before considering a pregnancy [8] to decrease their risk of a crisis. Women under good control can be reassured that they are likely to remain stable throughout pregnancy [3]. Young women with generalized AChR-Ab positive MG are typically advised to undergo thymectomy shortly after diagnosis. However, thymectomy can be a trigger for an exacerbation and its effect on disease activity takes months to years. Therefore, current guidelines recommend that thymectomy should be delayed in any women who is already pregnant or anticipating pregnancy in the next few months [3].

A discussion concerning the safety of therapies in MG is an essential part of pre-pregnancy counseling and is discussed in detail below. Mycophenolate mofetil and methotrexate increase the risk of teratogenicity and should not be used in pregnancy [3]. If there is an unplanned pregnancy on either of these medications, they should be slowly tapered off and in the case of methotrexate, the patient should start 5 mg of folic acid a day. Ideally, these medications should be stopped gradually prior to trying to conceive with a 3–6-month wash-out period.

Disease Management in Pregnancy

As previously discussed, pregnancy has a variable effect on myasthenia and each pregnancy may be different for a myasthenic patient. MG does not increase a women's risk of pre-eclampsia, fetal growth restriction, or spontaneous abortion but there may be an increased risk of preterm birth [9]. Pregnancy is associated with hemodynamic changes in the woman including an increase in blood volume and renal clearance as well as delayed gastric emptying and frequent emesis. These changes may interfere with absorption of medication, necessitating dose adjustments.

Oral acetylcholinesterase inhibitors such as pyridostigmine are standard first-line treatment for MG, including during pregnancy [3]. The available evidence does not suggest an increased risk of fetal malformation or adverse pregnancy outcomes [7]. Parenteral acetylcholinesterase inhibitors may produce uterine contractions and should not be used during pregnancy, outside of labor and delivery [6]. Pyridostigmine can be administered orally with usual doses of 60 mg every 4–6 h, up to 1500 mg a day. Abdominal cramps and diarrhea may limit the amount of pyridostigmine that a patient can tolerate. MuSk antibody-positive patients' are also less responsive to pyridostigmine and frequently need to start an immunosuppressant shortly after diagnosis.

If a pregnant women's myasthenic symptoms are inadequately controlled on pyridostigmine, prednisone is the immunosuppressant of choice [3]. Glucocorticoids should be started at a low dose and gradually increased to reduce the risk of transient worsening of symptoms that can occur when starting this class of medication. While older data suggested a slight risk of cleft palate in babies born to women receiving corticosteroids in the first trimester, newer, prospective data does not support this association [6]. Current thinking is that there are no known teratogenic effects from glucocorticoids. However, glucocorticoids increase the risk of premature delivery and increase the risk of developing hypertension and gestational diabetes [10]. Women maintained on steroids during pregnancy need careful glucose monitoring.

Azathioprine and cyclosporine can be used if a pregnant woman has failed acetylcholinesterase inhibitors and glucocorticoids or if glucocorticoids are not well tolerated [3]. Prior studies of these medications in transplant patients and patients with other autoimmune diseases have shown them to be relatively safe in pregnancy with no increased risk of congenital abnormalities [7]. However, use of azathioprine during pregnancy has been associated with a possible increased risk of fetal growth restriction and low birth weight [7]. If possible, the dose of azathioprine should be decreased at 32 weeks gestation to reduce the risk of neonatal leukopenia and thrombocytopenia [8]. Cyclosporine has been shown to cross the placenta readily but there is no increased risk of severe complications or malformations. There is, however, a risk of preterm delivery and lower birth weight in the neonate [7].

Rituximab is a newer therapy that has been demonstrated to improve disease control in MuSK antibody-positive patients [11]. By 16 weeks gestation, rituximab does cross the placenta. A recently published review of women with other autoimmune disease who received rituximab within 6 months of conception found no increased risk of major malformations [12]. However, there were some cases of decreased B-cell counts in infants born to women using rituximab that resolved within 6 months [12]. MuSK positive patients also respond well to plasmapheresis [3].

Plasmapheresis and IVIg therapy are used for treatment of a myasthenic crisis, for acute worsening of myasthenic symptoms, or for patients with refractory generalized myasthenia. These treatments may also be considered if there are intolerable side effects to the first- and second-line therapies previously discussed. There is a theoretical risk of causing premature labor with plasmapheresis, because of the removal of circulating hormones [8]. Fetal monitoring during plasmapheresis is recommended in the third trimester. Continuous fetal monitoring is also indicated during a myasthenic crisis if the fetus is at a viable gestational age, given risk of maternal and fetal hypoxia (UpToDate). IVIg is typically administered at a dose of 2 g/kg divided over 3–5 days as an initial loading dose. The safety of using IVIg during pregnancy has not been studied in MG but the obstetric literature contains many reports of IVIg being used safely in pregnancy for the treatment of other autoimmune conditions such as antiphospholipid syndrome. IVIg is generally well tolerated but common side effects include headache, nausea, and malaise. More serious risks of systemic side effects include aseptic meningitis, thromboembolic events, and anaphylactic reaction. Volume overloading associated with the infusion and hyperviscosity may carry an increased significance in pregnancy [8].

Other Considerations in Pregnancy

Even in an uncomplicated pregnancy, the growing fetus may restrict the diaphragm and cause impairment in respiratory function [8]. Women with MG who already have respiratory involvement may develop more respiratory symptoms in the later stages of pregnancy. Baseline pulmonary function testing and close follow-up of respiratory status should be considered in all pregnant women with generalized MG [9].

Globally, pre-eclampsia complicates 2–8% of pregnancies [13, 14]: while MG does not increase the risk of pre-eclampsia, if the two conditions are present together, careful management is needed. Magnesium sulfate is used as an anticonvulsant in pre-eclampsia and has been demonstrated to decrease maternal mortality [13, 14]. However, owing to the neuromuscular blocking effects of magnesium sulfate, a pregnant myasthenic patient with pre-eclampsia or eclampsia should not be treated with magnesium sulfate as its use could precipitate a myasthenic crisis [3]. Instead, levetiracetam or valproic acid can be used for seizure prophylaxis. Phenytoin can also worsen MG and should only be used for refractory seizures. For treatment of hypertension during pregnancy, beta-blockers and calcium channel blockers should be avoided when possible as both classes of medication can exacerbate myasthenic symptoms. Methyldopa or hydralazine should be used instead for the management of elevated blood pressure.

Fetal Assessment

MG is rarely associated with fetal abnormalities from the transplacental passage of AchR-Abs during pregnancy. The most severe finding in the fetus is arthrogryposis multiplex congenita, a condition characterized by multiple joint contractures from the lack of movement in utero [15]. Decreased fetal movement has been described in the setting of maternal MG, so women should be encouraged to monitor fetal movement starting at 24 weeks of gestation and if there is concern for reduced fetal movement, ultrasound scanning should be done [6]. Polyhydramnios from impaired fetal swallowing can also affect pregnancies secondary to transplacental passage of AchR-Abs [16].

Labor and Delivery

During the first stage of labor, uterine contraction is not affected by MG as the uterus is composed of smooth muscle, which lacks post-synaptic acetylcholine receptors [9]. However, the second stage of labor may be affected because it requires the use of voluntary straited muscles to ultimately deliver the baby. Even with this consideration, spontaneous vaginal delivery should be the goal for most myasthenic patients [3]. Assisted vaginal delivery with either forceps or vacuum can be considered if the woman develops significant fatigue or weakness [9]. Cesarean section should be reserved for obstetrical indications only as surgery has increased risk in myasthenic patients. Myasthenic fatigue during labor can be helped by the administration of cholinesterase inhibitors, which should be administered parentally during this time to avoid the unpredictable gastrointestinal absorption that occurs during labor. Pyridostigmine can be given intramuscularly or intravenously at approximately 1/30th the dose of an oral preparation, such as 2.0 mg every 3–4 h during labor. Neostigmine doses of 1.5 mg intramuscularly or 0.5 mg intravenously are equivalent to 60 mg of oral pyridostigmine [8];

however, this cholinesterase inhibitor has strong muscarinic and nicotinic side effects making parenteral pyridostigmine the preferred choice (Djelmis).

Maternal respiratory status (pulse oximetry and respiratory rate) should be monitored carefully during labor because stress and fatigue may precipitate worsening of disease. According to some experts, women who have been on prednisone for more than 2 weeks at a dose of more than 7.5 mg a day are recommended to receive stress-dose hydrocortisone during the intrapartum period [6].

Pregnant women with MG should consult with an anesthesiologist prior to labor to discuss options for analgesia and anesthesia, if needed. Regional anesthesia with an epidural or combined spinal-epidural is recommended when vaginal delivery is anticipated as it can reduce fatigue and allow for adequate anesthesia if assisted delivery is needed [6]. General endotracheal anesthesia is recommended for a patient with severe disease and compromised respiratory or bulbar status who needs a cesarean section. Nondepolarizing muscle relaxants, usually used for intubation, should be avoided, if possible. If these drugs are required, the dose should be lowered [6]. Sedatives and opioids should also be avoided due to the risk of respiratory depression. If opioids are used for pain, increased respiratory monitoring is recommended. Nonsteroidal anti-inflammatory drugs such as ibuprofen can be safely used in the postpartum period for pain control.

MG is generally thought to have an increased risk of complications and operative interventions during delivery [17]. A retrospective study in Norway of 127 births by mothers with MG compared to a reference group of 1.9 million births by mother without MG found that women with MG had a higher risk of complications at delivery (40.9% vs. 32.9%) [18]. In particular, the risk of preterm rupture of amniotic membranes was 5.5% in the MG group vs. 1.7% in the reference group. Additionally, the rate of interventions during birth (cesarean section or forceps/vacuum assisted vaginal delivery) was higher in the MG group 33.9% vs. 20% in the non-MG group [18]. In contrast, a Taiwanese population-based study of 163 women with MG compared to 815 matched population controls found no increased risk in myasthenic women of having preterm labor or giving birth to an infant that was small for gestational age or with a low birth weight [19]. Additionally, they found that women with MG also did not have a higher risk of cesarean delivery compared to unaffected women [19].

Neonatal Concerns

10–21% of infants born to myasthenic women will develop transient neonatal MG [5, 7] secondary to placental transfer of antibodies in the second and third trimesters. Typically, the baby will develop symptoms 1–4 days after birth including muscle weakness, feeding difficulty, ptosis, weak cry, and mild respiratory distress. It is recommended that all babies born to myasthenic mothers be monitored in the inpatient setting for 2 days after birth [6]. A symptomatic neonate will need to be monitored closely for a longer period, but treatment with oral or parenteral anticholinesterase agents will generally improve symptoms. Neonatal MG usually reverses after 3–8 weeks as the antibodies from the mother are degraded [5, 7]. It is important to note that the development of neonatal MG does not necessarily corelate with the severity of maternal symptoms and has occurred in babies born to myasthenic women whose disease was in remission [16]. Some data does suggest that babies born to mothers who have already undergone thymectomy prior to pregnancy have a lower incidence of neonatal myasthenia [9, 17, 18]. Even if the mother's myasthenia is well-controlled, all babies born to myasthenic mothers should be examined for evidence of weakness and have rapid access to neonatal critical care support [3].

Postpartum Management

Women should be monitored closely in the first few weeks after delivery because of a 30% increased risk for a crisis [9]. Since infection can trigger a crisis, women and their health care providers should be vigilant about monitoring for and treating common postpartum infections such as cystitis, mastitis, or a wound infection. Breastfeeding is an option for most myasthenic women if their disease is under good control and there is no concern for neonatal myasthenia [9]. Nursing can be physically exhausting for a mother and if her myasthenic symptoms are worsened by fatigue, bottle feedings may allow a partner to help more in infant care so that she can get additional rest. Glucocorticoids can be safely used in lactation and should not be abruptly stopped or started during this period when risk of a crisis is high. Low levels of azathioprine metabolites are found in breast milk of some women using this medication and there are conflicting opinions in the literature as to the safety of this drug in breastfeeding. A National Institutes of Health summary found no evidence of adverse effects on the health and development of infants exposed to azathioprine during breastfeeding for up to 3.5 years, however long-term follow up has not been performed (NIH/med lac website). Mycophenolate mofetil and methotrexate are contraindicated for a lactating mother. Anticholinesterase drugs are considered safe in lactation but some of the drug may be found in breast milk so higher doses should be avoided if possible.

Conclusion

While many myasthenic women have a safe and uneventful pregnancy, preconception planning is ideal. The course of the disease is variable during pregnancy with the first trimester and the postpartum period carrying the highest risk of a myasthenic crisis. Women need to be monitored closely during pregnancy and labor and delivery with a multidisciplinary approach involving obstetrics, neurology, pediatrics, and anesthesia.

Many commonly used medications to control the disease are generally still safe during pregnancy and lactation. When possible, myasthenic women should deliver at a hospital equipped to manage obstetrical complications in the mother and to provide advanced care for the infant, if needed.

References

1. Amato A, James R. Disorders of neuromuscular transmission. In: Neuromuscular disorders. China: McGraw-Hill; 2008. p. 457–528.
2. Wolfe GI, Kaminski HJ, Aban IB, et al. Randomized trial of thymectomy in myasthenia gravis. N Engl J Med. 2016;375:511–22.
3. Sanders DB, Wolfe GE, Benatar M, et al. International consensus guidance for management of myasthenia gravis: executive summary. Neurology. 2016;87:419–25.
4. Berrouschot J, Baumann I, Kalischewski P, Sterker M, Schneider D. Therapy of myasthenic crisis. Crit Care Med. 1997;25(7):1228–35.
5. Tellez-Zento JF, et al. Myasthenia gravis and pregnancy: clinical implications and neonatal outcome. BMV Musculosket Disord. 2004;5(42):1–5.
6. Norwood F, Dhanjal M, Hill M, et al. Myasthenia in pregnancy: best practice guidelines from a UK multispecialty working group. J Neurol Neurosurg Psychiatry. 2014;85(5):538–43.
7. Chaudhry S, Vignaraja B, Koren G. Myasthenia gravis during pregnancy. Can Fam Physician. 2012;58:1346–9.
8. Da Silva FC, do Cima LC, da Ram SA. Myasthenia gravis and pregnancy. In: Minagar A, editor. Neurological disorders and pregnancy. Burlington, MA: Elsevier; 2011. p. 55–68.
9. Varner M. Myasthenia gravis and pregnancy. Clin Obstet Gynecol. 2013;56(2):372–81.
10. Laskin CA, Bombardier C, Hannah ME, et al. Prednisone and aspirin in women with autoantibodies and unexplained recurrent fetal loss. N Engl J Med. 1997;337:148–53.
11. Hehir MK, Hobson-Webb LD, Benatar M. Rituximab as treatment for anti-MuSK myasthenia gravis. Multicenter blinded prospective review. Neurology. 2017;89(10):1069–77.
12. Das G, Damotte V, Gelfand JM, et al. Rituximab before and during pregnancy. A systematic review, and a case series in MS and NMOSD. Neurol Neuroimmunol Neuroinflamm. 2018;5(3):1–11.
13. Duley L, Gulmexoglu AM, Henderson-Smart DJ, Chou D. Magnesium sulphate and other anticonvulstans for women with pre-eclampsia. Cochrane Database Syst Rev. 2010;2010(11):CD000025.
14. Duley L. The global impact of pre-eclampsia and eclampsia. Semin Perinatol. 2009;33(3):130–7.

15. Vincent A, Newland C, Brueton L, et al. Arthrogryposis multiplex congenita with maternal autoantibodies specific for a fetal antigen. Lancet. 1995;346:24–5.

16. Verspyck E, Mandelbrot L, Dommergues M, et al. Myasthenia gravis with polyhydramnios in the fetus of an asymptomatic mother. Prenat Diagn. 1993;13:539–42.

17. Hoff JM, Daltveit AK, Gihus NE. Myasthenia gravis in pregnancy and birth: identifying risk factors, optimizing care. Eur J Neurol. 2007;14:38–43.

18. Hoff JM, Dalveit AK, Gihus NE. Myasthenia gravis consequences for pregnancy, delivery and the newborn. Neurology. 2003;61:1362–6.

19. Wen JC, Liu TC, Chen YH, et al. No increased risk of adverse pregnancy outcomes for women with myasthenia gravis: a nationwide population-based study. Eur J Neurol. 2009;16:889–94.

Peripheral Nerve Disorders in Pregnancy

Anna C. Filley and Christopher J. Winfree

Introduction

Peripheral neuropathy is a relatively common complication of pregnancy. Obstetric patients are at risk of sustaining peripheral nerve injuries directly related to pregnancy and parturition and may be predisposed to developing certain neuropathies, which often follow a different clinical course than what is seen in the general population. In fact, pregnancy is an established risk factor for the development of distal entrapment neuropathies like carpal tunnel syndrome (CTS) [1] and immune-mediated cranial neuropathies like Bell's Palsy [2]. The diagnostic workup and management of pregnant patients with peripheral neuropathy create unique and complex challenges for the clinician. Consideration must be made to pregnancy-specific risk factors and modifiers of disease as well as the implications of the disease course, workup, and treatment for the pregnancy. Certain diagnostic tests (computed tomography, contrast administration), medications classically used to treat neuropathic pain (anticonvulsants and antidepressants), and procedures (surgical intervention, general anesthesia) pose risks to the developing fetus, often placing functional constraints on the scope of diagnostic workup and management of these patients. As a result, a thorough understanding of the natural history and clinical course of pregnancy-associated neuropathies becomes more imperative in establishing an accurate clinical diagnosis, predicting recovery and functional outcomes, and minimizing the use of unnecessary tests or procedures that may have lasting consequences to the pregnancy.

Peripheral nerve disorders in pregnancy can be described as either an acute nerve injury or subacute neuropathy, though a spectrum does exist between the two categories. The importance in distinguishing between these two processes lies in the identification of pathologies that may necessitate acute intervention and differentiating them from those that may be safer and more appropriate to conservatively manage, particularly in a patient population in which risks of diagnostic testing and treatments to a developing fetus must be considered. Acute peripheral nerve injuries tend to be associated with an identifiable mechanism of injury and immediate onset of neurological deficits. In the obstetric population, these tend to be sustained as complications of childbirth and include procedure-related nerve injuries, labor-related nerve injuries, and positioning nerve injuries [3–6]. Autoimmune or inflammatory neuropathies, such as Parsonage-Turner syndrome and idiopathic lumbosacral plexopathy, may present after a triggering event such as parturition [4]. In these cases, neurological deficits typically occur in a delayed fashion

A. C. Filley · C. J. Winfree (✉)
Department of Neurological Surgery, Columbia University, New York, NY, USA
e-mail: cjw12@cumc.columbia.edu

after the inciting event and often after a prodrome of pain. Entrapment neuropathies occur secondary to a more chronic application of lower-intensity forces, usually at sites of pre-existing stenosis. They are classically associated with pregnancy and tend to present in a more subacute manner with gradual onset of symptoms in later trimesters [7].

Most cases of pregnancy-related peripheral neuropathy are mild compression or positioning-related neuropathies that develop as a direct or indirect result of local and systemic factors acting on vulnerable distal entrapment sites. During pregnancy, there are a multitude of hormonal, metabolic, and anatomic changes that may predispose women to the development of peripheral neuropathies. In later stages of pregnancy, fluid retention and tissue edema, together with the weight gain and increased abdominal girth associated with fetal growth, may progressively compress or stretch peripheral nerves at pre-existing stenotic locations [8]. Changes in immune status that occur during pregnancy may influence susceptibility to infection, strength and nature of immune responses, propensity for or protection against latent viral re-activation, and relative risk of autoimmune disease [2, 9]. Altered metabolism and energy utilization occurring during pregnancy to meet the needs of the developing fetus may lead to acute metabolic derangements that, in the setting of underlying systemic disorders (glucose metabolism in gestational or pre-pregnancy diabetes, thyroid dysfunction), may influence the development or progression of neuropathic symptoms. Women with pre-existing nerve damage or dysfunction are at greater risk for developing peripheral neuropathy in the setting of pregnancy, tend to experience more severe symptoms, and have a worse prognosis for recovery [10, 11]. Hereditary neuropathies including Charcot-Marie-Tooth (CMT), hereditary neuropathy with liability to pressure palsies (HNLPP), hereditary brachial plexopathy, and Isaac's syndrome may manifest for the first time during pregnancy and must be considered even in patients without prior diagnosis [12, 13].

Fortunately, most pregnancy-related neuropathies are caused by mild demyelinating injuries and spontaneously resolve in the months postpartum [4, 6]. Given this excellent prognosis, in the absence of concerning signs or symptoms, patients are initially managed conservatively and additional diagnostic workup in the form of imaging or electrodiagnostics is not pursued. A combination of patient history correlated with relevant clinical examination findings is often sufficient to localize the anatomic level of the lesion and form the basis for a differential diagnosis. Patients with atypical clinical presentation, prolonged disease course, refractory symptoms, or evidence of disproportionately significant nerve injury, however, should undergo a more extensive evaluation for possible underlying diagnoses that may directly or indirectly lead to nerve damage or augment susceptibility to the development of neuropathies [13, 14]. The presence of severe weakness, numbness in the groin area, incontinence, or other progressive deficits may be secondary to acute cord compression and should prompt immediate further evaluation to rule out compressive pathology (expanding hematoma, mass lesion, herniated disc, lacerating injury) that may require timely intervention [10, 15, 16].

Fundamentally underlying initial evaluation of suspected peripheral neuropathy is identification of clinical scenarios that may require surgical intervention in order to prevent permanent disability. The peripheral nerve surgeon plays a crucial role in this process, with procedures that remove compressive forces or restore anatomical continuity of healthy nerve segments that otherwise would be unable to independently recover. Operative management of peripheral nerve injury in both pregnant and non-pregnant patients therefore hinges on the crucial distinction between neuropathies with the capacity for independent regeneration and those in which no functional recovery could be expected without surgical intervention.

Patient Assessment

Physical Exam

Physical examination should involve testing of all muscle groups; the distribution of affected muscles can be used to localize the level of the lesion. Any muscular atrophy, asymmetry, or abnormal resting positions should be noted, taking care to look for any constellation of symptoms indicative of a specific injury pattern (Klumpke or Erb's palsy in brachial plexus avulsions). For suspected peripheral nerve entrapments, there is often pain and tenderness at the entrapment site which may be reproduced with focal palpation (e.g., reproduction of hand paresthesias in the distribution of the median nerve by tapping over the carpal tunnel entrapment site at the wrist, diagnostic of CTS). The examiner should attempt to reproduce symptoms with exaggerated limb movements or positions (straight leg raise, Phalen's sign, Tinel's test) [10].

Electrodiagnostic Studies

Electrodiagnostic evaluation with nerve conduction studies (NCSs) and electromyography (EMG) may be performed to localize the level of the lesion, characterize the involvement of demyelinating and axonal injury, and evaluate for evidence of functional recovery. Compression or entrapment neuropathies tend to cause local damage to the myelin sheath that manifest with decreased conduction velocity or focal conduction block of sensory nerve action potentials (SNAPs) across the demyelinated segment, thereby revealing the site of entrapment. Radiculopathies can be differentiated from plexopathies and peripheral neuropathies by the presence of early paraspinal muscle EMG abnormalities in the former. Paraspinal muscles are innervated by the most proximal nerve root branches that exit prior to plexus formation and are not typically affected in a peripheral neuropathy [4]. Abnormalities across several muscles innervated by different peripheral nerves suggest a more proximal cause; widespread, patchy involvement may also be due to systemic autoimmune or inflammatory process rather than a focal nerve injury.

Diagnostic Imaging

Ultrasound

Diagnostic ultrasound (US) is a non-invasive imaging modality that is commonly employed in the early workup of peripheral neuropathies in pregnant and non-pregnant patients. High-resolution ultrasonography allows visualization of peripheral nerves and surrounding structures within the superficial soft tissues that can both reveal the presence of structural causes of entrapment and detect changes in nerve morphology indicative of ongoing compression and injury. Static and dynamic views can be used to evaluate these relationships in various anatomical positions and may reveal pathology such as nerve tethering and symptomatic adhesions that may only be evident with motion. Ultrasound has proved to be particularly valuable in the evaluation of suspected entrapment syndromes and is helpful in differentiating between idiopathic and secondary disease [17]. Visualization of structural abnormalities such as tumors or other space-occupying mass lesions, fluid collections (hematoma, abscess, seroma), hypertrophied bony prominences, tendon synovitis, or restrictive scar tissue may provide clues to the etiology of symptoms. Anatomical variations predisposing to nerve entrapment such as accessory muscle bellies or abnormal nerve courses can also be readily detected with ultrasound imaging. Imaging along the course of a nerve can reveal sites of focal stenosis that may be correlated with structural changes in the nerve itself. Evaluation of nerve morphology may demonstrate changes consistent with nerve entrapment including fusiform swelling proximal to the site of compression, focal kinking or deformation, loss of normal fascicular architecture, or intraneural thickening and fibrosis; the addition of Doppler imaging may demonstrate alterations in microvascularity including intraneural and perineural hyperemia [18]. In settings of trauma and severe nerve damage, US can be used to assess neuronal continuity and the presence of surrounding tissue injury or edema.

Magnetic Resonance Imaging/MR Neurography

Magnetic resonance imaging (MRI) and MR neurography (MRN) allow high-resolution visualization of superficial and deep soft tissues without exposing the developing fetus to harmful radiation. Contrast agents are not routinely used in MR neurography, which is helpful in limiting the exposure of the fetus to unnecessary agents. These imaging modalities may be particularly useful in evaluation of spinal disease and can be used to rule out the presence of compressive pathology such as hematoma, inflammation, or infection [19], disc herniation [20], or malignancy [3]. Imaging may also be used in the setting of trauma to evaluate neuronal continuity, characterize any surrounding tissue disruption or edema [4], and evaluate for disruption of spinal elements [21]. MR neurography may provide evidence of neuronal injury. Injured, inflamed nerves often appear grossly edematous and exhibit increased signal on T2-weighted images. Eventually, chronic denervation leads to muscle atrophy and volume loss associated with fatty infiltration resulting in areas of T1 hyperintensity [22]. In addition to providing valuable diagnostic insights regarding anatomical integrity of a nerve and its relationship to surrounding structures, imaging can be used to guide additional diagnostic and therapeutic percutaneous procedures such as nerve blocks.

Differential Diagnosis

Acute Peripheral Nerve Injury

Acute peripheral nerve injuries tend to be associated with an identifiable mechanism of injury and immediate onset of neurological deficits. In the obstetric population, acute nerve injuries tend to be associated with events surrounding parturition and include procedure-related nerve injuries, labor-related nerve injuries, and positioning nerve injuries [3–6]. Symptoms are usually related to compression and stretch of the nerve by the fetal head, maternal positioning, or obstetric

care [3, 23–25]. A prolonged second stage of labor, particularly in the lithotomy position, has been established as an independent predictor of postpartum neuropathy [3, 23]. Other proposed risk factors include nulliparity [6, 16, 26], short stature [26, 27], excessive weight gain, fetal macrosomia [27] or malpresentation [27], and forceps-assisted delivery [6, 16, 26, 27]. Neuraxial anesthesia, in addition to prolonging the time spent in the second stage of labor, may contribute to the risk of compressive neuropathy by dulling pressure sensations that would otherwise prompt the patient to change positions to avoid impending injury [3, 6, 28, 29]. Rarely, administration of epidural anesthesia may cause neurologic injury secondary to acute development of a compressive epidural hematoma or delayed complication with abscess, chemical meningitis or arachnoiditis, or neurotoxicity from anesthetic agents [30].

Among the most frequently diagnosed pregnancy-related nerve injuries are postpartum lower extremity neuropathies, which are estimated to affect at least 1% of women [3, 27]. Most commonly affected in descending order of frequency are the lateral femoral cutaneous, femoral, peroneal, sciatic, and obturator nerves; injuries to the lumbosacral plexus have also been reported [3, 23]. Patients typically present in the immediate postpartum period with sensory or motor deficits. The prognosis for these injuries is excellent, and most mild cases completely resolve within 2–3 months [4–6, 23]. More severe palsies may recover over the course of a year and permanent deficits are exceedingly rare [6, 23, 26, 27]. Conservative management, including physical therapy, is the cornerstone of treatment [28, 31]. Surgical decompression is performed in the setting of persistent deficits and nerve entrapment. Nerve repair is appropriate if the patient shows no clinically significant recovery after 3 months.

Entrapment Neuropathy

Entrapment neuropathies are focal compressive neuropathies that occur within a confined space; they may arise anywhere along the course of a nerve, though are more common at sites of pre-existing stenosis that may be less accommodating to any further narrowing. Some patients are particularly prone to developing entrapment neuropathies due to congenitally narrowed nerve tunnels [32], variant anatomy or course (split nerves, course through slips of muscle), or abnormal nerves or nerve sheaths themselves [33]. Inflammation or swelling of surrounding structures may reduce the available space for the nerve and when the pressure in the surrounding space exceeds the perfusion pressure into the nerve, adequate perfusion and nutrient delivery can be compromised, leading to nerve damage. This risk may be augmented with certain lifestyle, occupational, or recreational risk factors including repetitive motions (keyboard typing, cycling, pitching, etc.) that may provoke or exacerbate existing injury.

In most cases, a definitive diagnosis can be made on the basis of classical patient history and clinical exam findings. Patients typically experience a gradual onset of symptoms in the third trimester of pregnancy that parallels the progressive fluid retention, focal or generalized edema, and increased abdominal girth accompanying the growing fetus [34–36]. Indeed, pregnancy is one of the strongest risk factors for the development of entrapment neuropathies, most commonly CTS [8]. On physical exam, patients often demonstrate a positive Tinel's sign at the location of entrapment. Symptoms typically spontaneously resolve after delivery, and complete recovery generally occurs over the course of days to months postpartum [25].

Radiculopathy

Key in the diagnostic evaluation of suspected compressive neuropathy is localization of the site of compression. The presence of neck (or back) pain deficits that extend across the territories of multiple peripheral nerves, or paraspinal involvement on electrodiagnostics should raise suspicion of a more proximal etiology of symptoms. It is important to consider as part of the differential diagnosis, lesions located more proximally or distally along the course of the nerve (e.g., clinical presentation with foot drop may be secondary to injury of the L5 nerve root, lumbar plexus, sciatic nerve, common peroneal nerve, deep peroneal nerve, or even more distally with neuromuscular pathology). At the most proximal level is a radiculopathy, which is caused by pathology at the level of the nerve root and often correlates with a visible mass lesion on MRI [4]. Although there is some degree of clinical overlap with peripheral neuropathies, the distribution of sensory, motor, and reflex abnormalities occurs in a dermatomal distribution. Patients classically complain of neck or back pain with characteristic radiating pain or paresthesias in a dermatomal distribution, often reproduced with specific physical exam maneuvers [37]. Electrodiagnostics reveal hallmark involvement of paravertebral muscles with normal sensory studies, as the site of compression is proximal to the DRG [4].

Systemic/Inflammatory Neuropathies

Peripheral neuropathy may also be secondary to inflammatory or autoimmune-mediated processes that may be hereditary or acquired. Systemic inflammation and metabolic derangements generally tend to cause diffuse, multifocal lesions that do not follow the distribution of a peripheral nerve. Autoimmune or inflammatory neuropathies, such as Parsonage-Turner syndrome and idiopathic lumbosacral plexopathy, may occur suddenly but in a delayed fashion after a triggering event such as parturition [4]. Neurological deficits typically occur after a prodrome of pain. Peripheral neuropathy is also a characteristic feature of many systemic inflammatory and vasculitis-related syndromes (systemic lupus erythematosus (SLE), rheumatoid arthritis (RA), polyarteritis nodosa, Churg-Strauss, other connective tissue disorders) and may also occur as a complication of infection (Guillain-Barré syndrome (GBS) and its chronic form chronic inflammatory demyelinating polyneuropathy (CIDP), Lyme disease and other tick-borne illnesses, HIV/AIDS).

Management Principles

Operative intervention, either with a decompressive procedure or direct nerve repair, has significant potential to restore lost function if performed in the appropriate setting and time frame. There are several well accepted principles that may function to guide indications for and timing of repair to optimize nerve healing and ultimate regenerative outcomes. Fundamental in this decision-making process is distinguishing between lesions that may be expected to independently recover over time and those that would require surgical intervention to preserve or restore function.

Acute Setting

Acute operative intervention may be performed in select instances of acute, severe nerve injury that would otherwise result in permanent disability. Sharp nerve transection should be repaired within 72 h, if possible, to enable repair prior to the nerve ends retracting too far apart to permit end-to-end repair. Demyelinating lesions and those with axonal damage but without severe structural derangement have potential for recovery if the injurious stimulus is removed. This principle underlies the role of decompression or surgical release of stenotic sites that may otherwise cause ongoing compression and continued nerve injury that may eventually lead to permanent deficits. Emergent operative intervention should be considered in patients with severe focal neurologic deficits or rapid progression of symptoms concerning for expanding mass lesion (hematoma, AV fistula, pseudoaneurysm) or other compressive pathology (herniated disc) [15, 37]. Decompressive procedures may safely be performed during pregnancy to relieve nerve or spinal cord compression [38].

0–3 Months

For nerve injuries caused by blunt trauma, stretch, or compression, the extent of total injury is rarely initially evident and is often unpredictable. In these cases, acute repair is not indicated. Even for those that will ultimately require surgical intervention for functional recovery, it is imperative that intervention be delayed in order to allow the development of scar tissue in the damaged segments; this allows delineation of damaged areas that should be excised prior to re-approximation of healthy tissue. Premature surgical intervention may result either in failure due to anastomosis of damaged ends or in unnecessary resection of tissue that would have otherwise recovered.

Instead, lesions are observed over a period of 3 months and monitored for evidence of spontaneous recovery. As symptoms are generally caused by transient forces applied during labor and delivery or due to physiologic changes of pregnancy that are expected to resolve postpartum, there is rarely the need for acute intervention. Most result in mild demyelinating injury and are expected to fully recover in the weeks to months postpartum. Management typically is with supportive therapy aimed at symptomatic relief during the recovery period. Progressive resumption of normal activities and physical therapy, avoiding aggravating activities, and the use of splints to limit the risk of contractures and falls may all be appropriate treatment options. Peripheral neuropathy associated pain has been shown to respond well to topical lidocaine patches [10]. Intractable pain may also be managed with nerve blocks, which may provide diagnostic confirmation and therapeutic relief [39–41]. Systemic pharmacologic options may be considered if other, more conservative, pain management strategies fail to provide adequate relief. However, possible teratogenic or other adverse effects of medications traditionally used to treat neuropathic pain in non-pregnant patients must be addressed when considering pharmacologic management options.

3 Months

Following a period of observation, peripheral nerve function can be assessed with electrodiagnostic studies to evaluate for electrical evidence of recovery, which often precedes the ability for voluntary contraction. If no recovery, surgical intervention should be considered. Surgical exploration with intra-operative electrodiagnostic evaluation of nerve action potential (NAP) recordings can more definitively indicate whether or not nerve regeneration is occurring. If performed at least 3 months after initial injury, NAP would be expected to be present to some degree and would be indicative of active regeneration that would be expected to lead to meaningful recovery. An absence of NAP when stimulating a presumed neuroma-in-continuity may prompt surgical excision of the non-conducting area and graft procedure.

Syndromes

Carpal Tunnel Syndrome

Carpal tunnel syndrome (CTS) is an entrapment neuropathy of the median nerve at the wrist that is classically associated with pregnancy. Similar to idiopathic CTS, the pain and paresthesias in the wrist and hand are classically worse at night [34, 42, 43] and may be reproduced clinically with sustained wrist flexion (Phalen's maneuver) [42] or by tapping the wrist over the carpal tunnel (Tinel's sign) [8]. In pregnant patients, symptoms are more often bilateral and onset in the later months of pregnancy in association with generalized edema or localized swelling of the hands or fingers [34–36]. Most patients experience spontaneous resolution of symptoms from both a clinical and neurophysiological standpoint in the immediate postpartum period [44–46], in some cases paralleling postpartum weight loss [45]. Splinting of the wrist, particularly at night, to limit hyperflexion leads to symptomatic improvement in most patients after 1–2 weeks of use [34, 36, 47]. Local injections of 1% lidocaine mixed with dexamethasone have been shown to reduce pain and significantly improve electrophysiological parameters in pregnant patients with persistent CTS [48]. Surgical intervention is typically reserved for patients with severe sensory loss or prolonged motor latencies on electrodiagnostic testing. Carpal tunnel release, performed by sectioning the transverse carpal ligament, can be safely done during pregnancy under local anesthesia with excellent, long-lasting results [34, 43].

Radial Neuropathy

Radial neuropathy presents with pain or paresthesias in the forearm or hand and impaired wrist and finger extension manifesting with a classical "wrist drop." Uncommonly injured during pregnancy, there have been reports of postpartum radial neuropathy attributed to inappropriate arm positioning with use of a birthing bar during labor [49].

Parsonage-Turner Syndrome

Parsonage-Turner syndrome (PTS), also known as idiopathic neuralgic amyotrophy, is a relatively uncommon cause of brachial plexopathy that may occur in association with pregnancy. PTS classically presents as pain, usually in the neck, shoulder, or arm, followed by patchy motor weakness, often involving the suprascapular nerve. Parsonage-Turner syndrome tends to occur in association with physiologic stressors (exercise, surgery, injury, vaccination), though often in a delayed fashion, in contrast to traumatic brachial plexus injuries, which tend to require a more significant force and tend to present in the immediate postpartum period [50]. Further differentiating PTS from neuropathies caused by pressure injuries or compressive lesions is a patchy distribution of symptoms throughout the brachial plexus, involvement of the phrenic or cranial nerves, and lack of chronic sensory changes. Recovery from PTS is variable, though typically occurs within 8–12 months; however, some patients are left with persistent symptoms. Patients with persistent symptoms at 3 months should undergo nerve imaging with some combination of ultrasound and/or MR neurography to screen for hourglass constrictions, which represent a neve entrapment potentially treatable with surgery.

Hereditary Brachial Plexus Neuropathy (HBPN)

Hereditary brachial plexus neuropathy (HBPN) is characterized by recurrent episodes of debilitating pain, multifocal weakness, atrophy, and abnormal sensation in the upper extremities [51]. The exact pathogenesis is unknown, but symptoms are thought to be secondary to inflammation that may be immune-mediated. Symptoms often follow an antecedent event, including infection, exercise, surgery, and pregnancy; recurrent attacks often occur during the postpartum period [13, 51]. Considered to be the hereditary variant of PTS, HBPN tends to present at an earlier age, tends to recur, and patients have an overall more severe disease course with poorer functional outcomes compared to PTS [52]. A family history and minor dysmorphic features such as hypotelorism, epicanthic folds, and a short stature are more consistent with HBPN [51]. Steroid treatment, with or without immunoglobulin, may provide symptomatic relief and prevent anticipated attacks in the setting of surgery or parturition [13, 51, 52]. However, recovery is often incomplete and most patients have some degree of permanent deficits [52].

Idiopathic Lumbosacral Plexopathy

The lumbosacral plexus originates from nerve roots L4 to S5 and provides motor function and sensation to the lower extremities as well as innervation of sphincter function allowing control of the bowels and bladder [53, 54]. Lumbosacral plexopathy during pregnancy may be related to progressive compression of plexal elements by an enlarging uterus [55]. Patients tend to present in later stages of pregnancy with slowly progressive symptoms [56]. Lumbosacral plexopathy should be suspected in the setting of deficits involving the territories of multiple peripheral nerves derived from the lumbar (obturator, femoral, etc.) or lumbosacral (sciatic, peroneal, tibial, superior and inferior gluteal nerves) plexus [4, 37]. EMG may show evidence of denervation that involves multiple peripheral nerve territories without paraspinal muscle involvement [56]. Urodynamic investigations may be performed in the setting of urinary symptoms [54]. MRI may be obtained to rule out underlying sources of compression such as a herniated disc or space-occupying mass lesion [54, 56]. In cases of idiopathic lumbosacral plexopathy, a clear causative etiology is never found [4, 56]. Nevertheless, the prognosis is generally good, with most patients experiencing resolution of symptoms with conservative management; symptoms have been reported to recur in subsequent pregnancies, with a similar spontaneous resolution [56].

Traumatic Lumbosacral Plexopathy

Lumbosacral plexopathy has been reported as a rare complication of delivery, usually secondary to the use of forceps [16, 57, 58]. Patients classically present with persistent perineal hypoesthesia and motor deficits, with or without urinary, anorectal, or sexual dysfunction, usually following vaginal delivery [54, 58]. Traumatic lumbosacral plexopathy may also result from direct compression by the fetal head as it descends through the pelvis; classically, this occurs in women of shorter stature with larger fetuses, prolonged labor, fetal malpresentation, and instrumented deliveries [27, 57, 58].

Lateral Femoral Cutaneous Neuropathy

Neuropathy of the lateral femoral cutaneous nerve (LFCN) of the thigh, also known as meralgia paresthetica (MP), is the most commonly diagnosed lower extremity neuropathy in the obstetric population [59]. MP is a focal sensory neuropathy characterized by numbness, tingling, burning discomfort, or pain over the anterolateral upper leg that may be exacerbated by ambulation or hip flexion or extension [2]; motor deficits and reflex changes are notably absent. Classically, the LFCN is compressed externally by belts or tight clothing as it travels down the lateral aspect of the thigh [39]. Surgical and cadaveric studies of the LFCN have established a high degree of anatomic variability and lead to the identification of several patterns that may be predisposed to entrapment neuropathy [39, 60, 61]. In later stages of pregnancy, the exaggerated lumbar lordosis that accompanies the growing abdomen may impact the angle between the LFCN and inguinal ligament, leading to nerve stretching [3]. Injury at this level may occur with prolonged pushing in positions with exaggerated thigh flexion during delivery [2]. Management primarily focuses on postpartum weight loss, avoiding aggravating positions and eliminating tight-fitting clothing or belts. MP is generally self-limited and conservative therapy is successful in managing over 90% of patients [40]. For those with refractory symptoms, surgical intervention can be considered, which may involve procedures such as neurolysis and/or transposition. Nerve transection may be indicated when decompression is ineffective [39, 40, 61]. Neuromodulation, including spinal cord stimulation, dorsal root ganglion stimulation, or peripheral nerve stimulation may also be considered salvage treatment options for medically and surgically refractory pain.

Femoral Neuropathy

The femoral nerve is the second most common site of lower extremity neuropathy, accounting for 35% of all cases [3]. Femoral neuropathy is more common after vaginal delivery and prolonged lithotomy positioning [10, 62–66]. Excessive positioning-related hip abduction and external rotation is postulated to cause nerve stretching and compression at the level of the inguinal ligament leading to nerve ischemia [64]. Compression from retroperitoneal hemorrhage and intrapelvic pathology are other rare causes of postpartum femoral neuropathy [37, 67]. Patients classically present with proximal lower extremity weakness manifesting as difficulty standing from seated position or walking upstairs and may complain of leg "buckling" and falls [65, 68]. Physical exam may reveal hypoesthesia of the anterome-

dial thigh and lower leg and diminished patellar reflexes; a positive Tinel sign over the inguinal ligament may be present [10]. Compression at the level of the inguinal ligament will produce isolated weakness of knee extension as motor branches to the psoas and iliacus muscles exit proximally, sparing hip flexion [68]. More commonly, weakness involves both hip flexion and knee extension due to nerve compression proximal to the inguinal ligament [69]. In either case, strength of hip abduction and adduction should remain normal; deficits in these groups may indicate a more proximal origin of injury [37]. Similarly, EMG may show abnormalities in the saphenous nerve and femoral nerve-innervated muscle(s), notably without abnormality in the tibialis anterior or other L4-innervated muscles. Management of most cases is conservative, with spontaneous recovery occurring over the subsequent days to weeks [3, 63, 65, 68]. A knee brace may be used to keep the leg extended and provide support during ambulation [66]. If nerve imaging reveals femoral nerve compression at the inguinal ligament in the setting of persistent symptoms, then nerve decompression is appropriate.

Peroneal Neuropathy

The common peroneal (fibular) nerve provides sensation to the lateral lower leg and foot and motor innervation of dorsiflexion and eversion and is particularly vulnerable to positioning-related injury due to its relatively superficial location near the lateral fibular head. Patients classically present with a characteristic "foot drop" secondary to dorsiflexion weakness [10, 28, 29, 70]. Physical exam may reveal a positive Tinel sign over the lateral fibular head [10]. Weakness should not involve foot inversion or plantarflexion, functions innervated by the tibial nerve, and ankle reflexes should be intact; dysfunction indicates a more proximal lesion [37]. EMG may show conduction slowing or reduced amplitudes at the level of the fibular head or lateral leg; abnormalities should be absent in the posterior tibialis, gluteus medius, and other L5-innervated muscles [4, 28]. In the obstetric patient, peroneal neuropathy has been associated with prolonged periods of time spent in the lithotomy position [53]. Injury may also result from sustained pressure on the lateral knees or posterior distal thigh by the hands of parturients or others assisting with delivery; ecchymosis of the lateral knee may provide evidence of the site of compression [28, 70, 71]. The nerve may also be compressed between the biceps femoris tendon and lateral head of the gastrocnemius muscle or fibular head by the weight of the body during labor in the squatting position; these patients commonly develop a bilateral palsy [28, 72, 73]. If nerve imaging reveals peroneal nerve compression at the fibular head (or elsewhere) in the setting of persistent symptoms, then nerve decompression is appropriate.

Obturator Neuropathy

Obturator neuropathy is a rare complication of pregnancy, accounting for <5% of postpartum lower extremity injuries [3]. It is more common in the setting of instrumented (forceps-assisted) deliveries [41, 74] or after cesarean section [22, 75, 76]. Rarely, the obturator nerve may be compressed by a hematoma or infection that develops during parturition or as a complication of a pudendal nerve block [3, 37]. Patients commonly present with pain or dysesthesias over the medial thigh and groin area; frank weakness of adduction is not commonly seen due to the redundant motor supply of thigh adductors. A diagnosis of obturator neuropathy is primarily clinical [26]; obturator nerve block may provide diagnostic confirmation and therapeutic relief [41]. If nerve imaging reveals peroneal nerve compression at the obturator foramen in the setting of persistent symptoms, then nerve decompression is appropriate.

Bell's Palsy

Bell's palsy is an inflammatory neuropathy of the facial nerve (cranial nerve VII) that may be more common in pregnant patients in the later stages of pregnancy [77–80]. Physiologic changes that become more pronounced in the third trimester like relative immunosuppression, hypercoagulability, and fluctuating hormone levels causing fluid retention and soft tissue edema can lead to ischemia or compression of the facial nerve through similar mechanisms proposed for pregnancy-related CTS [9, 81]. Chronic or gestational hypertension and obesity have also been identified as significant independent risk factors [9]. Management is with supportive therapy and corticosteroids to reduce inflammation, and most patients experience significant improvement over the course of weeks to months [82, 83]. Patients with incomplete paralysis generally have a good prognosis and are expected to achieve full recovery of facial nerve function [82]. However, some studies have found that pregnant patients are more likely to progress to complete facial paralysis [77]. Outcomes for these patients have been reported to be significantly worse than in the general population, including age matched controls and non-pregnant women [77, 84]. Recurrence in a subsequent pregnancy has been proposed as an unfavorable overall prognostic indicator, as is the development of bilateral disease [81]. Facial nerve reconstruction may be appropriate for patients with persistent facial paralysis.

Inflammatory Demyelinating Polyneuropathies

Guillain-Barré syndrome (GBS) is a severe, inflammatory autoimmune neuropathy characterized by acute onset of rapidly progressive, ascending paralysis [85]. In pregnancy, GBS is disproportionately more likely to occur in the second or third trimesters and immediate postpartum period [86]. Close observation of these patients for clinical deterioration and respiratory distress is imperative due to normal respiratory changes seen in pregnancy such as increased tidal volume and decreased residual volume; among pregnant patients with GBS, up to 35% require ICU admission for ventilatory support and maternal mortality has been reported up to 10% [85]. Also important in pregnant patients, particularly in the setting of parturition is the potential to develop autonomic dysfunction, which may manifest as flushing or diaphoresis, urinary retention, ileus, blood pressure changes, or arrhythmias, which may be fatal. Termination of pregnancy does not shorten disease duration or improve maternal outcomes [86]. Optimal treatment for all patients is with plasma exchange [87] or intravenous immune globulin (IVIG) initiated within the first 2 weeks of symptom onset [88, 89]. Persistence of symptoms of GBS after 8 weeks necessitates a diagnosis of *chronic* inflammatory demyelinating polyneuropathy (CIDP). Patients with CIDP tend to be older, and as such, CIDP is relatively rare in the obstetric population. Relapse in patients with recurrent CIPD has been tied to pregnancy, and worsening of existing symptoms has been noted to occur, particularly in the third trimester and postpartum periods [90].

Multifocal motor neuropathy (MMN) is another chronic immune-mediated neuropathy characterized by asymmetric, weakness primarily of the distal upper more than lower limbs, that is a classic mimic of amyotrophic lateral sclerosis (ALS). In pregnancy, weakness of affected muscles may worsen and new muscles may become involved. Treatment is with IVIG, and patients generally experience full recovery [91]. In-depth discussion of GBS in pregnancy is provided in Chap. 22.

Isaac's Syndrome

Isaac's syndrome is a disorder of peripheral nerve hyper-excitability caused by dysfunction of voltage-gated potassium channels (VGKC). It may either be hereditary or more commonly, acquired, usually in association with infection or inflammation, autoimmune disorders, or malignancy [92, 93]. Patients experience muscle cramping and stiffness, pseudomyotonia (delayed muscle relaxation), and myokymia (muscle twitching at rest). EMG classically shows myokymic and neuromyotonic discharges, fasciculations, and fibrillation potentials [92]. The clinical course for Isaac's syndrome in pregnancy tends to be benign; however, symptom management

may be complicated by the teratogenicity of standard pharmacologic therapy with anticonvulsants (carbamazepine, phenytoin). Plasma exchange may be considered in refractory cases [94].

Charcot-Marie-Tooth Disease

Charcot-Marie-Tooth (CMT) disease, the most common inherited neuropathy, encompasses a heterogeneous group of disorders caused by genetic mutations leading to defective peripheral nerve myelination. Patients present in the first two decades of life with slowly progressive, symmetric weakness, numbness, and classical foot deformities. Symptom exacerbation is relatively common during pregnancy, occurring in up to 50% of women with clinically significant CMT and nearly all have a recurrence in subsequent pregnancies [95]. Furthermore, these patients tend to experience a more prolonged course of disease and are at greater risk of sustaining permanent neurologic damage [95, 96]. Pregnant women with CMT may also be more likely to require operative deliveries (cesarean, forceps/vacuum assist). In one such study, women with CMT had nearly twice the risk of fetal malpresentation, emergent operative delivery, and postpartum bleeding [97].

Hereditary Neuropathy with Liability to Pressure Palsies (HNPP)

Hereditary neuropathy with liability to pressure palsies (HNPP) is a rare autosomal dominant disorder caused by a deletion in the PMP22 gene that diffusely reduces the stability of peripheral nerve myelin, predisposing nerve to breakdown with minor applied pressure. Beginning in early adulthood, patients develop recurrent episodes of focal, painless sensorimotor pressure-induced mononeuropathies at common entrapment sites (median nerve at the carpal tunnel, ulnar nerve at the elbow, peroneal nerve at the fibular head) or after minor trauma or compression. Electrodiagnostic evaluation shows conduction block and changes consistent with demyelination, which are notably present even in clinically unaffected nerves [98]. There have been case reports of pregnancy-related neuropathy exacerbations in women with HNPP [12, 99].

Conclusion

Peripheral neuropathies that occur in the setting of pregnancy present a unique set of challenges to the clinician. Pregnant patients may have an increased risk of developing certain peripheral neuropathies and may experience a different clinical course of disease as compared to the general population. Distinction between acute nerve injury and subacute neuropathy has significant implications for management, particularly in this patient population. To appropriately care for these patients, considerations must be made regarding pregnancy-specific risk factors and modifiers of disease as well as implications of the disease course, workup, and treatment for the pregnancy.

References

1. Padua L, et al. Systematic review of pregnancy-related carpal tunnel syndrome. Muscle Nerve. 2010;42(5):697–702.
2. Guidon AC, Massey EW. Neuromuscular disorders in pregnancy. Neurol Clin. 2012;30(3):889–911.
3. Wong CA, et al. Incidence of postpartum lumbosacral spine and lower extremity nerve injuries. Obstet Gynecol. 2003;101(2):279–88.
4. Richard A, et al. Good prognosis of postpartum lower limb sensorimotor deficit: a combined clinical, electrophysiological, and radiological follow-up. J Neurol. 2017;264(3):529–40.
5. Holdcroft A, et al. Neurological complications associated with pregnancy. Br J Anaesth. 1995;75(5):522–6.
6. Ong BY, et al. Paresthesias and motor dysfunction after labor and delivery. Anesth Analg. 1987;66(1):18–22.
7. Ritchie JR. Orthopedic considerations during pregnancy. Clin Obstet Gynecol. 2003;46(2):456–66.
8. Stolp-Smith KA, Pascoe MK, Ogburn PL Jr. Carpal tunnel syndrome in pregnancy: frequency, severity, and prognosis. Arch Phys Med Rehabil. 1998;79(10):1285–7.
9. Katz A, et al. Bell's palsy during pregnancy: is it associated with adverse perinatal outcome? Laryngoscope. 2011;121(7):1395–8.
10. Meier T, et al. Efficacy of lidocaine patch 5% in the treatment of focal peripheral neuropathic pain syndromes: a randomized, double-blind, placebo-controlled study. Pain. 2003;106(1–2):151–8.
11. Hebl JR, et al. Neurologic complications after neuraxial anesthesia or analgesia in patients with preexisting peripheral sensorimotor neuropathy or diabetic polyneuropathy. Anesth Analg. 2006;103(5):1294–9.
12. Peters G, Hinds NP. Inherited neuropathy can cause postpartum foot drop. Anesth Analg. 2005;100(2):547–8.
13. Klein CJ, et al. Surgical and postpartum hereditary brachial plexus attacks and prophylactic immunotherapy. Muscle Nerve. 2013;47(1):23–7.
14. Klein A. Peripheral nerve disease in pregnancy. Clin Obstet Gynecol. 2013;56(2):382–8.
15. LaBan MM, et al. The lumbar herniated disk of pregnancy: a report of six cases identified by magnetic resonance imaging. Arch Phys Med Rehabil. 1995;76(5):476–9.
16. Murray RR. Maternal obstetrical paralysis. Am J Obstet Gynecol. 1964;88:399–403.
17. Padua L, et al. Carpal tunnel syndrome: ultrasound, neurophysiology, clinical and patient-oriented assessment. Clin Neurophysiol. 2008;119(9):2064–9.
18. Koenig RW, et al. High-resolution ultrasonography in evaluating peripheral nerve entrapment and trauma. Neurosurg Focus. 2009;26(2):E13.
19. Liu XQ, et al. Postpartum septic sacroiliitis misdiagnosed as sciatic neuropathy. Am J Med Sci. 2010;339(3):292–5.
20. LaBan MM, Perrin JC, Latimer FR. Pregnancy and the herniated lumbar disc. Arch Phys Med Rehabil. 1983;64(7):319–21.
21. Karatas M, et al. Postpartum sacral stress fracture: an unusual case of low-back and buttock pain. Am J Phys Med Rehabil. 2008;87(5):418–22.
22. Nogajski JH, Shnier RC, Zagami AS. Postpartum obturator neuropathy. Neurology. 2004;63(12):2450–1.
23. Bademosi O, et al. Obstetric neuropraxia in the Nigerian African. Int J Gynaecol Obstet. 1980;17(6):611–4.
24. Brusse E, Visser LH. Footdrop during pregnancy or labor due to obstetric lumbosacral plexopathy. Ned Tijdschr Geneeskd. 2002;146(1):31–4.
25. Katirji B, et al. Intrapartum maternal lumbosacral plexopathy. Muscle Nerve. 2002;26(3):340–7.
26. Haas DM, et al. Postpartum obturator neurapraxia. A case report. J Reprod Med. 2003;48(6):469–70.
27. Brown JT, McDougall A. Traumatic maternal birth palsy. J Obstet Gynaecol Br Emp. 1957;64(3):431–5.
28. Sahai-Srivastava S, Amezcua L. Compressive neuropathies complicating normal childbirth: case report and literature review. Birth. 2007;34(2):173–5.
29. Bunch K, Hope E. An uncommon case of bilateral peroneal nerve palsy following delivery: a case report and review of the literature. Case Rep Obstet Gynecol. 2014;2014:746480.
30. Ruppen W, et al. Incidence of epidural hematoma, infection, and neurologic injury in obstetric patients

with epidural analgesia/anesthesia. Anesthesiology. 2006;105(2):394–9.

31. Kirdi N, et al. Physical therapy in a patient with bilateral obturator nerve paralysis after surgery. A case report. Clin Exp Obstet Gynecol. 2000;27(1):59–60.

32. Dekel S, et al. Idiopathic carpal tunnel syndrome caused by carpal stenosis. Br Med J. 1980;280(6227):1297–9.

33. Vazquez MT, et al. Femoral nerve entrapment: a new insight. Clin Anat. 2007;20(2):175–9.

34. Ekman-Ordeberg G, Salgeback S, Ordeberg G. Carpal tunnel syndrome in pregnancy. A prospective study. Acta Obstet Gynecol Scand. 1987;66(3):233–5.

35. Padua L, et al. Symptoms and neurophysiological picture of carpal tunnel syndrome in pregnancy. Clin Neurophysiol. 2001;112(10):1946–51.

36. Padua L, et al. Carpal tunnel syndrome in pregnancy: multiperspective follow-up of untreated cases. Neurology. 2002;59(10):1643–6.

37. O'Neal MA, Chang LY, Salajegheh MK. Postpartum spinal cord, root, plexus and peripheral nerve injuries involving the lower extremities: a practical approach. Anesth Analg. 2015;120(1):141–8.

38. Di Martino A, et al. How to treat lumbar disc herniation in pregnancy? A systematic review on current standards. Eur Spine J. 2017;26(Suppl 4):496–504.

39. Ivins GK. Meralgia paresthetica, the elusive diagnosis: clinical experience with 14 adult patients. Ann Surg. 2000;232(2):281–6.

40. Williams PH, Trzil KP. Management of meralgia paresthetica. J Neurosurg. 1991;74(1):76–80.

41. Warfield CA. Obturator neuropathy after forceps delivery. Obstet Gynecol. 1984;64(3 Suppl):47S–8S.

42. Phalen GS. The carpal-tunnel syndrome. Seventeen years' experience in diagnosis and treatment of six hundred fifty-four hands. J Bone Joint Surg Am. 1966;48(2):211–28.

43. Assmus H, Hashemi B. Surgical treatment of carpal tunnel syndrome in pregnancy: results from 314 cases. Nervenarzt. 2000;71(6):470–3.

44. Turgut F, et al. The management of carpal tunnel syndrome in pregnancy. J Clin Neurosci. 2001;8(4):332–4.

45. Finsen V, Zeitlmann H. Carpal tunnel syndrome during pregnancy. Scand J Plast Reconstr Surg Hand Surg. 2006;40(1):41–5.

46. Pazzaglia C, et al. Multicenter study on carpal tunnel syndrome and pregnancy incidence and natural course. Acta Neurochir Suppl. 2005;92:35–9.

47. Mondelli M, et al. Prospective study of positive factors for improvement of carpal tunnel syndrome in pregnant women. Muscle Nerve. 2007;36(6):778–83.

48. Moghtaderi AR, Moghtaderi N, Loghmani A. Evaluating the effectiveness of local dexamethasone injection in pregnant women with carpal tunnel syndrome. J Res Med Sci. 2011;16(5):687–90.

49. Roubal PJ, Chavinson AH, LaGrandeur RM. Bilateral radial nerve palsies from use of the standard birthing bar. Obstet Gynecol. 1996;87(5 Pt 2):820–1.

50. Ozaras N, et al. Brachial plexus injury complicating the labor: mother is the victim at this time. J Matern Fetal Neonatal Med. 2014;27(13):1382–4.

51. Klein CJ, et al. Inflammation and neuropathic attacks in hereditary brachial plexus neuropathy. J Neurol Neurosurg Psychiatry. 2002;73(1):45–50.

52. van Alfen N, van Engelen BG. The clinical spectrum of neuralgic amyotrophy in 246 cases. Brain. 2006;129(Pt 2):438–50.

53. Kowe O, Waters JH. Neurologic complications in the patient receiving obstetric anesthesia. Neurol Clin. 2012;30(3):823–33.

54. Ismael SS, et al. Postpartum lumbosacral plexopathy limited to autonomic and perineal manifestations: clinical and electrophysiological study of 19 patients. J Neurol Neurosurg Psychiatry. 2000;68(6):771–3.

55. Turgut F, Turgut M, Mentes E. Lumbosacral plexus compression by fetus: an unusual cause of radiculopathy during teenage pregnancy. Eur J Obstet Gynecol Reprod Biol. 1997;73(2):203–4.

56. Delarue MW, Vles JS, Hasaart TH. Lumbosacral plexopathy in the third trimester of pregnancy: a report of three cases. Eur J Obstet Gynecol Reprod Biol. 1994;53(1):67–8.

57. Feasby TE, Burton SR, Hahn AF. Obstetrical lumbosacral plexus injury. Muscle Nerve. 1992;15(8):937–40.

58. Park S, Park SW, Kim KS. Lumbosacral plexus injury following vaginal delivery with epidural analgesia -a case report. Korean J Anesthesiol. 2013;64(2):175–9.

59. van Slobbe AM, et al. Incidence rates and determinants in meralgia paresthetica in general practice. J Neurol. 2004;251(3):294–7.

60. de Ridder VA, de Lange S, Popta JV. Anatomical variations of the lateral femoral cutaneous nerve and the consequences for surgery. J Orthop Trauma. 1999;13(3):207–11.

61. Macnicol MF, Thompson WJ. Idiopathic meralgia paresthetica. Clin Orthop Relat Res. 1990;254:270–4.

62. Vargo MM, et al. Postpartum femoral neuropathy: relic of an earlier era? Arch Phys Med Rehabil. 1990;71(8):591–6.

63. Rowland C, Kane D, Eogan M. Postpartum femoral neuropathy: managing the next pregnancy. BMJ Case Rep. 2019;12(12):e232967.

64. Al Hakim M, Katirji B. Femoral mononeuropathy induced by the lithotomy position: a report of 5 cases with a review of literature. Muscle Nerve. 1993;16(9):891–5.

65. Dar AQ, Robinson A, Lyons G. Postpartum femoral neuropathy: more common than you think. Anaesthesia. 1999;54(5):512.

66. Cohen S, Zada Y. Postpartum femoral neuropathy. Anaesthesia. 2001;56(5):500–1.

67. Tokarz VA, et al. Femoral neuropathy and iliopsoas hematoma as a result of postpartum factor-VIII inhibitor syndrome. A case report. J Bone Joint Surg Am. 2003;85(9):1812–5.

68. Pham LH, Bulich LA, Datta S. Bilateral postpartum femoral neuropathy. Anesth Analg. 1995;80(5):1036–7.

69. Adelman JU, Goldberg GS, Puckett JD. Postpartum bilateral femoral neuropathy. Obstet Gynecol. 1973;42(6):845–50.

70. Radawski MM, Strakowski JA, Johnson EW. Acute common peroneal neuropathy due to hand positioning in normal labor and delivery. Obstet Gynecol. 2011;118(2 Pt 2):421–3.

71. Colachis SC 3rd, Pease WS, Johnson EW. A preventable cause of foot drop during childbirth. Am J Obstet Gynecol. 1994;171(1):270–2.

72. Babayev M, Bodack MP, Creatura C. Common peroneal neuropathy secondary to squatting during childbirth. Obstet Gynecol. 1998;91(5 Pt 2):830–2.

73. Reif ME. Bilateral common peroneal nerve palsy secondary to prolonged squatting in natural childbirth. Birth. 1988;15(2):100–2.

74. Sorenson EJ, Chen JJ, Daube JR. Obturator neuropathy: causes and outcome. Muscle Nerve. 2002;25(4):605–7.

75. Hong BY, et al. Intrapartum obturator neuropathy diagnosed after cesarean delivery. Arch Gynecol Obstet. 2010;282(3):349–50.

76. Hakoiwa S, et al. Case of bilateral obturator neuropathy after caesarean section. Masui. 2011;60(6):721–3.

77. Gillman GS, et al. Bell's palsy in pregnancy: a study of recovery outcomes. Otolaryngol Head Neck Surg. 2002;126(1):26–30.

78. Falco NA, Eriksson E. Idiopathic facial palsy in pregnancy and the puerperium. Surg Gynecol Obstet. 1989;169(4):337–40.

79. Hilsinger RL Jr, Adour KK, Doty HE. Idiopathic facial paralysis, pregnancy, and the menstrual cycle. Ann Otol Rhinol Laryngol. 1975;84(4 Pt 1):433–42.

80. Vrabec JT, Isaacson B, Van Hook JW. Bell's palsy and pregnancy. Otolaryngol Head Neck Surg. 2007;137(6):858–61.

81. Cohen Y, et al. Bell palsy complicating pregnancy: a review. Obstet Gynecol Surv. 2000;55(3):184–8.

82. Zandian A, et al. The neurologist's dilemma: a comprehensive clinical review of Bell's palsy, with emphasis on current management trends. Med Sci Monit. 2014;20:83–90.

83. Gronseth GS, Paduga R, American Academy of Neurology. Evidence-based guideline update: steroids and antivirals for bell palsy: report of the guideline development Subcommittee of the American Academy of Neurology. Neurology. 2012;79(22):2209–13.

84. Phillips KM, et al. Onset of bell's palsy in late pregnancy and early puerperium is associated with worse long-term outcomes. Laryngoscope. 2017;127(12):2854–9.

85. Pacheco LD, et al. Guillain-Barre syndrome in pregnancy. Obstet Gynecol. 2016;128(5):1105–10.

86. Chan LY, Tsui MH, Leung TN. Guillain-Barre syndrome in pregnancy. Acta Obstet Gynecol Scand. 2004;83(4):319–25.

87. Chevret S, Hughes RA, Annane D. Plasma exchange for Guillain-Barre syndrome. Cochrane Database Syst Rev. 2017;2:CD001798.

88. Randomised trial of plasma exchange, intravenous immunoglobulin, and combined treatments in Guillain-Barre syndrome. Plasma exchange/ Sandoglobulin Guillain-Barre syndrome trial group. Lancet. 1997;349(9047):225–30.

89. Hughes RA, Swan AV, van Doorn PA. Intravenous immunoglobulin for Guillain-Barre syndrome. Cochrane Database Syst Rev. 2014;9:CD002063.

90. McCombe PA, et al. Chronic inflammatory demyelinating polyradiculoneuropathy associated with pregnancy. Ann Neurol. 1987;21(1):102–4.

91. Chaudhry V, Escolar DM, Cornblath DR. Worsening of multifocal motor neuropathy during pregnancy. Neurology. 2002;59(1):139–41.

92. Morgan PJ. Peripartum management of a patient with Isaacs' syndrome. Can J Anaesth. 1997;44(11):1174–7.

93. Lide B, Singh J, Haeri S. Isaacs' syndrome in pregnancy. BMJ Case Rep. 2014;2014:bcr2014206704.

94. Basiri K, Fatehi F, Chitsaz A. Isaac's syndrome associated with CIDP and pregnancy. Arch Iran Med. 2011;14(3):206–8.

95. Rudnik-Schoneborn S, et al. Pregnancy and delivery in Charcot-Marie-tooth disease type 1. Neurology. 1993;43(10):2011–6.

96. Awater C, Zerres K, Rudnik-Schoneborn S. Pregnancy course and outcome in women with hereditary neuromuscular disorders: comparison of obstetric risks in 178 patients. Eur J Obstet Gynecol Reprod Biol. 2012;162(2):153–9.

97. Hoff JM, Gilhus NE, Daltveit AK. Pregnancies and deliveries in patients with Charcot-Marie-tooth disease. Neurology. 2005;64(3):459–62.

98. Chance PF. Overview of hereditary neuropathy with liability to pressure palsies. Ann N Y Acad Sci. 1999;883:14–21.

99. Simonetti S. Lesion of the anterior branch of axillary nerve in a patient with hereditary neuropathy with liability to pressure palsies. Eur J Neurol. 2000;7(5):577–9.

Peripheral Nerve Disorders in the Newborn

25

Anna C. Filley and Christopher J. Winfree

Introduction

Obstetrical nerve injuries can occur at any point during the birth process. The presence of intrauterine structural abnormalities may be associated with the development of peripheral nerve palsies due to ongoing compression, usually occurring in the later stages of pregnancy. Parturition involves fetal movement through a variety of positions within a confined space prior to expulsion from the birth canal. Birth trauma may cause neonatal nerve palsies, examples of which include forced extreme limb positions that occur during the birth process and focally applied pressures during assisted delivery (forceps, vacuum). Skeletal fractures and hematomas that result from the birth process can also injure peripheral nerves [1]. Mild nerve injury typically results from plexus contusion and reversible damage [2]. The actual mechanisms of injury variably include some combination of stretch and/or compression and often involve both.

An increased risk of obstetric palsy is present in situations of mismatch between fetal size and abdominopelvic parameters that cause fetal nerve injury directly or indirectly by necessitating the application of tractional or compressive forces to facilitate delivery. However, only half of the cases of traumatic nerve palsy can be associated with known risk factors [3]. Factors related to the fetus that predispose to nerve injury include macrosomia [4], shoulder dystocia, and breech presentation [5, 6]. The presence of shoulder dystocia, in which the mother's pubic symphysis physically blocks delivery of the fetus's upper shoulder, may result in an increase in the tractional forces applied to the fetal head, exacerbating stretching of the ipsilateral brachial plexus [5]. Maternal factors that predispose to nerve injury include obesity, gestational diabetes [7], and a prolonged second stage of labor [5, 6, 8]. Treatment of gestational diabetes has been shown to reduce the risk of fetal macrosomia and serious perinatal outcomes, including shoulder dystocia and nerve palsy [7]. Although there is a higher incidence of birth palsy with vaginal delivery, a cesarean section does not eliminate this risk [3].

The most frequently diagnosed childbirth-related traumatic nerve palsy in neonates is a traction injury of the brachial plexus, usually involving the upper trunk. Transient cranial nerve palsies may also be seen, usually in association with forceps deliveries [9]. The majority of palsies are transient and spontaneously resolve in the first few weeks to months of life and are therefore typically managed conservatively [9]. Operative intervention may be indicated in cases without improvement in the first few months and generally involves nerve grafts or transfers [1]. Tendon transfers, osteotomies, and other ortho-

A. C. Filley · C. J. Winfree (✉)
Department of Neurological Surgery, Columbia University, New York, NY, USA
e-mail: cjw12@cumc.columbia.edu

pedic procedures may be performed to address functional deficits, deformities, or fixed contractures [2]. Surgical reconstruction is ultimately performed in ~10 to 20% of cases in order to prevent development of permanent weakness or deformity [6].

Patient Evaluation

A thorough and efficient clinical exam is imperative in the neonatal population, given the limited patient history. In most cases of neonatal peripheral nerve palsy, the diagnosis is clinical. Additional imaging studies such as X-ray, ultrasound, CT, or MRI may be ordered in more complicated cases to evaluate for confounding factors or underlying pathology like fractures [2, 9].

Patients with traumatic peripheral nerve palsy tend to present at birth with loss of motor function in the affected nerve territory, for example, a flaccid upper extremity in patients with brachial plexus palsies [2]. The resting posture of the affected limb can help localize the injury and differentiate between palsies of the brachial plexus and upper extremity peripheral nerves. In upper plexus injuries (Erb's palsy), the arm is held in the classical "waiter's tip" position with the shoulder adducted and internally rotated, elbow extended, forearm pronated, and wrist and fingers in sustained flexion. This is in contrast to lower trunk palsies, in which the arm is supinated, elbow is flexed, and the wrist extended [9]. Additional damage at the C7 level leads to impairment of finger extension and a resting limb position with continuous finger flexion. Severe avulsion injuries involving the entire plexus (C5-T1) manifest with complete loss of upper extremity motor activity, termed a "flail arm" [1].

Asymmetric thoracic and abdominal expansion with breathing may be suggestive of a unilateral phrenic nerve palsy; this may occur in association with an upper plexus injury [1]. A winged scapula suggests long thoracic nerve injury, which is derived from C5–7 nerve roots [1]. The presence of a Horner's syndrome (ptosis, miosis, anhidrosis) indicates injury at the T1 level involving the sympathetic fibers [1, 2].

Diagnoses

Obstetric Brachial Plexus Palsy (OBPP)

Obstetric brachial plexus palsy (OBPP) is the most common congenital nerve palsy, estimated to affect 0.35 to 5 infants per 1000 live births [6]. Plexus injuries often result from an application of tractional forces to the fetal head leading to forced lateral cervical extension during delivery. Traumatic brachial plexus injuries are classically differentiated by the levels involved. Most commonly observed are upper trunk palsies (Erb's type) involving the fifth and sixth cervical nerve roots. Isolated lower trunk palsies (Klumpke's type) that involve the eighth cervical and first thoracic nerve roots are uncommonly associated with birth trauma; involvement of these levels is more often seen with mixed or total palsies that affect the entire plexus [2].

First descried by Erb and Duchenne, injury to the upper brachial plexus results in paresis of the supraspinatus, infraspinatus, deltoid, biceps, brachialis, and brachioradialis muscles. Injury is usually unilateral [10] and the affected limb demonstrates a classical resting position with the shoulder adducted and internally rotated, elbow extended, forearm pronated, and wrist and fingers flexed [9]. Erb's palsy is more common in larger fetuses and has been shown to be more frequently preceded by abnormal labor [10]. Across multiple studies, birth trauma or the presence of shoulder dystocia is noted in approximately half of cases of brachial plexus injury [4, 11, 12]. Initially thought to necessarily be a consequence of shoulder dystocia, a more recent review and understanding of neonatal Erb's palsy has revealed that a significant portion of neonatal Erb's palsy diagnoses occur in the absence of shoulder dystocia. The underlying mechanics and severity of injury between these two clinical situations appear to differ, reflected in the tendency for non-dystocia associated injuries to occur in the posterior, rather than anterior arm [13]. Furthermore, of infants who do develop Erb's palsy, the disease is deemed moderate to severe in 51% of those with shoulder dystocia and only 18% of those without documented labor problems [10].

Of note, regardless of mechanism, the vast majority of infants with OBPP make a full spontaneous recovery by age 1 year [14], with an average time to resolution of 4.5 months [2]. Although most cases are transient, some degree of residual deficits may be present in up to 20–30% of cases [5]. Persistent OBPP, defined as symptoms remaining after 12 months, is rare and estimated to occur in only 1.1–2.2 per 10,000 births [15].

Radial Nerve

Transient neonatal radial nerve palsy is an uncommon complication of childbirth, estimated to occur in 0.1%–4.0% of live births [9]. Infants exhibit wrist drop due to an inability to extend the wrist and fingers; external rotation and elbow flexion remain intact, distinguishing this condition from the more common brachial plexus palsy [16]. In most cases, a firm nodule can be found on the inferior posterolateral arm; this is thought to represent fat necrosis caused by sustained pressure exerted on the arm during prolonged labor. Symptoms resulting from birth trauma are usually unilateral; bilateral palsies have been reported and are more likely secondary to intra-uterine compression or abnormal arm positioning [9, 16]. Differential diagnosis should also consider other causes of decreased arm movement including intracranial disease, shoulder dislocation, clavicle or humerus fracture, Caffey's disease, and infection or septic arthritis of the shoulder [1, 16]. Management is supportive and may be aided by physiotherapy, orthoses, and taping [16]. Full recovery is most often seen in the first 2 months and should be expected by 6 months of age [17]. Diagnostic nerve imaging and surgical exploration for radial nerve decompression and/or repair are indicated when spontaneous recovery does not occur.

Phrenic Nerve

Neonatal phrenic nerve palsy may result from excessive cervical extension during childbirth and often occurs in the setting of upper brachial plexus injury [18]. More commonly observed on the right side, approximately 75% of cases are associated with an Erb's palsy [19]. Innervated by cervical roots C3–5, the phrenic nerve is the only motor supply of the diaphragm and injury results in diaphragmatic paralysis. Presentation is typically shortly after birth with profound dyspnea, irregular respirations, and cyanosis. Infants exhibit asymmetric chest expansion with respiration, and imaging may reveal unilateral diaphragmatic elevation [19, 20]. Bilateral paralysis results in respiratory insufficiency and failure that often requires prolonged mechanical ventilation [19]. Initial management is with expectant management and ventilatory support, as a minority may recover spontaneously [21]. Operative management should be considered in infants who cannot be weaned from the ventilator after 1 month, or earlier if there is clinical decompensation [19]. Definitive treatment is with surgical plication, ideally performed before 45 days of life [18].

Recurrent Laryngeal Nerve

Congenital vocal cord paralysis is an uncommon nerve palsy in the neonatal population that may present with noisy breathing, stridor, and cyanosis. Palsy may be secondary to birth trauma, which usually results in unilateral disease that spontaneously recovers over the first few months of life. CNS disorders such as Chiari malformation or other congenital syndromes may cause bilateral paralysis that is frequently permanent, often necessitating tracheostomy [22].

Cranial Nerves

Cranial nerve palsies secondary to birth trauma are rare, but documented complications of labor. Most commonly involved is the facial nerve (cranial nerve VII), usually occurring in the setting of forceps-assisted delivery [12, 23, 24]. Instrumented deliveries are also associated with neonatal abducens (cranial nerve VI) palsies [25]. These injuries are usually unilateral and may be associated with evidence of trauma such as facial swelling or ecchymosis [9]. Infants exhibit features including facial asymmetry, incomplete closure of the ipsilateral eye, and difficulty with feeding. When caused by birth trauma, spontaneous recovery is expected to occur in the first 2 months of life [12, 23, 24]. These cases must be differentiated from the less common, palsies that are manifestations of an underlying congenital disorder; these tend to cause bilateral symptoms, are often associated with other anomalies, and have a worse prognosis for recovery [26]. Among these is Moebius syndrome, a rare congenital disease characterized by unilateral or bilateral facial and abducens nerve palsies. In addition to oculomotor dysfunction and facial weakness, infants may exhibit other cranial nerve palsies, craniofacial malformations, and limb defects [27].

Management Principles

Nonoperative Management

Initial management of neonatal peripheral nerve injury is predominantly conservative. Early mobilization of affected limbs with passive range of motion exercises should be initiated in the first few weeks of life [2]. Key in the rehabilitation process is frequent mobilization to prevent the formation of contractures that will restrict motion and joint mobility [5]. With more severe injuries, absent innervation of distal muscles results in deformities and contractures [28]. The use of orthotic devices is not uncommon and may help to help maintain surgical correction and slow progression of deformity [2].

Operative Management

Microsurgical repair is indicated for neonatal patients with persistent nerve palsy with limited spontaneous recovery. Key in management of patients with OBPP and other neonatal nerve palsies is distinguishing the cases from those with similar deficits but potential for eventual recovery. Unfortunately, prognostication in the first few months of life is particularly difficult, as physical exams are often unreliable. Current clinical guidelines recommend close observation in the first few months of life, with re-evaluation after 3–6 months of age for determination of injury severity and need for surgical reconstruction [28–31]. In upper trunk lesions, persistent paralysis of the biceps after 3 months has been cited as a poor prognostic indicator for ultimate motor recovery, prompting many to advocate for early nerve reconstruction if severe disability remains by age 3 months [32]. Indeed, many studies support improved outcomes and overall function for these patients with early reconstruction [33–35]. Even in the setting of severe injury and nerve root avulsion, recovery of useful distal function occurs in most patients [35]. This potential benefit, however, must be weighed against the risks associated with performing an operative procedure, with inherent risk, in a child that may have otherwise independently recovered. In children who will ultimately spontaneously recover biceps motor function, resultant motor outcomes have been shown to be relatively equivalent in children who recovered biceps motor function between age 3 and 6 months and those with evidence of recovery prior to age 3 months [30]. In infants that may be expected to possibly recover spontaneously and in the absence of nerve root avulsion injury, some authors advocate a more delayed approach to operative intervention with consideration of surgery after 6 months of observation.

Prior to surgical intervention, imaging studies like CT-myelography and magnetic resonance imaging (MRI) may be obtained to better characterize the underlying pathology, providing valuable information regarding the mechanism, location, and type of injury, structures involved, extent of damage, and presence of neuromas or scar formation, all of which have functional implications for operative management [31, 36]. Both can be used to distinguish pathologies like nerve root avulsions that may prompt differential management, although MRI studies avoid risks associated with radiation exposure.

Operative intervention is reserved for severe injuries in which spontaneous recovery of function is thought to not be possible without surgical reconstruction. The type of procedure performed is largely based on surgeon preference and anatomical feasibility. Nerve grafting can be used to functionally bypass an injured segment of nerve, usually with a short segment of autograft [37]. In addition to the potential for donor site morbidity (autograft is usually harvested from the sural nerve), an important limitation of this procedure is that it requires an intact nerve stump and therefore is impossible to perform in settings of nerve root avulsions [36]. Fascicles may also be re-routed from another nerve to restore motor function of select de-innervated muscles. In patients with upper plexus injury, some studies have shown that nerve transfer may lead slightly better functional outcomes than nerve grafting [38, 39].

Nerve reconstruction with nerve grafts or transfers may be performed for persistent OBPP to restore core motor functions of shoulder abduction and elbow flexion [36]. Restoration of shoulder abduction and external rotation after C5 nerve root injury can be performed by procedures that target reinnervation of the suprascapular nerve and the supraspinatus or deltoid muscles [36]; functional results are better with earlier (prior to 3 months) reconstruction, but improvement may be seen even with more delayed palliative procedures [34]. Recovery of elbow flexion after C6 nerve root injury can be achieved by procedures that target the musculocutaneous nerve or biceps muscle [36]. One such procedure, termed an Oberlin transfer, involves re-routing ulnar nerve fascicles to anastomose with the biceps nerve in order to regain elbow flexion [40]. Elbow flexion may also be restored by medial pectoral to musculocutaneous nerve transfer; however, this approach is limited in the neonatal population by the small size of the medial pectoral nerve [41].

In addition to reinnervation procedures, tendon transfers may be performed to restore motor function by transposition of tendon origins to a more proximal location [37, 42]. Overall, the treatment of OBPP is complex and involves a comprehensive, multidisciplinary team of pediatric neurologists, neuroradiologists, neurosur-

geons, orthopedic surgeons, physiatrists, and physiotherapists. Even after surgical reconstruction, these patients require intensive physiotherapy to optimize their outcomes. It is common for patients with these injuries to be referred to tertiary care centers so that they may receive comprehensive care.

Conclusions

Neonatal nerve palsy secondary to birth trauma is an uncommon neurologic complication of pregnancy and childbirth. There is a higher risk of such injury for large infants born to obese or diabetic mothers and with prolonged or instrumented deliveries and fetal malpresentation. Nevertheless, up to half of cases are not associated with documented risk factors. Luckily, the vast majority of cases are transient and exhibit spontaneous, rapid recovery. Observation for a period of 3–6 months, even in the setting of severe deficits, is the recommended initial approach due to the high rate of recovery seen in most patients. Operative intervention in the form of nerve grafts or transfers may be performed in select situations to restore lost function if spontaneous recovery is deemed unlikely. Physiotherapy, both before and after surgical reconstruction, remains crucial for the optimization of outcomes following OBPP and other neonatal nerve injuries.

References

1. Borschel GH, Clarke HM. Obstetrical brachial plexus palsy. Plast Reconstr Surg. 2009;124(1 Suppl):144e–55e.
2. Jahnke AH Jr, et al. Persistent brachial plexus birth palsies. J Pediatr Orthop. 1991;11(4):533–7.
3. Hale HB, Bae DS, Waters PM. Current concepts in the management of brachial plexus birth palsy. J Hand Surg Am. 2010;35(2):322–31.
4. Graham EM, Forouzan I, Morgan MA. A retrospective analysis of Erb's palsy cases and their relation to birth weight and trauma at delivery. J Matern Fetal Med. 1997;6(1):1–5.
5. Malessy MJ, Pondaag W. Obstetric brachial plexus injuries. Neurosurg Clin N Am. 2009;20(1):1–14. v

6. Gosk J, Rutowski R. Obstetrical brachial plexus palsy—etiopathogenesis, risk factors, prevention, prognosis. Ginekol Pol. 2004;75(10):814–20.

7. Crowther CA, et al. Effect of treatment of gestational diabetes mellitus on pregnancy outcomes. N Engl J Med. 2005;352(24):2477–86.

8. Mehta SH, et al. What factors are associated with neonatal injury following shoulder dystocia? J Perinatol. 2006;26(2):85–8.

9. Malik S, Bhandekar HS, Korday CS. Traumatic peripheral neuropraxias in neonates: a case series. J Clin Diagn Res. 2014;8(10):PD10–2.

10. Weizsaecker K, Deaver JE, Cohen WR. Labour characteristics and neonatal Erb's palsy. BJOG. 2007;114(8):1003–9.

11. Vaquero G, et al. Obstetric brachial plexus palsy: incidence, monitoring of progress and prognostic factors. Rev Neurol. 2017;65(1):19–25.

12. Rehm A, Promod P, Ogilvy-Stuart A. Obstetric neonatal brachial plexus and facial nerve injuries: a 17 years single tertiary maternity hospital experience. Eur J Obstet Gynecol Reprod Biol. 2019;243:57–62.

13. Sandmire HF, DeMott RK. Erb's palsy without shoulder dystocia. Int J Gynaecol Obstet. 2002;78(3):253–6.

14. Hardy AE. Birth injuries of the brachial plexus: incidence and prognosis. J Bone Joint Surg Br. 1981;63-B(1):98–101.

15. McLaren RA Jr, et al. Persistence of neonatal brachial plexus palsy among nulliparous versus parous women. AJP Rep. 2019;9(1):1–5.

16. Carsi MB, Clarke AM, Clarke NP. Transient neonatal radial nerve palsy. A case series and review of the literature. J Hand Ther. 2015;28(2):212–5; quiz 216.

17. Alsubhi FS, et al. Radial nerve palsy in the newborn: a case series. CMAJ. 2011;183(12):1367–70.

18. Rizeq YK, et al. Diaphragmatic paralysis after phrenic nerve injury in newborns. J Pediatr Surg. 2020;55(2):240–4.

19. Murty VS, Ram KD. Phrenic nerve palsy: a rare cause of respiratory distress in newborn. J Pediatr Neurosci. 2012;7(3):225–7.

20. Shiohama T, et al. Phrenic nerve palsy associated with birth trauma—case reports and a literature review. Brain and Development. 2013;35(4):363–6.

21. Stramrood CA, et al. Neonatal phrenic nerve injury due to traumatic delivery. J Perinat Med. 2009;37(3):293–6.

22. Ada M, Isildak H, Saritzali G. Congenital vocal cord paralysis. J Craniofac Surg. 2010;21(1):273–4.

23. Falco NA, Eriksson E. Facial nerve palsy in the newborn: incidence and outcome. Plast Reconstr Surg. 1990;85(1):1–4.

24. Al Tawil K, et al. Traumatic facial nerve palsy in newborns: is it always iatrogenic? Am J Perinatol. 2010;27(9):711–3.

25. Galbraith RS. Incidence of neonatal sixth nerve palsy in relation to mode of delivery. Am J Obstet Gynecol. 1994;170(4):1158–9.

26. Smith JD, Crumley RL, Harker LA. Facial paralysis in the newborn. Otolaryngol Head Neck Surg. 1981;89(6):1021–4.

27. Picciolini O, et al. Moebius syndrome: clinical features, diagnosis, management and early intervention. Ital J Pediatr. 2016;42(1):56.

28. Vekris MD, et al. Management of obstetrical brachial plexus palsy with early plexus microreconstruction and late muscle transfers. Microsurgery. 2008;28(4):252–61.

29. O'Brien DF, et al. Management of birth brachial plexus palsy. Childs Nerv Syst. 2006;22(2):103–12.

30. Philandrianos C, et al. Management of upper obstetrical brachial plexus palsy. Long-term results of non-operative treatment in 22 children. Ann Chir Plast Esthet. 2013;58(4):327–35.

31. Buterbaugh KL, Shah AS. The natural history and management of brachial plexus birth palsy. Curr Rev Musculoskelet Med. 2016;9(4):418–26.

32. Smith NC, et al. Neonatal brachial plexus palsy. Outcome of absent biceps function at three months of age. J Bone Joint Surg Am. 2004;86(10):2163–70.

33. Soucacos PN, et al. Secondary reanimation procedures in late obstetrical brachial plexus palsy patients. Microsurgery. 2006;26(4):343–51.

34. Terzis JK, Kokkalis ZT. Primary and secondary shoulder reconstruction in obstetric brachial plexus palsy. Injury. 2008;39(Suppl 3):S5–14.

35. Gilbert A, Pivato G, Kheiralla T. Long-term results of primary repair of brachial plexus lesions in children. Microsurgery. 2006;26(4):334–42.

36. Malessy MJ, Pondaag W. Neonatal brachial plexus palsy with neurotmesis of C5 and avulsion of C6: supraclavicular reconstruction strategies and outcome. J Bone Joint Surg Am. 2014;96(20):e174.

37. Bertelli JA. Brachialis muscle transfer to the forearm muscles in obstetric brachial plexus palsy. J Hand Surg Br. 2006;31(3):261–5.

38. Chang KWC, et al. Oberlin transfer compared with nerve grafting for improving early supination in neonatal brachial plexus palsy. J Neurosurg Pediatr. 2018;21(2):178–84.

39. Manske MC, et al. Reconstruction of the suprascapular nerve in brachial plexus birth injury: a comparison of nerve grafting and nerve transfers. J Bone Joint Surg Am. 2020;102(4):298–308.

40. Noaman HH, Shiha AE, Bahm J. Oberlin's ulnar nerve transfer to the biceps motor nerve in obstetric brachial plexus palsy: indications, and good and bad results. Microsurgery. 2004;24(3):182–7.

41. Wellons JC, et al. Medial pectoral nerve to musculocutaneous nerve neurotization for the treatment of persistent birth-related brachial plexus palsy: an 11-year institutional experience. J Neurosurg Pediatr. 2009;3(5):348–53.

42. Al-Qattan MM. Elbow flexion reconstruction by Steindler flexorplasty in obstetric brachial plexus palsy. J Hand Surg Br. 2005;30(4):424–7.

Ira Goldstein

Epidemiology

The incidence of low back pain (LBP), pelvic girdle pain (PGP), or sciatica during pregnancy exceeds two-thirds of women [1–4]. In one study, 80% of pregnant women experienced low back pain, but that number decreased to 40% in the postpartum period [5]. 75% of pregnant women take analgesics for their musculoskeletal pain during pregnancy, although 85% report not being offered medical assistance for this pain [4]. Pain carries implications beyond maternal discomfort—greater back and pelvic pain during the third trimester has been found to be associated with an increased incidence of delivery via cesarean section, assisted delivery, and a longer duration of labor [6]. It should be concluded then that greater attention should be given to the identification and treatment of maternal pain.

Back pain as well as the incidence of sick leave increases throughout the course of pregnancy. Of 566 women, 3 out of 4 reported back pain at 20 weeks, which increased to 9 out of 10 at 32 weeks [7]. In another 200 women, most cases of back pain began between the fifth and seventh months of pregnancy [8]. Pain also intensified later in pregnancy—it was moderate to severe in 1 of 3 at 20 weeks and in one half at 32 weeks. Sick leave and physical disability increased with greater low back pain scores. The prevalence of sick leave has been reported as 56% of employed pregnant women during the first 32 weeks of gestation, and inability to perform activities of daily living increased from 58% to 78% over the course of pregnancy [9–11]. In addition, greater than 25% reported sick leave of greater than 20 days. The most common reason for leave was low back pain.

In 45.5% of cases of low back pain the pain radiated to the lower extremities. Of these, one-third of patients had pain increased over the course of the day and one-third had pain which increased at night and woke them from sleep. Pain was generally exacerbated by standing, sitting, forward bending, lifting, and walking [8].

Additional factors have been found to influence the reporting of back pain in pregnancy. A prior history of back pain [7, 11–14], mechanically demanding jobs [12], lower degrees of educational attainment [7, 9], and multiparity [7, 9, 11, 13–15] have been found to be the strongest predictors of back pain. In addition, a history of anxiety or depression [9, 13], lower job satisfaction [13], younger maternal age [11, 14], and stress [13] contributed to the reporting of pain. Interestingly, Ostgaard et al. found younger age to be principally associated with greater incidence of back pain ($p < 0.001$) as well as greater pain intensity during the first trimester ($p < 0.05$) [14]. Ostgaard et al. also noted that back pain and

I. Goldstein (✉)
Department of Neurological Surgery, Rutgers New
Jersey Medical School, Newark, NJ, USA

© The Author(s), under exclusive license to Springer Nature Switzerland AG 2023
G. Gupta et al. (eds.), *Neurological Disorders in Pregnancy*,
https://doi.org/10.1007/978-3-031-36490-7_26

pelvic pain were common during pregnancy with greater pain generally noted from the posterior pelvis during pregnancy [14]. Pelvic pain has been found to improve much faster than low back pain following delivery [1, 16, 17]. Greater pain during pregnancy was correlated with persistent pain following delivery. Pain was also more likely to persist postpartum when experienced from multiple sites during pregnancy [1, 17, 18].

Much as is the case with low back pain, pelvic girdle pain and sacroiliac pain in pregnancy are disabling and are predicted by many similar factors. Risk factors for developing pelvic girdle or sacroiliac pain in pregnancy include previous low back pain and trauma to the back or pelvis, multiparae, lower job satisfaction, and greater stress [13]. Greater weight contributed to pelvic girdle pain but not to sacroiliac pain [13, 15]. In a cohort of 371 women, long-term pelvic girdle pain was predicted by greater number of pain provocation tests during pregnancy (OR = 1.79) and a prior history of low back pain (LBP) (OR = 2.28) [18]. They were significantly less able to independently perform activities of daily living ($p < 0.001$), experienced lower self-esteem ($p = 0.046$), decreased health-related quality of life ($p < 0.001$), greater levels of anxiety and depression ($p < 0.001$), and worked significantly fewer hours per week ($p = 0.032$) than did women without pelvic girdle pain. Accordingly, they concluded that the presence of truncal pain during pregnancy was associated with long-term social, economic, and health concerns for many women and treatment for this should be pursued.

Role of Scoliosis

Dewan et al. conducted a systematic literature review of pregnancy related outcomes in patients with adolescent idiopathic scoliosis (AIS). 22 articles with 3125 patients were included in this review. Patients with AIS patients demonstrated somewhat higher rates of nulliparity and more often sought infertility treatments. Prepartum back pain was more common in women with

AIS. Back pain in pregnancy was more severe in these patients than in healthy women. Progression of the scoliotic curve was often seen, however minor and of unclear permanence. AIS was not associated with an increase in perinatal complications to either the mother or child [19].

In a single-center retrospective review of 59 pregnant women with the diagnosis of AIS, 14 had previously undergone posterior spinal fusion [20]. Obstetric complications included preterm birth in 21.4%, induction of labor in 23.8%, and emergency cesarean section in 14%. None of these was associated with scoliotic curve severity or with prior spinal fusion. Spinal anesthesia was successful in 70 of 71 attempts, including in 13 patients with prior fusion. 11 patients underwent postpartum scoliosis imaging with no statistically significant change in curve seen during or shortly after pregnancy. Other studies have found a modest progression of scoliotic curves during pregnancy but not when surgery had been performed [21, 22]. It can be concluded then that AIS does not increase the risk of complication with regional anesthesia or with delivery and the scoliotic curve does not progress significantly during pregnancy.

In a study with an average of 5 years follow-up of 108 nulliparous women who had scoliosis surgery, 97 women with scoliosis surgery and pregnancy, 91 pregnant controls and 82 nulliparous controls found a greater degree of back pain during pregnancy when prior scoliosis surgery was performed (48% vs. 34%) [23]. The prevalence of low back pain after childbirth was equal in the two groups (43% vs. 42%). An important finding was the importance of the lowest instrumented segment: women with surgery above L3 demonstrated less frequent back pain during pregnancy than those whose fusions extended to L3 or L4 ($p < 0.05$). Moreover, cesarean (C)-section was significantly more likely in women with surgery (64% vs. 33%), and the likelihood of C-section was greater when the surgery extended to or below L4 ($p < 0.05$). Anesthesia for C-section was more often via general, rather than spinal, anesthesia for fusions to L4 or below

($p < 0.05$). Quality of life after pregnancy was the same for women who had scoliosis surgery as for healthy controls. Accordingly, the lowest instrumented segment of a spinal fusion carries far greater significance during pregnancy than does the presence of a fusion itself.

Influence of Prior Anterior Spinal Surgery

A history of anterior lumbar fusion raises the concern of difficulty with pregnancy due to prior surgery with scarring and instrumentation near the woman's growing uterus. In one single institution study of 67 women who underwent previous anterior spinal surgery, 19 later attempted to become pregnant [24]. All succeeded in becoming pregnant and in bearing a child. 37% underwent delivery by cesarean section, consistent with the general population. Anterior spinal fusion poses no increase in risk of delivery complication or of difficulty with conception.

Influence of Prior Diskectomy

A history of prior lumbar diskectomy potentially could increase the risk of back pain encountered during pregnancy as well as an increase in risk of recurrent disk herniation from the mechanical stresses upon the low back. A retrospective evaluation of 26 women who gave birth an average of 3 1/2 years after lumbar microdiscectomy found an increased prevalence of back pain, leg pain, and motor and sensory deficits during pregnancy [25]. The majority of patients noted improvement in back pain, leg pain, motor and sensory deficits following delivery. No case of recurrent lumbar disk herniation was seen by 6 months following delivery. Three patients (11%) underwent surgery for recurrent disk herniation at an average of 7.7 years following delivery, consistent with historical controls. The authors surmised that venous compression from the uterus, along with an increasing body fluid volume during pregnancy could account for some of the symptoms encountered during pregnancy [8, 26].

Diagnosis

A challenge with discussion of back pain in pregnancy is the overlapping symptoms and classification of the nature of pain. Sciatica, pelvic pain, and radiculopathy may not be appreciated to be distinct entities and their diagnoses may be mistaken by clinicians. Likewise, back pain and sacroiliac pain may be difficult to distinguish. Each entity may be sought on the basis of the patient's history and physical examination. Unfortunately, physical examination of the pregnant woman is complicated by the apprehensions of clinicians who do not routinely work with pregnant women as well as by difficulty with certain examination techniques. In some cases diagnostic studies may be necessary to fully appreciate the underlying pathology. As a result of the difficulty in understanding or identifying the source of pain, patients may be subjected to greater period of pain or seek treatment for longer periods as different solutions are attempted [27]. Clinical diagnosis as well as research would benefit from agreed upon diagnostic criteria for these diagnoses.

Low back pain during pregnancy does not differ significantly from its clinical presentation at other times in life. Back pain generally increases toward the end of the day, consistent with patients with mechanical pain generation. Pain is often exacerbated by prolonged standing or walking. Distinct from typical back pain, more than 1/3 of pregnant women report nighttime low back pain suggestive of contribution other than mechanical strain [8]. In addition, a larger proportion of the pregnant women have pain over the sacroiliac joint than is generally seen in nonpregnant women with low back pain. The relative proportion of patients with pain near the sacroiliac joint increased as pregnancy progressed. The use of pain drawings helps clinicians differentiate between low back pain, sacroiliac pain, and pelvic girdle pain [16].

Nonspinal Neuropathic Pain

Meralgia paresthetica (MP), the symptom of numbness and paresthesias to the anterolateral thigh, is the result of compression of the lateral femoral cutaneous nerve. MP is commonly seen with conditions that result in increased intraabdominal pressure and from direct compression at the level of the inguinal ligament. It is commonly seen in police and linesmen who wear heavy utility belts, as well as following prone surgery and in patients with obesity, pregnancy, and pelvic or abdominal masses [28]. It needs to be kept in the differential diagnosis of radicular pain during pregnancy. A comprehensive history and pertinent physical examination is essential in arriving at the diagnosis; point tenderness over the lateral femoral cutaneous nerve is expected. Response to anesthetic block of the nerve is diagnostic.

Sacroiliac Pain

The sacroiliac (SI) joints serve as the interface between the pelvis and the spinal column. They transmit load from the lumbar spine to the lower extremities. It does not have much stability of its own against shear loads. The joint maintains its resistance to shear stress by the ligaments traversing the sacrum and hips as well as by the tight fit between the sacrum and the posterior pelvis. It demonstrates a limited range of motion—3° in flexion/extension, 0.8° to lateral bend, and 1.5° of axial rotation. The pelvis of women is wider and shallower than that of men, creating a broader and less stable SI joint interface. In addition, the ligamentous laxity and broadening of the pelvic joints during pregnancy contribute further to a destabilization of the joint in gravid females. The SI joint is believed to be the etiology of pain in up to 25% of healthy adults complaining of low back pain [29]. That number is far higher in postpartum women—the SI joint is believed to be the source of posterior pelvic girdle pain in 75% of women with persistent postpartum pain [30]. In a prospective study of 1500 primigravid women between ages 25 and 35 who experienced low back pain without prior symptoms of sacroiliac pain, 79% were ultimately diagnosed with SI joint pain [31]. Pain attributed to the SI joint worsened from the first through the third trimes-

ter ($P < 0.001$) as did the degree of disability assessed by the pain motility index ($P < 0.001$). Accordingly, it may be concluded that SI joint dysfunction is an important contributor to pain and mobility difficulty during pregnancy, as well as a contributor to the symptom of low back pain.

Examination for sacroiliac pain includes many methods. Some of the more common techniques are the pelvic compression test, pelvic distraction, thigh thrust, Gaenslen's test, Patrick's Flexion, Abduction and External Rotation (FABER) test, sacral thrust test, and the drop test. The physical examination findings for back pain and sacroiliac pain suffer from poor inter-rater reliability and as such the predictive accuracy of an individual test cannot be relied upon [32]. Subsequently, clinicians have utilized composites of diagnostic tests for the evaluation of sacroiliac pain. An examination demonstrating 3 of 6 positive diagnostic provocative tests or 2 of any 4 tests produced a reliable positive predictive value for SI joint pain as confirmed by diagnostic intraarticular SI joint block [33, 34].

Although radiography of the sacroiliac joint has been found to be of little diagnostic value, MRI may hold greater promise. An evaluation of 93 hip and pelvis MRIs of pregnant and < 6 month postpartum women to look for SI joint changes and compared to the responses of 52 patients regarding pain and clinical outcomes [35]. SI joint bone marrow edema correlated with gestational age or postpartum time. This edema was correlated with greater sacroiliac pain and was predictive of a slower clinical improvement of sacroiliac pain and of the development of spondyloarthropathy and chronic pain.

Diagnostic Studies

Physical examination for low back pain and pelvic pain is not specific for identifying the presence of pathology. When back or sacroiliac region pain is not intractable and disabling and when significant neurologic deficit is not present, diagnostic imaging studies are not warranted as management should be conservative. In those instances in which pain is incapacitating, it is of sudden onset, or when significant and progressive neurological symptoms are present, diagnostic studies are indicated to identify serious pathology.

In light of the concern for radiation exposure to the fetus, utilizing electrodiagnostic studies in lieu of an imaging modality may have merit. Electrodiagnostic studies have been shown to demonstrate greater correlation with muscle weakness on physical examination for lumbar disk herniation and lumbar stenosis than MRI [36]. Although structural lesions cannot be identified by EMG, it has demonstrated utility in localizing dysfunction of muscle and nerve and therefore can help eliminate unnecessary imaging studies.

When imaging is warranted, ultrasound is of limited value for evaluation of the adult spinal canal. Sonography cannot traverse solid bone, limiting the utility of this modality as a purely diagnostic study, but its application is actively explored. Compression of the spinal canal has been identified through ultrasound [37]. Ultrasound has also been used to identify changes to the spinal cord itself, as demonstrated by the diagnosis of syringomyelia [38]. It should be emphasized that ultrasound is very operator dependent and produces images that spine surgeons are generally less familiar with than radiographs, CT, or MRI.

MRI has been shown to be a safe diagnostic modality at all time points throughout pregnancy [6, 39, 40].

Fetal exposure to strong magnetic fields has not demonstrated a risk for fetal demise, neoplasm, hearing loss, or teratogenesis [41]. Thus, noncontrasted MRI offers the safest imaging modality for evaluation of the spinal canal in pregnant women with no demonstrated reports of harm to the fetus. The risk with the use of gadolinium contrast on the other hand is less clear. Gadolinium is known to accumulate within amniotic fluid which then can be swallowed by the fetus, resulting in absorption into fetal tissues [42]. The potential for harm from gadolinium build-up has not been established [41, 43, 44].

Unlike ultrasound and MRI, diagnostic CT and intraoperative fluoroscopy place both mother and fetus at risk from radiation exposure. In some instances, such modalities are required for diagnosis or for interventions. A fair appraisal of the risk from these studies, and the treatments which require their use, must include an assessment of the risk from the radiation involved. Estimated conceptus doses and adult effective doses for various X-ray based modalities are summarized in Tables 26.1 and 26.2.

Radiation risk depends on the state of development perhaps as much as the radiation dosage. Prior to implantation of the zygote, roughly from fertilization to day 14 of gestation, the cell mass is undifferentiated and DNA damage is either

Table 26.1 Estimated conceptus doses from various X-ray-based examinations

Examination	Estimated conceptus dose (mSv)
Head CT	0
Chest CT	0.2
Abdominal CT	4
Abdominal/pelvic CT	25
CTA of the chest, abdomen, pelvis	34

Source: McCollough CH, Schueler BA, Atwell TD, et al. Radiation exposure and pregnancy: when should we be concerned? Radiographics 2007;27:909–917

Table 26.2 Adult effective doses for various neuroimaging examinations

Examination	Average effective dose (mSv)	Days of equivalent background radiation
Skull radiograph	0.1	12
Cervical spine radiograph	0.2	24
Thoracic spine radiograph	1	118
Lumbar spine radiograph	1.5	177
Head CT	2	240
Neck CT	3	350
Spine CT	6	710
Neuroangiography	30–150	10–50 years

Adapted from Mettler FA Jr., Huda W, Yoshizumi TT, Mahesh M. Effective doses in radiology and diagnostic nuclear medicine: a catalog. Radiology 2008;248:254–263 and Gkanatsios NA, Huda W, Peters KR. Adult patient doses in interventional neuroradiology. Med Phys 2002;29: 717–723 repaired or the cells die. It is believed that radiation exposure of <50 mGy will have little effect during this stage [45]. The embryonic stage (weeks 3–8) involves much of the differentiation of organs and limbs. During this period radiation exposure carries the greatest risk for developmental malformation or CNS defect. Exposure to >100 mGy is believed to place the embryo at risk for teratogenic effects from radiation [45, 46]. Radiation exposure continues to pose risk to cerebral development or growth retardation until the end of the first trimester. Thereafter, the risk from radiation exposure for miscarriage or malformation is not believed to be significant at radiation doses of <150 mGy [47]. Likewise, the risk for subsequent cancer risk from radiation exposure to the fetus deters many physicians from obtaining CT imaging later in pregnancy. However, this risk has been estimated at an increase of 1/1000 from CT scanning [48].

The effects of radiation and exposure magnitude for a given study are relevant when the conceptus lies within the direct field of the scan, such as CT of the pelvis, abdomen, and lumbar spine which typically confer doses <50 mGy. CT imaging of the abdomen and lumbar spine in a series of pregnant women was shown to confer no increase in poor fetal or neonatal outcomes [49]. The effective dose to the uterus is far less for studies outside of this region, such as imaging of the head, cervical and thoracic spine. Although the radiation exposure of a CT scan may carry low to negligible risk, it is still prudent to utilize CT imaging only when clearly indicated. Further, when this modality is required, such as cases in which MRI is precluded by ferromagnetic metallic implants or by the presence of spinal implants marring the local image quality, CT neuroimaging should not be withheld.

Pathogenesis

The etiology of low back pain during pregnancy cannot be ascribed to a single issue. The contributing factors include an increase in the woman's body weight by 15–25% with an accompanying increase in mechanical demand on the joints, tendons, and ligaments [50]. Weight gain alone is not likely to increase the risk of back pain during pregnancy. Maternal weight gain and the baby's weights were not associated with an increased risk of backache during pregnancy [51]. Furthermore, most studies fail to demonstrate a continuous increase in pain throughout pregnancy which would have been expected if maternal weight was the principal contributor.

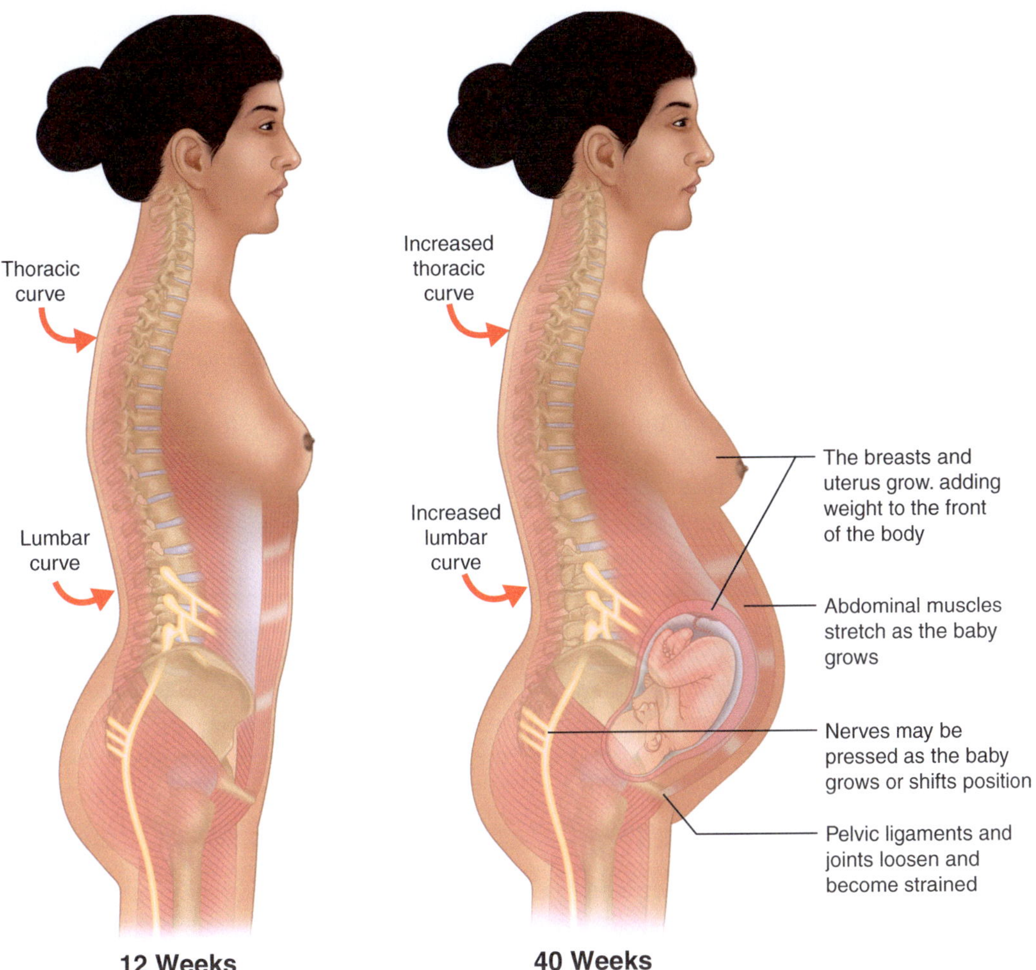

Would be nice to have an image of a pregnant woman with her spinal column showing through the 'skin' side-by-side with a nonpregnant woman, to depict the difference in standing posture between the two

The spine and pelvis undergo many changes during pregnancy as well, with an increase in ventral load throughout pregnancy from the expanding uterus as well as an increase in breast mass resulting in an increase in lumbar lordosis and an increase in pelvic tilt [50]. Lordosis and pelvic tilt alone should not be considered an adequate explanation for pain as these do not correlate with pain measures in nonpregnant adults [52]. Levels of relaxin increase by ten-fold during pregnancy, reaching a peak between the 38th and 42nd weeks [53]. Ligamentous laxity as a result of elevated levels of estrogen and relaxin will destabilize joints and increase the risk for pain and injury [53–55]. As back pain does not increase throughout pregnancy, this would also not seem to be a principal contributor, however, the marked increase in sacroiliac pain in the latter stages of pregnancy would be explained well by the decrease in collagen stiffness—and therefore of joint stability—as a result of these hormones.

Muscular disability has been raised as a key contributor to back and pelvic pain during and following pregnancy [56]. In a 3 year prospective cohort study of 799 women, pain persisting 3 years after pregnancy was more disabling when it involved both the low back and the posterior pelvis ($p < 0.05$) and these women experienced significantly impaired endurance of the lumbar paraspinal and hip abduction musculature

($P < 0.01$). Benefits were noted from a structured physiotherapy program during pregnancy for the reduction of low back and posterior pelvis pain and these benefits could last for several years. Poor truncal muscle function was concluded to be a major contributor to lumbopelvic pain during and after pregnancy.

The impact of muscular dysfunction on pain was also investigated through measures of truncal muscle endurance, gait speed, and hip muscle strength [57]. Lower values of truncal muscle endurance, hip extension, and gait speed were observed in women experiencing truncal pain compared to women without low back pain both in pregnancy and postpartum ($p < 0.001$–0.04). Levels of physical activity were observed to decrease throughout pregnancy ($p < 0.0001$) and limitations to activity increased throughout pregnancy ($p < 0.0001$) [58]. Severity of lumbopelvic pain was positively correlated with activity limitations ($r = 0.51$ to 0.55) and negatively correlated to levels of physical activity ($r = -0.39$ to -0.41). Evaluation of pain as a function of general fitness has been investigated as well [5]. Peak oxygen uptake during cycle ergometer testing, as a measure of aerobic fitness, did not seem to affect the incidence of back pain during or after pregnancy. It did, however, demonstrate an inverse relationship with the intensity of back pain. Self-reported assessments of physical fitness have also been associated with less body pain, lumbar pain, and disability (all $p < 0.05$) at 16 weeks of gestation and with lower degrees of body and sciatic pain at 34 weeks [59]. Women who engage in regular recreational physical activity for a longer period before pregnancy encountered lower risk of back pain and pelvic pain during pregnancy [15]. Physical deconditioning was felt to be a consequence, not a cause, of back pain associated with pregnancy but better pre-pregnancy fitness seemed to improve the degree of pain encountered.

Beyond the increased demand of added gestational mass on the mother's musculature, clear stressors are placed on the spine during the advancing pregnancy. A significant increase is seen by the third trimester for back pain ($p < 0.05$), lumbar lordosis ($p < 0.01$), pelvic sagittal tilt ($p < 0.05$), and posterior head position ($p < 0.01$) but no significant association was found between the change in lumbar lordosis or pelvic tilt and back pain [60, 61]. EMG evaluation of the erector spinae and biceps femoris muscles in pregnant women in their third trimester demonstrated significantly increased muscular activity, decreased degrees of truncal flexion permitted, and decreased endurance of maximal flexion in pregnant women compared to nonpregnant controls as well as to themselves 2 months after birth [62]. The extensors of the trunk demonstrate an increase in effort in response to the increased anterior loads encountered in pregnancy. Increasing activation of the spinal extensors seems to counter the ligamentous laxity and increasing mechanical demands during pregnancy.

In addition to the change in orientation of the lumbar spine as a result of increased ventral mass and the accompanying increase in pelvic tilt, the pelvis undergoes further structural change during pregnancy. An increase in both the anterior and posterior width of the pelvis as pregnancy progresses has been demonstrated [63]. The anterior width of the pelvis remains wider 1 month after childbirth than at 12 weeks of pregnancy ($p < 0.001$). This malalignment of the pelvic bones can be considered a contributor to lumbopelvic pain and to dysfunction of load transfer between the torso and legs as a broadened and destabilized sacroiliac joint will be the consequence of decreased wedging between the sacrum and the ilium and the ligamentous laxity during pregnancy.

Vascular phenomena have been implicated in back pain of pregnancy as well. In one study, 67% of women reported experiencing back pain at night during the second half of their pregnancy [64]. The authors hypothesized that the enlarging uterus obstructed the inferior vena cava leading to venous engorgement of the lumbar vertebral bodies. These changes could then result in hypoxemia and irrigation of unmyelinated nerves, leading to nighttime backache. Supporting this vascular hypothesis, a review of MRIs of 9640 adult patients with back pain or sciatica yielded 13 with radicular symptoms who did not demonstrate lumbar pathology but instead demonstrated obstruction or occlusion of the inferior vena cava resulting in distention of the epidural venous system and spinal nerve root compression [26]. Two patients experienced inferior vena cava compression from pregnancy. All of the patients presented with the acute onset of low back pain which was soon followed by the onset of acute radicular symptoms. Symptoms were relieved in all patients following treatment or delivery.

Structural Pathology

Symptoms of severe and unremitting back pain should prompt further evaluation with diagnostic imaging studies. More so, the presence of neurologic deficits, particularly motor weakness, myelopathy, or cauda equina syndrome, is an indication to obtain advanced spinal imaging in anticipation of possible surgical intervention. Clinical diagnosis may be possible on the basis of physical examination alone or with the use of electrophysiologic evaluation, but pathology amenable to decompression or stabilization may only be identified with appropriate radiographic examination.

The most common surgical lumbar pathology in pregnancy is the herniated disk. The presence of a symptomatic disk herniation in pregnancy has been reported at 1 in 10,000 [65]. Evaluation of MRIs of pregnant women and that of asymptomatic nonpregnant women of childbearing age demonstrated no difference in the incidence of lumbar disk herniations, suggesting against an increase in frequency of disk herniation associated with pregnancy [66].

Another compressive spinal pathology in pregnancy is spontaneous epidural hematoma. Of 16 cases reported in two series, 14 patients presented during the third trimester and the other two during the second trimester [67, 68]. All patients initially presented with back pain, and 15 of 16 subsequently developed spinal cord deficits. All cases were diagnosed by MRI. Hematoma was most commonly found in the cervicothoracic region. Surgery is recommended urgently in the presence of spinal cord dysfunction but a period of observation and possibly delivery can be considered when deficits are modest.

Aggressive vertebral hemangiomas during pregnancy have been reported in the literature [69, 70]. Hemangiomas of the vertebral bodies can become more aggressive during pregnancy, resulting in neurologic deficit. Treatment consisting of decompression and possible vertebroplasty is advocated. In some instances, spinal fusion consisting of posterior decompression and fusion during pregnancy and corpectomy with anterior fusion postpartum has been performed for large vertebral hemangiomas [71].

Spinal meningioma has been reported in pregnancy as well. A case of meningioma resulting in spinal cord compression in the third trimester of pregnancy with continued neurologic deficit following delivery which led to MRI, diagnosis, and ultimately to surgical resection several months following birth was previously described [72]. Additional cases have been reported [73]. Meningiomas may harbor estrogen and progesterone receptors and demonstrate rapid growth during pregnancy [74].

Other spinal tumors have been encountered during pregnancy as well me. Meng et al. reported a series of 21 women diagnosed with tumors during pregnancy (5 giant cell tumor, 5 hemangioma, 4 schwannoma, 3 metastatic, 2 eosinophilic granuloma, 1 neurofibroma, 1 multiple myeloma) [75]. Hemangioblastoma growth during pregnancy has been found as well [76]. Spinal metastases from breast cancer have also been diagnosed during pregnancy [77]. Surgery for benign tumors was typically postponed until after delivery unless the patient suffered a significant neurologic deterioration. Aggressive lesions underwent surgery during pregnancy. In these cases, the risk to the fetus from surgery was felt to be less than the risk from radiation or chemotherapy.

Spinal fracture from pregnancy-induced osteoporosis is uncommon but generally occurs during the third trimester or postpartum, particularly from continued calcium loss due to [78, 79]. In a series of 535 patients with osteoporotic vertebral compression fractures, two were believed to be due to pregnancy-induced osteoporosis [80]. In another group of 52 women with osteoporotic fracture diagnosed within 2 months of pregnancy, the majority had poor bone density prior to pregnancy and all demonstrated osteoporosis via dual-energy X-ray absorptiometry (DEXA) scan (spinal T-score—3.4, hip T-score—2) [79]. All patients received medical therapy with bisphosphones or teriparatide. In these cases, imaging to diagnose the fracture and dual-energy X-ray absorptiometry scan to assess for presence of osteoporosis is warranted.

Treatment

Conservative Therapy

Ostgaard et al. conducted a prospective randomized study of women with back pain during pregnancy to evaluate the effect of a physiotherapy and patient education program [81] 352 women were randomly assigned to a control group or to two intervention groups and followed throughout pregnancy and at 3 months and 6 years following delivery. Back pain was reported by 18% before pregnancy, 71% during pregnancy, and 16% at 6 years' follow-up. Pain severity was greatest at 36 weeks of pregnancy (VAS 5.4) and declined by 6 years (VAS 2.5). Recovery from pain was slower in women who experienced back pain before pregnancy ($p < 0.05$) and was of greater intensity during pregnancy ($p < 0.01$). For the women in the two treatment groups, pain during pregnancy resolved faster and long-term pain was not present. Likewise, sick leave frequency was reduced ($p < 0.01$). Education and physiotherapy did not prevent the subsequent development of back pain in women who did not experience LBP during pregnancy but good fitness and regular exercise prior to pregnancy reduced the risk of developing back pain during pregnancy [81].

Other studies assessing the effect of physiotherapy on pregnancy-associated back pain have found benefit for pain reduction during pregnancy, improved balance, truncal activation, and stability but without an improvement in disability [82]. The goal of therapy to improve fitness, core strength, and functional adaption to the changes of pregnancy is clear, but the absence of a correction between postural change in pregnancy and back pain suggests against the utility of exercise programs which focus on postural correction [60].

Pelvic and sacroiliac pain of pregnancy has been shown to be improved by training the transversus abdominis muscles which cross the sacroiliac joint and the pelvic floor muscles which stabilize the sacrum [83]. There is also evidence for some pain relief in 82% of women with posterior pelvic pain from the use of a non-elastic sacroiliac belt [84].

One review of treatments for pregnancy-associated lumbopelvic pain found strong benefit from the use of acupuncture and pelvic belts [85]. Lower quality evidence supports the use of exercise therapy in general and stabilizing exercises. Little evidence could be provided to support the use of osteopathic manipulation, yoga, muscle relaxation, or electrotherapy. Adverse events were not reported with any of these interventions. Additionally, transcutaneous electrical nerve stimulation (TENS) during pregnancy is safe but its efficacy is unclear [86].

Perhaps the broadest evaluation of treatments for low back and pelvic pain in pregnancy is the Cochrane review by Pennick and Liddle [87]. They reviewed randomized controlled trials of treatments intended to prevent or mitigate the incidence or severity of low back or pelvic pain in pregnancy. They noted that trials for the treatment of low back pain offered low-quality evidence with the findings that exercise significantly reduced pain and disability. The use of pelvic support belts did not offer significant benefit compared to osteopathic manipulation or to usual care. Pelvic pain was improved with acupuncture more than with exercise for evening pain and both were an improvement over usual care. Acupuncture was also found to improve function but not daily pain. Rigid sacroiliac belts with an exercise program improved pain compared to exercise alone but did not improve function. Exercise was also beneficial for reducing lumbopelvic-related sick leave and for improving function. A physical training program significantly reduced pain and disability from low back pain but this was not beneficial for preventing the onset of lumbar or lumbopelvic pain.

Cultural norms may influence the reporting of low back pain (LBP) and pelvic girdle pain (PGP), as well as the likelihood of women to seek treatment. Gutke et al. evaluated 869 women in their third trimester of pregnancy in the USA (214), the UK (220), Norway (220), and Sweden (215) for the presence and severity of LBP and/or PGP [2]. Significant differences in reporting between countries were observed ($p < 0.001$), with the greatest pain reported by U.K. women and the least by U.S. women. In addition, women were most likely to receive treatment for these afflictions in Norway (53%) and least likely in the U.S. (15–24%) ($p < 0.001$) [2, 4]. Of those women who received treatment, 68%–87% reported a positive effect.

In other surveys of women during and after pregnancy, poor utilization of healthcare resources for the treatment of back pain during pregnancy is a recurring theme. In one study, 67.7% of women experienced back pain during pregnancy, 57.7% found it severe enough to prevent them from performing daily activities, but only 7.0% received treatment [10]. Another survey reported 68.5% of women experienced low back pain during their current pregnancy but only 32% sought help for their pain and then only one of four of those providers recommended treatment [11]. Treatment for low back pain and pelvic girdle pain related to pregnancy is underutilized due to a combination of poor understanding of management options and the fear of causing harm to the fetus and mother [88].

It can be concluded that the heterogeneity of pain disorders which result in back pain during pregnancy and the variety of underlying etiologies contributing to pain likely lead to the inconsistent benefit appreciated from its treatment. Several underlying themes are clear: the role of social support for the pregnant woman, the role of fitness and exercise prior to pregnancy, the need for healthcare providers to proactively inquire about her pain and her ability to perform regular activities, and the role of an individualized exercise program to maintain her level of function throughout pregnancy. It is of great import for the medical professional to distinguish between typical lumbopelvic pain and that which could represent a surgical emergency.

Surgery

Lumbar spine surgery during pregnancy can be performed safely but as the perioperative course has implications for both mother and child, the surgeon should be judicious with the decision to proceed with operative intervention. Special consideration must be taken with patient positioning, the amount of radiation exposure with intraoperative fluoroscopy, blood loss, blood pressure stability, and consultation with obstetrics prior to surgery for fetal monitoring in advanced pregnancies.

Positioning of the pregnant woman for surgery has raised concerns due to the potential for impairment of perfusion to the uterus when prone or with side-lying [89]. Positioning begins to take on special consideration during the second trimester as the increasing size of the uterus creates risk for aortocaval compression. In the third trimester, fetal viability raises the prospect of urgent delivery prior to surgery as well as the use of fetal monitoring during surgery. Prone positioning on a table with generous abdominal freedom, such as a Jackson spine table, may be utilized safely during the second trimester. The increasing abdominal habitus during the third trimester may deter prone surgery, whereas a lateral decubitus or three-quarter prone position may remain reasonable options.

The treatment of lumbar disk herniation in pregnant women should generally begin with conservative therapy. Surgery must be considered when progressive neurologic deficits arise or when intractable radicular pain has proven unresponsive to appropriate medical therapy. Cauda equina syndrome and acute foot drop represent clear indications for emergent surgery at any stage of pregnancy. Consultation with the obstetrician should be sought prior to surgery and anesthesia [39, 40].

Surgery for lumbar disk herniation with progressive neurologic deficit or for cauda equina syndrome was performed safely with patients in the prone position on a 4-poster frame under epidural anesthesia [90]. In one retrospective series, nine pregnant women underwent emergency spine surgery, six for lumbar disk herniation resulting in severe sciatica or foot drop and an additional three patients with thoracic lesions with cauda equina syndrome or myelopathy [91]. C-sections were performed in three women prior to surgery and the pregnancies were carried to term in the other 6 patients. The eight children who were born healthy demonstrated a normal subsequent course.

A review of cases of lumbar diskectomy during pregnancy yielded 17 papers representing 22 cases [92]. Most cases of surgery in the first and early second trimester were performed prone. In the third trimester the majority of patients underwent C-section prior to prone surgery. Left lateral position was utilized in the late second trimester and third trimester when surgery was indicated and delivery could not be performed.

Similarly, the role of surgery for the treatment of spinal oncology and spinal fracture reflects a balance of the risk of surgery to both mother and fetus against the risk of delayed intervention. Larger procedures with greater intraoperative fluoroscopy, surgical duration, and blood loss should involve consultation of the obstetric service. In some cases, preterm delivery or therapeutic abortion may need to be considered [93]. Particular concern should be given to procedures involving the lumbar spine as the conceptus will lie near or within the collimated radiation field and receive far greater exposure than for cervical, thoracic, or upper lumbar procedures.

Theocharopoulos et al. demonstrated this issue with a series of anterior–posterior and lateral fluoroscopic shots at 5 spinal levels performed on anthropomorphic phantoms simulating the 3 trimesters of gestation to estimate the radiation exposure to the conceptus from a typical pedicle screw fixation and kyphoplasty procedure—assuming pedicle screw fixation to require 3.3 min of fluoroscopy, and a kyphoplasty to require 10.1 min of fluoroscopy [94]. They found the conceptus doses from fluoroscopically guided pedicle screw fixation and kyphoplasty to be smaller than 4 mGy during all three trimesters of pregnancy *if the conceptus lies outside the primarily irradiated region*. Accordingly, the risk of fatal cancer during childhood or congenital malformation on the progeny was estimated to be at least 2 and 1500 times, respectively, lower than the spontaneous incidence rates. When the embryo is primarily irradiated, mean conceptus dose can be as high as 105 mGy from a nonoptimized exposure (Table 26.3). They noted a marked increase in exposure to the embryo from AP fluoroscopy compared to lateral views, with replacing AP with lateral views enabling a 90% reduction in radiation exposure, which would amount to a 3 and 12 mGy exposure to an embryo within the irradiated region. With typical imaging, they conclude that at least 35 min of fluoroscopy time is required for the induction of deterministic effects.

An alternative to the use of intraoperative fluoroscopy is to utilize neuronavigation with an intraoperative cone-beam CT. In a series of 73 patients who underwent CT-navigated spinal instrumentation with 73 controls who underwent

Table 26.3 Conceptus doses from typical fluoroscopically guided surgical treatments of the spine during pregnancy[a]

	First trimester		Second trimester		Third trimester	
	Pedicle screw	Kyphoplasty	Pedicle screw	Kyphoplasty	Pedicle screw	Kyphoplasty
T5	0.0187	0.0835	0.0124	0.0491	0.0337	0.120
T9	0.0546	0.256	0.205	0.660	0.395	2.55
L1	0.113	0.460	0.714	4.05	6.88	60.4
L3	0.658	4.05	2.76	18.6	11.8	105
L5	3.88	28.8	4.63	31.8	11.7	104

[a]Expressed in mGy

Adapted from: Nicholas Theocharopoulos N, Damilakis J, Perisinakis K, Papadokostakis G, Hadjipavlou A, Gourtsoyiannis N. Fluoroscopically Assisted Surgical Treatments of Spinal Disorders: Conceptus Radiation Doses and Risks. Spine 2006 Jan 15;31(2):239–44 fluoroscopically guided spinal instrumentation, Mendelsohn et al. found the average CT exposure to be 6.93 mSv, 2.8 times greater than the value for case-matched fluoroscopic procedures and similar to that of a diagnostic CT scan [95]. Noteworthy, in their series navigation did not reduce the number of X-rays or CT scans obtained in the postoperative period. Despite the advantages offered by intraoperative CT-based neuronavigation, with enhanced accuracy, decreased radiation exposure to the surgical team, and potentially a decrease in operative time, the patient is subject to an increased radiation exposure.

As noted previously with diagnostic studies, ultrasonography offers the promise of radiation-free spinal localization. This modality is more user-dependent than are fluoroscopy and intraoperative CT. Cases of use in the USA for localization of spinal level via spinous process identification have been reported with greater accuracy than by palpation [96, 97]. Ultrasound has also been used to count the correct vertebral level in a post-laminectomy patient [98]. One study utilized ultrasound to identify articular processes and pedicles as well as to serve as the guidance for percutaneous pedicle screw insertion [99].

In conclusion, intraoperative imaging is safe for CT and fluoroscopy when the conceptus lies outside of the irradiated field. For procedures of the lower lumbar spine (L3 to sacrum), greater consideration should be offered regarding the possibility of preoperative delivery of the late-term fetus and the surgeon should be thoughtful with regard to minimizing the radiation exposure, in particular minimizing the use of AP fluoroscopy, narrow collimation, and low-dose fluoroscopy for procedures which require multiple images.

Conclusions

Back pain is a common complaint reported during pregnancy. Indeed, the majority of expectant women will experience truncal pain during their pregnancy. This risk is greater in women with a previous history of back pain or history of spinal fusion below the L3 level and in women who are younger, multiparous, have greater social stressors, lower job satisfaction, and who have not engaged in regular exercise prior to pregnancy. In most cases, pain is bothersome and limits the patient's ability to perform their daily activities. In far too many cases, it is not treated. Exercise programs, including physical therapy, can help maintain the pregnant woman's level of function and help decrease their level of pain, as well as lead to a faster postpartum recovery. Rarely, this pain is the result of fracture, tumor, or neurologic compression. In these cases, diagnostic imaging should not be withheld as the risk to the developing child is minimal. Surgery, too, may be performed safely with appropriate precautions. When urgent surgery is warranted, the surgeon should consult with anesthesia and obstetrics to ensure appropriate care will be provided for both mother and her future child.

References

1. Dunn G, Egger MJ, Shaw JM, et al. Trajectories of lower back, upper back, and pelvic girdle pain during pregnancy and early postpartum in primiparous women. Womens Health (Lond). 2019;15:1745506519842757.
2. Gutke A, Boissonnault J, Brook G, et al. The severity and impact of pelvic girdle pain and low-back pain in pregnancy: a multinational study. J Womens Health (Larchmt). 2018;27(4):510–7.
3. Borg-Stein J, Dugan SA, Gruber J. Musculoskeletal aspects of pregnancy. Am J Phys Med Rehabil. 2005;84(3):180–92.
4. Skaggs CD, Prather H, Gross G, et al. Back and pelvic pain in an underserved United States pregnant population: a preliminary descriptive survey. J Manip Physiol Ther. 2007;30(2):130–4.
5. Thorell E, Kristiansson P. Pregnancy related back pain, is it related to aerobic fitness? A longitudinal cohort study. BMC Pregnancy Childbirth. 2012;12:30.
6. Brown A, Johnston R. Maternal experience of musculoskeletal pain during pregnancy and birth outcomes: significance of lower back and pelvic pain. Midwifery. 2013;29(12):1346–51.
7. Backhausen MG, Bendix JM, Damm P, et al. Low back pain intensity among childbearing women and associated predictors. A cohort study. Women Birth. 2019;32(4):e467–e76.
8. Fast A, Shapiro D, Ducommun EJ, et al. Low-back pain in pregnancy. Spine (Phila Pa 1976). 1987;12(4):368–71.

9. Backhausen M, Damm P, Bendix J, et al. The prevalence of sick leave: reasons and associated predictors—a survey among employed pregnant women. Sex Reprod Healthc. 2018;15:54–61.

10. Mota MJ, Cardoso M, Carvalho A, et al. Women's experiences of low back pain during pregnancy. J Back Musculoskelet Rehabil. 2015;28(2):351–7.

11. Wang SM, Dezinno P, Maranets I, et al. Low back pain during pregnancy: prevalence, risk factors, and outcomes. Obstet Gynecol. 2004;104(1):65–70.

12. Ng BK, Kipli M, Abdul Karim AK, et al. Back pain in pregnancy among office workers: risk factors and its impact on quality of life. Horm Mol Biol Clin Investig. 2017;32(3)

13. Albert HB, Godskesen M, Korsholm L, et al. Risk factors in developing pregnancy-related pelvic girdle pain. Acta Obstet Gynecol Scand. 2006;85(5):539–44.

14. Ostgaard HC, Andersson GB, Karlsson K. Prevalence of back pain in pregnancy. Spine (Phila Pa 1976). 1991;16(5):549–52.

15. Mogren IM, Pohjanen AI. Low back pain and pelvic pain during pregnancy: prevalence and risk factors. Spine (Phila Pa 1976). 2005;30(8):983–91.

16. Ostergaard M, Bonde B, Thomsen BS. Pelvic insufficiency during pregnancy. Is pelvic girdle relaxation an unambiguous concept? Ugeskr Laeger. 1992;154(50):3568–72.

17. Albert HB, Godskesen M, Westergaard JG. Incidence of four syndromes of pregnancy-related pelvic joint pain. Spine (Phila Pa 1976). 2002;27(24):2831–4.

18. Elden H, Gutke A, Kjellby-Wendt G, et al. Predictors and consequences of long-term pregnancy-related pelvic girdle pain: a longitudinal follow-up study. BMC Musculoskelet Disord. 2016;17:276.

19. Dewan MC, Mummareddy N, Bonfield C. The influence of pregnancy on women with adolescent idiopathic scoliosis. Eur Spine J. 2018;27(2):253–63.

20. Chan EW, Gannon SR, Shannon CN, et al. The impact of curve severity on obstetric complications and regional anesthesia utilization in pregnant patients with adolescent idiopathic scoliosis: a preliminary analysis. Neurosurg Focus. 2017;43(4):E4.

21. Betz RR, Bunnell WP, Lambrecht-Mulier E, et al. Scoliosis and pregnancy. J Bone Joint Surg Am. 1987;69(1):90–6.

22. Orvomaa E, Hiilesmaa V, Poussa M, et al. Pregnancy and delivery in patients operated by the Harrington method for idiopathic scoliosis. Eur Spine J. 1997;6(5):304–7.

23. Grabala P, Helenius I, Buchowski JM, et al. Back pain and outcomes of pregnancy after instrumented spinal fusion for adolescent idiopathic scoliosis. World Neurosurg. 2019;124:e404.

24. Lavelle WF, Demers E, Fuchs A, et al. Pregnancy after anterior spinal surgery: fertility, cesarean-section rate, and the use of neuraxial anesthesia. Spine J. 2009;9(4):271–4.

25. Berkmann S, Fandino J. Pregnancy and childbirth after microsurgery for lumbar disc herniation. Acta Neurochir. 2012;154(2):329–34.

26. Paksoy Y, Gormus N. Epidural venous plexus enlargements presenting with radiculopathy and back pain in patients with inferior vena cava obstruction or occlusion. Spine (Phila Pa 1976). 2004;29(21):2419–24.

27. Prather H, Spitznagle T, Hunt D. Benefits of exercise during pregnancy. PM R. 2012;4(11):845–50; quiz 50.

28. Harney D, Patijn J. Meralgia paresthetica: diagnosis and management strategies. Pain Med. 2007;8(8):669–77.

29. Sembrano JN, Polly DW Jr. How often is low back pain not coming from the back? Spine (Phila Pa 1976). 2009;34(1):E27–32.

30. Capobianco R, Cher D, Group SS. Safety and effectiveness of minimally invasive sacroiliac joint fusion in women with persistent post-partum posterior pelvic girdle pain: 12-month outcomes from a prospective, multi-center trial. Springerplus. 2015;4:570.

31. Filipec M, Jadanec M, Kostovic-Srzentic M, et al. Incidence, pain, and mobility assessment of pregnant women with sacroiliac dysfunction. Int J Gynaecol Obstet. 2018;142(3):283–7.

32. van Tilburg CWJ, Groeneweg JG, Stronks DL, et al. Inter-rater reliability of diagnostic criteria for sacroiliac joint-, disc- and facet joint pain. J Back Musculoskelet Rehabil. 2017;30(3):551–7.

33. Laslett M. Evidence-based diagnosis and treatment of the painful sacroiliac joint. J Man Manip Ther. 2008;16(3):142–52.

34. Robinson HS, Brox JI, Robinson R, et al. The reliability of selected motion- and pain provocation tests for the sacroiliac joint. Man Ther. 2007;12(1):72–9.

35. Eshed I, Miloh-Raz H, Dulitzki M, et al. Peripartum changes of the sacroiliac joints on MRI: increasing mechanical load correlating with signs of edema and inflammation kindling spondyloarthropathy in the genetically prone. Clin Rheumatol. 2015;34(8):1419–26.

36. Lee JH, Lee SH. Physical examination, magnetic resonance image, and electrodiagnostic study in patients with lumbosacral disc herniation or spinal stenosis. J Rehabil Med. 2012;44(10):845–50.

37. Mueller LA, Degreif J, Schmidt R, et al. Ultrasound-guided spinal fracture repositioning, ligamentotaxis, and remodeling after thoracolumbar burst fractures. Spine (Phila Pa 1976). 2006;31(20):E739–46; discussion E47.

38. Provoost V, Geusens E, Brys P, et al. A special case on the use of ultrasonography for evaluation of the spinal canal and its contents in adults. Emerg Radiol. 2005;11(3):150–2.

39. Ahern DP, Gibbons D, Johnson GP, et al. Management of herniated lumbar disk disease and cauda equina syndrome in pregnancy. Clin Spine Surg. 2019;32(10):412–6.

40. Di Martino A, Russo F, Denaro L, et al. How to treat lumbar disc herniation in pregnancy? A systematic review on current standards. Eur Spine J. 2017;26(Suppl 4):496–504.

41. Ray JG, Vermeulen MJ, Bharatha A, et al. Association between MRI exposure during pregnancy and fetal and childhood outcomes. JAMA. 2016;316(9):952–61.

42. Oh KY, Roberts VH, Schabel MC, et al. Gadolinium chelate contrast material in pregnancy: fetal biodistribution in the nonhuman primate. Radiology. 2015;276(1):110–8.

43. Chansakul T, Young GS. Neuroimaging in pregnant women. Semin Neurol. 2017;37(6):712–23.

44. De Santis M, Straface G, Cavaliere AF, et al. Gadolinium periconceptional exposure: pregnancy and neonatal outcome. Acta Obstet Gynecol Scand. 2007;86(1):99–101.

45. McCollough CH, Schueler BA, Atwell TD, et al. Radiation exposure and pregnancy: when should we be concerned? Radiographics. 2007;27(4):909–17; discussion 17–8.

46. Patel SJ, Reede DL, Katz DS, et al. Imaging the pregnant patient for nonobstetric conditions: algorithms and radiation dose considerations. Radiographics. 2007;27(6):1705–22.

47. Brent RL, Bolden BT. Indirect effect of x-irradiation on embryonic development: utilization of high doses of maternal irradiation on the first day of gestation. Radiat Res. 1968;36(3):563–70.

48. Radiological Society of North America. CT safety during pregnancy. 2020. https://www.radiologyinfo. org/en/info/safety-ct-pregnancy.

49. Choi JS, Han JY, Ahn HK, et al. Foetal and neonatal outcomes in first-trimester pregnant women exposed to abdominal or lumbar radiodiagnostic procedures without administration of radionucleotides. Intern Med J. 2013;43(5):513–8.

50. Korsten-Reck U. Physical activity in pregnancy and in breast-feeding period in obese mothers. Z Geburtshilfe Neonatol. 2010;214(3):95–102.

51. Mantle MJ, Greenwood RM, Currey HL. Backache in pregnancy. Rheumatol Rehabil. 1977;16(2):95–101.

52. Youdas JW, Garrett TR, Egan KS, et al. Lumbar lordosis and pelvic inclination in adults with chronic low back pain. Phys Ther. 2000;80(3):261–75.

53. Kristiansson P, Svardsudd K, von Schoultz B. Reproductive hormones and aminoterminal propeptide of type III procollagen in serum as early markers of pelvic pain during late pregnancy. Am J Obstet Gynecol. 1999;180(1 Pt 1):128–34.

54. Hartmann S, Bung P. Physical exercise during pregnancy—physiological considerations and recommendations. J Perinat Med. 1999;27(3):204–15.

55. Artal R, O'Toole M. Guidelines of the American College of Obstetricians and Gynecologists for exercise during pregnancy and the postpartum period. Br J Sports Med. 2003;37(1):6–12; discussion.

56. Noren L, Ostgaard S, Johansson G, et al. Lumbar back and posterior pelvic pain during pregnancy: a 3-year follow-up. Eur Spine J. 2002;11(3):267–71.

57. Gutke A, Ostgaard HC, Oberg B. Association between muscle function and low back pain in relation to pregnancy. J Rehabil Med. 2008;40(4):304–11.

58. Lardon E, St-Laurent A, Babineau V, et al. Lumbopelvic pain, anxiety, physical activity and mode of conception: a prospective cohort study of pregnant women. BMJ Open. 2018;8(11):e022508.

59. Marin-Jimenez N, Acosta-Manzano P, Borges-Cosic M, et al. Association of self-reported physical fitness with pain during pregnancy: the GESTAFIT project. Scand J Med Sci Sports. 2019;29(7):1022–30.

60. Franklin ME, Conner-Kerr T. An analysis of posture and back pain in the first and third trimesters of pregnancy. J Orthop Sports Phys Ther. 1998;28(3):133–8.

61. Schroder G, Kundt G, Otte M, et al. Impact of pregnancy on back pain and body posture in women. J Phys Ther Sci. 2016;28(4):1199–207.

62. Bivia-Roig G, Lison JF, Sanchez-Zuriaga D. Effects of pregnancy on lumbar motion patterns and muscle responses. Spine J. 2019;19(2):364–71.

63. Morino S, Ishihara M, Umezaki F, et al. Pelvic alignment changes during the perinatal period. PLoS One. 2019;14(10):e0223776.

64. Fast A, Weiss L, Parikh S, et al. Night backache in pregnancy. Hypothetical pathophysiological mechanisms. Am J Phys Med Rehabil. 1989;68(5):227–9.

65. LaBan MM, Perrin JC, Latimer FR. Pregnancy and the herniated lumbar disc. Arch Phys Med Rehabil. 1983;64(7):319–21.

66. Weinreb JC, Wolbarsht LB, Cohen JM, et al. Prevalence of lumbosacral intervertebral disk abnormalities on MR images in pregnant and asymptomatic nonpregnant women. Radiology. 1989;170(1 Pt 1):125–8.

67. Soltani S, Nogaro MC, Jacqueline Kieser SC, et al. Spontaneous spinal epidural hematomas in pregnancy: a systematic review. World Neurosurg. 2019;128:254–8.

68. Jea A, Moza K, Levi AD, et al. Spontaneous spinal epidural hematoma during pregnancy: case report and literature review. Neurosurgery. 2005;56(5):E1156; discussion E.

69. Wang B, Jiang L, Wei F, et al. Progression of aggressive vertebral hemangiomas during pregnancy: three case reports and literature review. Medicine (Baltimore). 2018;97(40):e12724.

70. Moles A, Hamel O, Perret C, et al. Symptomatic vertebral hemangiomas during pregnancy. J Neurosurg Spine. 2014;20(5):585–91.

71. Vijay K, Shetty AP, Rajasekaran S. Symptomatic vertebral hemangioma in pregnancy treated antepartum. A case report with review of literature. Eur Spine J. 2008;17 Suppl 2(Suppl 2):S299–303.

72. Pikis S, Cohen JE, Rosenthal G, et al. Spinal meningioma becoming symptomatic in the third trimester of pregnancy. J Clin Neurosci. 2013;20(12):1797–9.

73. Cioffi F, Buric J, Carnesecchi S, et al. Spinal meningiomas in pregnancy: report of two cases and review of the literature. Eur J Gynaecol Oncol. 1996;17(5):384–8.

74. Cahill DW, Bashirelahi N, Solomon LW, et al. Estrogen and progesterone receptors in meningiomas. J Neurosurg. 1984;60(5):985–93.

75. Meng T, Yin H, Li Z, et al. Therapeutic strategy and outcome of spine tumors in pregnancy: a report of 21 cases and literature review. Spine (Phila Pa 1976). 2015;40(3):E146–53.

76. Frantzen C, Kruizinga RC, van Asselt SJ, et al. Pregnancy-related hemangioblastoma progression and complications in von Hippel-Lindau disease. Neurology. 2012;79(8):793–6.

77. El-Safadi S, Wuesten O, Muenstedt K. Primary diagnosis of metastatic breast cancer in the third trimester of pregnancy: a case report and review of the literature. J Obstet Gynaecol Res. 2012;38(3):589–92.

78. Yun KY, Han SE, Kim SC, et al. Pregnancy-related osteoporosis and spinal fractures. Obstet Gynecol Sci. 2017;60(1):133–7.

79. Laroche M, Talibart M, Cormier C, et al. Pregnancy-related fractures: a retrospective study of a French cohort of 52 patients and review of the literature. Osteoporos Int. 2017;28(11):3135–42.

80. Krishnakumar R, Kumar AT, Kuzhimattam MJ. Spinal compression fractures due to pregnancy-associated osteoporosis. J Craniovertebr Junction Spine. 2016;7(4):224–7.

81. Ostgaard HC, Zetherstrom G, Roos-Hansson E. Back pain in relation to pregnancy: a 6-year follow-up. Spine (Phila Pa 1976). 1997;22(24):2945–50.

82. Fontana Carvalho AP, Dufresne SS, Rogerio de Oliveira M, et al. Effects of lumbar stabilization and muscular stretching on pain, disabilities, postural control and muscle activation in pregnant woman with low back pain. Eur J Phys Rehabil Med. 2020;56(3):297–306.

83. Pel M. Pelvic pain caused by pregnancy. Ned Tijdschr Geneeskd. 1995;139(49):2586–7.

84. Ostgaard HC, Zetherstrom G, Roos-Hansson E, et al. Reduction of back and posterior pelvic pain in pregnancy. Spine (Phila Pa 1976). 1994;19(8):894–900.

85. Gutke A, Betten C, Degerskar K, et al. Treatments for pregnancy-related lumbopelvic pain: a systematic review of physiotherapy modalities. Acta Obstet Gynecol Scand. 2015;94(11):1156–67.

86. Simkin P, Bolding A. Update on nonpharmacologic approaches to relieve labor pain and prevent suffering. J Midwifery Womens Health. 2004;49(6):489–504.

87. Liddle SD, Pennick V. Interventions for preventing and treating low-back and pelvic pain during pregnancy. Cochrane Database Syst Rev. 2015;2015:CD001139.

88. Vermani E, Mittal R, Weeks A. Pelvic girdle pain and low back pain in pregnancy: a review. Pain Pract. 2010;10(1):60–71.

89. Bongetta D, Versace A, De Pirro A, et al. Positioning issues of spinal surgery during pregnancy. World Neurosurg. 2020;138:53–8.

90. Brown MD, Levi AD. Surgery for lumbar disc herniation during pregnancy. Spine (Phila Pa 1976). 2001;26(4):440–3.

91. Esmaeilzadeh M, Hong B, Polemikos M, et al. Spinal emergency surgery during pregnancy: contemporary strategies and outcome. World Neurosurg. 2020;139:e421–e7.

92. Ardaillon H, Laviv Y, Arle JE, et al. Lumbar disk herniation during pregnancy: a review on general management and timing of surgery. Acta Neurochir. 2018;160(7):1361–70.

93. Han IH, Kuh SU, Kim JH, et al. Clinical approach and surgical strategy for spinal diseases in pregnant women: a report of ten cases. Spine (Phila Pa 1976). 2008;33(17):E614–9.

94. Theocharopoulos N, Damilakis J, Perisinakis K, et al. Occupational gonadal and embryo/fetal doses from fluoroscopically assisted surgical treatments of spinal disorders. Spine (Phila Pa 1976). 2004;29(22):2573–80.

95. Mendelsohn D, Strelzow J, Dea N, et al. Patient and surgeon radiation exposure during spinal instrumentation using intraoperative computed tomography-based navigation. Spine J. 2016;16(3):343–54.

96. Schlotterbeck H, Schaeffer R, Dow WA, et al. Ultrasonographic control of the puncture level for lumbar neuraxial block in obstetric anaesthesia. Br J Anaesth. 2008;100(2):230–4.

97. Halpern SH, Banerjee A, Stocche R, et al. The use of ultrasound for lumbar spinous process identification: a pilot study. Can J Anaesth. 2010;57(9):817–22.

98. Yamauchi M, Honma E, Mimura M, et al. Identification of the lumbar intervertebral level using ultrasound imaging in a post-laminectomy patient. J Anesth. 2006;20(3):231–3.

99. Ungi T, Moult E, Schwab JH, et al. Tracked ultrasound snapshots in percutaneous pedicle screw placement navigation: a feasibility study. Clin Orthop Relat Res. 2013;471(12):4047–55.

Part V

Functional Neurological, Neuro-Otological, and Psychological Disorders in Pregnancy

Ian Hakkinen and Pengfei Zhang

Introduction

Headache is one of the most common complaints in neurology [1]. In order to avoid harm to the fetus and the patient, headaches in pregnancy pose unique challenges in diagnosis and treatment for clinicians in both inpatient and outpatient settings. Despite these challenges, however, the key to successful headache treatment remains the same: a detailed and carefully taken history can often allow clinicians to differentiate between primary headaches versus secondary headache.

Negro and colleagues in a 2017 review of headaches in pregnancy offer an excellent classification paradigm—a headache patient who is pregnant can only really present in three ways:

- The patient has a history of headaches presenting with her typical headaches.
- The patient without any prior headache history presenting with a first time headache.
- The patient with a prior history of headaches presenting with new type of headache [2].

In the case of those with new onset headache or one that is different from their typical, the focus of a clinician's investigation should be to rule out commonly occurring peripartum/intrapartum secondary headaches. Conversely, while vigilance should be practiced, the focus for a patient with her typical headache during pregnancy will most likely be on potential treatments. This chapter is organized around this theme: we will first introduce the natural progression of primary headaches. Then we will offer a list of secondary headaches commonly occurring in pregnancy. Finally we will discuss treatment options during pregnancy.

Primary Headaches in Pregnancy

Migraine

Migraine has a global prevalence of 14.7% and female migraine sufferers outnumber their male counter parts by a factor of 3:1 [3, 4]. The International Criteria for Headache Disorders (ICHD3) provides comprehensive diagnostic criteria for various types and subtypes of migraine, highlighting the importance of photo/phonophobia and/or nausea as features of migraine diagnosis in addition to two of the following: unilateral location, pulsating quality, moderate or severe pain, and aggravation by routine physical activity [5].

The natural progression of disease for migraine sufferers during pregnancy has been frequently studied: in a 2003 prospective study of

I. Hakkinen · P. Zhang (✉)
Department of Neurology, Rutgers Robert Wood Johnson Medical School, New Brunswick, NJ, USA
e-mail: ish14@rutgers.edu;
pz124@rwjms.rutgers.edu

© The Author(s), under exclusive license to Springer Nature Switzerland AG 2023
G. Gupta et al. (eds.), *Neurological Disorders in Pregnancy*,
https://doi.org/10.1007/978-3-031-36490-7_27

pregnant migraine patients, 50% showed a general improvement in migraine frequency and intensity during pregnancy [6]. The improvement of migraine symptoms follows a trend with relief of migraine symptoms and reduced frequency as the pregnancy progresses toward the third trimester. The improvement continues until the day of delivery when many, including those without a migraine diagnosis, experience a worsening or increase in headache frequency [6, 7]. With each subsequent pregnancy the improvement in headache frequency and intensity diminishes [8]. Migraines with aura patients, however, tend to have a worsening of their symptoms starting in the first trimester [8]. Menstrual-related migraine patients were reported to have no improvement with pregnancy [8].

Onset of a first migraine during pregnancy can occur in up to 10% of women. This frequently occurs in the first trimester [7]. The normal temporal pattern of a patient's migraines returns around 4–5 weeks following delivery. There can be some further prevention of migraines by breastfeeding but this is controversial [6, 7].

Tension-Type Headaches

Tension-type headache (TTH) has a global prevalence of approximately 42%; gender proportion tends to be equally distributed [9]. According to ICHD3 criteria, TTH should not be associated with nausea and should not have both photophobia and phonophobia. Two of the following features of headache should also be present: bilateral location, pressing or tightening quality, mild to moderate pain, and no aggravation of pain with physical activity [5].

Tension-type headaches make up about a quarter of headaches during pregnancy [8]. A study by Maggioni et al. suggests that tension-type headaches improve during pregnancy and rarely have a worsening of intensity or frequency [8]. Patients who suffer from migraines can also suffer from tension-type headaches and it may be hard to distinguish between the two if symptoms are mild.

Trigeminal-Autonomic Cephalalgias

Trigeminal-autonomic cephalalgias (TAC) are a group of headaches sharing clinical features of side-locked headaches with parasympathetic autonomic features. TAC include five primary headache disorders: cluster headache, paroxysmal hemicranias, hemicranias continua, short lasting unilateral neuralgiform headache with conjunctival injection and tearing (SUNCT), and short lasting unilateral neuralgiform headache with autonomic features (SUNA) [5]. A rare variant, LASH, has not yet been classified into the ICHD3 criteria [10].

TAC are rare; the most common of them, cluster headache, has a prevalence of approximately 0.1% [11]. Typical autonomic features include conjunctival injection, tearing, nasal congestion. Restlessness is also considered a cardinal feature [5]. There is limited data concerning TAC evolution during pregnancy. Available data does not show cluster headache as having a clear trend in pregnancy [12]. In some studies, it has been suggested that those who have suffered from cluster headaches were less likely to conceive due to the severity of their illness [12, 13].

Secondary Headaches

Physiological changes in pregnancy predispose patients to a number of neurological disorders. Indeed, secondary headaches account for approximately 33% of headaches in pregnancy [14]. The most common etiology of secondary headache is hypertensive related complications and of those pre-eclampsia is the most common [14].

The popular acronym for remembering headache red flags, SNOOP, remains as a good entry point in thinking about potential causes of secondary headaches in pregnancy [15]. SNOOP is an acronym for "Systemic symptoms," "Neurological symptoms," "Onset: sudden, abrupt," "Older: age > 50," "Previous headache history: either first headache or different, papilledema, precipitated by valsalva, postural." Abnormal neurological symptoms, for example, should alert physicians to posterior reversible encephalopathy syndrome (PRES). Sudden onset headache in pregnancy, for example, should alert clinicians to diagnoses such as pre-eclampsia, RCVS, CVT, pituitary apoplexy, and SAH. Papilledema should alert the practitioner to idiopathic intracranial hypertension (IIH). Postural headaches in the postpartum should put CSF leak on the differential.

Pre-eclampsia and Eclampsia

Pre-eclampsia is a well-known complication occurring in up to 8% of all pregnancies [16]. It is a leading cause of maternal and fetal morbidity worldwide. Onset most often occurs after the 20-week mark and can occur in the puerperium period up to 4 weeks following delivery. Presenting features include severe headache, elevated blood pressure, proteinuria, and can progress to eclampsia if the patient develops seizures [16]. ICHD 3 characterizes the headache as bilateral, pulsating, and worsened by physical activity [5]. Pregnant women presenting with headache in the middle of the second trimester and onward should be worked up for pre-eclampsia. Immediate treatment of blood pressure and seizure prophylaxis should be started [17]. Women presenting with headache following delivery should be treated for pre-eclampsia but also considered for cerebral venous thrombosis [13]. Pre-eclampsia and eclampsia are discussed in detail in Chap. 14.

Posterior Reversible Encephalopathy Syndrome

Posterior reversible encephalopathy syndrome (PRES) is a condition related to hypertension and is especially common in those with eclampsia. Elevated blood pressure is thought to cause changes in cerebral autoregulation that results in vasogenic edema [18]. Patients most often will have headache associated with confusion, visual disturbance that can be cortical blindness, nausea and vomiting, and seizures. PRES responds well to treatment of the underlying hypertension. MRI will show T2 FLAIR hyperintensities that can be seen on imaging for weeks after improvement of symptoms [19].

Cerebral Venous Thrombosis

Pregnancy predisposes patients to an increased risk of thrombotic events due to the underlying prothrombotic state. Pregnant women are 6 times more likely to develop a venous embolism compared to nonpregnant women [20]. Thrombotic events in the cerebral venous system are a rare form of stroke and occur at a rate of 11.6 per 100,000 in developed countries and up to 450 per 100,000 in developing countries [21]. There is an 11% mortality rate [21]. Cerebral venous thrombosis presents with a headache in 80–90% of cases. The headache can mimic many primary headaches without any definitive characteristics: The phenotype can be unilateral or diffuse, can have a rapid onset or progression, and can have symptoms of intracranial hypertension such as nausea and vomiting with papilledema. Other common associated symptoms are a focal neurological deficit or new onset seizures [5]. CVT treatment choice is with heparin or low molecular weight heparin [20]. CVST is discussed in detail in Chap. 13.

Subarachnoid Hemorrhage

It was previously thought that pregnancy carries a five-fold increase for risk of subarachnoid hemorrhage of a prevalence of 1 per 10,000 with typical onset occurs in the third trimester or in the puerperium period [22]. However recent study suggests that there may not be an increased risk of aneurysmal SAH in women, during pregnancy, in labor, or in the puerperium time [23]. Most common etiology is secondary to an underlying aneurysm presenting classically as "thunderclap headache"—an acute onset headache that peaks within seconds to minutes [5]. Aneurysms and SAH are discussed in detail in Chap. 10.

Reversible Cerebral Vasoconstriction Syndrome

Headache associated with reversible cerebral vasoconstriction syndrome (RCVS) generally has a thunderclap onset and is concerning for more sinister pathology such as subarachnoid hemorrhage. The vasoconstrictive effects can lead to ischemic or hemorrhagic strokes and patients can develop long term neurological deficits [5]. Etiology of RCVS is not well understood but there is a connection between drugs that are sympathomimetics or have serotonergic effects. Patients can also have symptoms brought on by straining, taking hot showers, or sex [24]. Classically, imaging studies with MRA or CT-A will show a "string of beads" sign. However this sign can be elusive if imaging study is done early on in the disease course. Symptoms are self-limited, and most patients have resolution of their headache within 4 weeks [24]. ICHD3 criteria maintain that there must be resolution within 3 months [5]. RCVS and its variant postpartum angiopathy are discussed in detail in Chaps. 15 and 16.

Idiopathic Intracranial Hypertension

Idiopathic intracranial hypertension (IIH), or pseudotumor cerebri, disproportionally affects women more commonly than men. Obesity is correlated with an increased incidence: the baseline incidence is 0.9 per 100,000, whereas in obese patients the incidence is 19.3 per 100,000 [25]. The headache is characterized as pulsating that is worsened with activity and maneuvers that raise intracranial pressure (ICP) such as coughing or valsalva. There can be visual disturbance that is transient initially and becomes permanent and associated with painful eye movements. On exam patients can have papilledema. Diagnosis is made by exclusion from other etiology and is confirmed with imaging (i.e., MRI) and lumbar puncture to look for elevated ICP. IIH can worsen in pregnancy which is thought to be due to weight gain [5, 25]. IIH is discussed in detail in Chap. 35.

Pituitary Apoplexy

The pituitary swells during pregnancy due to hypertrophy and hyperplasia of lactotrophs reaching a peak in the few days following delivery. The swelling predisposes the pituitary to ischemia and increases the risk of converting hemorrhage [26, 27]. Patients will often present with a sudden onset headache that is followed by visual disturbance and signs of hypopituitarism [5].

Imaging Choice when Evaluating Headache

Imaging in pregnancy poses a complex issue because of the risks to the developing fetus. Neurological emergencies pose a particular dilemma where acute imaging must be done in order to exclude various pathologies and narrow the differential. The image modalities used most commonly are CT and MRI [28]. In the American College of Obstetricians and Gynecologists 2017 opinion piece on the use of both CT and MRI, MRI is preferred over CT due to radiation risk. However, it is worth noting that CT imaging of the head will likely pose little risk to the fetus. Therefore, should there be high suspicion for emergency requiring a CT (for example, a subarachnoid hemorrhage), the clinician should not delay such an intervention [28].

However, in general, CT should be avoided in pregnancy: CT imaging utilizes ionizing radiation which at high levels can pose a risk to a developing fetus. The amount of radiation exposure and impact depends upon the location of imaging and fetus' developmental timeline. Theoretically, CT imaging of the head and neck poses a low risk of ionizing radiation to the fetus since the fetus is not directly in the scanner. There are other techniques to reduce the radiation exposure including using the lowest amount of radiation necessary to obtain imaging and applying a lead shield [28]. The use of contrast with CT remains controversial. Contrast used in CT is iodinated and can pose a risk for thyroid disease and should only be used if there is an absolute need. Following delivery there is no contraindication to CT with contrast and there should be no interruption of breastfeeding. CT imaging especially of the head should not be withheld as an imaging modality for patients where there is an acute need [28].

MRI use in pregnancy has shown no contraindication or precautions that need to be taken at any trimester. Human and animal studies have shown no increased risk or harm to the fetus. The use of gadolinium contrast in MRIs is debated but there is some evidence to suggest it can be harmful. Following delivery there is no contraindication to the use of gadolinium contrast and there should be no interruption of breastfeeding. MRI is one of the most useful imaging modalities for evaluating headaches in pregnant women since there is no radiation exposure and it provides high diagnostic quality of images [28, 29].

Considerations for neuroimaging during pregnancy are described in detail in Chap. 5.

Treatment of Headache in Pregnancy

Nonpharmacological Treatment

In recent years, neuromodulation has become a commonly utilized technique in migraine treatment. The most frequently used neuromodulation devices include: Cefaly, eNeura TMS, GammaCore, and Nerivio. The efficacies of these devices for both migraine abortive and/or prophylaxis have been demonstrated in clinical trials [30–35]. Since these devices are non-systemic, it would be logical to assume that they do not affect the fetus. Indeed, while evidence for safety in neuromodulation devices are lacking, it is standard teaching that they are safe in pregnancy. For example, Continuum, an often-used educational series for neurology residents, recommends it [36]. These techniques have also received treatment endorsement from experts [37].

At the individual device level, claims of safety are ambivalent, likely due to legal concerns. The Cefaly device, a supraorbital transcutaneous stimulator, and Nerivio, a remote electrical neu-

romodulation device, did not offer any advice in regard to pregnancy on their official websites [38, 39]. eNeura TMS, a single pulse transcranial magnetic stimulation device, has produced a single poster advocating for the lack of adverse events in pregnancy [40]. GammaCore, a vagal nerve stimulator, is more cautious, suggesting in its package insert that "Safety and efficacy of gammaCore have not been evaluated in the following patients, and therefore is NOT indicated for: …. pregnant women" [41].

Nerve Blocks

Peripheral nerve blocks have been established as effective for treatments of migraine [42, 43]. Indeed, it has so convinced headache practitioners of its efficacy that the American Headache Society (AHS) put forth a consensus statement in 2013 [44].

Given nerve block's local effect and low level of distribution the body, it is logical to consider nerve block as an appropriate option for headache treatment in pregnancy. Indeed, in a small study conducted by Govindappagari et al., nerve block does appear to be an effective and safe treatment in refractory headaches during pregnancy [45].

Although specific mixtures are practitioner dependent, the most common ingredients used in peripheral nerve block tend to be lidocaine, bupivacaine, and steroids. Lidocaine has usually been considered safe in pregnancy, given its category B status. However, bupivacaine is category C in pregnancy and standard teaching (as shown by AHS guidelines) suggests that bupivacaine should be avoided. This avoidance of bupivacaine from pain and family medicine literature is due to bioavailability data, which showed a 4: 1 increase in toxicity when compared to lidocaine [46]. Avoidance of bupivacaine in pregnancy has been challenged. And indeed, in the article by Govindappagari et al., it is noted that there was a lack of adverse events related to nerve block while using both lidocaine and bupivacaine.

Steroid use in nerve blocks suffers from similar controversy. AHS guidelines argue against the use of steroids. In the pain literature, however, we do have evidence that local steroid injection is safe in pregnancy; it is used in the treatment of carpal tunnel during pregnancy, for example [47, 48].

Behavioral Therapy

A number of behavioral therapy strategies have been proposed for migraine. Indeed, the US Headache Consortium, when attempting to evaluate evidence for these practices, counted up to 355 varieties [49]. The most well known of these are progressive relaxation, biofeedback, and cognitive-behavioral therapy. Since no medications are involved, these techniques are usually considered safe (it is difficult to imagine why they would not be). The US Headache Consortium found that relaxation training, including progressive muscle relaxation, autogenic training, meditation/passive relaxation, EMG biofeedback therapy, and cognitive-behavioral therapy display some evidence for headache improvement [49].

Summary for Non-pharmacological Interventions

There exist a wide range of nonpharmacological options available for pregnant headache sufferers. As with any medical treatments in pregnancy, although evidence of safety is scarce, it is logical for these techniques to not produce adverse effect in both the fetus and the mother. The lack of evidence of adverse effects for many of these treatments seems to at least corroborate this latter statement. In the author's practice, this view is offered to pregnant patients and a decision regarding which treatment to pursue is then made on an individual basis with the patient.

Pharmacological Treatment

Medications for headache treatments are separated into abortive medications, which abort headache, and prevention medications, which act as headache prophylaxis. We will describe the safety of a selection of the most commonly used medications in pregnancy:

Acetaminophen

Acetaminophen is a commonly used over the counter analgesic that is well tolerated by patients. The use of acetaminophen in headaches has shown efficacy including in the treatment of migraine [50]. In the hospital setting, acetaminophen is the drug of choice for pregnant women with headaches as it is believed to have very few side effects and is category B by the FDA [51]. However, maternal use of Tylenol has recently been suspected to be associated with development of ADHD and the risk increases with duration of use [52].

Aspirin

Aspirin works as an analgesic and antiplatelet that is used to prevent cardiovascular and stroke complications. There has been a benefit shown in pregnant women for secondary prevention of pre-eclampsia [53]. The use of aspirin during pregnancy or in the puerperium period poses a risk of premature closure of the ductus arteriosus and in breastfeeding can cause Reye's syndrome. Aspirin is category D and is generally not used in the treatment of headache in the pregnant population [51].

Nonsteroidal Anti-Inflammatory Drugs

Nonsteroidal anti-inflammatory drugs (NSAIDs) are one of the most widely used treatments for both primary and secondary headaches. In the third trimester there is a higher risk of vaginal bleeding, premature closure of the ductus arteriosus, and concern for an increase in asthma in the newborn [54]. There is some controversy with regard to use in the first trimester where there may be an increased risk of cardiac malformation

[55]. Regardless of the controversy, the FDA has labeled NSAIDs as category B in the first and second trimester and category D in the third trimester [51].

Triptans

Triptans are an effective abortive medication used in the treatment of migraine. Their mechanism of action is serotonin receptor agonism which helps to modulate the blood flow in order to abort migraine symptoms [56]. Triptans can cross the placenta but at a low rate and result in low serum levels in the fetus and are unlikely to adversely impact the fetus. Triptans can be used during pregnancy but there is the risk of preterm delivery [56]. Some advocate for its use, however [57].

Opiates

Opiate based pain medications can be very effective in the treatment of pain during pregnancy. Opiates bind to the Mu opiate receptor in the brain and body producing an analgesic and euphoric effect [58]. However, fetal exposure to opioids can be a serious concern and they of course carry significant abuse potential.

Ergotamine

Ergotamine has a strong vasoconstrictive effect and has been used to treat migraines. In pregnancy the use of ergotamine is contraindicated. There are numerous side effects that include neural tube defects, low birth weight, and preterm delivery [59].

Antiemetics

Antiemetics such as ondansetron and metoclopramide are used for the treatment of nausea during pregnancy [13]. Of these medications, metoclopramide has been shown to treat both headache and nausea [60].

Beta-Blockers

Antihypertensive medication is commonly used in pregnancy. Beta-blockers are used for prophylactic treatment of migraines and a number of practitioners would consider its use during pregnancy as long bradycardia and hypotension are avoided [61]. However, it has been noted that beta-blocker exposure is related to small size for gestational age in a large Scandinavian study [62].

Antiepileptic Medication

Antiseizure medication is contraindicated in pregnancy since there are many teratogenic effects to the fetus [13]. Valproic acid is associated with neural tube defects. Topiramate has a risk of cleft palate [13]. Gabapentin has limited data but it may be one of the few anticonvulsants that does not have a teratogenic effects [63]. Nevertheless gabapentin is category C in pregnancy [64].

Tricyclic Antidepressants

All of the tricyclic antidepressants (TCA) are category C in pregnancy [65].

Botox

Botulinum toxin is an effective and FDA approved medication for migraine prevention. Pregnancy is listed as a contraindication in the product's package insert [66]. It has been argued, however, that botox is too big (150 kDa) to cross the placenta. However, given that botox is category C, it is not the standard of care in pregnancy. Indeed, in a 2006 survey of 396 physicians who used commercial botox, only 12 reported using botox for pregnant women [67].

Supplements Used in Headache

There are a broad range of other medications which have been reported to relive the symptom of headache. Magnesium appears to be a relatively safe medication in pregnancy. In a Cochrane review on magnesium supplementation, for example, there was no benefit but also no harm for the infant nor the mother [68]. The doses included in the review ranged from 128 mg to 4 g daily. The evidenced-based dose for migraine prevention is approximately 400–600 mg [69]. Of note, magnesium sulfate injections (for the purpose of stopping preterm labor) is category D by the FDA [70]. Caffeine is one of the oldest and most commonly used treatments for headaches [1]. In pregnant women with headache, caffeine can be consumed and acceptable up to 200 mg per day [71]. Short periods of high dose oxygen therapy via a nasal cannula are also a safe option for pregnant women with headache [1].

Summary for Pharmacological Interventions

It is worth noting that of the number of prescription medication we have discussed so far, only acetaminophen, metoclopramide, ondansetron remain in category B in pregnancy. NSAIDs are category B in early pregnancy as discussed above, but their use is nevertheless controversial.

It is often taught that, in general, prevention medication should be avoided in pregnancy due to fetal interactions. This is the authors' view and recommendation. This is also in part due to the positive improvement that often accompanies pregnancy, as well as that any oral medication adjustment takes approximately 3 months, or 1 trimester, to take effect.

This dogma of avoiding any prevention mediation has been challenged in recent years. It is curious, therefore, to see whether this dogma actually translates to standard of care in the headache community: Hamilton and colleagues conducted precisely such a study of the members of the American Headache Society between October 2018 and December 2018. In this study they offered practitioners a number of abortives and preventives and asked how comfortable the headache specialist would be in prescribing each medication. Of the acute treatments, more than 80% are comfortable with nonpharmacological treatments and acetaminophen. More than 70% are comfortable with nerve blocks. More than 50% are comfortable with neuromodulation and dopamine. Less than 50% of all responders feel very comfortable with the remainder of medications: NSAIDs, caffeine, steroids, opioids, butalbital, triptans, and muscle relaxants. Of those surveyed, >60% feel very uncomfortable with butalbital use. Similarly, >50% of responders feel "very comfortable" with non-pharmacologics, neuromodulation, and nerve blocks as preventives only. Over 50% of practitioners feel very uncomfortable with prescribing topiramate, valproic acid, CGRP antagonists, memantine (despite it is category B designation), Butterbur, calcium channel blockers, ACE inhibitors, and ARBs. The remainder of medications have mixed review. The authors note that there is "less consensus about the use of triptans for acute treatment and onabotulinumtoxin A for preventive treatment of migraine in pregnancy" [72]. However, it is always the best practice for any headache physician to consult with the patient on risks and benefits of each intervention. If possible, the intervention with the lowest risk but maximum benefit should be tried first.

Conclusion

Headaches in pregnancy are a complicated scenario for any practicing physician. The clinician must decide whether to pursue the patient's headache symptoms further and do so in a manner that will have the least risk to the fetus. Ultimately, the clinician may decide about imaging and treatment based upon their experience and how comfortable they are with treating pregnant women. There is no algorithmic approach as of yet for the management of headache in pregnancy but following the advice of Negro et al. and the SNOOP model can help to guide the clinician's differential and management. When imaging is warranted it should not be withheld from the pregnant woman and, if possible, MRI should be the preferred imaging modality.

In the treatment of headache there are many conflicting studies with regard to medications and their side effects. The clinician should gauge the woman's desire for treatment and provide informed consent regarding the treatment options. When non-pharmacologic options fail, there are many pharmacologics that can provide relief of the headache with little to no risk for the fetus. Likely the best treatment approach is that of a conservative one.

References

1. Rizzoli P, Mullally WJ. Headache. Am J Med. 2018;131:17–24.
2. Negro A, Delaruelle Z, Ivanova TA, et al. Headache and pregancy: a systematic review. J Headache Pain. 2017;18:106. https://doi.org/10.1186/s10194-017-0816-0.
3. Steiner TJ, Stovner LJ, Birbeck GL. Migraine: the seventh disabler. J Headache Pain. 2013;14:1.
4. Robbins MS, Lipton RB. The epidemiology of primary headache disorder. Semin Neurol. 2010;30(2):107–19.
5. International Headache Society. The international classification of headache disorders, 3rd edition. Cephalalgia. 38(1):1–211.
6. Sances G, Granella F, Nappi RE, Fignon A, Ghiotto N, Polatti F, Nappi G. Course of migraine during pregnancy and postpartum: a prospective study. Cephalalgia. 2003;23(3):197–205.
7. Kvisvik EV, Stovner LJ, Helde G, et al. Headache and migraine during pregnancy and puerperium: the MIGRA-study. J Headache Pain. 2011;12(4):443–51.
8. Maggioni F, Alessi C, Maggino T, Zanchin G. Headache during pregnancy. Cephalalgia. 1997;17(7):765–9.
9. Ferrante T, Manzoni GC, Russo M, Camarda C, et al. Prevalence of tension-type headache in adult general population: the PACE study and review of literature. Neurol Sci. 2013;34:137–8.
10. Kingston W, Halker R. LASH: a review of current literature. Curr Pain Headache Rep. 2017;21(8):36. https://doi.org/10.1007/s11916-017-0636-6.
11. Matharu MS, Goasby PJ. Trigeminal autonomic Cephalgias. J Neurol Neurosurg Psychiatry. 2002;72:ii19–26.
12. Van Vilet JA, Favier I, Helmerhorst FM, et al. Cluster headache in women: relation with menstruation, use of oral contraceptives, pregnancy, and menopause. J Neurol Neurosurg Psychiatry. 2006;77(5):690–2.
13. Pearce CF, Hansen WF. Headache and neurological disease in pregnancy. Clin Obstet Gynecol. 2012;55(3):810–28.
14. Robbins MS, Farmakidis C, Dayal AK, Lipton RB. Acute headache diagnosis in pregnant women: a hospital-based study. Neurology. 2015;85(12):1024–30.
15. Dodick DW. Pearls: headache. Semin Neurol. 2010;30(1):74–81.
16. Uzan J, Ayoubi CM. Pre-eclampsia: pathophysiology diagnosis and management. Vasc Health Risk Manag. 2011;7:467–74.
17. The American College of Obstetricians and Gynecologist. Emergent therapy for acute-onset, severe hypertension during pregnancy and the post-partum period. Washington, DC: ACOG Committee Opinion; 2018. https://www.acog.org/Clinical-Guidance-and-Publications/Committee-Opinions/Committee-on-Obstetric-Practice/Emergent-Therapy-for-Acute-Onset-Severe-Hypertension-During-Pregnancy-and-the-Postpartum-Period. Accessed 29 Feb 2020.
18. Hobson EV, Craven I, Blank SC. Posterior reversible encephalopathy syndrome: a truly treatable neurologic illness. Perit Dial Int. 2012;32(6):590–4.
19. Nielsen LH, Gron BS, Ovesen PG. Posterior reversible encephalopathy syndrome postpartum. Clin Case Rep. 2015;3(4):266–70.
20. Kupferminc MJ. Thrombophilia and pregnancy. Reprod Biol Endocrinol. 2003;1:111. https://doi.org/10.1186/1477-7827-1-111.
21. Liang ZW, Gao WL, Feng LM. Clinical characteristics and prognosis of cerebral venous thrombosis in Chinese women during pregnancy and puerperium. Sci Rep. 2017;7:43866. https://doi.org/10.1038/srep43866.
22. Guida M, Altieri R, Platucci V, et al. Aneurysmal subarachnoid Haemorrhage in pregnancy: a case series. Transl Med UniSa. 2012;2:59–63.
23. Groenestege AT, Rinkel G, Van der Bom J, Algra A, Klijn C. The risk of aneurysmal subarachnoid hemorrhage during pregnancy, delivery, and the puerperium in the Utrecht population: case-crossover study and standardized incidence ratio estimation. Stroke. 2009;40(4):1148–51.
24. Chen SP, Fuh JL, Wang SJ. Reversible cerebral vasoconstriction syndrome: an under-recognized clinical emergency. Ther Adv Neurol Disord. 2010;3(3):161–71.
25. Thirumalaikumar L, Ramalingam K, Heafield T. Idiopathic intracranial hypertension in pregnancy. Obstet Gynaecol. 2014;16:93–7.
26. Grand'Maison S, Weber F, Bedard M, et al. Pituitary apoplexy in pregnancy: a case series and literature review. Obstet Med. 2015;8(4):177–83.
27. Hayes AR, O'Sullivan AJ, Davies MA. A case of pituitary apoplexy in pregnancy. Endocrinol Diabetes

Metab Case Rep. 2014;2014:140043. https://doi.org/10.1530/EDM-14-0043.

28. Kanekar S, Bennett S. Imaging of neurologic conditions in pregnant patients. Radiographics. 2016;36(7):2102–22.

29. American College of Obstetricians and Gynecologists. Guidelines for diagnostic imaging during pregnancy and lactation. Committee Opinion. https://www.acog.org/Clinical-Guidance-and-Publications/Committee-Opinions/Committee-on-Obstetric-Practice/Guidelines-for-Diagnostic-Imaging-During-Pregnancy-and-Lactation. Accessed 29 Feb 2020. 2017

30. Chou DE, Shnayderman Yugrakh M, Winegarner D, et al. Acute migraine therapy with external trigeminal neurostimulation (ACME): a randomized controlled trial. Cephalalgia. 2019;39(1):3–14.

31. Schoenen J, Vandersmissen B, Jeangette S, et al. Migraine prevention with a supraorbital transcutaneous stimulator. Neurology. 2013;80(8):697–704.

32. Lipton RB, Dodick DW, Silberstein SD, et al. Single-pulse transcranial magnetic stimulation for acute treatment of migraine with aura: a randomised, double-blind, parallel-group, sham-controlled trial. Lancet Neurol. 2010;9(4):373–80.

33. Starling AJ, Tepper SJ, Marmura MJ, et al. A multicenter, prospective, single arm, open label, observational study of sTMS for migraine prevention (ESPOUSE study). Cephalalgia. 2018;38:1038–48.

34. Yarnitsky D, Dodick DW, Grosberg BM, et al. Remote electrical neuromodulation (REN) relieves acute migraine: a randomized, double-blind, placebo-controlled, multicenter trial. Headache. 2019;59(8):1240–52.

35. Grazzi L, Tassorelli C, de Tommaso M, et al. Practical and clinical utility of non-invasive vagus nerve stimulation (nVNS) for the acute treatment of migraine: a post hoc analysis of the randomized, sham-controlled, double-blind PRESTO trial. J Headache Pain. 2018;19:98.

36. Robbins MS. Headache in pregnancy. Continnum. 2018;24(4):1092–107.

37. Sheikh H. Noninvasive neuromodulation: finding its place in your practice. NeurologyLive. https://www.neurologylive.com/journals/neurologylive/2019/september-2019/noninvasive-neuromodulation-migraine-finding-its-place-in-your-practice. Accessed 20 Feb 2020.

38. Cefaly Technology https://www.cefaly.us/en/questions. Accessed 20 Feb 2020.

39. Theranica Bio-electronic Ltd. https://theranica.com/homepage/. Accessed 20 Feb 2020.

40. Bhola R, Giffin N, Ahmed F. Single pulse transcranial magnetic stimulation (sTMS) as a non-drug treatment option for pregnant patients with migraine. http://www.eneura.com/wp-cotent/uploads/2017/03/SpringTMS_Abstract_IHC2013_Pregnancy_data_Mini_Poster-2.pdf. Accessed 20 Feb 2020.

41. Electrocore Inc. GammaCore Package Insert. https://gammacore.com/wp-content/themes/gammacore-p2/pdf/gammacore_IFU.pdf. Accessed 20 Feb 2020.

42. Zhang H, Yang X, Lin Y, Chen L, Ye H. The efficacy of greater occipital nerve block for the treatment of migraine: a systematic review and meta-analysis. Clin Neurol Neurosurg. 2018;165:129–33.

43. Allen SM, Mookadam F, Cha SS, et al. Greater occipital nerve block for acute treatment of migraine headache: a large retrospective cohort study. J Am Board Fam Med. 2018;31(2):211–8.

44. Blumenfeld A, Ashkenazi A, Napchan U, et al. Expert consensus recommendations for the performance of peripheral nerve blocks for headache—a narrative review. Headache. 2013;53(3):437–46.

45. Govindappagari S, Grossman T, Dayal A, Grosberg B, et al. Peripheral nerve blocks in the treatment of migraine in pregnancy. Obstet Gyncecol. 2014;124(6):1169–74.

46. Lathan J, Martin SN. Infiltrative anesthesia in office practice. Am Fam Physician. 2014;89(12):956–62.

47. Greengrass RA, Isenhower MW, Rospigliosi K, et al. Continuous peripheral nerve catheters and regional analgesia in pregnancy—a brief review of safety. J Rom Anest Ter Intensivă. 2013;20(2):121–4.

48. Sax TW, Rosenbaum RB. Neuromuscular disorders in pregnancy. Muscle Nerve. 2006;34(5):559–71.

49. Campbell JK, Penzien DB, Wall EM. Evidenced-based guidelines for migraine headache: behavioral and physical treatments. Mt Royal, NJ: US Headache Consortium; 2000. p. 2000.

50. Lipton RB, Baggish JS, Stewart WF. Efficacy and safety of acetaminophen in the treatment of migraine results of a randomized, double-blind, placebo-controlled, population-based study. Arch Intern Med. 2000;160(22):3486–92.

51. Black RA, Hill DA. Over-the-counter medications in pregnancy. Am Fam Physician. 2003;67(12):2517–24.

52. Lew Z, Ritz B, Rebordosa C, et al. Acetaminophen use during pregnancy, behavioral problems, and hyperkinetic disorders. JAMA Pediatr. 2014;168(4):313–20.

53. Atallah A, Lecarpentier E, Goffinet F, et al. Aspirin for prevention of preeclampsia. Drugs. 2017;77(17):1819–31.

54. Negro A, Delaruelle Z, Ivanova TA, Khan S, Ornello R, Raffaelli B, Terrin A, Reuter U, Mitsikostas DD. Headache and pregnancy: a systematic review. J Headache Pain. 2017;18(1):106.

55. Nezvalova-Henriksen K, Spigset O, Nordeng H. Effects of ibuprofen, diclofenac, naproxen, and piroxicam on the course of pregnancy and pregnancy outcome: a prospective cohort study. BJOG. 2013;120(8):948–59.

56. Soldin O, Dahlin J, Mara D. Triptans in pregnancy. Ther Drug Monit. 2008;30(1):5–9.

57. Hamilton KT, Robbins MS. Migraine treatment in pregnant women presenting to the acute care: a retrospective observational study. Headache. 2018;59(2):173–9.

58. Lind JN, Interrante JD, Ailes EC, et al. Maternal use of opioids during pregnancy and congenital malformations: a systematic review. Pediatrics. 2017;139(6):e20164131. https://doi.org/10.1542/peds.2016-4131.

59. Banhidy F, Acs N, Puho E, et al. Ergotamine treatment during pregnancy and a higher rate of low birthweight and preterm birth. Br J Clin Pharmacol. 2007;64(4):510–6.

60. Friedman BW, Mulvey L, Esses D, et al. Metoclopramide for acute migraine: a dose-finding randomized clinical trial. Ann Emerg Med. 2011;57(5):475–82.

61. Bergman JEH, Lutke LR, Gans ROB, et al. Beta-blocker use in pregnancy and risk of specific congenital anomalies: a European case-malformed control study. Drug Saf. 2018;41(4):415–27.

62. Petersen KM, Jimenez-Solem E, Andersen JT. Beta-blocker treatment during pregnancy and adverse pregnancy outcomes: a nationwide population-based cohort study. BMJ Open. 2012;2(4):e001185. https://doi.org/10.1136/bmjopen-2012-001185.

63. Fujii H, Goel A, Bernard N, et al. *Pregnancy outcomes following gabapentin use*: result of a prospective comparative cohort study. Neurology. 2013;80(17):1565–70.

64. Gabapentin. Package Insert. https://www.accessdata.fda.gov/drugsatfda_docs/label/2011/020235s036,020882s022,021129s022lbl.pdf Accessed Mar 1 2020.

65. Armstrong C. Practice guidelines: ACOG guidelines on psychiatric medication use during pregnancy and lactation. Am Fam Physician. 2008;78(6):772–8.

66. Botox. Package insert. https://www.accessdata.fda.gov/drugsatfda_docs/label/2011/103000s5236lbl.pdf a. Accessed 1 Mar 2020.

67. Morgan JC, Iyer SS, Moser ET, et al. Botulinum toxin a during pregnancy: a survey of treating physicians. J Neurol Neurosurg Psychiatry. 2006;77(1):117–9.

68. Makrides M, Crosby DD, Shepard E. Magnesium supplementation in pregnancy. Cochrane Database Syst Rev. 2014;2014:CD000937. https://doi.org/10.1002/14651858.CD000937.pub2.

69. Yablon LA, Mauskop A. Magnesium in headache. In: Vink R, Nechifor M, editors. Magnesium in the central nervous System. Adelaide: University of Adelaide Press; 2011.

70. FDA. Safety announcement. 2013. https://www.fda.gov/media/85971/download. Accessed 1 Mar 2020.

71. American College of Obstetrician and Gynecologists. ACOG Committee Opinion No. 462: moderate caffeine consumption during pregnancy. Obstet Gynecol. 2010;116:467–8.

72. Hamilton KT, Singh RH, Ailani A et al. A survey of American headache society members on treatment of migraine in pregnancy. Poster presentation at American headache Society's 61st annual scientific meeting, Philadelphia convention center. July 12 to 13, 2019. 2019.

Management of Epilepsy During Pregnancy

28

Stephen Wong

Issues Relating to Conception Reduction in Fertility

Women with epilepsy (WWE) experience up to 2–3 times higher infertility rates than the general population [1]. The problem of reduced fertility in WWE is complex and multifactorial and includes both biological and social factors. Age, education, seizure frequency, seizure types, and anticonvulsant usage are likely to play significant roles. Additionally, social inhibition, poor self-esteem, fear of having seizures during relationships, and consequent later age of marriage may contribute to a reduction in fertility.

Reduction in libido is reported in a third of patients with epilepsy, particularly in focal, temporal lobe epilepsy relative to generalized epilepsy [2]. Hyposexuality is a component of Geschwind syndrome [3], which is a constellation of behavioral phenomena in patients with temporal lobe epilepsy that includes hyperreligiosity and reduced sexuality. Lower libido in WWE may also be related to chronic anticonvulsant usage. Enzyme-inducing antiepileptic drugs (AEDs) and valproic acid induce the liver to produce higher levels of sex-hormone binding globulin [4], leading over time to lowered testosterone and estradiol levels which consequently may negatively affect libido and fertility.

WWE may have a more difficult time with conception as they can experience greater menstrual irregularity and anovulatory cycles. This is estimated to occur at up to 2.5 times the rate of the general population [5]. Menstrual irregularity is potentially due to a greater incidence of polycystic ovarian syndrome (PCOS). PCOS affects roughly 5–10% of reproductive-age women and is characterized by hyperandrogenism, ovarian cysts, anovulatory cycles, hirsutism, and obesity. WWE have higher rates of PCOS ranging between 12 and 26% [6, 7], with higher risks in patients taking valproic acid [8, 9]. Menstrual irregularity may possibly be due to the influence of seizures on brain endocrine centers, inducing aberrant hormone secretion.

In contrast to the above, Pennell et al. conducted a recent prospective cohort study demonstrating that WWE, without a history of infertility or PCOS, had a similar likelihood of achieving pregnancy compared to those without epilepsy [10]. This cohort of women was largely on monotherapy, with roughly half being seizure free during the prior 9 months of enrollment, implying perhaps a less severe burden of epileptic seizures.

S. Wong (✉)
Department of Neurology, Rutgers Robert Wood
Johnson Medical School, New Brunswick, NJ, USA

Contraceptives and Anticonvulsants

In addition to fertility problems, there are contraception issues with many AEDs. Hepatic enzyme induction (EI) by anticonvulsants is known to accelerate the metabolism of bystander drugs. Circulating estrogens and progestins are substrates for the hepatic cytochrome p450 enzyme CYP3A4, which catalyzes chemical reactions leading to their inactivation. As a result, WWE taking enzyme-inducing AEDs (EIAEDs) that induce the hepatic isozyme CYP3A4 may experience reduced effectiveness of COCs (combined oral contraceptives), resulting in increased contraception failure rates. Among anticonvulsants, strong inducers of CYP3A4 include phenytoin, carbamazepine, and phenobarbital/primidone. Weak or dose-dependent inducers include eslicarbazepine, oxcarbazepine, topiramate, rufinamide, and felbamate. WWE on EIAEDs may be counseled to take COCs with a higher dose of estrogen (e.g., 50 μg of ethinyl estradiol), though care should be taken due to pro-convulsant effects of estrogen. Because depot injections avoid hepatic first-pass effects, they are not susceptible to this phenomenon. Other methods such as the IUD or barrier methods to prevent unforeseen pregnancy are also recommended.

One major interaction in the reverse direction involves estrogenic components of COCs that induce UGT (uridine-diphosphate glucuronosyltransferase) to increase glucuronidation, the major metabolic inactivation pathway for lamotrigine. Lamotrigine levels may thus decline up to 50%, resulting in breakthrough seizures. Other AED levels affected to a lesser degree include valproic acid, whose levels may be reduced by 20–40%. This effect can be remedied by avoiding estrogen-containing COCs (e.g., the "minipill," or progestin-only COC) or by checking susceptible AED levels before and after oral contraceptive initiation and adjusting the AED dosage accordingly.

Issues Relating to Pregnancy Changes in Seizure Rate

Changes in seizure rate during pregnancy may be a question on the minds of patients. Pregnancy is typically a fairly uneventful process with respect to their seizures, and most children are delivered healthy without obstetric complications. Statistically, there is no change in seizure rate in approximately 70% of women with epilepsy; among the remainder, there are equal numbers who experience improvement and exacerbation of seizures. The reasons are likely related to a complex mix of physiological changes that render the direction of change difficult to predict. Reassuringly, WWE who are seizure free for the 9 months prior to pregnancy are 84–92% likely to remain seizure-free during pregnancy and should be counseled as such to allay any fears [11].

Worsening of seizures during pregnancy may be related to anticonvulsant level fluctuation, in turn due to metabolic changes associated with pregnancy, medical nonadherence, and hyperemesis gravidarum. A monitoring plan should be made to frequently check serum levels of anticonvulsants that are likely to decline during the course of pregnancy. Notably, glucuronidation becomes more efficient during pregnancy, resulting in reduction of lamotrigine and oxcarbazepine levels. WWE on these medications require higher doses and may have more clinical seizures [12, 13]. After delivery, AED levels can be adjusted back to their prepregnancy doses to avoid developing toxicity.

Maternal Mortality in WWE

Alarmingly, several studies have found that maternal mortality in WWE is significantly higher than that of the general population. Sampled hospital data from the USA [14] imply a ten-fold increase in maternal death in WWE during hospitalization for delivery. Similarly, data from the UK examining all maternities during successive 2-year periods suggest a ten-fold increase in maternal death in WWE during pregnancy and up to 42 days after delivery [15]. Most deaths were from SUDEP (sudden unexplained death in epilepsy) among women taking lamotrigine, though the high numbers associated with lamotrigine may have simply correlated to prescribing practice. A five-fold increase in mortality during and up to 42 days after delivery was found in Denmark [16]. Speculative reasons include possibly stoppage of AEDs (antiepileptic drugs) or increased clearance of AEDs during pregnancy, resulting in severe seizures.

In addition to mortality, increased maternal complications such as preeclampsia, preterm labor, hemorrhage, increased cesarean utilization, and prolonged length of stay [14, 17]. Given these issues, WWE who are pregnant are placed in a high-risk obstetrical category and are often referred to neurology for consultation.

Teratogenicity of Anticonvulsants

A significant concern of hopeful parents is the influence of medications on the developing fetus. The background rate of major congenital malformations (MCMs) in the general population is 1.5–3%, and anticonvulsant therapy in general can raise that risk on average two-fold. Over the past few decades, data regarding the teratogenicity of specific anticonvulsants have been gathered in several pregnancy registries run in different countries (North America, Europe, the UK, and Australia). All registries have consistently shown a three- to five-fold increase in MCM rates by valproic acid, as well as increased rates with polytherapy. Other agents associated with significantly higher rates of MCMs include topiramate and phenobarbital. In general, polytherapy and higher anticonvulsant doses [18] are associated with higher teratogenicity. Anticonvulsants that are regarded as safer and associated with a low rate of MCMs include lamotrigine and levetiracetam. These results can be seen in the North American Pregnancy Registry (www.aedpregnancyregistry.org); the NAPR publishes their results on monotherapy and major congenital malformations (MCMs) on a biennial basis and their tabulated data are downloadable from their website.

Most MCMs related to anticonvulsants include craniofacial defects such as oral clefts, cardiac abnormalities, hypospadias, microcephaly, and neural tube defects (e.g., spina bifida, encephaloceles); specific anticonvulsants are more associated with particular deformities. In the absence of obvious malformations, there may be cognitive and neurobehavioral deficits induced by AED exposure. In the NEAD (Neurodevelopmental Effects of Antiepileptic Drugs) study, over 300 children born to women on four anticonvulsants (phenytoin, carbamazepine, valproic acid, and lamotrigine) were followed after birth, and IQ tested at age 3 and 6. A 10-point reduction in IQ was found associated with in utero exposure to valproic acid, particularly in the verbal domain [19, 20].

Low folate levels are associated with increased risk of spontaneous abortion and MCMs. Whether administration of folic acid will reduce AED-related MCMs is debatable, with a prospective study from the UK revealing no difference in MCMs with folate supplementation [21]. Other studies have found that treatment with supplemental folate may help attenuate teratogenicity and improve neurocognitive outcomes [20, 22].

Careful planning is essential to a healthy neonatal outcome. Transition from polytherapy to monotherapy at the lowest dose possible should be considered. Ideally, switching from agents such as valproic acid, topiramate, and phenobarbital, to safer drugs such as lamotrigine and levetiracetam, should occur prior to conception. Many neural tube defects will have occurred prior to a women's awareness of her pregnancy following a missed menstruation if AED switching is not done prior to conception. Additionally, maternal seizures can have equally deleterious effects on pregnancy outcome. Falls related to seizure can cause direct trauma to the uterus. Even focal seizures without tonic-clonic evolution may result in hemodynamic changes [23] or injury due to loss of awareness that may be harmful for the developing fetus. Given this risk–benefit ratio, women with epilepsy should be counseled to continue treatment for their seizures, as sudden stoppage may lead to status epilepticus. Furthermore, the best medication for any specific patient is one which will control the seizures, even if it is one that has been associated with a higher rate of teratogenesis.

Issues Relating to the Peri- and Post-Partum Period Vitamin K

Neonates are at risk for vitamin K deficiency due to low vitamin K stores, poor placental transfer of vitamin K, and hepatic immaturity which precludes efficiently utilization vitamin K. The American Academy of Pediatrics recommends that all newborn infants should receive vitamin K at birth as an intramuscular dose of 0.5–1 mg to prevent bleeding. It is surmised that more severe vitamin K deficiency may occur in infants whose mothers are taking EIAEDs; as such, it has been recommended that mothers take 10–20 mg of oral vitamin K daily for 1 month prior to delivery. However, there appears to be insufficient evidence that hemorrhagic complications exist in higher frequencies among mothers taking EIAEDs; likewise, there is insufficient evidence to support or refute the use of supplemental vitamin K supplementation in WWE [11].

Breastfeeding

Anticonvulsants are measurable in breastmilk. Factors that are correlated with higher presence in breastmilk include increased lipophilicity, lower molecular weight, and lower protein binding. However, gaps in the mammary alveolar cells early post-partum may allow medications to pass through in higher amounts than mature milk. Timing of serum levels relative to breastfeeding or breastmilk pumping and the amount of breastmilk consumed by the infant also play a role. Finally, infant metabolism and elimination changes as the newborn grows. These factors explain why infant and maternal serum levels of anticonvulsants are complex and not simply proportionate.

Though AED levels in breastmilk vary widely (from 5 to 10% with valproate and up to 100% with levetiracetam), measurable levels in breastfeeding infants tend to be much lower [24]. Certain sedating medications such as barbiturates or benzodiazepines may accumulate due to slow metabolism and are anecdotally associated with sedation after feeding. Despite these particular cases, there is little evidence on the whole to support adverse events on the baby from AED exposure through breastmilk [11, 25]. It is recommended to avoid breastfeeding if there is significant sedation correlated to nursing, or the mother is taking anticonvulsants with higher potential for severe idiosyncratic side effects (e.g., felbamate or vigabatrin). AED polypharmacy and prematurity (with likely reduced neonatal metabolism and increased accumulation) also represent potentially increased risk. For the majority of cases, however, the general recommendation is to continue with breastfeeding due to the known benefits of nursing on neurodevelopment [26], though WWE appear less likely to breastfeed overall [27].

References

1. Sukumaran SC, Sarma PS, Thomas SV. Polytherapy increases the risk of infertility in women with epilepsy. Neurology. 2010;75(15):1351–5. https://doi.org/10.1212/WNL.0b013e3181f73673.
2. Shukla GD, Srivastava ON, B.C. Katiyar sexual disturbances in temporal lobe epilepsy: a controlled study. Br J Psychiatry. 1979;134:288–92.
3. Tebartz Van Elst L, Krishnamoorthy ES, Bäumer D, Selai C, von Gunten A, Gene-Cos N, Ebert D, Trimble MR. Psychopathological profile in patients with severe bilateral hippocampal atrophy and temporal lobe epilepsy: evidence in support of the Geschwind syndrome? Epilepsy Behav. 2003;4(3):291–7. https://doi.org/10.1016/S1525-5050(03)000842. PMID 12791331. S2CID 34974937.
4. Barragry JM, Makin HL, Trafford DJ, Scott DF. Effect of anticonvulsants on plasma testosterone and sex hormone binding globulin levels. J Neurol Neurosurg Psychiatry. 1978;41(10):913–4. PubMed PMID: 569688; PubMed Central PMCID: PMC493193.
5. Herzog AG. Menstrual disorders in women with epilepsy. Neurology. 2006;66(6 Suppl 3):S23–8. https://doi.org/10.1212/wnl.66.66_suppl_3.s23d.
6. Bilo L, Meo R. Epilepsy and polycystic ovary syndrome: where is the link? Neurol Sci. 2006;27:221–30 [PubMed] [Google Scholar].
7. Herzog AG, Schachter SC. Valproate and the polycystic ovarian syndrome: final thoughts. Epilepsia. 2001;42:311–5 [PubMed] [Google Scholar].
8. Gastaut H, Collomb H. Sexual behavior in psychomotor epileptics. Ann Med Psychol. 1954;112(2(5)):657–96.

9. Hu X, Wang J, Dong W, Fang Q, Hu L, Liu C. A meta-analysis of polycystic ovary syndrome in women taking valproate for epilepsy. Epilepsy Res. 2011;97(1–2):73–82. https://doi.org/10.1016/j.eplepsyres.2011.07.006.

10. Pennell PB, French JA, Harden CL, Davis A, Bagiella E, Andreopoulos E, Lau C, Llewellyn N, Barnard S, Allien S. Fertility and birth outcomes in women with epilepsy seeking pregnancy. JAMA Neurol. 2018;75(8):962–9. https://doi.org/10.1001/jamaneurol.2018.0646. PMID: 29710218; PMCID: PMC6142930.

11. Harden CL, Pennell PB, Koppel BS, Hovinga CA, Gidal B, Meador KJ, Hopp J, Ting TY, Hauser WA, Thurman D, Kaplan PW, Robinson JN, French JA, Wiebe S, Wilner AN, Vazquez B, Holmes L, Krumholz A, Finnell R, Shafer PO, Le Guen C, American Academy of Neurology; American Epilepsy Society. Practice parameter update: management issues for women with epilepsy—focus on pregnancy (an evidence-based review): vitamin K, folic acid, blood levels, and breastfeeding: report of the Quality Standards Subcommittee and Therapeutics and Technology Assessment Subcommittee of the American Academy of Neurology and American Epilepsy Society. Neurology. 2009;73(2):142–9. https://doi.org/10.1212/WNL.0b013e3181a6b325. Epub 2009 Apr 27. PMID: 19398680; PMCID: PMC3475193.

12. Vajda FJ, Hitchcock A, Graham J, et al. Foetal malformations and seizure control: 52 months data of the Australian pregnancy registry. Eur J Neurol. 2006;13(6):645–54. https://doi.org/10.1111/j.1468-1331.2006.01359.x.

13. EURAP Study Group. Seizure control and treatment in pregnancy: observations from the EURAP epilepsy pregnancy registry. Neurology. 2006;66(3):354–60. https://doi.org/10.1212/01.wnl.0000195888.51845.80.

14. MacDonald SC, Bateman BT, McElrath TF, Hernández-Díaz S. Mortality and morbidity during delivery hospitalization among pregnant women with epilepsy in the United States. JAMA Neurol. 2015;72(9):981–8. https://doi.org/10.1001/jamaneurol.2015.1017.

15. Edey S, Moran N, Nashef L. SUDEP and epilepsy-related mortality in pregnancy. Epilepsia. 2014;55(7):e72–4. https://doi.org/10.1111/epi.12621.

16. Christensen J, Vestergaard C, Hammer BB. Maternal death in women with epilepsy: Smaller scope studies. Neurology. 2018;91(18):e1716. https://doi.org/10.1212/WNL.0000000000006426. Epub 2018 Sep 26. PMID: 30258019; PMCID: PMC6207413.

17. Borthen I, Eide MG, Daltveit AK, Gilhus NE. Obstetric outcome in women with epilepsy: a hospital-based, retrospective study. BJOG. 2011;118(8):956–65. https://doi.org/10.1111/j.1471-0528.2011.03004.x.

18. Tomson T, Battino D, Bonizzoni E, Craig J, Lindhout D, Sabers A, Perucca E, Vajda F, EURAP Study Group. Dose-dependent risk of malformations with antiepileptic drugs: an analysis of data from the EURAP epilepsy and pregnancy registry. Lancet Neurol. 2011;10(7):609–17. https://doi.org/10.1016/S1474-4422(11)70107-7. Epub 2011 Jun 5. PubMed PMID: 21652013.

19. Cohen MJ, Meador KJ, May R, Loblein H, Conrad T, Baker GA, Bromley RL, Clayton-Smith J, Kalayjian LA, Kanner A, Liporace JD, Pennell PB, Privitera M, Loring DW, NEAD Study Group. Fetal antiepileptic drug exposure and learning and memory functioning at 6 years of age: the NEAD prospective observational study. Epilepsy Behav. 2019;92:154–64. https://doi.org/10.1016/j.yebeh.2018.12.031. Epub 2019 Jan 17. PubMed PMID: 30660966.

20. Meador KJ, Baker GA, Browning N, Cohen MJ, Bromley RL, Clayton-Smith J, Kalayjian LA, Kanner A, Liporace JD, Pennell PB, Privitera M, Loring DW, NEAD Study Group. Fetal antiepileptic drug exposure and cognitive outcomes at age 6 years (NEAD study): a prospective observational study. Lancet Neurol. 2013;12(3):244–52. https://doi.org/10.1016/S1474-4422(12)70323-X. Epub 2013 Jan 23. PubMed PMID: 23352199; PubMed Central PMCID: PMC3684942.

21. Morrow JI, Hunt SJ, Russell AJ, Smithson WH, Parsons L, Robertson I, Waddell R, Irwin B, Morrison PJ, Craig JJ. Folic acid use and major congenital malformations in offspring of women with epilepsy: a prospective study from the UK epilepsy and pregnancy register. J Neurol Neurosurg Psychiatry. 2009;80(5):506–11. https://doi.org/10.1136/jnnp.2008.156109. Epub 2008 Oct 31. PMID: 18977812.

22. Meador KJ, Pennell PB, May RC, Brown CA, Baker G, Bromley R, Loring DW, Cohen MJ, NEAD Investigator Group. Effects of periconceptional folate on cognition in children of women with epilepsy: NEAD study. Neurology. 2019;94(7):e729–40. https://doi.org/10.1212/WNL.0000000000008757.

23. Sahoo S, Klein P. Maternal complex partial seizure associated with fetal distress. Arch Neurol. 2005;62(8):1304–5. PubMed PMID: 16087773.

24. Birnbaum AK, Meador KJ, Karanam A, Brown C, May RC, Gerard EE, Gedzelman ER, Penovich PE, Kalayjian LA, Cavitt J, Pack AM, Miller JW, Stowe ZN, Pennell PB, MONEAD Investigator Group. Antiepileptic drug exposure in infants of breastfeeding mothers with epilepsy. JAMA Neurol. 2020;77(4):441–50. https://doi.org/10.1001/jamaneurol.2019.4443. PMID: 31886825; PMCID: PMC6990802.

25. Meador KJ, Baker GA, Browning N, Clayton-Smith J, Combs-Cantrell DT, Cohen M, Kalayjian LA, Kanner A, Liporace JD, Pennell PB, Privitera M, Loring DW, NEAD Study Group. Effects of breastfeeding in children of women taking antiepileptic drugs. Neurology. 2010;75(22):1954–60. https://doi.org/10.1212/WNL.0b013e3181ffe4a9. Epub 2010 Nov 24. PMID: 21106960; PMCID: PMC3014232.

26. Meador KJ, Baker GA, Browning N, Cohen MJ, Bromley RL, Clayton-Smith J, Kalayjian LA, Kanner A, Liporace JD, Pennell PB, Privitera M, Loring DW. Neurodevelopmental effects of antiepileptic drugs (NEAD) study group. Breastfeeding in children of women taking antiepileptic drugs: cognitive outcomes at age 6 years. JAMA Pediatr. 2014;168(8):729–36. https://doi.org/10.1001/jamapediatrics.2014.118. PMID: 24934501; PMCID: PMC4122685.

27. Al-faraj AO, Wigton R, Pang, TD. Factors affecting breastfeeding patterns in women with epilepsy. AES 2019 Annual meeting Abstract database. AESNet.org. 2019.

Sleep Disorders and Their Management in Pregnancy

Aesha Jobanputra, Vandan Kumar Patel, Renuka Rajagopal, Krithika Namasivayam, and Jag Sunderram

Sleep Architecture in Pregnancy

It is well known that adequate quantity and quality of sleep are important for a feeling of wellness and overall health. However, changes in sleep architecture including changes in sleep latency, duration, and depth of sleep occur during pregnancy due to various physiological and anatomical reasons. These alterations have an impact on the well-being of the mother as well as the baby and have been reported using both subjective, self-reported data and with objective testing such as actigraphy and polysomnography.

Subjective Data

Various questionnaires have been utilized to study changes in sleep that occur throughout the perinatal period [1–3]. Some of the commonly used questionnaires include Pittsburgh Sleep Quality Index (PSQI), Epworth Sleepiness Scale (ESS), Berlin questionnaire, and General Sleep Disturbance Scale (GSDS). Similarly, a sleep diary is another form of subjective method used to assess sleep prospectively. For a sleep diary, an individual is asked to complete several questions about their sleep from the night prior upon awakening in the morning.

A study by Mindell et al. that assessed a total of 2427 women over the entire duration of pregnancy reported poor sleep based on PSQI scores, especially in the later months of the pregnancy [1]. The study noted that among other factors, sleep worsens as the pregnancy progresses [1]. Increased sleep latency and fragmented sleep was also reported in this study with 33.1% of the women with sleep latency of >30 min and at least one nocturnal awakening throughout the pregnancy [1]. Similarly, other studies have found poor sleep based on higher GSDS scores in the third trimester and in the first postpartum month [4, 5]. Several studies that assessed women using PSQI have also demonstrated increase in PSQI score or worsening sleep from early to late pregnancy and in the postpartum period [6].

Similarly, studies utilizing sleep diaries demonstrate poor sleep as measured by wake after sleep onset (WASO), a measure of sleep fragmentation [7–10]. WASO has been shown to worsen from approximately 30 min at the beginning of the pregnancy to up to 2 h in the first postpartum month [7–10]. However, total sleep time (TST), or total duration of sleep remained between 7 and 8 h. Similarly, sleep onset latency (SOL), the amount of time required to fall asleep, demonstrated little variability and remained between 10 and 25 min [7–10]. Studies have also

A. Jobanputra · V. K. Patel · R. Rajagopal ·
K. Namasivayam · J. Sunderram (✉)
Division of Pulmonary and Critical Care Medicine,
Department of Medicine, Rutgers, Robert Wood
Johnson Medical School, New Brunswick, NJ, USA
e-mail: sunderja@rwjms.rutgers.edu

G. Gupta et al. (eds.), *Neurological Disorders in Pregnancy*,
https://doi.org/10.1007/978-3-031-36490-7_29

shown that compared to control individuals, women had the most disturbed sleep in the first postpartum week. These women had more fragmented sleep, longer wake periods, and more naps during the day compared to the control group [11, 12].

Objective Data

Actigraphy and polysomnography are objective tests used to characterize sleep. Actigraphy is a method of measuring movement over a period of days using a noninvasive accelerometer. Actigraphy provides an accurate estimate of sleep patterns and has been validated to be used in normal, healthy adults as well as in patients with certain sleep disorders [13].

Actigraphy has been utilized to objectively measure sleep in pregnancy and in the perinatal period. The majority of the studies using actigraphy confirm findings from subjective testing such as from sleep diaries that demonstrated increase in WASO [4, 14–16]. However, the major difference between sleep diaries and actigraphy findings was the decrease seen in TST with actigraphy [4, 14–16]. Total sleep time was decreased from average of 7–8 h to 5.5–7 h per night from late pregnancy to the first postpartum month [4, 14–16].

Polysomnography (PSG) is the gold standard for evaluation of various sleep disorders. There are a limited number of studies utilizing PSGs due to the cost, inconvenience, and time intensiveness. These studies have reached similar conclusions as studies utilizing subjective methods. In a study by Lee et al., two consecutive nights of PSG were done in each trimester as well as at the first and third months postpartum. They demonstrated decrease in TST from an average of 446 min during the first trimester to an average of 372 min at 1 month postpartum [17]. Similarly, sleep efficiency (defined as total sleep time over time in bed) decreased as well from 93% prior to pregnancy to 81% during the first month postpartum [17]. Other longitudinal studies also show

decreased sleep efficiency and increased WASO [18–21]. There was also a decrease in deep sleep throughout pregnancy compared with baseline and postpartum [17]. No significant change was seen in latency to the first REM cycle and the percentage of total sleep time spent in REM [17].

In summary, subjective and objective methods of assessing sleep in pregnant women both demonstrate decreased total sleep time and increased WASO. All methods of assessing sleep are consistent with increased sleep fragmentation through the progression of the pregnancy and into the postpartum period. Although sleep diaries demonstrate no change in total sleep time, the objective PSG data demonstrates decreased total sleep time (see Table 29.1).

Table 29.1 Change in sleep architecture during pregnancy as determined by subjective and objective methods

Methods to identify changes in sleep architecture	Changes noted in sleep throughout pregnancy
Sleep questionnaires	• Overall poor sleep [1, 4–6] • ↑ sleep latency [1] • ↑ sleep fragmentation [1]
Sleep diary	• ↑sleep fragmentation (as measured by WASO) [7–10] • Unchanged total sleep time [7–10] • Unchanged sleep onset latency [7–10]
Actigraphy	• ↑sleep fragmentation (as measured by WASO) [4, 14–16] • ↓ total sleep time [4, 14–16]
Polysomnography	• ↓ total sleep time [17] • ↓ sleep efficiency [17–21] • ↑ sleep fragmentation as measured by WASO [17–21] • ↓ N3 sleep [17] • Unchanged latency to REM [17] • Unchanged percentage of total sleep time in REM [17]

Changes During Pregnancy that Can Affect and Alter Sleep Patterns

The above described changes in sleep quantity and quality are attributable to changes in melatonin, hormones, as well as to physiological changes that manifest as nocturnal symptoms leading to disrupted sleep. In addition, sleep may be disrupted due to the physical discomfort from a growing baby and finally from emotional and/or psychological stress regarding pregnancy and childbirth.

Changes in Melatonin and Sleep Onset in Pregnancy

Melatonin has been described as the "Dark Hormone" secreted by the pineal gland. The onset of melatonin secretion and peak serum concentrations are responsible for the timing of sleep, especially sleep onset [22]. Melatonin secretion peaks in the night and is lowest during mid-day. While the onset of melatonin secretion has not been studied during pregnancy, the concentration of melatonin changes during each trimester of pregnancy [23]. For example, the serum melatonin concentration measured at 2 AM decreases slightly between the first and second trimester and then begins to increase after 24 weeks, reaching maximum levels by the end of pregnancy before returning to pre-pregnancy values by the second day postpartum [23]. These changes in melatonin concentration may occur as a result of changes in the level of vasoactive intestinal peptide (VIP), a neuropeptide that controls melatonin synthesis not only in the pineal gland but also in the placenta and the growing fetus [24–26].

During pregnancy, women tend to sleep earlier during their first two trimesters and then return to pre-pregnancy levels during the third trimester. Additionally, women have longer sleep duration but have more activity in sleep during pregnancy than they did before or after pregnancy [27]. These changes in sleep onset and duration during pregnancy suggest a relationship with changes in the onset of melatonin secretion, although this has so far not been studied.

Hormonal Changes During Pregnancy and Their Effect on Sleep

Among the many hormonal changes that occur during pregnancy, the hormones of significance to sleep are cortisol, estrogen, progesterone, and prolactin.

Cortisol is a hormone with significant circadian rhythmicity with an early morning peak and evening dip. This rhythmicity is maintained during pregnancy, but the amplitude of the peak is higher with serum cortisol levels being elevated overall [28]. This increase in cortisol levels is said to be important to fetal lung and brain growth [29]. Increased evening levels of serum cortisol are known to be associated with sleep fragmentation and insomnia.

Conversely, increased levels of serum progesterone are associated with increased sleep duration and N3 sleep, while increased estrogen levels are associated with decreased REM sleep [30]. Both these hormones gradually increase during pregnancy [30].

The Growing Baby

Sleep during pregnancy may be disturbed just by the physical discomfort related to the growing fetus [1]. Additionally, the growing fetus puts increasing pressure on the maternal bladder resulting in frequent urination and nocturia as the pregnancy progresses [31].

Gastroesophageal reflux (GER) occurs early in pregnancy due to relaxation of the lower esophageal sphincter and delayed gastric emptying. As pregnancy progresses, with increase in fetal size, the diaphragm and stomach are displaced upward thus worsening GER symptoms. Worsened symptoms, especially in the recumbent position, result in poor sleep.

Sleep Disorders During Pregnancy

Sleep Disordered Breathing (SDB) and Pregnancy

Sleep disordered breathing refers to conditions that lead to abnormal breathing patterns and gas exchange during sleep. The commonest form of sleep disordered breathing is obstructive sleep apnea (OSA), where there is obstruction of the upper airway during sleep resulting in progressive asphyxia. The obstruction is relieved following a brief arousal. Repeated obstructive events leads to sleep fragmentation and intermittent hypoxia. Common symptoms include snoring and excessive daytime sleepiness.

Pregnancy results in the elevation of the diaphragm as the growing uterus pushes it upwards, resulting in smaller total lung volume, tracheal shortening, and a greater predisposition to upper airway obstruction [32]. Additionally, fluid shifts and increase in neck circumference at night, especially in the second trimester of pregnancy, increase the likelihood of OSA [33]. Increased levels of estrogen during pregnancy contribute to vasomotor rhinitis leading to inflammation and narrowing of the upper airway further predisposing individuals to OSA. Snoring is the most commonly reported symptom of OSA in pregnant women. In longitudinal studies the frequency of regular snoring increases from about 7 to 11% in the first trimester to approximately 16–25% in the third trimester [34, 35]. Similarly, OSA has been shown to worsen across pregnancy with an increase from 7% in the first trimester to 27% later in pregnancy [36]. The prevalence of OSA increases with the presence of obesity in pregnancy. In fact, a direct correlation was found between higher BMI and increased risk of developing OSA in a recent UK study [37, 38]. In developed countries the incidence of obesity in pregnant women is greater than 20% [37, 38]. In the third trimester, 40% of obese women have OSA, compared to 14.5% of their normal and overweight cohorts [36]. Another risk factor for OSA is advanced age. There is a rising number of women that are of advanced maternal age which significantly increases the risk of developing OSA. The development of OSA in pregnancy can predispose the mother to unfavorable outcomes including gestational hypertension, pre-eclampsia, and gestational diabetes due to the associated sleep fragmentation and chronic intermittent hypoxia.

SDB in Pregnancy and GDM

Sleep disturbances, short sleep duration, and SDB are associated with increased risk of developing metabolic and cardiovascular risks in the general population. Shorter nocturnal sleep has been associated with higher plasma glucose concentrations during the non-fasting glucose challenge test. Sleep disordered breathing, which affects sleep quality, may also play integral role in glucose intolerance during pregnancy. SDB is associated with increased incidence of type II diabetes in the general population and, similarly, SDB during pregnancy is correlated with increased propensity of developing gestational diabetes mellitus (GDM). Pregnant women with SDB were three times more likely to develop gestational diabetes based on a meta-analysis of six studies [39]. Studies have also shown that frequent snoring greater than three times a week is associated with increased odds of GDM when adjusted for maternal age, race/ethnicity, pre-pregnancy BMI, and short sleep duration and may be associated with greater than three-fold odds of GDM when adjusted for BMI [34, 40]. However, there are limitations to self-reported frequent snoring or Berlin Questionnaire data as these cannot be used to diagnose OSA. Polysomnogram diagnosed OSA can, therefore, better establish the correlation between SDB with GDM. In the analysis of the United States Nationwide Inpatient Sample database of over 55 million gravid women, after adjusting for maternal age, obesity, ethnicity, and other comorbidities, PSG diagnosed OSA was associated with a two-fold increase in the odds of developing GDM compared to women who were not diagnosed with OSA [34, 41]. However, in a prospective study exposure to OSA (Apnea Hypopnea Index, AHI ≥5) was not associated with GDM or hyperglycemia [42]. This study was limited by small sample size and underscoring the need for more prospective and longitudinal studies with more robust numbers. Additionally, there are no prospective studies demonstrating whether the treatment of SDB or OSA leads to improvement in glycemic control in pregnant women.

Pathophysiological Mechanism of GDM with SDB in Pregnancy

Sleep fragmentation and intermittent hypoxia cause greater oxidative stress and generate reactive oxygen species (ROS). [43] Even in healthy pregnancies, markers of oxidative stress increase during the first and second trimesters relative to non-pregnant women [44]. The concentration of ROS is higher in women with gestational diabetes compared to women with normal glucose tolerance [34, 45]. The increased oxidative stress exposure due to SDB may potentiate the development of maternal hyperglycemia [46]. In normal individuals, hyperglycemia can induce release of pro-inflammatory markers such as IL-6, CRP, and TNF-α [46]. Sleep deprivation also induces similar release of inflammatory markers, and decrease in leptin, a hormone critical in appetite regulation and metabolism [47]. Normal pregnancy is associated with increased levels of TNF-α, CRP, and leptin, and these levels of TNF-α and leptin correlate inversely with insulin sensitivity [34, 48]. Women with GDM have higher levels of TNF-α and leptin compared to pregnant women with euglycemia when adjusted for BMI [34, 49]. SDB can lead to increased oxidative stress and insulin resistance contributing to hyperglycemia which in turn leads to more ROS, thus creating a deleterious feedback loop.

Additionally, insufficient sleep and SDB can lead to enhanced sympathomimetic activity with increased catecholamine and cortisol levels [50]. During pregnancy, plasma noradrenaline levels during the night are higher compared with levels in non-gravid women [28]. These changes during pregnancy in addition to SDB and sleep deprivation could promote gluconeogenesis and susceptibility to developing GDM. Furthermore, persistently elevated cortisol can alter glucose metabolism by suppressing insulin secretion from pancreatic β-cells, preventing glucose absorption, and enhancing gluconeogenesis [34, 51]. Finally, the lack of sleep and stress of pregnancy alone can induce high levels of cortisol and lead to glucose dysregulation.

SDB in Pregnancy and Hypertensive Disorders of Pregnancy (HDP)

Women with SDB have a significantly increased risk of entering pregnancy with chronic hypertension and/or developing hypertensive disorders of pregnancy (HDP), a group of conditions that include chronic hypertension, gestational hypertension, pre-eclampsia, and eclampsia. As a class, HDP represents a major cause of maternal morbidity and mortality, including serious complications such as postpartum hemorrhage, hemorrhagic stroke, cardiomyopathy, acute renal insufficiency, myocardial infarction, and pulmonary edema [52]. Notably, pre-eclampsia and eclampsia can increase the risk of cardiovascular disease later in life [53, 54]. The pathophysiological mechanism by which OSA can lead to pre-eclampsia is via common pathways of oxidative stress, systemic inflammation, sympathetic dysregulation, and eventually endothelial dysfunction.

Pre-eclampsia and OSA share many comorbidities such as chronic hypertension, diabetes mellitus, obesity, and advanced maternal age. Only recently OSA has been considered as a potential risk factor for pre-eclampsia and other HDP [53]. Two recent meta-analyses have indicated that gravid women with OSA are at increased risk of developing pre-eclampsia, and that women with HDP are at increased risk for having SDB during pregnancy [55, 56]. The nuMom2b-SDB sub-study of 3702 nulliparous women who underwent sleep studies during pregnancy found that women with mild OSA (AHI <15 per hour) had twice the odds of developing pre-eclampsia. This risk was significantly increased with greater than four times odds of developing pre-eclampsia with moderate and severe OSA (AHI ≥15 per hour) [53, 57].

In pregnancy, OSA seems to be an important co-morbidity for chronic hypertension. The recent prospective study of over 3000 women postulated that chronic hypertension is significantly more common among pregnant women with OSA, and that this prevalence increases with OSA severity [53]. A smaller prospective cohort study confirmed that pregnant women with chronic hypertension had 43% incidence of OSA compared to 19% in their normotensive counterparts [58]. There was correlation between chronic snoring and the development of chronic hypertension, and gestational onset snoring with development of gestational hypertension [53, 58]. A prospective study of 248 pregnant women who underwent home sleep studies in the third trimester had a combined incidence of chronic and gestational hypertension of 57% among women with AHI ≥5 per hour compared to 23% among women with AHI < 5 per hour [53, 59]. Finally, approximately 20–30% of women with chronic hypertension will develop pre-eclampsia during pregnancy [60].

Pathophysiological Mechanism of Pre-Eclampsia with SDB in Pregnancy

SDB can lead to intermittent hypoxia and catecholamine surge. It is postulated that hypoxemia may be an upstream mediator in the development of pre-eclampsia. Women who live at high altitude regions with lower partial pressures of oxygen have higher incidences of pre-eclampsia [61]. Hypoxia inducible factors 1 and 2 (HIF 1 and 2) are transcription factors found to be overexpressed in the placentas of women living at

high altitude [61]. HIFs have been connected to OSA and hypertension by being mediators of inflammation, sympathetic activation, oxidative stress, and endothelial dysfunction [53, 62]. One study has shown that placental hypoxia was present in women with SDB and habitual snoring when compared to the placentas of non-OSA and non-snoring controls [63]. The SDB mothers' placentas had increased normoblasts which is a sign of fetal hypoxia and increased expression of calcium-exchanger 1 (CAX1), an indirect cellular marker of HIF-1 activation [53, 64]. Pro-inflammatory markers such as tumor necrosis factor-alpha (TNF-α), C-reactive protein (CRP), interlukin-6, and interleukin-8 are significantly increased in pre-eclampsia [65]. These same markers are also found to be increased in OSA [66]. Release of these pro-inflammatory cytokines along with oxidative stress can cause endothelin dysregulation with fluctuations of vascular-derived endothelial growth factor (VEGF) and placental growth factor (PlFG), thus increasing the risk of pre-eclampsia [53, 67].

Figure 29.1 describes the common pathophysiological pathways between shortened sleep,

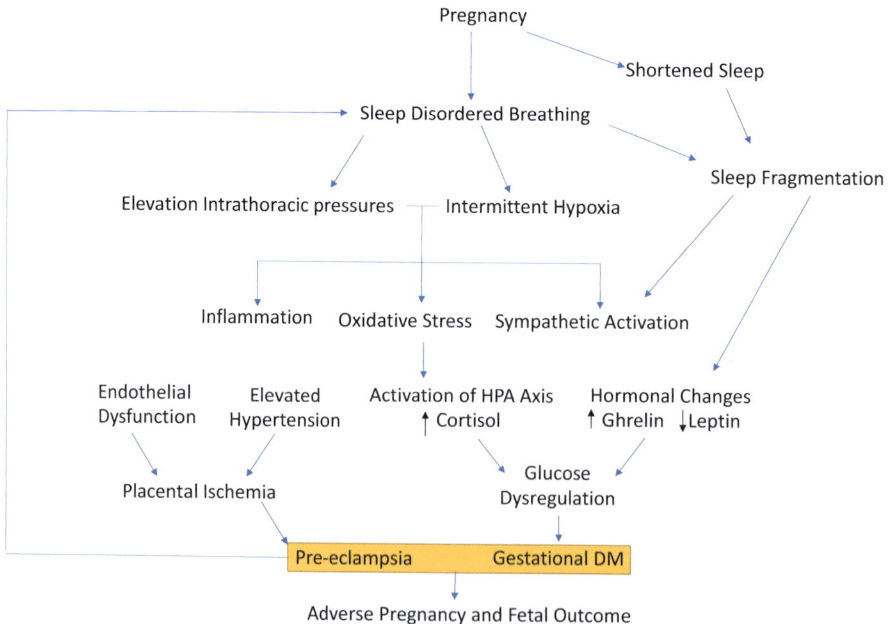

Fig. 29.1 Pathogenesis of pre-eclampsia and gestational DM as a result of short sleep and sleep disordered breathing during pregnancy

sleep fragmentation, and sleep disordered breathing that lead to GDM and pre-eclampsia which can ultimately lead to adverse fetal outcomes.

In many studies of non-gravid adults, the treatment of OSA with continuous positive airway pressure (CPAP) has improved daytime sleepiness, quality of life, mood, hypertension, sympathetic dysregulation, and endothelial function [68–70]. However, in pregnant women more studies are needed to support the utility of CPAP therapy in the prevention of HDP. A recent case report describes a pregnant female with severe pre-eclampsia and diagnosed OSA who was started on nocturnal CPAP therapy ultimately delaying the need for induction of labor for 30 days after the diagnosis of severe pre-eclampsia [71]. One week of CPAP treatment not only improved the blood pressure but proteinuria and uric acid level were also significantly improved. This report also demonstrated lower levels of soluble fms-like tyrosine kinase 1 (sFlt-1, a VEGF receptor) after the commencement of CPAP therapy [71]. Further studies are needed to evaluate the efficacy of CPAP therapy to mitigate adverse pregnancy outcomes due to HDP.

Restless Leg Syndrome in Pregnancy

Restless leg syndrome (RLS) or Willis-Ekbom disease is a sensorimotor disorder that is associated with a near irresistible urge to move the limbs which gets worse at the end of the day and is relieved with movement. RLS symptoms often lead to difficulty initiating sleep. RLS is associated with periodic limb movements in sleep (PLM), which is a polysomnographic diagnosed condition. If PLMs lead to difficulty maintaining sleep, this is termed PLM disorder. Iron deficiency anemia and chronic kidney disease are often associated with RLS symptoms [72]. Pregnancy can worsen RLS or can lead to new onset RLS. Some of the mechanisms implicated include the relative iron deficiency of pregnancy and hormonal changes. The prevalence of RLS is three fold higher in pregnancy at 20–25% when compared to the general population [73].

Pregnancy-related RLS peaks in the third trimester of gestation and usually remits around delivery. Reported prevalence rates of RLS are 8% in the first, 16% in the second and 22% in the third trimester, and rates decrease to 4% prevalence after delivery [74, 75]. RLS during pregnancy can be detrimental and lead to complications that can contribute to SDB, insomnia, birth complications, and mood disorders [74].

RLS and Insomnia

The prevalence of insomnia in pregnancy is greatly increased with the presence of RLS [73]. RLS during gestation leads to excessive daytime sleepiness, poor daytime function, diminished concentration, and poor sleep quality [74]. Most women will report difficulty in initiating sleep with RLS during pregnancy. The diagnosis of insomnia can make it difficult to diagnose RLS in pregnancy. In most questionnaires and studies women are found to be under diagnosed with RLS [74].

Mood Disorders with RLS

The direct correlation between poor sleep and depression during pregnancy has been greatly studied. Perception of sleep deficiency via questionnaires and sleep diaries is strongly correlated with depressive symptomatology [6]. RLS causes psychological distress and, when present in pregnant women, it increases the risk of developing perinatal depression [76]. In a longitudinal survey of 1428 pregnant women, mid-pregnancy and postpartum depression were associated with pre-pregnancy RLS rather than pregnancy onset RLS [76, 77].

RLS and Gestational Diabetes

RLS can lead to poor sleep and there is an association between RLS and SDB [78]. In an Appalachian primary care population, one study reported increased likelihood of RLS symptoms in pregnant women with GDM [79]. Daily RLS symptoms in the later part of pregnancy were associated with poor glycemic control and worsening severity of RLS was linked to greater likelihood of GDM and SDB [79].

RLS and Hypertensive Disorders of Pregnancy

In a cross-sectional study of 1000 women immediately postpartum, those who reported daily RLS symptoms in the last 3 months of pregnancy had a higher likelihood of gestational hypertension with adjusted odds ratios of 3.7 and 2.1 for chronic hypertension and pre-eclampsia, respectively [77, 80]. RLS has increased association with OSA leading to increased risk of HDP [74]. RLS and poor sleep have similar pro-inflammatory cytokine release and oxidative stress on the pregnant woman leading to risk of pre-eclampsia and eclampsia [74].

Insomnia and Pregnancy

Peripartum Mood Disorders: Depression and Anxiety

Perinatal depression can affect both the mother and newborn. Sleep deprivation, quality of sleep, and insomnia can potentiate the development of peripartum mood disorders such as depression. Perinatal depression has prevalence of 6.5%–12.9% among childbearing women [81]. These women have increased risk of recurrence of depression later in life of 20–40% [82]. The symptoms of depression in the mother include apathy, decreased appetite, anxiety, sleep disturbance, irritability, feelings of guilt, suicidal ideations, memory impairment, poor concentration, and decreased engagement with their infant [83]. These symptoms can present during pregnancy and persist up to one-year postpartum [84]. Many of the physiological changes in pregnancy, physical discomfort, and altered endogenous progesterone levels can lead to insomnia during pregnancy and in the postpartum months as well [84]. A study that included 1480 healthy mothers demonstrated that insomnia and short sleep duration were frequent symptoms prior to and after pregnancy [85]. Another large longitudinal, population-based study of 2088 gravid women found that insomnia may be a contributing risk factor for perinatal depression [86]. Depression in pregnancy can be attributed to fluctuations in hormone levels; however, one study found that poor sleep quality, but not the measured hormones (estradiol, prolactin or cortisol), was associated with recurrence of perinatal depression at 17 weeks postpartum [87]. In post-menopausal women the decrease in sleep and onset of insomnia are related to a decrease in annual estradiol levels [88]. When hormonal replacement therapy was implemented, women reported better sleep quality, decreased arousals, and longer duration of sleep [84]. This suggests there is interplay between poor sleep/insomnia and the dramatic decrease in hormones following delivery which may increase risk of perinatal depression. There is a need for more studies to elucidate the effect of insomnia on peripartum depression.

Postpartum Weight Retention

The role of sleep fragmentation in the peripartum is related to multiple variables including socio-economic factors and obesity. Postpartum weight retention (PPWR) is worsened by these factors and poor sleep quality [89]. In a study of over 500 women, a short sleep duration of 5 h or less predicted greater PPWR at 3 months [90]. Another study of 90 overweight and obese women ages 25–65 who completed a 7-month weight loss program found that those with greater sleep fragmentation displayed less weight loss [91]. It is postulated that during sleep the release of leptin, a satiety hormone, is increased and modulates metabolism. During periods of sleep fragmentation there is a decrease of leptin in the serum resulting in increased caloric intake and lowered adipose tissue metabolism in mouse models [89]. During pregnancy there is an increase in leptin levels; however, after delivery the leptin levels precipitously drop which may lead to more caloric intake and weight retention in postpartum women.

Consequences of Sleep Disorders During Pregnancy on the Fetus and Child

The adverse impact of sleep disorders during pregnancy on fetal outcomes is less defined compared to the maternal consequences. However, there is growing evidence to suggest that sleep disorders in pregnancy may have serious implications on the short- and long-term health of the neonate.

Maternal sleep disordered breathing (SDB) is associated with a 1.5–2 times increased risk of low birth weight (<tenth percentile) and small for gestational age infants [92]. The developing fetus needs a constant supply of nutrients, including oxygen. It is hypothesized that the intermittent episodes of hypoxemia and reoxygenation from SDB reduce the placental oxygen delivery to the fetus, causing fetal growth restriction (FGR). Some studies demonstrate that mothers with OSA who experienced nocturnal episodes of apnea also had concomitant prolonged fetal decelerations [93]. Moderate to severe SDB in pregnancy is linked to higher rates of preterm deliveries and admissions to neonatal intensive care units [92]. A recent retrospective study of 672 women identified by chart review showed a 1.3 and 1.5 times greater odds of preterm births in patients diagnosed with insomnia and sleep apnea, respectively [89].

On the other side of the spectrum of sleep disorders, restless leg syndrome (RLS) and insomnia also have a direct and indirect effect on fetal outcomes. Studies show an inverse relationship between severity of RLS and insomnia symptoms and neonatal birth weight and age of birth [77].

Sleep, specifically slow-wave sleep (SWS), is a physiologic necessity that is thought to be "restorative" in nature; it is an anabolic process that is essential for tissue and cell regeneration and is upregulated in times of stress like pregnancy. This theory is supported by the linear relationship between the amount of growth hormone (GH) secretion and the amount of slow-wave non-rapid-eye-movement (NREM) sleep one receives [77]. It is further demonstrated by the gradual decrease in SWS over an organism's lifespan, correlating with the decreased capacity to repair and regenerate cells as we age [77]. Understanding this, it is no surprise that poor sleep, either in quality, quantity, or continuity is associated with the negative health outcomes as described above [94]. Women who sleep less than 8 h a night during pregnancy have a 2.2 fold

increased risk of caesarian sections, preterm births, and low gestational weight when compared to women with unimpaired sleep patterns [95]. In addition, RLS and insomnia can indirectly impact the child by increasing the risk for perinatal depression, which can begin within pregnancy and persist up to 12 months postpartum [74]. Maternal depression has repeatedly been shown to have negative consequences on the overall cognitive and socioemotional development of an infant [81].

Clinical observations suggest sleep disorders in pregnancy are also associated with longer labor, higher risk pregnancies, and increased mortality risk; though, these claims have yet to be substantiated [95]. The long-term physiologic impact of sleep disorders in pregnancy on the child is still not well known and additional prospective evidence is needed to further investigate.

Nonpharmacological and Pharmacological Management of Sleep Disorders during Pregnancy

Management of Pre-Existing Sleep Disorders

Narcolepsy

Narcolepsy is a primary sleep disorder that affects the sleep-wake cycle with intrusion of REM and REM related muscle atonia into wakefulness which manifests as excessive daytime sleepiness (EDS), and episodes of muscle paralysis or loss in muscle tone while awake termed cataplexy. Narcolepsy with cataplexy or type 1 Narcolepsy is due to a deficiency in the neurotransmitter Orexin [96]. Onset of narcolepsy is usually in early teens and therefore can commonly be seen in young women of child-bearing age. Management of narcolepsy is usually with stimulant medications such as modafinil and amphetamines for the excessive daytime sleepiness, while cataplexy is treated with sodium oxybate and selective serotonin reuptake inhibitors (SSRI) or tricyclic antidepressants (TCA) that act to suppress REM episodes [96]. Due to the concerns for the teratogenicity of the medications, non-pharmacological treatment, discussed below, remains first line of treatment of symptoms in patients with narcolepsy [97].

1. Scheduled naps: EDS, the main symptom of narcolepsy, leads to impaired daytime performance [97]. A scheduled nap can help to alleviate the EDS. The exact duration and number of naps varies throughout the literature. Two afternoon scheduled naps of 15–30 minutes duration improves mean wakefulness time, increases alertness, and promotes sleep latency times. Similarly, an hour-long nap about 180 degree out of phase with nocturnal midsleep results in improved performance [98].
2. Sleep hygiene: Restful nocturnal sleep is promoted by good sleep hygiene. Sleep hygiene includes:
   (a) Avoiding stimulants like caffeine close to bedtime and
   (b) Limiting use of electronic devices and blue light exposure close to bedtime.

Pharmacological Management

Pharmacological treatment for narcolepsy during pregnancy is challenging. There are limited data on the safety of the medications available. In about 60–80% of cases the physicians elect to discontinue the treatment during pregnancy [99]. All the groups of medications are pregnancy category C. Thus, all the medications remain second line of treatment. Medications used for narcolepsy is divided into wakefulness promoting agents and medications for cataplexy.

Wakefulness Promoting Agents

1. Caffeine: Caffeine can be used to promote wakefulness. Caffeine is equivalent to Modafinil in efficacy [100].
2. Amphetamines and similar agents:
   This group includes methylphenidate, amphetamines, and methylamphetamine. These stimulant group of drugs act at presynaptic dopamine (DA) transporters by competing with DA for uptake or transport into vesicles, thus increasing synaptic dopamine levels. At higher concentration, they can increase monoamine oxidase (MAO) levels by inhibiting its degradation.

   Amphetamines were traditionally used for narcolepsy in the past. Methamphetamine is derived by addition of a methyl group to amphetamine, which facilitates penetration across the blood–brain barrier. Methylphenidate is a derivative of amphetamine and is considered less potent than amphetamines.

   The adverse effects include higher potential for abuse and tachycardia, hypertension, and major cardiovascular side effects. There are conflicting reports on teratogenicity of the amphetamine groups. There have been reports of an increase in cardiac malformation with methylphenidate [101]. However, population-based epidemiological data from a Danish registry failed to show an increased risk of congenital malformation with these agents [102]. Although the risk described in other studies might have been falsely elevated due to confounding factors, there still remains a lack of safety data.
3. Non-amphetamine stimulant group
   Modafinil is the drug of choice for narcolepsy for treatment of EDS in non-pregnant patients [103]. Modafinil is a non-amphetamine wakefulness promoting agent. The drug blocks uptake of dopamine by acting on dopamine receptors. The drug also releases histamine from the tuberomammillary nucleus and increases hypocretin release from the hypothalamus. The drug has lesser abuse potential than amphetamine. The medication is normally started at 100–200 mg once per day with a maximum dose up to 400 mg/day.

   While there have been earlier reports that modafinil exposure in the first trimester leads to increased congenital abnormalities, a more recent report from Sweden did not show this association [104, 105]. Therefore, a decision with regard to the use of modafinil in pregnancy should be made after careful discussion with the patient, especially in the first trimester.

Armodafinil belongs to the same class as modafinil and has same mechanism of action. However, it is more potent and has a longer duration of action with a delayed peak onset. The main side effects of these non-amphetamines include nausea, headache, and insomnia.

Medications for Cataplexy

Gamma-hydroxybutyrate (GHB) Group:

Sodium Oxybate: The mechanism of action is unclear but it is said to act on the GHB and GABA-B receptors. It is the only FDA approved medication to treat cataplexy. It has effects on cataplexy, sleep paralysis, and nighttime sleep disturbances [106].

Other non-FDA Approved Medications

Tricyclic Antidepressants (TCAs)
The medications in this group are imipramine, protriptyline, clomipramine. This group of medications acts by increasing norepinephrine, serotonin, and dopamine concentration by reducing their uptake. TCAs in addition can also decrease sleep paralysis and hypnagogic hallucinations [107].

Selective Serotonin Reuptake Inhibitors (SSRIs)
SSRIs are less efficacious than TCAs. Fluoxetine is the commonly used SSRI and has less adverse effects compared to TCAs [108].

Management of Pregnancy Induced Sleep Disorders

Insomnia

Nonpharmacological Interventions

Nonpharmacological interventions remain the first line of treatment. Promotion of sleep hygiene, control of stimulation, and cognitive behavior therapy are some of the commonly employed nonpharmacological treatments.

Pharmacological Interventions

Medications are reserved for resistant cases. Medications used include:

1. Benzodiazepines (BZDs)
2. Non-BZD hypnotic agents
3. Melatonin receptor agonist: Ramelteon
4. Antidepressants
5. Antihistamines

BZDs are classified as group D and non-BZD hypnotics are classified as group C in terms of risk with regard to teratogenicity [109]. Although population-based studies failed to show increased major congenital risk with BZD and non-BZD, there are reports of preterm birth, cesarean delivery, small for gestational age, and low birth weight infants. Infant withdrawal syndrome has been reported with all of the above groups [109].

Melatonin has been reported to have protective effects on fetus, but the safety is yet to be determined [110].

Although used widely the safety profile of antihistamines is not clearly established.

Restless Leg Syndrome

Nonpharmacological Treatment

Although there is lack of data from controlled studies, the following nonpharmacological measures are recommended during pregnancy prior to pharmacological interventions [111].

While there is stronger evidence in the literature for some of these measures, others are recommended as part of general practice guidelines.

1. Exercise: Light to moderate exercise seems to alleviate the symptoms [112]
2. Yoga [74]
3. Stretches [74]
4. Sleep Hygiene: Promoting sleep hygiene measures [74]
5. Pneumatic Compression Stockings (PCP): PCP has shown to improve symptoms of

RLS. Thought to function through stimulation of endothelial cells and release of modulating mediators and promoting perfusion by relieving venous and lymphatic congestion [113].

6. Acupuncture [74]
7. Repetitive transcranial magnetic stimulation [74]

Pharmacological Intervention

Iron supplementation is recommended in all patients with low ferritin [74]. There is limited evidence supporting supplementation of iron if patient does not have low ferritin.

Other Medications

1. Dopaminergic agents.
   (a) Non-Ergot Dopaminergic Agents: These are first line agents in treatment of RLS [114]. Ropinirole and pramipexole have not shown to increase fetal malformations based on few case reports. However, there is insufficient safety data on use of these medications in pregnancy [111].
   (b) Levodopa: Levodopa/carbidopa combination therapy can be useful in refractory cases. Levodopa taken during the pregnancy did not show increased risk of teratogenicity [111].
   (c) Ergot-Derived Dopaminergic Agents: Includes drugs such as bromocriptine and cabergoline. This group of medications is not reported to have adverse effects on the fetus [111].

   Adverse effects of dopaminergic agonists include transient lightheadedness, fatigue, insomnia, increased impulse control disorder, and augmentation. Augmentation refers to worsening or increasing symptoms or decreased latency of symptom appearance. It is important to rule out other causes of worsening symptoms such as iron deficiency and lifestyle changes. The treatment options for augmentation include splitting the medication into two doses, using an extending release medication, or switching to an alpha-2-delta calcium channel ligand [114].

2. Benzodiazepines: Clonazepam is the commonest benzodiazepine prescribed for RLS. However, there is a risk of neonatal withdrawal and issues related to medication tolerance limit long-term use [115].

3. Alpha-2-Delta Calcium Ligands: Includes drugs such as gabapentin and pregabalin. These medications may be particularly helpful if patient has concurrent neuropathy or chronic pain syndrome or in patients with impulse control disorders. However, there are some reports of developmental delay/impairment in animal studies. The risks during human pregnancy are unknown [116].

Table 29.2 summarizes all of the nonpharmacological and pharmacological approaches to management of sleep disorders during pregnancy.

Management of SDB

Pregnant patients with symptoms suspicious of OSA should be referred for sleep study and should be treated appropriately. Although there are no randomized trials on the safety of CPAP in pregnancy, it is generally considered safe [117]. Patients with diagnosed OSA should be treated with CPAP with goal of normalizing the AHI and sleep patterns. Peripartum care should include close observation for opioid-induced respiratory depression and hypoventilation. In patients with severe OSA, comorbid cardiovascular disease should be ruled out.

Table 29.2 Management of sleep disorders in pregnancy, pregnancy risk category of pharmacological agents, and reported pregnancy and fetal risk

Insomnia		Pregnancy category	Pregnancy and fetal risk
Nonpharmacological measures	Cognitive behavioral therapy		
	Sleep hygiene		
Benzodiazepines	Oxazepam Lorazepam Flurazepam Temazepam	C	May increase risk of cleft palate, cleft lip Increased preterm delivery
	Zolpidem-B	B	Increased preterm delivery, low birth weight
Non-benzodiazepine hypnotics	Cyclopyrrolones: Zopiclone Eszopiclone	C	
Antidepressants	Trazadone	C	Unknown
	Fluoxetine	C	Cardiovascular defects Cranial abnormalities

Restless leg syndrome		Pregnancy category	Teratogenicity
Nonpharmacological measures	Aerobic exercises Pneumatic compression stockings Stretches Acupuncture Transcranial magnetic stimulation Sleep hygiene		
Non-ergot dopaminergic agents	Levodopa	B	
	Ropinirole Pramipexole Rotigotine	C	Insufficient data
Ergot dopaminergic agents	Bromocriptine Pergolide Cabergoline	B	Fibrotic reactions
Benzodiazepine	Clonazepam	C	Newborn hypotonia Fetal distress
Antiepileptic agents	Gabapentin Carbamazepine	C	Low birth weight

References

1. Mindell JA, Cook RA, Nikolovski J. Sleep patterns and sleep disturbances across pregnancy. Sleep Med. 2015;16(4):483–8.
2. Lee KA. Self-reported sleep disturbances in employed women. Sleep. 1992;15(6):493–8.
3. Buysse DJ, Reynolds CF 3rd, Monk TH, Berman SR, Kupfer DJ. The Pittsburgh sleep quality index: a new instrument for psychiatric practice and research. Psychiatry Res. 1989;28(2):193–213.
4. Gay CL, Lee KA, Lee SY. Sleep patterns and fatigue in new mothers and fathers. Biol Res Nurs. 2004;5(4):311–8.
5. Lee KA, Gay CL. Sleep in late pregnancy predicts length of labor and type of delivery. Am J Obstet Gynecol. 2004;191(6):2041–6.
6. Kamysheva E, Skouteris H, Wertheim EH, Paxton SJ, Milgrom J. A prospective investigation of the relationships among sleep quality, physical symptoms, and depressive symptoms during pregnancy. J Affect Disord. 2010;123(1–3):317–20.

7. Okun ML, Hall M, Coussons-Read ME. Sleep disturbances increase interleukin-6 production during pregnancy: implications for pregnancy complications. Reprod Sci. 2007;14(6):560–7.
8. Greenwood KM, Hazendonk KM. Self-reported sleep during the third trimester of pregnancy. Behav Sleep Med. 2004;2(4):191–204.
9. Dorheim SK, Bondevik GT, Eberhard-Gran M, Bjorvatn B. Subjective and objective sleep among depressed and non-depressed postnatal women. Acta Psychiatr Scand. 2009;119(2):128–36.
10. Matsumoto K, Shinkoda H, Kang MJ, Seo YJ. Longitudinal study of mothers' sleep-wake behaviors and circadian time patterns from late pregnancy to postpartum—monitoring of wrist Actigraphy and sleep logs. Biol Rhythm Res. 2003;34(3):265–78.
11. Swain AM, O'Hara MW, Starr KR, Gorman LL. A prospective study of sleep, mood, and cognitive function in postpartum and nonpostpartum women. Obstet Gynecol. 1997;90(3):381–6.
12. Signal TL, Gander PH, Sangalli MR, Travier N, Firestone RT, Tuohy JF. Sleep duration and quality in healthy nulliparous and multiparous women across pregnancy and post-partum. Aust N Z J Obstet Gynaecol. 2007;47(1):16–22.
13. Morgenthaler T, Alessi C, Friedman L, Owens J, Kapur V, Boehlecke B, et al. Practice parameters for the use of actigraphy in the assessment of sleep and sleep disorders: an update for 2007. Sleep. 2007;30(4):519–29.
14. Coo S, Milgrom J, Trinder J. Mood and objective and subjective measures of sleep during late pregnancy and the postpartum period. Behav Sleep Med. 2014;12(4):317–30.
15. Bei B, Milgrom J, Ericksen J, Trinder J. Subjective perception of sleep, but not its objective quality, is associated with immediate postpartum mood disturbances in healthy women. Sleep. 2010;33(4):531–8.
16. Berndt C, Diekelmann S, Alexander N, Pustal A, Kirschbaum C. Sleep fragmentation and false memories during pregnancy and motherhood. Behav Brain Res. 2014;266:52–7.
17. Lee KA, Zaffke ME, McEnany G. Parity and sleep patterns during and after pregnancy. Obstet Gynecol. 2000;95(1):14–8.
18. Driver HS, Shapiro CM. A longitudinal study of sleep stages in young women during pregnancy and postpartum. Sleep. 1992;15(5):449–53.
19. Brunner DP, Munch M, Biedermann K, Huch R, Huch A, Borbely AA. Changes in sleep and sleep electroencephalogram during pregnancy. Sleep. 1994;17(7):576–82.
20. Schorr SJ, Chawla A, Devidas M, Sullivan CA, Naef RW 3rd, Morrison JC. Sleep patterns in pregnancy: a longitudinal study of polysomnography recordings during pregnancy. J Perinatol. 1998;18(6 Pt 1):427–30.
21. Ekholm EM, Polo O, Rauhala ER, Ekblad UU. Sleep quality in preeclampsia. Am J Obstet Gynecol. 1992;167(5):1262–6.
22. Dunlap JC, Loros JJ, DeCoursey PJ. Chronobiology: biological timekeeping. Sunderland, MA: Sinauer Associates; 2004.
23. Nakamura Y, Tamura H, Kashida S, Takayama H, Yamagata Y, Karube A, et al. Changes of serum melatonin level and its relationship to feto-placental unit during pregnancy. J Pineal Res. 2001;30(1):29–33.
24. Graf AH, Nutter W, Hacker GW, Steiner H, Anderson V, Staudach A, et al. Localization and distribution of vasoactive neuropeptides in the human placenta. Placenta. 1996;17(7):413–21.
25. Simonneaux V, Kienlen-Campard P, Loeffler JP, Basille M, Gonzalez BJ, Vaudry H, et al. Pharmacological, molecular and functional characterization of vasoactive intestinal polypeptide/pituitary adenylate cyclase-activating polypeptide receptors in the rat pineal gland. Neuroscience. 1998;85(3):887–96.
26. Swaab DF, Zhou JN, Ehlhart T, Hofman MA. Development of vasoactive intestinal polypeptide neurons in the human suprachiasmatic nucleus in relation to birth and sex. Dev Brain Res. 1994;79(2):249–59.
27. Martin-Fairey CA, Zhao P, Wan L, Roenneberg T, Fay J, Ma X, et al. Pregnancy induces an earlier Chronotype in both mice and women. J Biol Rhythm. 2019;34(3):323–31.
28. Nolten WE, Lindheimer MD, Rueckert PA, Oparil S, Ehrlich EN. Diurnal patterns and regulation of cortisol secretion in pregnancy*. J Clin Endocrinol Metabol. 1980;51(3):466–72.
29. Matthews SG, Owen D, Kalabis G, Banjanin S, Setiawan EB, Dunn EA, et al. Fetal glucocorticoid exposure and Hypothalamo-pituitary-adrenal (HPA) function after birth. Endocr Res. 2004;30(4):827–36.
30. Bourjeily G. Sleep disorders in pregnancy. Obstet Med. 2009;2(3):100–6.
31. Sedov ID, Cameron EE, Madigan S, Tomfohr-Madsen LM. Sleep quality during pregnancy: a meta-analysis. Sleep Med Rev. 2018;38:168–76.
32. Izci BB. Sleep disordered breathing in pregnancy. Breathe. 2015;11(4):268–77.
33. Robertson NT, Turner JM, Kumar S. Pathophysiological changes associated with sleep disordered breathing and supine sleep position in pregnancy. Sleep Med Rev. 2019;46:1–8.
34. Gooley JJ, Mohapatra L, Twan DCK. The role of sleep duration and sleep disordered breathing in gestational diabetes mellitus. Neurobiol Sleep Circadian Rhythms. 2018;4:34–43.
35. Sarberg M, Svanborg E, Wiréhn A-B, Josefsson A. Snoring during pregnancy and its relation to sleepiness and pregnancy outcome—a prospective study. BMC Pregnancy Childbirth. 2014;14:15.

36. Pien GW, Pack AI, Jackson N, Maislin G, Macones GA, Schwab RJ. Risk factors for sleep-disordered breathing in pregnancy. Thorax. 2014;69(4):371–7.

37. Johns EC, Denison FC, Reynolds RM. Sleep disordered breathing in pregnancy: a review of the pathophysiology of adverse pregnancy outcomes. Acta Physiol. 2020;229(2):e13458.

38. Heslehurst N, Rankin J, Wilkinson JR, Summerbell CD. A nationally representative study of maternal obesity in England, UK: trends in incidence and demographic inequalities in 619 323 births, 1989-2007. Int J Obes. 2010;34(3):420–8.

39. Luque-Fernandez MA, Bain PA, Gelaye B, Redline S, Williams MA. Sleep-disordered breathing and gestational diabetes mellitus a meta-analysis of 9,795 participants enrolled in epidemiological observational studies. Diabetes Care. 2013;36(10):3353–60.

40. Reutrakul S, Zaidi N, Wroblewski K, Kay HH, Ismail M, Ehrmann DA, et al. Sleep disturbances and their relationship to glucose tolerance in pregnancy. Diabetes Care. 2011;34(11):2454–7.

41. Louis JM, Mogos MF, Salemi JL, Redline S, Salihu HM. Obstructive sleep apnea and severe maternal-infant morbidity/mortality in the United States, 1998-2009. Sleep. 2014;37(5):843–9.

42. Xu T, Feng Y, Peng H, Guo D, Li T. Obstructive sleep apnea and the risk of perinatal outcomes: a meta-analysis of cohort studies. Sci Rep. 2014;4(1):6982.

43. Wieser V, Moschen AR, Tilg H. Inflammation, cytokines and insulin resistance: a clinical perspective. Arch Immunol Ther Exp. 2013;61(2):119–25.

44. Fialová L, Malbohan I, Kalousová M, Soukupová J, Krofta L, Stípek S, et al. Oxidative stress and inflammation in pregnancy. Scand J Clin Lab Invest. 2006;66(2):121–7.

45. Karacay O, Sepici-Dincel A, Karcaaltincaba D, Sahin D, Yalvaç S, Akyol M, et al. A quantitative evaluation of total antioxidant status and oxidative stress markers in preeclampsia and gestational diabetic patients in 24-36 weeks of gestation. Diabetes Res Clin Pract. 2010;89(3):231–8.

46. Esposito K, Nappo F, Marfella R, Giugliano G, Giugliano F, Ciotola M, et al. Inflammatory cytokine concentrations are acutely increased by hyperglycemia in humans. Circulation. 2002;106(16):2067–72.

47. Spiegel K, Leproult R, L'Hermite-Balériaux M, Copinschi G, Penev PD, Van Cauter E. Leptin levels are dependent on sleep duration: relationships with sympathovagal balance, carbohydrate regulation, cortisol, and thyrotropin. J Clin Endocrinol Metab. 2004;89(11):5762–71.

48. Kirwan JP, Hauguel-De Mouzon S, Lepercq J, Challier J-C, Huston-Presley L, Friedman JE, et al. TNF-α is a predictor of insulin resistance in human pregnancy. Diabetes. 2002;51(7):2207–13.

49. Xu J, Zhao YH, Chen YP, Yuan XL, Wang J, Zhu H, et al. Maternal circulating concentrations of tumor necrosis factor-alpha, leptin, and adiponectin in gestational diabetes mellitus: a systematic review and meta-analysis. ScientificWorldJournal. 2014;2014:926932.

50. Nedeltcheva AV, Kessler L, Imperial J, Penev PD. Exposure to recurrent sleep restriction in the setting of high caloric intake and physical inactivity results in increased insulin resistance and reduced glucose tolerance. J Clin Endocrinol Metab. 2009;94(9):3242–50.

51. Rizza RA, Mandarino LJ, Gerich JE. Cortisol-induced insulin resistance in man: impaired suppression of glucose production and stimulation of glucose utilization due to a postreceptor detect of insulin action. J Clin Endocrinol Metab. 1982;54(1):131–8.

52. Say L, Chou D, Gemmill A, Tunçalp Ö, Moller AB, Daniels J, et al. Global causes of maternal death: a WHO systematic analysis. Lancet Glob Health. 2014;2(6):e323–33.

53. Dominguez JE, Habib AS, Krystal AD. A review of the associations between obstructive sleep apnea and hypertensive disorders of pregnancy and possible mechanisms of disease. Sleep Med Rev. 2018;42:37–46.

54. Bellamy L, Casas JP, Hingorani AD, Williams DJ. Pre-eclampsia and risk of cardiovascular disease and cancer in later life: systematic review and meta-analysis. BMJ. 2007;335(7627):974.

55. Bourjeily G, Danilack VA, Bublitz MH, Lipkind H, Muri J, Caldwell D, et al. Obstructive sleep apnea in pregnancy is associated with adverse maternal outcomes: a national cohort. Sleep Med. 2017;38:50–7.

56. Champagne K, Schwartzman K, Opatrny L, Barriga P, Morin L, Mallozzi A, et al. Obstructive sleep apnoea and its association with gestational hypertension. Eur Respir J. 2009;33(3):559–65.

57. Facco FL, Parker CB, Reddy UM, Silver RM, Louis JM, Basner RC, et al. NuMoM2b sleep-disordered breathing study: objectives and methods. Am J Obstet Gynecol. 2015;212(4):542.e1–127.

58. O'Brien LM, Bullough AS, Chames MC, Shelgikar AV, Armitage R, Guilleminualt C, et al. Hypertension, snoring, and obstructive sleep apnoea during pregnancy: a cohort study. BJOG. 2014;121(13):1685–93.

59. Lockhart EM, Ben Abdallah A, Tuuli MG, Leighton BL. Obstructive sleep apnea in pregnancy: assessment of current screening tools. Obstet Gynecol. 2015;126(1):93–102.

60. Milne F, Redman C, Walker J, Baker P, Bradley J, Cooper C, et al. The pre-eclampsia community guideline (PRECOG): how to screen for and detect onset of pre-eclampsia in the community. BMJ. 2005;330(7491):576–80.

61. Zamudio S, Wu Y, Ietta F, Rolfo A, Cross A, Wheeler T, et al. Human placental hypoxia-inducible factor-1alpha expression correlates with clinical outcomes in chronic hypoxia in vivo. Am J Pathol. 2007;170(6):2171–9.

62. Nanduri J, Peng Y-J, Yuan G, Kumar GK, Prabhakar NR. Hypoxia-inducible factors and hypertension:

lessons from sleep apnea syndrome. J Mol Med (Berl). 2015;93(5):473–80.

63. Ravishankar S, Bourjeily G, Lambert-Messerlian G, He M, De Paepe ME, Gündoğan F. Evidence of placental hypoxia in maternal sleep disordered breathing. Pediatr Dev Pathol. 2015;18(5):380–6.

64. Leon-Garcia SM, Roeder HA, Nelson KK, Liao X, Pizzo DP, Laurent LC, et al. Maternal obesity and sex-specific differences in placental pathology. Placenta. 2016;38:33–40.

65. Sharma S, Norris WE, Kalkunte S. Beyond the threshold: an etiological bridge between hypoxia and immunity in preeclampsia. J Reprod Immunol. 2010;85(1):112–6.

66. de Lima FF, Mazzotti DR, Tufik S, Bittencourt L. The role inflammatory response genes in obstructive sleep apnea syndrome: a review. Sleep Breath. 2016;20(1):331–8.

67. Venkatesha S, Toporsian M, Lam C, Hanai J, Mammoto T, Kim YM, et al. Soluble endoglin contributes to the pathogenesis of preeclampsia. Nat Med. 2006;12(6):642–9.

68. Ciccone MM, Favale S, Scicchitano P, Mangini F, Mitacchione G, Gadaleta F, et al. Reversibility of the endothelial dysfunction after CPAP therapy in OSAS patients. Int J Cardiol. 2012;158(3):383–6.

69. Campos-Rodriguez F, Queipo-Corona C, Carmona-Bernal C, Jurado-Gamez B, Cordero-Guevara J, Reyes-Nunez N, et al. Continuous positive airway pressure improves quality of life in women with obstructive sleep apnea. A randomized controlled trial. Am J Respir Crit Care Med. 2016;194(10):1286–94.

70. Antic NA, Catcheside P, Buchan C, Hensley M, Naughton MT, Rowland S, et al. The effect of CPAP in normalizing daytime sleepiness, quality of life, and neurocognitive function in patients with moderate to severe OSA. Sleep. 2011;34(1):111–9.

71. Whitehead C, Tong S, Wilson D, Howard M, Walker SP. Treatment of early-onset preeclampsia with continuous positive airway pressure. Obstet Gynecol. 2015;125(5):1106–9.

72. Aurora RN, Kristo DA, Bista SR, Rowley JA, Zak RS, Casey KR, et al. The treatment of restless legs syndrome and periodic limb movement disorder in adults—an update for 2012: practice parameters with an evidence-based systematic review and meta-analyses: an American Academy of Sleep Medicine Clinical Practice Guideline. Sleep. 2012;35(8):1039–62.

73. Manconi M, Govoni V, De Vito A, Economou NT, Cesnik E, Mollica G, et al. Pregnancy as a risk factor for restless legs syndrome. Sleep Med. 2004;5(3):305–8.

74. Garbazza C, Manconi M. Management strategies for restless legs syndrome/Willis-Ekbom disease during pregnancy. Sleep Med Clin. 2018;13(3):335–48.

75. Chen SJ, Shi L, Bao YP, Sun YK, Lin X, Que JY, et al. Prevalence of restless legs syndrome during pregnancy: a systematic review and meta-analysis. Sleep Med Rev. 2018;40:43–54.

76. Wesström J, Skalkidou A, Manconi M, Fulda S, Sundström-Poromaa I. Pre-pregnancy restless legs syndrome (Willis-Ekbom disease) is associated with perinatal depression. J Clin Sleep Med. 2014;10(5):527–33.

77. Bazalakova M. Sleep disorders in pregnancy. Semin Neurol. 2017;37(6):661–8.

78. Terzi H, Terzi R, Zeybek B, Ergenoglu M, Hacivelioglu S, Akdemir A, et al. Restless legs syndrome is related to obstructive sleep apnea symptoms during pregnancy. Sleep Breath. 2015;19(1):73–8.

79. Innes KE, Kandati S, Flack KL, Agarwal P, Selfe TK. The Association of Restless legs syndrome to history of gestational diabetes in an appalachian primary care population. J Clin Sleep Med. 2015;11(10):1121–30.

80. Lawson A, Parmar R, Sloan EP. Sleep disorders. In: Uguz F, Orsolini L, editors. Perinatal psychopharmacology. Cham: Springer; 2019. p. 341–76.

81. Emamian F, Khazaie H, Okun ML, Tahmasian M, Sepehry AA. Link between insomnia and perinatal depressive symptoms: a meta-analysis. J Sleep Res. 2019;28(6):e12858.

82. Gaynes BN, Gavin N, Meltzer-Brody S, Lohr KN, Swinson T, Gartlehner G, et al. Perinatal depression: prevalence, screening accuracy, and screening outcomes. Evid Rep Technol Assess (Summ). 2005;119:1–8.

83. Behrendt HF, Konrad K, Goecke TW, Fakhrabadi R, Herpertz-Dahlmann B, Firk C. Postnatal mother-to-infant attachment in subclinically depressed mothers: dyads at risk? Psychopathology. 2016;49(4):269–76.

84. Okun ML. Sleep and postpartum depression. Curr Opin Psychiatry. 2015;28(6):490–6.

85. Sivertsen B, Hysing M, Dorheim SK, Eberhard-Gran M. Trajectories of maternal sleep problems before and after childbirth: a longitudinal population-based study. BMC Pregnancy Childbirth. 2015;15:129.

86. Dorheim SK, Bjorvatn B, Eberhard-Gran M. Can insomnia in pregnancy predict postpartum depression? A longitudinal, population-based study. PLoS One. 2014;9(4):e94674.

87. Okun ML, Luther J, Prather AA, Perel JM, Wisniewski S, Wisner KL. Changes in sleep quality, but not hormones predict time to postpartum depression recurrence. J Affect Disord. 2011;130(3):378–84.

88. Hachul H, Bittencourt LR, Andersen ML, Haidar MA, Baracat EC, Tufik S. Effects of hormone therapy with estrogen and/or progesterone on sleep pattern in postmenopausal women. Int J Gynaecol Obstet. 2008;103(3):207–12.

89. Christian LM, Carroll JE, Teti DM, Hall MH. Maternal sleep in pregnancy and postpartum part I: mental, physical, and interpersonal consequences. Curr Psychiatry Rep. 2019;21(3):20.

90. Siega-Riz AM, Herring AH, Carrier K, Evenson KR, Dole N, Deierlein A. Sociodemographic, perinatal, behavioral, and psychosocial predictors of weight retention at 3 and 12 months postpartum. Obesity (Silver Spring). 2010;18(10):1996–2003.

91. Wang Y, Carreras A, Lee S, Hakim F, Zhang SX, Nair D, et al. Chronic sleep fragmentation promotes obesity in young adult mice. Obesity (Silver Spring). 2014;22(3):758–62.

92. Dominguez JE, Street L, Louis J. Management of Obstructive Sleep Apnea in pregnancy. Obstet Gynecol Clin N Am. 2018;45(2):233–47.

93. Johnson SM, Randhawa KS, Epstein JJ, Gustafson E, Hocker AD, Huxtable AG, et al. Gestational intermittent hypoxia increases susceptibility to neuroinflammation and alters respiratory motor control in neonatal rats. Respir Physiol Neurobiol. 2018;256:128–42.

94. Bacaro V, Benz F, Pappaccogli A, De Bartolo P, Johann AF, Palagini L, et al. Interventions for sleep problems during pregnancy: a systematic review. Sleep Med Rev. 2020;50:101234.

95. Silva-Perez LJ, Gonzalez-Cardenas N, Surani S, Etindele Sosso FA, Surani SR. Socioeconomic status in pregnant women and sleep quality during pregnancy. Cureus. 2019;11(11):e6183.

96. Thorpy MJ, Bogan RK. Update on the pharmacologic management of narcolepsy: mechanisms of action and clinical implications. Sleep Med. 2020;68:97–109.

97. Miller MA, Mehta N, Clark-Bilodeau C, Bourjeily G. Sleep pharmacotherapy for common sleep disorders in pregnancy and lactation. Chest. 2020;157(1):184–97.

98. Mullington J, Broughton R. Scheduled naps in the management of daytime sleepiness in narcolepsy-cataplexy. Sleep. 1993;16(5):444–56.

99. Thorpy M, Zhao CG, Dauvilliers Y. Management of narcolepsy during pregnancy. Sleep Med. 2013;14(4):367–76.

100. Wesensten NJ, Killgore WD, Balkin TJ. Performance and alertness effects of caffeine, dextroamphetamine, and modafinil during sleep deprivation. J Sleep Res. 2005;14(3):255–66.

101. Huybrechts KF, Bröms G, Christensen LB, Einarsdóttir K, Engeland A, Furu K, et al. Association between methylphenidate and amphetamine use in pregnancy and risk of congenital malformations: a cohort study from the international pregnancy safety study consortium. JAMA Psychiat. 2018;75(2):167–75.

102. Pottegård A, Hallas J, Andersen JT, Løkkegaard EC, Dideriksen D, Aagaard L, et al. First-trimester exposure to methylphenidate: a population-based cohort study. J Clin Psychiatry. 2014;75(1):e88–93.

103. Kallweit U, Bassetti CL. Pharmacological management of narcolepsy with and without cataplexy. Expert Opin Pharmacother. 2017;18(8):809–17.

104. Cesta CE, Engeland A, Karlsson P, Kieler H, Reutfors J, Furu K. Incidence of malformations after early pregnancy exposure to Modafinil in Sweden and Norway. JAMA. 2020;324(9):895–7.

105. Damkier P, Broe A. First-trimester pregnancy exposure to modafinil and risk of congenital malformations. JAMA. 2020;323(4):374–6.

106. Abad VC. An evaluation of sodium oxybate as a treatment option for narcolepsy. Expert Opin Pharmacother. 2019;20(10):1189–99.

107. De la Herrán-Arita AK, García-García F. Current and emerging options for the drug treatment of narcolepsy. Drugs. 2013;73(16):1771–81.

108. Gowda CR, Lundt LP. Mechanism of action of narcolepsy medications. CNS Spectr. 2014;19(Suppl 1):25–33; quiz 25–7, 34.

109. Shyken JM, Babbar S, Babbar S, Forinash A. Benzodiazepines in Pregnancy. Clin Obstet Gynecol. 2019;62(1):156–67.

110. Wilkinson D, Shepherd E, Wallace EM. Melatonin for women in pregnancy for neuroprotection of the fetus. Cochrane Database Syst Rev. 2016;3(3):Cd010527.

111. Picchietti DL, Hensley JG, Bainbridge JL, Lee KA, Manconi M, McGregor JA, et al. Consensus clinical practice guidelines for the diagnosis and treatment of restless legs syndrome/Willis-Ekbom disease during pregnancy and lactation. Sleep Med Rev. 2015;22:64–77.

112. Giannaki CD, Sakkas GK, Karatzaferi C, Hadjigeorgiou GM, Lavdas E, Kyriakides T, et al. Effect of exercise training and dopamine agonists in patients with uremic restless legs syndrome: a six-month randomized, partially double-blind, placebo-controlled comparative study. BMC Nephrol. 2013;14:194.

113. Lettieri CJ, Eliasson AH. Pneumatic compression devices are an effective therapy for restless legs syndrome: a prospective, randomized, double-blinded, sham-controlled trial. Chest. 2009;135(1):74–80.

114. Silber MH, Becker PM, Earley C, Garcia-Borreguero D, Ondo WG. Willis-Ekbom disease foundation revised consensus statement on the management of restless legs syndrome. Mayo Clin Proc. 2013;88(9):977–86.

115. McElhatton PR. The effects of benzodiazepine use during pregnancy and lactation. Reprod Toxicol. 1994;8(6):461–75.

116. Patorno E, Hernandez-Diaz S, Huybrechts KF, Desai RJ, Cohen JM, Mogun H, et al. Gabapentin in pregnancy and the risk of adverse neonatal and maternal outcomes: a population-based cohort study nested in the US Medicaid analytic eXtract dataset. PLoS Med. 2020;17(9):e1003322.

117. Blyton DM, Skilton MR, Edwards N, Hennessy A, Celermajer DS, Sullivan CE. Treatment of sleep disordered breathing reverses low fetal activity levels in preeclampsia. Sleep. 2013;36(1):15–21.

Otologic and Neurotologic Disorders in Pregnancy

David Y. Goldrich, Seth J. Barishansky, and P. Ashley Wackym

Introduction

This chapter is important because of the overlap in otologic and neurotologic symptoms during pregnancy and need for co-management. The physiologic changes during pregnancy altering metabolism, autonomic function, hormonal changes, and emotional stress can impact the hearing and balance systems and manifest as audiologic and vestibular symptoms such as hearing loss, aural fullness, tinnitus, and vertigo [1]. However, the obstetrician acting as primary care provider during pregnancy may be less familiar with diagnosis and management of otologic and neurotologic disorders; for example, morning sickness is a common disorder in first trimester pregnancy, yet may be challenging to distinguish from nausea associated with an acute vertigo attack. Conversely, while the otologist and neurotologist are familiar with diagnosing and treating hearing and balance disorders as well as cranial nerve pathologies, they may be less familiar with their association with physiologic changes of pregnancy or safety guidelines for therapeutic options during pregnancy [2]; many may default to opt against treatment altogether out of consideration for the challenges of maternal and fetal risk. Therefore, it is important to review select otologic and neurotologic disorders and complaints that may present during pregnancy and examine available treatment options. The highest prevalence of up to 22% is seen among the <29 age group [3].

Menière Disease/Endolymphatic Hydrops

Menière disease is an otologic disorder characterized by the classic triad of spontaneous bouts of true rotational vertigo associated with low-frequency sensorineural hearing loss and tinnitus. A fourth symptom is aural pressure and fullness, which reflects endolymphatic hydrops. Menière disease most commonly presents in adults between ages 40 and 60, with U.S. prevalence approximately 190 per 100,000. Increased incidence is seen with aging and female gender, with one study reporting a 1.9:1 female:male ratio [4]. Menière disease is typically unilateral, though 24% of patients may be diagnosed with

D. Y. Goldrich
Department of Otolaryngology–Head and Neck Surgery, The Pennsylvania State University College of Medicine, Hershey, PA, USA

S. J. Barishansky
Department of Obstetrics and Gynecology, George Washington University School of Medicine and Health Sciences, Washington, DC, USA

P. A. Wackym (✉)
Department of Otolaryngology–Head and Neck Surgery, Rutgers Robert Wood Johnson Medical School, New Brunswick, NJ, USA
e-mail: ashley.wackym@rutgers.edu

bilateral Menière disease and 11% at presentation [5]. Bilateral disease is more common with family history of Menière disease and earlier age of disease onset [6]. The degenerative disease course can lead to permanent sensorineural hearing loss. Vertigo may spontaneously cease in over half of cases after 2 years and 71% at 8 years [7]. There is a great deal of clinical overlap between Menière disease and vestibular migraine which will be discussed later. It was in 1861 that Prosper Menière made the connection between the inner ear and vertigo with hearing loss; however, this was the same year that Abraham Lincoln was inaugurated as the 16th President of the USA. It has been suggested that Menière disease is actually vestibular migraine [8].

The pathogenesis of Menière disease remains unclear. Endolymphatic hydrops, or distention of the endolymphatic space within the inner ear, is observed in virtually all cases of Menière disease and degree of endolymphatic hydrops has been correlated to symptom severity, yet not all causes of endolymphatic hydrops develop Menière disease, leading to belief that it is a necessary but not sufficient component of Menière disease (Fig. 30.1) [9–11]. One theory holds that hydrops distension of the endolymphatic duct causes membrane rupture, allowing potassium-rich endolymph to leak in to the perilymphatic space and contact basilar hair cells, causing excitation and episodic vertigo due to rotational receptor asymmetric afferent input, while repeat exposure

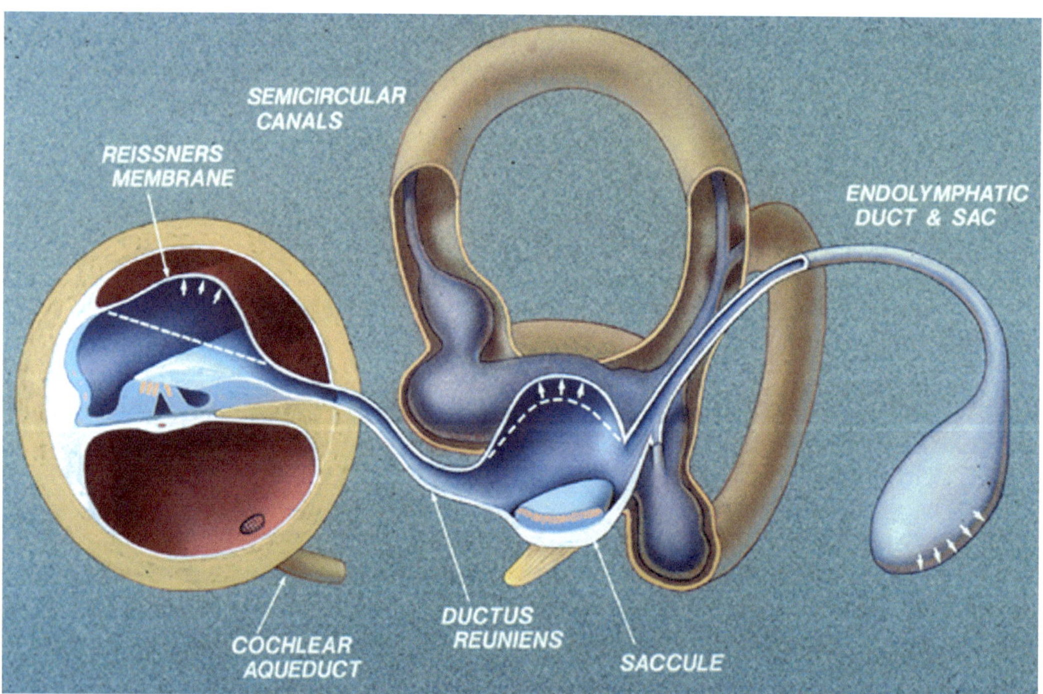

Fig. 30.1 Endolymphatic hydrops. The central compartment of the inner ear, the scala media, and endolymphatic duct is filled with a unique fluid of the body. It is high in potassium and low in sodium, whereas every other fluid in the body is high in sodium and low in potassium. This fluid composition is essential for the function and survival of the hair cells of the hearing and balance end-organs. With endolymphatic hydrops, Reissner membrane is distended from the normal position (dotted line) as highlighted by the small arrows within the cochlea. In addition, within the vestibular portion of the inner ear, in the vestibule where the gravitational (otolithic) receptors are located, endolymphatic hydrops results in distention as well (small arrows). The endolymphatic sac is both the site of the immunologic interface between the inner ear and the rest of the body, as well as being responsible for the absorption of endolymph produced within the inner ear. (Published with permission, Copyright © P.A. Wackym)

of vestibular hair cells to toxic levels of potassium-rich endolymph may cause longitudinal progressive hearing loss. However, more recent in vivo studies indicate this model may not adequately explain attacks and suggest a different theory involving excess endolymph forcing open the utriculo-endolymphatic valve due to high pressures, causing vertigo with fluid entry into the vestibule, cochlear fluid shift causing hearing symptoms, and oxidative stress causing long-term damage to inner ear structures [12]. A number of different contributing factors, including infection, autoimmunity, genetics, ischemia, vasospasm, mechanical dysfunction, and trauma have also been implicated in Menière disease, suggesting multifactorial etiology [12–15].

Typical clinical presentation of Menière disease consists of acute attacks of true vertigo (96.2%) lasting 20 min to 12 h, associated with unilateral hearing loss (87.7%) and ipsilateral non-pulsatile tinnitus (91.1%), as well as possible aural fullness [16]. Nausea, vomiting, perspiration, and diarrhea may accompany attacks, and intensification of tinnitus may precede attacks. Patients may initially present with only auditory or vestibular symptoms, though both are needed for eventual diagnosis [12]. Caffeine, sodium intake, stress, and changes in barometric pressure have been suggested as triggers of Menière disease attacks [17, 18]. Attacks may vary in frequency and severity, with normalized auditory and vestibular function between attacks. Symptoms may greatly affect quality of life, especially among patients with bilateral symptoms and progression to permanent hearing loss [19]. Less frequently and later in disease course, approximately 5% of patients may have dangerous "drop attacks," termed an otolithic crisis of Tumarkin, in which sudden otolithic asymmetry occurs and can result in falls [20].

Diagnosis can be made with clinical history fitting pattern of Menière disease, and physical exam, audiometric and vestibular testing can confirm diagnosis. Definitive diagnostic criteria include: (A) 2+ spontaneous vertigo episodes lasting 20 min to 12 h; (B) documented low-frequency sensorineural hearing loss >30 dB; (C) fluctuating aural symptoms in the affected ear;

and, (D) not better explained by another vestibular disorder (probable diagnostic criteria include A, C, and D).

Careful history-taking should distinguish Menière disease from alternative causes of episodic vertigo. Benign paroxysmal positional vertigo, third window syndrome, or perilymph fistula vertigo attacks should last only seconds-minutes; vestibular migraine attacks should be variable duration and have migraine features without hearing loss, although one-third of vestibular migraine patients have endolymphatic hydrops and some can also have sensorineural hearing loss caused by vestibular migraine attacks (see section "Vestibular Migraine"); vestibular neuritis (no hearing loss) or labyrinthitis (with hearing loss) should last >24 h; acoustic neuroma (vestibular schwannoma) or trauma can present with chronic symptoms. Bilateral vestibular loss is more common in ototoxicity, autoimmune inner ear disease, or familial disorders. Audiometric testing should be performed in all suspected Menière disease patients and shows a characteristic pattern of normal mid-frequency hearing with low-frequency or low- and high-frequency sensorineural hearing loss [21]. Physical examination should include cardiovascular and orthostatic blood pressure examination to rule out cardiogenic or hypovolemic-related dizziness, cranial nerve, cerebellar and gait examinations to rule out non-vestibular causes of vertigo, and otoscopy to rule out external or middle ear pathology. Weber and Rinne testing can identify patterns of hearing loss before audiometric studies are completed. Dix-Hallpike testing can rule out BPPV (Fig. 30.2). In Menière disease, physical exam findings are minimal between attacks and early in disease course. Vestibular testing via videonystagmography or video head-impulse testing may show weakened caloric response or decreased gain in the ipsilateral ear between attacks late in disease course. Though rarely presenting during active attacks, 60–70% of these patients exhibit head-shaking nystagmus and altered vestibulo-ocular reflexes on head-impulse tests (HIT) [22, 23]. Electrocochleography (ECoG) is highly specific for endolymphatic hydrops, which is also seen in Menière disease, and can be useful in confirming diagnosis in the

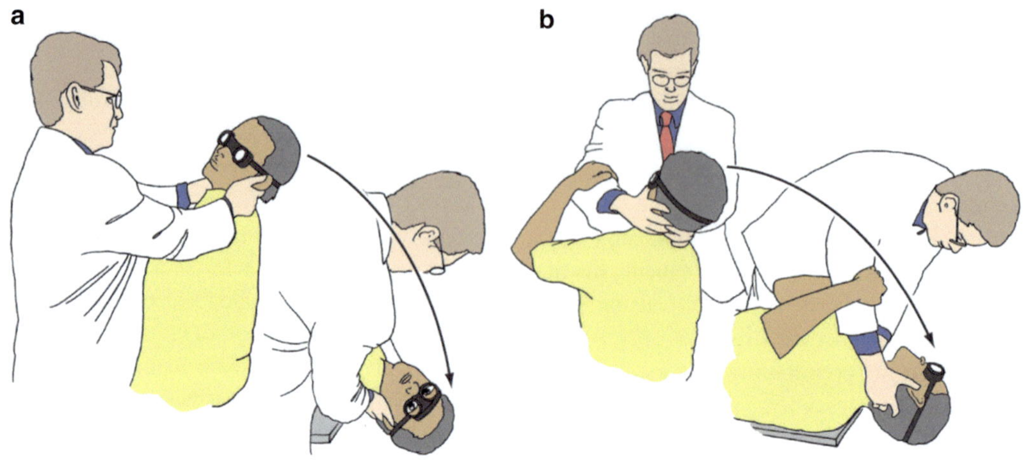

Fig. 30.2 Dix-Hallpike maneuver for the physical diagnosis of benign paroxysmal positional vertigo. In performing the Dix-Hallpike maneuver, the patient is taken rapidly from the sitting to the left head-hanging (**a**) and right head-hanging (**b**) positions. This maneuver elicits nystagmus characteristic of benign paroxysmal positional vertigo. (Published with permission, Copyright © P.A. Wackym)

setting of less clear findings [24]. Imaging is not routinely indicated, but MRI of the internal auditory canal with and without contrast may be indicated in the setting of unilateral tinnitus and/or asymmetric sensorineural hearing loss and/or sudden sensorineural hearing loss to rule out alternate diagnoses such as vestibular schwannoma (acoustic neuroma), aneurysm, multiple sclerosis, or Chiari malformation [25]. High resolution MRI after injection of gadolinium into the middle ear is sensitive for visualizing endolymphatic hydrops in Menière disease patients, but is not approved for this specific use by the United States Food and Drug Administration (FDA) [12]. Recently, 3T MRI with intravenous contrast has been reported to demonstrate endolymphatic hydrops and distention of the endolymphatic space that correlates with treatment and resolution of symptoms in Menière disease patients [26].

Due to unclear pathologic basis of Menière disease, treatment of Menière disease consists of symptomatic control rather than curative therapy. First-line therapy consists of lifestyle modification such as dietary sodium restriction (<1500 mg daily), adequate sleep, and trigger avoidance such as caffeine, stress, and barometric pressure changes [27]. Diuretics targeting fluid volume of endolymphatic hydrops are effective at limiting vertigo frequency, with possible benefits for long-term hearing deterioration [28]; common options include hydrochlorothiazide (HCTZ)-triamterene, acetazolamide, and spironolactone. Betahistine is commonly used in Europe to decrease vertigo attacks but is not approved for use by the FDA in the USA [29]. In the USA, betahistine is commonly prepared at compounding pharmacies or obtained from Canadian pharmacies. Symptoms of vertigo with acute Menière disease attacks can be treated with short-onset vestibular suppressants including benzodiazepines as a first-line treatment (diazepam, lorazepam, clonazepam), anticholinergics (scopolamine), and phenothiazine (promethazine) [27]. Meclizine, an antihistamine, should not be used due to lack of efficacy and adverse side effects. Nausea and vomiting can be treated with antiemetics including ondansetron and promethazine. Oral corticosteroids may be intermittently used for symptom exacerbation, though this is largely based on expert opinion without significant clinical trials [30, 31]. Due to association and increased incidence of migraine and allergy among Menière disease patients, adequate avoidance and prophylactic treatment of these disorders in comorbid patients can reduce frequency and severity of Menière disease attacks [12, 27, 32–35]. Vestibular rehabilitation therapy may be helpful as well, especially in later stages of Menière disease [36]. Hearing loss later in disease progression can be treated with hearing aids or cochlear implantation versus contralateral routing of signal (CROS) hearing aid system, depending on hearing preserved versus poor word recognition. Tinnitus can be managed as in other disorders with emotional distress reduction via cognitive behavioral therapy (CBT), yoga, biofeedback, and meditation [37], and sound therapy options including tinnitus maskers, white noise generators, hearing amplification, and cochlear implantation.

For patients with Menière disease symptoms uncontrolled with conservative medical therapy, vestibular and hearing preservation techniques (intratympanic steroid injection, endolymphatic sac decompression) and secondarily with vestibular ablation techniques (intratympanic gentamicin injection, labyrinthectomy, and vestibular nerve section) are potential options [38]. Patients may escalate through these options as needed, but with careful decision-making emphasizing hearing preservation in bilateral Menière disease [38]. Like oral corticosteroid treatment, intratympanic corticosteroid injection is an available outpatient option for use while maintaining medical therapy to decrease Menière disease symptoms, but without systemic side effects; injections have been shown some efficacy in improving Menière disease symptoms and can be repeated as needed. Endolymphatic sac decompression, in which a transmastoid craniectomy is performed to expose the posterior fossa dura and isolate the extradural endolymphatic sac, reduces endolymphatic pressure by removing the bony covering and allowing expansion or opening of the endolymphatic sac and perfusing corticosteroids. Historically, endolymphatic sac shunt placement for drainage was popular before ultrastructural study revealed that the endolymphatic sac is a series of tubules rather than a sac with a single lumen [39–41]. A meta-analysis showed endolymphatic sac decompression is effective in controlling vertigo in 75% of medication refractory Menière disease patients with good preservation of hearing in most patients

[42]; quality of life improved for 87% of patients undergoing endolymphatic sac decompression [43]. For patients refractory to these procedures, vestibular ablative techniques can be used to eradicate Menière disease symptoms by eliminating remaining vestibular function in the affected ear. Intratympanic gentamicin injection, or chemical labyrinthectomy, acts as deliberate ototoxicity to the vestibular system; it may be even more effective in combination with intratympanic steroid injection [44]. Gentamicin is more vestibulotoxic than ototoxic. While curative for vestibular symptoms in 83–90% of patients, outcomes have shown complication of worsened hearing in 25–32% of patients [45, 46]. Next, neurectomy of the vestibular nerve via a middle cranial fossa, translabyrinthine, retrolabyrinthine, or retrosigmoid approach can relieve vertigo symptoms. While each approach controls vertigo in >90% of patients, the retrosigmoid approach carries the lowest rate of hearing loss, facial nerve injury, and CSF leak. Finally, labyrinthectomy can be the last definitive treatment for refractory vertigo in Menière disease through destruction of the inner ear, with up to 99% control of vertigo following transmastoid labyrinthectomy [47, 48]. As it destroys natural hearing in the operative ear, patients with disabling unilateral Menière disease and poor hearing are ideal candidates; CROS, Baha, Osio, BoneBridge, and cochlear implantation are potential hearing rehabilitation options following labyrinthectomy.

Pregnancy

Isolated complaint of ringing or tinnitus is a common finding in pregnancy. Normal physiologic changes of pregnancy, including raised perilymphatic fluid pressure, hyperdynamic circulation, and hormonal changes can all contribute to development of tinnitus [49]. As many as 33% of women complain of tinnitus during pregnancy compared to 11% of non-pregnant women, with transient course that is relieved with delivery [50, 51]. While the symptom itself in isolation is temporary, benign, and often tolerable, tinnitus can be an early warning sign for preeclampsia or gestational hypertension and may warrant further monitoring [52]. Rarely, isolated tinnitus has proved severe enough to warrant caesarian delivery at 34 weeks' gestation [53].

Unlike isolated tinnitus, Menière disease is a rare finding in pregnancy. Wu et al.'s study of otologic presentations among 68 pregnant women found only 3 cases of Menière disease (4.4%), while Swain et al. documented only 1 among 82 patients (1.2%) [1, 49]. Worsening in existing Menière disease can be seen early during pregnancy due to water retention causing reduced serum osmolarity, altering osmotic gradients in the membranous labyrinth [50, 54]. However, as serum osmolarity can normalize after the fourth month, Menière disease attacks may actually decline through gestation. Uchide et al. described a patient with Menière disease who experienced up to 10 attacks per month in first trimester, resolving during later gestation [54]; likewise, all three reported cases in Wu et al. had vertiginous episodes prior to the fourth month, supporting this hypothesis [1]. One case even reported a Menière disease patient with comorbid vestibular migraine who saw audiometry-confirmed objective hearing improvement following her first trimester, followed by decrease to baseline after delivery, with repeated pattern in a second pregnancy [55]. Stevens et al. proposed the hormonal changes of pregnancy may actually be *protective* against Menière disease attacks, citing studies showing decreased attacks while on estrogen birth control and leuprolide [55]. Andrews and Honrubia similarly discussed how Menière disease can be exacerbated by premenstrual (late luteal) phase of the menstrual cycle and presented a case of Menière disease relieved by pregnancy and postpartum period on estrogen birth control [56]. Significant Menière disease vertigo improvement was seen in women with premenstrual syndrome upon postmenses [57].

Few studies of Menière disease treatment in pregnancy have been conducted. Diazepam, though effective for vertigo in Menière disease, is contraindicated as a Class D medication during pregnancy [54]. Diuretic use should be avoided during pregnancy, especially during second and third trimester due to risk of hyponatremia, hyperbilirubinemia, thrombocytopenia, placental hypoperfusion, and preeclampsia [58, 59]. Vlastarakos et al. and Wu et al. recommend dimenhydrinate and B6 (Class B) for Menière disease attacks to decrease fetal risk [1, 60]. Sherlie et al. also recommended meclizine for acute attacks, and metoclopramide (Class B) for intractable vomiting [2]. Treatment of the underlying disorder should wait until the pregnancy has been completed and delivery achieved.

Since migraine disorders including vestibular migraine have elevated incidence in pregnancy, treatment and control of comorbid migraine is important to limiting Menière disease attacks, which may actually represent vestibular migraine.

Vestibular Migraine

Vestibular migraine, alternately known as migrainous vertigo, migraine-associated dizziness, or benign positional vertigo of childhood (unfortunate term as it is not associated with benign positional vertigo), is a disorder consisting of bouts of vertigo directly caused by migraine mechanisms. Clinical symptoms of vestibular migraine include vertigo associated with migraine-type headache (unilateral, pulsatile headache of varying severity) with associated photophobia, phonophobia, and/or visual aura, accompanied by nausea, motion sensitivity, and/or imbalance. However, migraine headache only occurs with vestibular migraine episodes 10–30% of the time. Onset of vertigo is variable; it may present antecedent to the headache as an aura, beginning with headache, appear later in headache phase, or even without headache. Hearing loss and tinnitus are not often seen but have been reported [61]. Unlike benign paroxysmal positional vertigo or Menière disease, which can often be diagnosed by specific duration of vertigo, vestibular migraine-associated vertigo is quite variable and can last seconds, minutes, hours or even days. Often if a patient can sleep the symptoms are resolved upon awakening. Like migraine, vestibular migraine may be triggered by stress, dehydration, irregular sleep, menstruation, caffeine, and certain foods such as aged cheeses, red wine, monosodium glutamate (MSG), and chocolate. Many patients may also have a family history of vestibular migraine or family members with similar symptoms [62]; the high female:male ratio suggests the possibility of an autosomal dominant inheritance pattern with decreased penetrance in males [62, 63]. Wackym et al. have reported that migraine headaches and vestibular migraine can also be associated with third window syndrome and resolve or improve after surgical management [64–66].

Pathophysiology

While the pathophysiology of vestibular migraine and migraine in general is not fully understood, because many migraine patients report high rates of episodic vertigo (20–33%) [67–71], motion sickness [70, 72, 73], and peripheral (25%) [74] or central vestibular abnormalities [75, 76], vestibular involvement may be a characteristic part of migraine disorders. Like migraine, vestibular migraine may have multiple potential mechanisms of action that are not mutually exclusive.

- Vestibular migraine may represent **migraine aura** when preceding headache or lasting for a short duration (<60 min); whereas typical migraine aura is understood as cortical spreading depression (a wave of neuronal/glial depolarization), vestibular migraine may be either a "brainstem aura" of noncortical spreading depression, or alternatively a projection of cortical spreading depression to vestibular nuclei via the posterior parietal cortex [74, 76]. Only 10–30% of the time are vestibular migraine and migraine headaches concurrent.
- Vestibular migraine may be due to **stimulation of the trigeminovascular system** when vestibular symptoms are longer-lasting. This proposed mechanism involves stimulation of trigeminal nucleus neurons causing vasodilation and release of inflammatory neuropeptides such as substance P, neurokinin A, and calcitonin gene-related peptide (CGRP); this

pathway has been shown to cause migraine headache, and vestibular receptors for CGRP are distributed within the inner ear. Likewise, connections between vestibular and trigeminal nuclei linked to migraine may also connect vestibular and trigeminal processes [74]. The vestibular efferent system is largely based upon CGRP as the neuromodulator innervating the primary afferent neurons for type I and type II hair cells, directly innervating type II hair cells and rarely directly innervating the type I hair cells in the vestibular periphery [77].

- **Channelopathies** may play a role in vestibular migraine pathogenesis; 50% of patients with episodic ataxia type 2 have migraine, and familial hemiplegic migraine is due to abnormality of the same calcium channel [78, 79].
- **Migraine-induced ischemia** of the inner ear can cause cochlear/labyrinth injury and vestibular migraine symptoms as well as hearing loss [74, 80].
- For some, vestibular migraine attacks may be due to **sensory sensitivity**; migraine patients have been shown to have reduced threshold to light, sound, smell, and tactile stimuli, as well as motion, optokinetic, and vestibular stimuli [74, 81].
- Vertigo may act as a **migraine trigger**; in one study, 49% of patients with migraine history experienced migraine attack with vestibular testing, compared to 5% of controls [72].
- **Hormonal changes** are often associated with the onset of, change of, or resolution of migraine headaches or the three variants of migraine: vestibular migraine, ocular migraine, or hemiplegic migraine. These changes can occur at four physiologic changes in hormones for both sexes: (1) children affected can have improvement or resolution transitioning through puberty; (2) young women, classically during a first pregnancy, can have the onset of migraine headaches and variants; (3) at menopause the migraine headaches and variants can start, or the character of the migraine headaches can change, or the migraine headaches may resolve and the variants can start; and (4) men in their 50s and 60s

as their testosterone levels decline may also have changes in their migraine headaches or variants.

Like migraine, diagnosis of vestibular migraine relies largely on patient history and clinical symptoms; vestibular migraine patients are usually asymptomatic in the symptom-free period, although 10–20% of vestibular migraine patients may exhibit hyperactivity to unilateral caloric stimulation, and mild central oculomotor deficits may be seen [76, 82]. Diagnostic criteria per International Classification of Headache Disorders, third ed., include a current or past his-tory of migraine with or without aura, and ≥5 episodes consisting of: (1) vestibular symptoms of moderate-severe intensity lasting 5 min–72 h, and (2) at least half of episodes associated with migraine headache features, photophobia and phonophobia, or visual aura (Table 30.1) [83].

Treatment of vestibular migraine consists of avoidance of migraine triggers, such as sleep and diet modification, and may include acute and prophylactic therapy for treatment of vestibular migraine attacks. Because most available data on vestibular migraine treatment comes from case reports and retrospective studies, the efficacy of these treatments is not well-evaluated. As a 2015

Table 30.1 Diagnostic criteria for vestibular migraine

Vestibular migraine: ICHD-3 diagnostic criteria
A. At least five episodes fulfilling criteria C and D
B. A current or past history of 1.1 *Migraine without aura* or 1.2 *Migraine with aura*[a]
C. Vestibular symptoms[b] of moderate or severe intensity,[c] lasting between 5 min and 72 h[d]
D. At least half of episodes are associated with at least one of the following three migrainous features:[e]
1. Headache with at least two of the following four characteristics:
(a) Unilateral location
(b) Pulsating quality
(c) Moderate or severe intensity
(d) Aggravation by routine physical activity
2. Photophobia and phonophobia[f]
3. Visual aura
E. Not better accounted for by another ICHD-3 diagnosis or by another vestibular disorder

ICHD-3 International Classification of Headache Disorders, 3rd ed

[a]Code also for the underlying migraine diagnosis

[b]Vestibular symptoms, as defined by the Bárány Society's Classification of Vestibular Symptoms and qualifying for a diagnosis of A1.6.6 *Vestibular migraine*, include:

  (a) spontaneous vertigo

    • internal vertigo (a false sensation of self-motion)

    • external vertigo (a false sensation that the visual surround is spinning or flowing)

  (b) positional vertigo, occurring after a change of head position

  (c) visually induced vertigo, triggered by a complex or large moving visual stimulus

  (d) head motion-induced vertigo, occurring during head motion

  (e) head motion-induced dizziness with nausea (dizziness is characterized by a sensation of disturbed spatial orienta-tion; other forms of dizziness are currently not included in the classification of vestibular migraine)

[c]Vestibular symptoms are rated *moderate* when they interfere with but do not prevent daily activities and *severe* when daily activities cannot be continued

[d]Duration of episodes is highly variable. About 30% of patients have episodes lasting minutes, 30% have attacks for hours and another 30% have attacks over several days. The remaining 10% have attacks lasting seconds only, which tend to occur repeatedly during head motion, visual stimulation, or after changes of head position. In these patients, episode duration is defined as the total period during which short attacks recur. At the other end of the spectrum, there are patients who may take 4 weeks to recover fully from an episode. However, the core episode rarely exceeds 72 h

[e]One symptom is sufficient during a single episode. Different symptoms may occur during different episodes. Associated symptoms may occur before, during, or after the vestibular symptoms

[f]History and physical examinations do not suggest another vestibular disorder *or* such a disorder has been considered but ruled out by appropriate investigations *or* such a disorder is present as a comorbid condition but episodes can be clearly differentiated. Migraine attacks may be induced by vestibular stimulation. Therefore, the differential diagnosis should include other vestibular disorders complicated by superimposed migraine attacks

Cochrane review found insufficient randomized clinical trials of pharmacotherapy in vestibular migraine, treatment options are drawn from efficacy in migraine or vestibular migraine studies of small sample size [84]. Considerations in tailoring therapy include frequency/duration of attacks, medication side effects, and patient comorbidities.

Acute attacks with significant nausea or vertigo symptoms can be treated with vestibular suppressants including benzodiazepines (diazepam, lorazepam), antiemetics (prochlorperazine, meclizine, dimenhydrinate, metoclopramide, cyclizine), or antihistamines (promethazine) [61, 70, 85, 86]. Triptans (sumatriptan, zolmitriptan, rizatriptan) are commonly used for acute migraine treatment and have been shown efficacious in vertigo in some smaller vestibular migraine studies, but are not routinely used to treat acute vestibular migraine attacks unless the attacks precede or include headache symptoms [87–90]; paradoxically, a case series noted triptans may alleviate vertigo but actually trigger or exacerbate headache [91]. Intravenous methylprednisolone has also been used to abort prolonged attack [92].

Prophylactic therapy also lacks evidence from large randomized clinical trials and is largely drawn from migraine and vestibular disorder treatments. It can be considered in patients with frequent or severe symptoms not adequately treated with acute therapy and can be tailored based on individual risk profiles and patient comorbidities. Options include beta-blockers (propranolol, metoprolol) [76, 93, 94], tricyclic antidepressants (amitriptyline, nortriptyline) [70, 87, 95–97], or antiepileptics (topiramate, lamotrigine, valproate) [98–101]; Serotonin and norepinephrine reuptake inhibitors (SNRIs) such as venlafaxine may be useful especially with predominant vestibular symptoms or comorbid anxiety or depression, though they may worsen headaches [94, 102]. Calcium channel blockers (verapamil, flunarizine, betahistine) may be useful with vestibular aura or aura-predominant symptoms [95, 103]. Antihistamines can reduce headache and vertigo symptoms [104]. Non-pharmacologic options such as meditation, cognitive behavioral therapy (CBT), and vestibular rehabilitation may also be helpful in managing vestibular migraine attacks [105–107].

Age has been shown to be a risk factor for development of vestibular migraine [74]; one study found vestibular migraine to occur more often among individuals <40 years of age [108]. Benign paroxysmal vertigo of childhood (which has nothing in common with benign paroxysmal positional vertigo) is vestibular migraine in children, and some may develop more intense migraine disorders and vestibular migraine in adulthood [98, 109]. Migraine disorders generally follow a pattern of female preponderance following puberty, with women 2–3 times more likely than men to be affected. With high lifetime expected prevalence of migraine (16%) and vertigo (7%) in the general population, expected comorbidity of the two is 1.1%. However, the actual comorbidity rate seen is higher, at 3.2%, as individuals with migraine have been shown to be likelier to have occurrence of vertigo [61, 110]. Definite diagnosis of vestibular migraine has been estimated at 0.98% of the general population, and as high as 9% among migraine patients [110, 111]. Vestibular migraine has been previously reported to have a predilection for female gender among adolescents [112–115], and this gender disparity is seen among adult females as well, with women 1.5–5 times more likely to be diagnosed with vestibular migraine [70, 76, 111, 116]. Migraine disorders appear to have an even higher predilection during pregnancy, with as many as 23.8% of women reporting migraines during their first trimester [117]. Women with pre-existing headaches are also more likely to experience migraines during pregnancy. Because many women (63.6%) also experience first trimester dizziness, most frequently vertigo (35.7%), a portion of individuals in this population may be expected to meet vestibular migraine criteria [118]. While no large cohort studies have been conducted regarding vestibular migraine in pregnancy, a number of case reports and case series discuss vestibular migraine in pregnancy. A study of Taiwanese patients presenting to a neurotology clinic for new-onset complaints during pregnancy found vestibular migraine to account for 50% of cases

[1]. Based on risk factors of age and sex, child-bearing-age females may be at higher risk of vestibular migraine independent of pregnancy. However, as neuroactive steroids modulate the neurotransmitter system involved in the pathogenesis of migraine disorders, women have been shown to experience higher rates of migraine headache during times of unstable hormonal fluctuation such as peripartum or perimenopausal periods [119]; this pathophysiology may play a role in the increased rates of vestibular symptoms and vestibular migraine seen in pregnant patients as well [1, 50].

Though non-pharmacologic options such as diet, sleep, meditation, and trigger modifications are generally preferable for migraine treatment in pregnancy to avoid fetal risk, untreated or inadequately treated migraine can cause poor oral intake, poor sleep, or dehydration, increasing both maternal and fetal risk [120, 121]. Therefore, symptom relief versus fetal risk should be weighed for therapeutic options. Clinicians should consult professional society guidelines or FDA pregnancy and lactation labeling for up-to-date information on risk–benefit counseling. For acute attacks, a number of safe options exist. H1 antihistamines are effective for vestibular nausea [122]. Meclizine and dimenhydrinate (Category B) are antiemetics with lowest risk of teratogenicity; metoclopramide is also safe for use for continuous vomiting, and ondansetron second line due to less evidence [60]. Vitamin B6 also appears effective and safe, while betahistine should be avoided [123, 124]. For prophylaxis, beta-blockers and tricyclic antidepressants are considered safest during pregnancy, especially post-first trimester [121]. Antiepileptics like topiramate, zonisamide, and valproic acid carry significant fetal risks and are contraindicated.

While one study of headache in pregnancy found migraine headache to be by far the most common (65%), a number of serious causes of headache secondary to hypertension can present in pregnancy (18%), including preeclampsia or eclampsia, posterior reversible encephalopathy syndrome (PRES), acute hypertension, hemolysis/elevated liver enzymes/low platelet count syn-drome (HELLP), or reversible cerebral vasoconstriction syndrome (RCVS) [125]. Less common etiologies include pituitary adenoma/apoplexy (4%), intercurrent infection (2%), pneumocephalus (2%), cerebral venous thrombosis (1%), ictal headache (1%), intracranial hemorrhage (1%), and others (5%) [121]. Because of this significant minority of non-migraine headaches arising during pregnancy, patients presenting for suspected vestibular migraine or vertiginous complaints including symptoms of headache should undergo adequate history and workup to rule out more serious underlying conditions. The approach to evaluation and management of the pregnant patient with headache is discussed in detail in Chap. 27.

Vestibular migraine carries high comorbidity with psychiatric disorders, with comorbid anxiety seen in as high as 65% of patients among the general population [126]. Since pregnancy carries unique risks for additional psychiatric comorbidity, including peripartum depression and anxiety in as high as 20% of women, clinicians treating vestibular migraine in particular should consider screening for comorbid anxiety and depression among their patients [127]. Likewise, clinicians may opt for vestibular migraine treatment effective for comorbid anxiety and depression, including CBT, selective serotonin reuptake inhibitors (SSRIs), SNRIs, and tricyclic antidepressants [95, 102, 128, 129]. Considerations for managing mental health disorders during pregnancy are described in Chap. 31.

Otosclerosis

Otosclerosis is a disease process resulting in slow, progressive conductive hearing loss due to osseous dyscrasia within the temporal bone. The disease is found in up to 12% of Caucasians, though only 0.3–0.4% of these patients present with symptoms, and has a 2:1 female predominance [130]. Typical presentation consists of gradual onset, progressive hearing loss worse at low frequencies, with or without associated tinnitus (50%) [131]. Vertigo occurs infrequently (10%) with semicircular canal involvement [130]. Though often initially presenting unilaterally early in the disease process, otosclerosis can be found bilaterally in 80% of cases [132].

In terms of pathophysiology, the otosclerotic process consists of normal bone being replaced with spongiotic sclerotic bone. In normal humans, endochondral ossification forms the otic capsule during embryonic development. Compared to the rest of the bony skeleton, the otic capsule undergoes relatively little bone remodeling or turnover. However, in the setting of otosclerosis, dysregulation of bone remodeling occurs solely within the otic capsule, giving rise to otosclerotic foci. Areas of the otic capsule with highest propensity for development of these foci include the fissula ante fenestram and oval window, round window, and adjacent to the cochlea [133]. In early disease, bony resorption occurs and becomes replaced with spongy bone. Osteolytic osteocytes then appear at the leading edge of the lesion, and sheets of connective tissue slowly replace the bone. Finally, dense sclerotic bone forms in previously resorbed areas. On histologic exam, one can see disorganized bone, overpopulation of osteocytes, and enlarged marrow spaces replaced with dense sclerotic bone. This replacement appears pleomorphic as multiple stages of otosclerosis can co-occur.

The majority of otosclerotic lesions are limited to the anterior oval window or stapes footplate (80%), although some may occur near the round window (30%), pericochlear region (21%), or anterior segment of the internal auditory canal (19%) [134]. Eight percent of patients have cochlear or labyrinthine involvement (labyrinthine otosclerosis) causing sensorineural hearing loss, while the remaining 2% may have both labyrinthine and ossicular involvement. Although the etiology of the disease has yet to be fully understood, a number of environmental and genetic risk factors have been identified for development of otosclerosis, including family history (30–70%), female gender, prior measles virus infection, fluoride in drinking water, and certain connective tissue disorders [135].

Diagnosis

Diagnosis can be made with clinical history, physical exam, and audiometry. Proper history should seek to rule out other possible causes of conductive hearing loss, including external auditory canal obstruction, tympanic membrane perforation, tympanosclerosis, cholesteatoma, or other middle ear mass, ossicular chain discontinuity with trauma or incus necrosis associated with recurrent chronic otitis media; with vertigo symptoms, vestibular disorders like Menière disease, or third window syndrome should be excluded. Because there is a strong and frequent (60%) familial component to otosclerosis, exams should include a detailed family history of hearing loss [135]. Otoscopic exam is typically normal in otosclerosis, other than a possible Schwartze sign (redness along the cochlear promontory seen through the tympanic membrane) seen inconsistently [136]. Whisper voice testing shows decreased hearing on the affected side, and Weber and Rinne tuning fork testing should demonstrate conductive hearing loss on the affected side. Formal audiogram should be completed in suspected otosclerosis. A characteristic bone-conduction loss at 2000 Hz (Carhart notch) is historically diagnostic and often appreciable on audiometry [134]. Comprehensive audiograms can also monitor disease progress and localization: ossicular stiffening and stapes-oval window changes will show low-frequency mild conductive loss; stapes fixation to oval window will increase the conductive component of the loss and begin to involve additional frequencies; cochlear involvement will add high-frequency sensorineural hearing loss, resulting in a mixed pattern; significant cochlear progression will show a mixed pattern of hearing loss at all frequencies [134]. Tympanometry is typically normal, with tympanogram flattening only in extensive cases with significant ossicular chain fixation. There is loss of the stapedial reflex because of the stapes fixation. While imaging is not required for diagnosis, high-resolution temporal bone CT can rule out third window syndrome, ossicular fixation to the temporal bone, middle ear masses, reveal anatomic involvement of otosclerosis with "halo sign" of radiolucent areas in and around the cochlea, and be useful for surgical planning [134].

Treatment

Surgery is considered first-line management for otosclerosis, provided the air-bone gap is large enough. Options include stapes surgery as well as wearable or implantable hearing aid. Stapedectomy, opening the stapes footplate and removal of the crurae with replacement using a prosthesis attached to the long process of the incus and extending into the vestibule of the inner ear, is a minimally invasive same-day surgical procedure that can restore mechanical transmission of sound through the middle ear and successfully correct the conductive loss of otosclerosis, although not sensorineural loss with cochlear extension of disease, in over 94% of patients [137]. Indications include conductive hearing loss with air-bone gap >20 dB, speech discrimination score > 60% and healthy patients; the converse along with additional symptoms such as endolymphatic hydrops and vertigo are contraindications. Ten to 20% will require surgical revision due to progressive disease [138]. Despite surgery, long-term outcomes are unpredictable and hearing loss may progress; one study found at 30 years postsurgery, 88% of patients had bilateral disease involvement, and 66% had developed moderate-profound sensorineural hearing loss [139].

For patients with sensorineural loss or otherwise not candidates for stapes surgery with hearing loss >25 dB, air-conduction hearing aids are an option for sound amplification. Middle ear implants can be placed concurrently with or following stapes surgery and can be fixated to the ossicles to act in mechanical vibration [140]; they provide compensation for sensorineural hearing loss to a degree of improvement comparable to traditional hearing aids. Bone-conduction implants are used for conductive or mixed hearing loss and transmit directly to the cochlea by attachment to the temporal bone and bypass of the external and middle ear. Traditional air-conduction hearing aids should be tested before undergoing bone-conduction implant due to their much cheaper cost. Finally, cochlear implants bypass sound transmission through the ear by delivering electrical stimulation to the primary afferent neurons of the cochlear nerve via an implantable prosthetic device and can be used in the setting of moderate-to-severe mixed hearing loss. Because cochlear implantation in the setting of otosclerosis carries increased risk of post-implantation facial nerve stimulation and is associated with loss of residual hearing, and stapedectomy with hearing aids has good outcomes in severe mixed hearing loss with preserved speech discrimination ability, the latter remains first-line treatment before cochlear implantation [141, 142]. However, if the speech discrimination ability falls below 50%, cochlear implantation would be the better option.

There is currently no definitive pharmacologic therapy for otosclerosis. Some countries such as France use sodium fluoride treatment in otosclerosis for its effects against bone absorption and promoting bone calcification to reduce hearing deterioration, though evidence for its use and adequate dosage is limited [143, 144]. Similarly, there is research in the use of bisphosphonates and vitamin D, but no large-scale clinical trials have been conducted to date.

Pregnancy

Because otosclerosis has a tendency to occur in women of childbearing age, endocrine factors have been hypothesized to play a role in the pathophysiology [145–148]. Anecdotally, acceleration of the stapes fixation and associated widening of the air-bone gap is often seen with otosclerosis during pregnancy. However, while estrogen has been established as a factor in osteoblastic function by inhibiting osteoclast maturation and inhibiting bone resorption [149, 150], the role of osteoblasts is unclear in the pathogenesis of otosclerosis, and no studies have yet directly implicated sex hormones in this disease process [151, 152]. While estrogen receptors have been identified on otosclerotic cells, their specific regulatory function is not well understood [153]. Similarly, clinical studies examining clinical association and impact of pregnancy upon otosclerosis have conflicting results [154].

In a recent study examining the impact of pregnancy on age at stapedectomy, Qian et al. theorize that the discrepancy between studies measuring subjective versus objective hearing loss can be explained by the overlap between the ages at which otosclerosis progression occurs and the ages at which women bear children leading to identification of hearing loss during pregnancy or nursing, as well as increased healthcare utilization during parenthood [154].

However, other studies seem to indicate a more definitive link between pregnancy and development of otosclerosis. For instance, a 2019 study found significantly increased maternal serum IGF-1 and placental growth hormone variant (GHV) concentrations at 34 weeks' gestation in otosclerotic patients as compared to controls, suggesting that the GH-IGF axis may contribute to the development of this condition during pregnancy [133]. One British epidemiologic study of otosclerosis found that while no significant differences were observed in the age of onset, family history, bilateral disease, or incidence of tinnitus or vertigo between pregnant and non-pregnant women developing otosclerosis, 33% of pregnant women reported a subjective change in hearing during pregnancy [135]. As compared to women with no reported hearing change during pregnancy, these women were an average of 4 years younger at diagnosis. Additionally, a significantly higher proportion of women who reported change in hearing during pregnancy breastfed after pregnancy as compared to those who did not report hearing change (90% versus 78%). These findings led Crompton et al. to conclude that pregnancy may lead to reported hearing deterioration and acceleration of otosclerosis in a minority of patients. Likewise, some studies have indicated that women with pre-existing otosclerosis may have worsening symptoms and disease progression during pregnancy [146, 155, 156]. Though additional research is needed to identify the exact mechanism of hormonal influence on hearing loss, Batson et al. consider it prudent to suspect pre-existing otosclerosis in patients who develop hearing loss during times of increased sex hormonal production [134].

Sodium fluoride treatment is contraindicated during pregnancy due to adverse fetal effects [2].

Vestibular Schwannoma/Acoustic Neuroma

Vestibular schwannomas (VS), or acoustic neuromas, are rare slow-growing benign tumors of Schwann cell origin that can arise from the vestibular portion of the eighth cranial nerve. They represent 80–90% of cerebellopontine angle (CPA) tumors. While rare (incidence of 1 per 100,000 nationally) [157], vestibular schwannoma has been incidentally diagnosed with CT and MRI with increased frequency since imaging has become more prevalent [158, 159]. Vestibular schwannomas occur more frequently in women and may present with larger size and increased vascularity in females as well [160]. These slow-growing tumors have a median age of diagnosis later in life, at age 55 [161]. While occurring unilaterally in >90% of patients, bilateral VS is commonly seen in syndromic patients with neurofibromatosis type 2 (NF2) [161]. Neurofibromatosis type 2 patients usually develop bilateral VS as well as other tumors and present at a younger age (<30). Sporadic VS commonly presents with complaint of chronic hearing loss (95%) and tinnitus (63%), with less frequent involvement of vestibular (61%) complaints such as unsteadiness or vertigo, or trigeminal (17%) or facial nerve (6%) symptoms like facial numbness/pain, paresis, or taste disturbance; sudden sensorineural hearing loss may also occasionally be seen [162]. Gradual tumor growth can lead to mass effect on posterior cranial fossa structures, affect cerebellar or even brainstem function, and cause severe impairment. With increased tumor size, patients are proportionally likelier to report hearing loss and dizziness [163]. Due to the chronic effect on hearing, many patients experience hearing loss and tinnitus for years before presenting with an observable deficit.

Vestibular schwannomas develop from Schwann cells of the superior or inferior vestibular nerves, in a fashion similarly to peripheral schwannomas in other anatomic locations. Pathologic examination shows characteristic Antoni A and B regions consisting of alternate areas of dense spindle cells and scant disorganized cellularity. Immunohistochemical staining is usually positive for S100 protein, and other markers such as CD-34, EMA, and NFTP may help distinguish VS from a neurofibroma [164]. Vestibular schwannomas are nearly always benign, with malignant degeneration only reported in a handful of cases, including poststereotactic radiosurgery. In syndromic NF2, hereditary abnormality in the NF2 gene responsible for producing merlin (or schwannomin), a cell membrane-related protein with tumor suppressor function, can cause development of schwannomas and other tumors such as meningiomas and spinal tumors. In patients with sporadic VS, biallelic inactivation of the NF2 gene is similarly seen. Risk factors for sporadic VS include childhood radiation, and some studies implicate cellphone use and chronic noise exposure, although an equal number of opposing findings have been reported [157, 165–171].

Diagnosis of VS relies on patient history of asymmetric or unilateral hearing loss or cranial nerve deficit, often with tinnitus and/or unexplained vestibulopathy. History-taking should seek to rule out alternate causes of hearing loss. Physical exam can show abnormality on Weber and Rinne tuning fork tests suggestive of unilateral or asymmetric hearing loss. Neurologic exam including cranial nerves I–XII should be performed as facial, trigeminal, and other cranial neuropathies are sometimes seen with VS. Gait and vestibular testing, including Romberg and Dix-Hallpike maneuvers are typically normal; however, the sharpened Romberg is often abnormal. Audiometry is an important screening for VS patients, which typically shows asymmetric sensorineural hearing loss on the affected side, most noticeably at higher frequencies; down-sloping pattern versus flat type and differences in pure tone thresholds, pure tone averages, and in particular asymmetrically impaired speech discrimination ability can also help distinguish VS from non-VS CPA tumors [172]. Auditory brainstem response (ABR) testing can show delayed conduction on the affected side, and vestibular testing can show decreased or absent caloric response for superior vestibular nerve tumors and reduced cVEMP responses for inferior vestibular nerve tumors; these tests are useful in the setting of perioperative counseling but are not be adequate for confirmatory diagnosis [173, 174]. MRI with gadolinium contrast is the gold standard screening choice for suspected VS in the setting of asymmetric hearing loss, with reported sensitivity of up to 98% [175, 176]. High resolution CT with contrast is an alternative if MRI is contraindicated. On imaging, VSs appear as an enhancing mass in the internal auditory canal (IAC), extending into the CPA with larger tumors. On preoperative imaging, widening of the IAC and tumor extension anterior/caudal to the IAC can predict postoperative hearing loss [177].

Treatment of sporadic VS consists of three main options: surgery, radiotherapy, or conservative observation. Except in NF2, where bevacizumab may play a role in treatment, pharmacotherapy is not an adequate option for VS treatment [178]. Treatment choice can depend on clinical presentation, tumor size, expertise of the treating center, and patient choice. A 2014 study of VS management showed approximately 49% of patients were treated primarily with surgery, 24% with radiotherapy, and only 2% with combination therapy [161]. Younger patients and those with larger tumor size were likelier to be treated surgically. Racial disparities were also seen, with African American patients twice as likely to be treated conservatively despite large tumor size. Recent guidelines suggest smaller VS are best managed with observation versus radiosurgery, while large tumors should be treated with surgery and possibly followed with radiosurgery [178].

Surgical resection consists of either suboccipital (retrosigmoid), translabyrinthine, or middle fossa approach. The middle fossa approach is best for small tumors (<1.5 cm) with attempted hearing preservation [179]. The translabyrinthine approach is recommended for large tumors >3 cm, or small tumors when hearing preservation is not necessary [180]. Favorable outcomes are seen among most patients undergoing complete VS resection, with good long-term survival and low rates of recidivism [181–183]. One study of 2400 cases found 0.05%–1.8% recidivism based on surgical approach [184]. Postoperative complications can include CSF leakage (1–8.5%), infection (4%), bleeding (1%), as well as risk of hearing loss, facial weakness, vestibular symptoms, and headache depending on surgical approach [185, 186] Advanced patient age can also lead to higher rates of in-hospital complications [187]. Where subtotal microsurgical resection is performed for anatomic preservation, recurrence is up to 11 times more likely than with gross total resection [183]; however, it may still be acceptable strategy based on patient goals and functional preservation. High-volume hospitals and co-surgeons (neurotologist and neurosurgeon) have been shown to have lower rate of postoperative complications [188].

Radiation therapy, including stereotactic radiosurgery (SRS), stereotactic radiotherapy (SRT), proton beam therapy, and conventional fractionated radiation therapy have all been used in VS treatment. Though lacking adequate equivalent studies, these modalities all appear to have excellent tumor control rates of 91–100% [189]. SRS delivers a single high dose of radiation to a discrete treatment area via Gamma Knife radiosurgery or linear accelerator. SRS is a good treatment option for smaller tumors (<3 cm) or patients who are not surgical candidates. Complications of SRS include postradiation tumor expansion (14–22%) [190, 191], cystic degeneration (2%) [192], malignant transformation (0.3–0.5%) [192, 193], and local tissue scarring that can complicate salvage surgery, particularly with facial nerve preservation, in recurrence. Unlike SRS, SRT, e.g., CyberKnife, uses multiple radiation fractions over a series of treatment sessions. SRS and SRT both preserve

cranial nerves V and VII in >95% and have similar rates of hearing preservation as well [189, 194, 195]. Proton beam therapy, a newer modality that maximizes radiation delivery to target volume and tissue depth with minimal scatter, has also been shown to preserve cranial nerve function among many patients, though further study is needed to determine long-term hearing outcomes relative to other radiotherapy modalities [196]. Loss of hearing should be expected, particularly if the cochlear dose exceeds 4 Gy [197]. Likewise, changes in vestibular function occur over time after Gamma Knife radiosurgery [198].

Because VS are slow-growing benign tumors, observation with serial MRI imaging is a conservative management technique that should be considered for appropriate patients. This group includes patients who are asymptomatic, >60 years old, those with medical comorbidities, patient preference, or other factors precluding surgery, and small tumor size [178]. One meta-analysis found an average VS growth rate of 1.9 mm per year, with only 43% of patients experiencing growth, while 57% showed no growth or tumor regression; 20% of patients failed conservative management and eventually required interventional treatment due to tumor or symptom progression [199]. As one study of observational management found 59% of patients had VS growth <1 mm per year, such conservative treatment may be warranted in patients with small tumor size and slow progression [200]. Because non-intervention is associated with risk of progressive hearing loss, conservative observation should not be conducted for patients with larger or rapidly growing VS (<2.5 mm per year) [201]. Likewise, since hearing outcomes following interventional treatment are generally better among patients with normal baseline hearing, patients who prioritize hearing preservation may also benefit from early treatment and avoiding watchful waiting [202].

Due to potential for recurrence and slow tumor progression, patients managed for VS should receive regular follow-up and MRI screening for at least 15 years following treatment [184].

Pregnancy

The diagnosis of VS is rare during pregnancy; a retrospective study examining 68 pregnant patients presenting to neurotology clinic for new-onset inner ear symptoms diagnosed VS in only one patient [1]; other observational studies of general array of otolaryngologic symptoms (150 and 82 patients) did not diagnose any women with VS [49, 203]. Likewise, a major maternal-fetal medicine center reviewing head and neck cancer management during pregnancy over a 27-year period reported only 2 cases of VS, 1 new onset and 1 patient with previous history [204]. A 2014 review identified only 31 cases of VS diagnosed in pregnancy [205]. Nonetheless, due to VS female predilection and growth during pregnancy that can lead to serious maternal complications, it remains an important entity to understand.

Among pregnant patients, the most common presenting symptom is unilateral hearing loss. However, other presenting symptoms such as tinnitus, headache, nausea, and vomiting may be nonspecific, physiologic, and/or frequent in pregnancy, confounding a correct diagnosis. Likewise, headache and hypertension may be identified with preeclampsia rather than VS. Because accelerated tumor growth seen in some patients during pregnancy can cause hearing loss, these patients may have a greater proportion of acute hearing complaints than typical VS patients, and VS should be ruled out as an etiology in pregnant patients presenting with unilateral sensorineural hearing loss (see section "Hearing Loss") [206]. In the vast majority of cases, patients with VS present during the second or third trimester [205].

VS have been shown to occur primarily or with worsening symptoms during pregnancy [205]. Early case series noted this association, especially in later trimesters, and suggested hormonal factors could affect VS vascular supply and tumor growth [207]. Hypothesized mechanisms of accelerated tumor growth in pregnancy include increased blood volume causing vascular engorgement, directly increasing VS size, or growth mediated by progesterone and estrogen receptors [205, 208, 209]. Gestational hyperten-sion, preeclampsia, and fluid retention during pregnancy may also predispose to cerebral edema or increased intracranial pressure, leading to symptomatic VS [208]. Increased size and vascularity can also lead to complication of intratumor hemorrhage [208, 210]. While the impact of pregnancy on VS pathophysiology continues to be studied, a growing body of evidence supports the implication of hormonal effects of pregnancy in VS. Acoustic neuromas have been shown to grow faster in mice exposed to estrogen, while the estrogen receptor-blocking tamoxifen has been shown to decrease tumor volume [211]. Subsets of sporadic VS have been shown to exhibit estrogen receptor activity [212, 213]. Due to presence of this signaling pathway, Brown et al. suggested antiestrogen therapy might prove effective in VS inhibition [214]; mifepristone, an anti-progesterone and anti-glucocorticoid medication has also been explored for potential use in VS [215].

Management

Unlike non-pregnant patients, pregnant patients are limited in treatment modalities to observation and surgery. Radiotherapy is generally contraindicated due to risk of fetal radiation exposure [204, 216]. Pharmacologic treatment plays no role in pregnant VS management including NF2 patients, as bevacizumab lacks sufficient safety information during pregnancy [217]. Small, asymptomatic, and slow-growing pre-existing VS can undergo observation and continued follow-up after pregnancy. Management of large VS diagnosed or presenting with worsening symptoms during pregnancy requires balance of maternal benefits and fetal risk. Optimal treatment strategy consists of close observation with subsequent surgical resection following delivery and adequate postpartum recovery [205, 208, 209, 214, 218, 219]. However, severe presentation or exacerbation during pregnancy may preclude observational management. Since surgery during first trimester presents the highest fetal risk due to anesthesia exposure, VS surgery should be deferred to second trimester if possible to decrease risk of spontaneous abortion [212, 220]. Obstructive hydrocephalus secondary to VS mass effect can be managed with ventriculoperitoneal shunt placement, a lower-risk procedure than tumor resection which can allow continued CSF flow in order to delay surgery to a later trimester or the postpartum period. Nonetheless, surgical resection during the first trimester may be required with urgent indications such as increased intracranial pressure, neurologic symptoms, and/or signs of intracranial hemorrhage; despite surgical therapy, severe intracranial bleeds secondary to tumors carry high rate of maternal mortality and can still lead to nonviable pregnancy despite treatment [221]. The second trimester remains the safest time for surgical treatment in terms of both maternal and fetal risk [208, 212, 220]; one retrospective cohort study of skull base meningioma and schwannoma resection during pregnancy ($n = 9$) showed successful emergent surgery during the second trimester [222]. Conservative versus interventional management for VS presenting during the second trimester should be dictated by urgency and likelihood of surgical resection later in pregnancy if deferred. Third trimester resection carries the highest maternal risk due to cumulative effects of pregnancy, including hemodilution, decreased functional residual respiratory capacity, predisposition to hypoxemia, and venous engorgement of the airway [205]. Nonetheless, successful cases of third trimester VS resection have been reported [208, 223]. If late enough in the third trimester, caesarian delivery can be performed and followed by tumor resection [208]; though successful vaginal deliveries have been reported, caesarian delivery avoids potential risks of increased intracranial pressure with vaginal delivery [217, 220]. Ben Adani et al. recommend an optimal strategy of CSF drainage prior to caesarian delivery followed by immediate tumor resection, though resection may be delayed days-to-weeks in the postpartum period to restore hemodynamic stability. Shah et al. offer a useful management algorithm for symptomatic VS in pregnancy [205].

Patients with a history of NF2 or pre-existing VS should be counseled regarding potential for high-risk pregnancy due to tumor progression. Coordination between otolaryngology, neurosurgery, anesthesia, and high-risk obstetrics or maternal-fetal medicine is important throughout the pregnancy period to ensure proper maternal and fetal care [217]. Audiogram and MRI should be repeated periodically during pregnancy and the postpartum period to follow existing tumor progression and help guide patient management.

The general approach to management of intracranial tumors during pregnancy is discussed in Chap. 36.

Bell Palsy

Idiopathic facial paralysis, or Bell palsy, is a disorder involving acute-onset unilateral peripheral facial nerve weakness. Annual incidence is between 11 and 40 per 100,000 population [224]. While the disorder carries no gender preference, pregnant patients are three times as likely to be affected, especially in the peripartum period [225]. Incidence among the pregnant population contributes to the disease peak seen in younger adults under 40 years old [226]. Comorbid diabetes, obesity, and hypertension may also be present in a large subset of Bell palsy patients [226–229].

Typical symptoms consist of sudden onset (hours-days) of unilateral facial paresis or paralysis; this can include absence of ipsilateral forehead wrinkling, eyelid droop, and inability to close the eye, dry eye, epiphora (excessive tearing of the eye), drooping of the ipsilateral corner of the mouth and associated dribbling. Female patients may be more likely to have ocular symptoms [226]. Patients with Bell palsy can also experience loss of taste in the ipsilateral anterior two-thirds of the tongue because of chorda tympani nerve involvement (branch of the facial nerve). Many also present with understandable anxiety and distress [230]. Polycranial neuropathy can also be associated with Bell Palsy with trigeminal, glossopharyngeal, and hypoglossal nerve involvement [231]. Infrequently, patients may present with bilateral facial neuropathy.

While the etiology of Bell palsy remains unclear, herpes simplex virus type 1 (HSV-1) recrudescence is the suspected cause of Bell palsy in many cases via mechanism of axonal viral spread and causing facial nerve inflammation and edema within a bone surrounded space, leading to demyelination and clinical symptoms of weakness and paralysis [232]. Histopathologic findings corroborate the mechanism of viral neuritis, with maximal nerve damage in areas of the bony facial canal most susceptible to edema-related compression [233, 234]. Despite evidence of HSV-1 viral presence in a majority of cases, Bell palsy remains an idiopathic disorder because there is no established confirmatory testing for HSV-1 in the clinical setting of Bell palsy [235–238].

While not Bell palsy, less frequently other infectious etiologies have been associated with subsets of acute facial paralysis, including herpes zoster oticus (Ramsay Hunt syndrome), Epstein–Barr virus, cytomegalovirus, coxsackievirus, influenza B, mumps, and rubella [239–241].

Bell palsy has been alternately hypothesized to be a mononeuritic autoimmune response [242]; one study showed Bell palsy developed as an induced immune reaction to an inactivated influenza vaccine in a manner similar to HSV recrudescence [243]. Genetic predisposition may play a role in Bell palsy as well [244]. Facial nerve ischemia has also been postulated as potential etiology in Bell palsy, as evidenced by nocturnal onset and higher incidence in diabetic and pregnant populations with ischemic microcirculatory changes [227, 245, 246].

Diagnosis of Bell palsy can be made with clinical findings of acute onset, progressively worsening diffuse facial muscle paralysis or paresis in association with/without other symptoms such as altered taste and natural history of acute onset of hours-days, worsening within 3 weeks, and variable recovery within 6–18 months. Physical exam should include full cranial nerve testing and neurologic exam and head and neck exam including otoscopy. Though 60–75% of peripheral facial nerve palsy is idiopathic, central nervous system disease or alternative disorder causing peripheral facial nerve palsy should be ruled out [247]. Differential diagnosis should include other causes of peripheral facial nerve palsy including infections like Lyme disease, Ramsay Hunt syndrome (herpes zoster oticus), otitis media, HIV, autoimmune disorders including Sjögren syndrome and sarcoidosis, facial nerve trauma, Guillain-Barré syndrome (GBS), or Melkersson-Rosenthal syndrome; a mass present at various sites along the course of facial nerve, including cholesteatoma, facial neuroma, metastatic disease to the petrous apex or parotid tumor, may also cause unilateral facial paresis or paralysis. Wackym et al. used molecular temporal bone pathology approaches to demonstrate latent herpes varicella-zoster (VZV) DNA in archival temporal bone sections [240, 241]. Herpes VZV DNA was identified, using the polymerase chain reaction, in archival celloidin-embedded temporal bone sections from two patients who clinically had Ramsay Hunt syndrome (herpes zoster oticus). The presence of VZV was confirmed by sequencing the PCR products. These experiments demonstrated that VZV genomic DNA was present in the geniculate ganglion of the side with facial paralysis and cutaneous recrudescence in both patients and in the clinically unaffected side in patient 1. In addition, patient 2 had a sudden hearing loss and was found to have VZV genomic DNA in sections from the affected side containing the spiral ganglion, Scarpa ganglion, organ of Corti, and macula of the saccule. No VZV genomic DNA was identified in temporal bone sections from five patients with Bell palsy and ten patients without evidence of otologic disease [240, 241]. While ischemic or hemorrhagic cerebral stroke causing upper motor neuron (UMN) unilateral facial paralysis will often spare forehead muscles, strokes affecting brainstem facial nerve nuclei or tracts may present as lower motor neuron (LMN) lesions. While Bell palsy diagnosis can be made without further testing in the setting of typical clinical history, physical signs, and disease course, further testing may be needed with atypical symptoms or suspicion of alternative causes. MRI imaging may be indicated with atypical features such as nystagmus, hyperacusis or hearing changes, diplopia or other cranial neuropathies to rule out mass lesion of cerebellopontine angle, petrous bone, parotid gland, or brainstem [248].

Borrelia or VZV serology can be performed if indicated by clinical history, and other suspected viral etiologies can be detected with lumbar puncture and CSF PCR testing [247]. Transcranial canalicular magnetic stimulation is an ancillary neurophysiologic test that can help differentiate between central and peripheral pathology [247].

The House-Brackmann Facial Nerve Grading Scale (H-B) rates severity of facial nerve palsy on a six-point scale and is an important tool for BP clinical severity grading, serial tracking, and prognostication [249]. Electroneurography (ENOG) and electromyography (EMG) testing is not necessary for Bell palsy diagnosis but can be used for prognostication and decision-making regarding facial nerve decompression. Axonal injury can be demonstrated on ENOG as early as 10–14 days of symptom onset, and < 90% amplitude reduction is associated with favorable prognosis [247]. On EMG testing, potential generation with voluntary contraction in the setting of facial paralysis and reinnervation potentials later in disease course indicate nerve continuity and increased likelihood of recovery, while early pathologic spontaneous EMG activity 10–14 days after symptom onset carries unfavorable prognosis [247]. While patients with comorbid diabetes are likelier to present with more severe Bell palsy, Riga et al. found it did not impact recovery at 6 months [227].

Bell palsy management consists primarily of medical therapy and symptom supportive treatment. Early oral corticosteroid treatment within 3 days of symptom onset remains first-line therapy, with number to treat of 10. Use can reduce risk of incomplete facial nerve function recovery by 30–40% and increase speed of recovery [250–252]. Regimens include prednisolone 25 mg twice daily for 10 days, or prednisolone 60 mg daily for 5 days followed by taper [253, 254]. Despite HSV-1 suspected etiology, studies of antiviral therapy (acyclovir, valacyclovir) in Bell palsy have shown variable findings, preventing adequate recommendation [252, 255–258]; however, treatment is indicated in the setting of Ramsay Hunt syndrome [247]. Symptomatic treatment for incomplete lid closure can include artificial tears, dexpanthenol ophthalmic ointment, and a nocturnal moisture-retaining eye shield. Physical therapy may be mildly beneficial in synkinesis and function in partial paralysis for more severe Bell palsy patients [259–261]. Surgical therapy including facial nerve decompression is not regularly performed in acute Bell palsy treatment, though select severe Bell palsy patients may benefit from treatment [262, 263]. Facial nerve reanimation, static reanimation procedures, and facial cosmetic procedures are reserved for patients with inadequate nerve regeneration or severe residual weakness, usually 6–15 months after symptom onset.

Bell palsy prognosis is related to severity, as determined most commonly by the H-B grading scale. House-Brackmann grades I–II have best outcomes, H-B III–IV moderate function, and H-B V–VI indicate severe compromise and poor recovery prognosis. Without treatment, 85% of patients have partial recovery in 3 weeks from symptom onset, and 71% have complete recovery [264]; better prognosis is seen with less severe grade and with partial recovery occurring during the initial 3 week period [265]. Patients should be seen for several months following Bell palsy onset to monitor recovery and potential need for further treatment for residual symptoms, sequelae, or recurrence. Recurrence is seen in up to 12% of patients, most likely within the first 2 years [266].

Pregnancy

Among pregnant patients, Bell palsy most frequently presents in third trimester or early postpartum period. The etiologies responsible for the disease do not appear to be different among pregnant patients as compared to the general population; however, many physiologic factors of pregnancy may be responsible for its occurrence among affected patients. Edema and hypercoagulability can be contributory to nerve ischemia and compression. Insulin resistance and gestational diabetes may act as similar risk factors to those of diabetics seen in Bell palsy [267]. Immunosuppression and increased susceptibility to viral infection and reactivation, especially later in pregnancy, also correspond with the postulated HSV-mediated pathogenesis of Bell palsy and may help explain the predominance of Bell palsy incidence later in pregnancy [226]; HSV is commonly acquired or reactivated during pregnancy and has greater incidence among pregnant women [268, 269]. Additional association has been found with preeclampsia among pregnant patients, further signifying the role of extracellular edema in Bell palsy pathogenesis [52, 270, 271]. Bell palsy has not been shown to affect perinatal outcomes [226].

Treatment is generally similar to in the general population. Clinician knowledge of appropriate corticosteroid use during pregnancy is paramount due to worse Bell palsy outcomes seen in delayed or missed treatment, especially with more severe grade (see section "Hearing Loss" for further discussion of corticosteroids in pregnancy). Oral corticosteroids may be used in the third trimester, with prednisone or methylprednisolone preferred to betamethasone or dexamethasone, but should be avoided earlier in pregnancy; Hussain et al. recommend the same regimens as treatment of the general population above [226]. If HSV-1 is suspected as etiology, acyclovir (Category B) may be used [272]. Blood pressure, weight, and blood sugar should be monitored during treatment, and fetal monitoring should be considered during treatment duration as well. Pregnant women with poorly controlled comorbid or gestational diabetes or hypertension that may be exacerbated by corticosteroid administration require risk–benefit conversation regarding potential impact of treatment on general health and Bell palsy recovery.

The prognosis for pregnant patients with Bell palsy is significantly worse than the general population; one study found only 55% of patients with complete paralysis had adequate recovery within 10 days as compared to 77–88% of non-pregnant patients [272]. Similarly, pregnant women with BP may be more likely to develop complete paralysis than non-pregnant patients [272]. Additionally, treatment bias is evident in the pregnant population via hesitancy to administer corticosteroids, as one study demonstrated only 33% of pregnant patients received cortico-

steroid therapy as compared to 52% of controls [272]. With appropriate treatment, outcomes in pregnancy approach those in the general population [273]. Overall, these findings further reinforce the need for improvement in appropriate and timely BP management in pregnancy by obstetricians and otologists alike.

Hearing Loss

Change in hearing is a frequent complaint during pregnancy. One Brazilian study of pregnant women found 24.9% experienced new auditory complaints during the duration of pregnancy, as compared to 3.9% among a non-pregnant female control group [50]. Benign hearing changes may be commonly encountered among pregnant patients. Studies have demonstrated a gradual decrease in low-frequency air-conduction hearing acuity (125, 250, 500, 1000 Hz) from first trimester through the third trimester associated with normal ABR and other audiologic testing that returned to normal in the postpartum period [274–277]. This characteristic hearing change, while statistically significant, remains within physiologic limits and is not classified as hearing loss according to the American National Standards Institute (ANSI) [274]. Pregnant patients have been shown to have decreased middle ear resonance frequency on multifrequency tympanometry (MFT) [276]. As the low-frequency pattern mimics that of Menière disease, this change has been hypothesized to relate to excessive salt and water retention that worsens through pregnancy, inducing endolymphatic hydrops (Fig. 30.1) in a manner similar to Menière disease. Due to postpartum normalization in most patients without intervention, this hearing change can be managed expectantly through the postpartum period once appropriate audiometric testing confirms the diagnosis [274]. Likewise, hormone variation during pregnancy can also frequently cause transient symptoms of aural fullness that can be managed expectantly [278].

Sudden sensorineural hearing loss is defined as hearing loss ≥30 dB in ≥3 contiguous frequencies lasting ≥3 days and is considered a medical emergency. As an acute inner ear pathologic process, sudden sensorineual hearing loss should be urgently/emergently be evaluated with a comprehensive audiometric study and evaluation by an otologist-neurotologist. Incidence ranges from 27 to 160 per 100,000 population [279, 280]; however, it is a rarer incidence during pregnancy, with one Taiwanese study reporting as low as 2.71 per 100,000 pregnancies [281]. Nonetheless, as mean age of sudden sensorineural hearing loss in pregnancy is less than in the average population (age 32 versus 40–60), pregnancy may play a role in precipitating hearing loss among these patients [1]; sudden sensorineural hearing loss of pregnancy has been described as a separate disease entity [282]. Likewise, with sudden sensorineural hearing loss accounting for 21% new-onset otologic complaints in pregnancy, it is important to diagnose and treat within this population [1].

Sudden sensorineural hearing loss occurs at similar rates between men and women [283]. While there are many identifiable causes for sudden sensorineural hearing loss (neoplastic, infectious, autoimmune, neurologic, otologic, metabolic disorders, vascular diseases, ototoxic drugs, trauma), the majority of sudden sensorineural hearing loss cases are idiopathic. Numerous risk factors and etiologies have been proposed for general sudden sensorineural hearing loss, including viral cochleitis, microvascular events related to hypercoagulable state, and autoimmune disorders [284–286]. However, certain etiologies and physiologic changes may be more likely to cause sudden sensorineural hearing loss during pregnancy.

- **Hormonal changes** of increased estrogen and progesterone can cause salt and water retention, resulting in extracellular fluid volume increase [274, 287, 288]. As studies have shown widespread expression of estrogen receptors in the cochlea, this hormonal fluctuation may similarly affect endolymph and perilymph composition [289, 290]. Endolymphatic sodium and volume retention may be associated with endolymphatic hydrops, and in similar fashion to Menière disease, sudden sensorineural hearing loss can occur with vestibular membrane rupture [206]. Other studies have suggested these sex steroid hormones may interrupt cochlear microcirculation causing sudden hearing loss, though this correlation is uncertain [281].

- **Cardiovascular and hematologic changes** are common beginning in the second month of pregnancy through the second and third trimesters [291]; elevated coagulation factors (VII, VIII, IX, X, XII, and fibrinogen) can cause a hypercoagulable state during pregnancy [282]. Increased plasma viscosity and erythrocyte aggregation may lead to increased risk of thromboembolism in the labyrinth artery and vascular occlusion of cochlear microcirculation, evoking sudden sensorineural hearing loss [206, 282, 291]. Importantly, preeclampsia and its end-organ ischemic changes have been shown to be a risk factor for cochlear damage and permanent hearing loss [292, 293].

- **Autoimmune disorders** may play a role in sudden sensorineural hearing loss in pregnancy. Antiphospholipid syndrome, diagnosed by presence of autoimmune antiphospholid or anticardiolipin antibodies in association with thrombosis and/or miscarriages and pregnancy-related complications, has been implicated in some cases of sudden sensorineural hearing loss [294–296]. Antiphospholipid syndrome can cause thrombosis in the placenta and vessels leading abortion, or in the cochlea leading to sudden sensorineural hearing loss [206].

- **Acoustic neuroma (vestibular schwannoma)** may be a cause of sudden sensorineural hearing loss in some patients (See section "Vestibular Schwannoma/Acoustic Neuroma"). These benign neoplasms are found in up to 15% of patients with sudden sensorineural hearing loss [297]; in pregnancy, they may rapidly enlarge with hormonal changes. Increased neuroma growth and vestibular myelin sheath vascularization can cause worsen symptoms or cause sudden sensorineural hearing loss [220].

Studies of sudden sensorineural hearing loss in pregnancy have shown that most cases occur in the second and third trimester, and that it has an increased rate of occurrence among older pregnant women [281, 295, 298]. Trends in severity of sudden sensorineural hearing loss in pregnancy vary; while some studies found most of these patients to have moderate hearing loss, more recent studies have shown a majority to have severe or profound deafness [206, 298, 299].

Patients with acute hearing loss suspected to have sudden sensorineural hearing loss should be evaluated rapidly within days of symptom onset. Though all sudden hearing loss should be evaluated, sudden sensorineural hearing loss may have improved prognosis with early diagnosis and treatment [300]. Thorough clinical history should evaluate for recent head trauma, barotrauma or noise exposure, exposure to ototoxic medications, ophthalmic symptoms (suggestive of Cogan syndrome), focal neurologic symptoms (suggestive of cerebrovascular or neoplastic causes), history or symptoms of autoimmune or vasculitis disorders, risk factors for Lyme disease or other infectious etiologies, ear pain, drainage or fever (suggestive of acute otitis media, chronic otitis media, or mastoiditis), or prior history of hearing loss plus or minus associated vertigo or tinnitus (suggestive of Menière disease or other existing disorder). Physical examination should include neurologic exam, otoscopic exam, a whisper test to grossly examine hearing, and Weber and Rinne tests to confirm sensorineural versus conductive hearing loss. Formal audiometric testing should be used to accurately diagnose sudden sensorineural hearing loss and track changes over time but should not delay treatment if unavailable. For patients without identifiable sudden sensorineural hearing loss etiology, MRI may be used to evaluate for retrocochlear pathology [301]. As preeclampsia has been shown to increase maternal and fetal risk of hearing loss in pregnancy, patients with comorbid hearing loss and preeclampsia should receive careful examination [293, 302–304]. Likewise, since other pregnancy complications such as gestational diabetes and HELLP syndrome (Hemolysis, Elevated Liver enzymes, and a Low Platelet count) have also been shown to carry higher risk of hearing impairment, prophylactic hearing screening should be considered for the preeclamptic, gestational diabetic, and other complicated pregnancy populations [292, 293, 304–306].

With identifiable cause for sudden sensorineural hearing loss, treatment is targeted at corrective treatment of the underlying etiology; in addition, and as primary treatment for the remaining idiopathic sudden sensorineural hearing loss, treatment consists of intratympanic or oral corticosteroids. Systemic treatment is initially preferred as standard of care in non-pregnant patients, but intratympanic injection may be preferable in patients with medical comorbidity or systemic corticosteroid intolerance or pregnancy, in addition to use as salvage therapy for those unresponsive to initial systemic treatment [307]. Oral treatment consists of 60 mg prednisone daily for 10 days. Intratympanic treatment consists of 0.5 mL dexamethasone 10 mg/mL injected weekly for 3 weeks. Greatest likelihood of response occurs if treatment is started within 2 weeks of hearing loss onset [301]. Hyperbaric oxygen therapy (HBOT) has also been explored as adjuvant to steroid treatment and has been associated with a higher rate of hearing recovery when used in combination [308, 309]. Patients should undergo repeat audiometry evaluations to measure treatment response. Failure to improve >6 months following treatment may indicate permanent hearing loss and may require an assistive hearing device.

In the pregnant population, glucocorticoid use may increase fetal risk via premature rupture of membranes (PROM) or intrauterine growth restriction (IUGR) [310, 311], can affect fetal organ development at high doses especially in the first trimester [312], and can increase maternal risk of gestational diabetes and hypertension, osteoporosis, and infection [313]. Likewise, as in normal adult sudden sensorineural hearing loss, in some cases sudden sensorineural hearing loss of pregnancy has resolved spontaneously or after delivery without treatment [282, 297, 314]; however, some studies of the impact of preeclampsia and hearing loss found that hearing damage persisted beyond postpartum resolution of pre-eclampsia [292]. Likewise the course of sudden sensorineural hearing loss in pregnancy has not been well-defined in large studies. To balance the desire to limit maternal and fetal exposure high-dose corticosteroids with achieving treatment efficacy, intratympanic steroid administration may be preferred, as smaller studies among pregnant patients have shown satisfactory rates of complete or partial recovery without side effects [298, 299]. Medication choice may be relevant as well, since methylprednisolone (FDA category B) may be safer than dexamethasone (FDA category C) during pregnancy. Nonetheless, during third trimester, systemic steroid use has been thought to be safe following proscribing guidelines [315]. During lactation, breast milk should be discarded for the first 4 h following oral corticosteroid treatment of >20 mg. In regard to HBOT, use during pregnancy may be controversial due to risk of fetal adverse effects such as retinopathy of prematurity, cardiovascular effects, and teratogenicity. However, the short duration of HBOT seems to be well-tolerated with no adverse neonatal outcomes reported in animal and limited human studies [206, 282, 316, 317]. While no definitive prognostic studies of sudden sensorineural hearing loss in pregnancy have been conducted, most patients with sudden sensorineural hearing loss in pregnancy appear to achieve partial or complete recovery following treatment [206].

Eustachian Tube Dysfunction

The Eustachian tube connects the middle ear with the nasopharynx, acting to clear mucous from and aerate the middle ear. The Eustachian tube consists of a lateral bony component (12 mm) and a longer medial fibrocartilaginous section (24 mm). A normally functioning Eustachian tube equalizes atmospheric pressure with the middle ear when patent and can protect the middle ear from undesirable pressure fluctuation or noise when closed. Additionally, proper mucociliary drainage prevents middle ear infection. Eustachian tube dysfunction can occur with abnormal or impaired function and has a national prevalence of 0.9–4.6% [318, 319].

The etiology of Eustachian tube dysfunction can vary based on pathophysiology of those three normal physiologic functions: middle ear pressure regulation, mucociliary clearance, and protection.

- **Pressure dysregulation** can occur with either functional or anatomic obstruction. Functional obstruction occurs when Eustachian tube function is impaired without physical obstruction, seen with mucosal inflammation/edema and secretions, muscular deficiency impairing valve function, or barotrauma-induced following diving or air travel. Anatomic obstruction occurs less frequently with severe mucosal swelling, congenital stenosis, nasopharyngeal cancer, or adenoid hypertrophy.
- **Mucociliary clearance** can be impeded with defects in ciliary function or impaired elimination of middle ear secretions. Infections, toxins, allergies, smoking, and other inflammatory disorders can all impair proper clearance [320]. Primary ciliary dysmotility disorders (cystic fibrosis, Kartagener syndrome) or ciliary dysmotility secondary to inflammation can also impede clearance.
- **Impaired protective function** occurs when gastric reflux, nasopharyngeal pathogens, and other substances inappropriately enter the Eustachian tube. This can occur with congenitally patent Eustachian tube or flaccid, truncated Eustachian tube seen in younger children. Abnormal positive nasopharyngeal pressure can also transmit substances into the Eustachian tube, as in nasal blowing, obstruction, or crying. Chronic gastric secretions can also impair Eustachian tube mucosal protection and pathogen clearance as well as mucosal edema.

Patients with Eustachian tube dysfunction typically present with complaint of aural fullness, otalgia, "popping," and/or discomfort. They may also have tinnitus, autophony, or muffled hearing impairment [321] Symptoms may be acute (<3 months) or chronic (>3 months). Acute

Eustachian tube dysfunction will often be preceded by recent upper respiratory infection or allergy exacerbation. Patients should also be questioned regarding activities such as travel or diving that may induce barometric-associated Eustachian tube dysfunction. Patulous Eustachian tube dysfunction (abnormal Eustachian tube patency) has a 2:1 female predominance, often presents with aural fullness and autophony, may improve with supine position or worsen with exercise, and may be precipitated by recent weight loss [321, 322]. Physical exam should include otoscopic exam, tympanometry, Rinne and Weber tuning fork testing, and nasopharyngoscopy to assess Eustachian tube patency. Diagnosis can be made with clinical symptoms along with otoscopic evidence of tympanic membrane retraction and/or tympanogram demonstrating abnormal negative middle ear pressure. Pure tone audiometry may show mild to moderate conductive hearing loss. Nasopharyngoscopy may reveal inflammation adjacent to the Eustachian tube orifice or obstructive cause of Eustachian tube dysfunction. Barotrauma-induced Eustachian tube dysfunction may initially have normal findings and rely on clinical history alone, while patulous Eustachian tube dysfunction may demonstrate otoscopic or tympanogram evidence of tympanic membrane excursion with breathing [323]. The Eustachian Tube Dysfunction Questionnaire (ETDQ-7) is a clinically validated patient-reported outcomes tool that can be used [324]. A number of Eustachian tube ventilatory function tests including tubomanometry have been developed but are not yet widely available [325]. Chronic untreated Eustachian tube dysfunction can lead to complications and sequelae such as otitis media, tympanic membrane perforation or atelectasis, cholesteatoma and/or hearing loss, making proper diagnosis and management imperative.

Treatment of Eustachian tube dysfunction varies based on etiology. For obstructive dysfunction, underlying chronic rhinosinusitis can be medically managed with an array of medications including saline sprays, oral/topical glucocorticoids, antibiotics, leukotriene inhibitors, and/or antifungal medications. Underlying allergic rhinitis can be treated with antihistamines, nasal steroid sprays, or leukotriene inhibitors. Smoking cessation may aid relief, as can allergy testing and avoidance of triggering agents. Underlying reflux disorders should be controlled with diet and behavioral modifications and proton pump inhibitor therapy for gastroesophageal reflux disorder (GERD). Anatomic obstruction usually requires procedural intervention beyond medical therapy; adenoid hypertrophy can be treated with adenoidectomy, whereas nasopharyngeal carcinoma is often treated with radiation or chemoradiation therapy rather than surgical resection [326, 327]. While Eustachian tube dysfunction is often treated—on the short-term—with decongestants like phenylephrine or pseudoephedrine, or intranasal corticosteroids for symptom relief, these medications are not FDA-approved for nonspecific Eustachian tube dysfunction due to limited evidence of benefit, and focus should remain on identifying an underlying etiology [323, 328]. Eustachian tube dysfunction refractory to medical therapy can be treated with a number of surgical options as well [329]. In addition to adenoidectomy for adenoid hypertrophy, tympanostomy tube placement can be useful for relieving chronic negative middle ear pressure and sequelae in Eustachian tube dysfunction. Endonasal laser eustachian tuboplasty and endonasal microdebrider tuboplasty can be used to reduce the bulky posterior-medial wall of the tubal orifice and have shown modest efficacy [330–332]. Eustachian tube balloon dilation has recently emerged as a popular and efficacious therapeutic option in select populations, though additional study of its proper indications is required [318, 333]. For patulous Eustachian tube dysfunction, in addition to humidified air and ventilating tube placement, additional procedures such as shim placement or Eustachian tube reconstruction with calcium hydroxyapatite, circumferential cauterization, fat graft packing, cartilage grafting, endoscopic ligation, and/or bone wax occlusion have been performed [323, 334–337].

Pregnancy

Eustachian tube dysfunction is a disorder commonly associated with pregnancy. One study of otolaryngology disorders during pregnancy found Eustachian tube dysfunction to be the most common otologic manifestation, with 37% of otology patients diagnosed with Eustachian tube dysfunction confirmed by impedance audiometry with Type-C tympanometry [49]. Another study surveying otologic symptoms in pregnancy found 41% of pregnant patients complaining of ear fullness or blockage were diagnosed with Eustachian tube dysfunction [203]. Likewise, the female predominance of patulous Eustachian tube dysfunction has been linked to up to one-third of diagnoses coinciding with pregnancy or estrogen replacement therapy [338].

There are multiple etiologies of Eustachian tube dysfunction in pregnancy. Obstructive Eustachian tube dysfunction can be seen with increased Eustachian tube dysfunction mucosal edema secondary to fluid retention associated with pregnancy [2]. Obstruction may also be exacerbated by nasal obstruction and rhinitis of pregnancy, a well-documented physiologic change of pregnancy due to effects of sex hormone effects on nasal epithelia, vasodilation, and glandular secretion with associated clear rhinorrhea and edematous nasal mucosa [339, 340]. It occurs in up to 40% of women, most commonly during the first trimester, typically resolving at or in the weeks following delivery [340]. This condition may cause or exacerbate Eustachian tube dysfunction in the pregnant population [341]. Smoking and previous otologic problems are also risk factors for obstructive Eustachian tube dysfunction in pregnancy [341]. In addition to obstructive Eustachian tube dysfunction, patulous Eustachian tube may also be seen, particularly among women with inadequate weight gain during pregnancy [342].

In terms of treatment of both obstructive and patulous Eustachian tube dysfunction, reassurance of the transient nature of these symptoms is important. With demonstrable etiologies of Eustachian tube dysfunction in pregnancy linked to normal physiologic changes, studies have shown resolution of obstructive and patulous Eustachian tube dysfunction symptoms by 3 months postpartum in most patients [341]. Further treatment is largely supportive, with humidified air, hydration, supine positioning, and Valsalva maneuver beneficial in patulous Eustachian tube dysfunction symptoms [2]. Nasal saline drops and potassium iodide can aid in mucous thickening to relieve symptoms [335]. For obstructive symptoms where medical therapy is indicated, intranasal topical corticosteroids, particularly budesonide, is a safe choice (FDA Category B) [60]. Oral decongestants such as phenylephrine or oxymetazoline are not indicated due to teratogenicity in animals; the American College of Obstetrics and Gynecology (ACOG) recommends pseudoephedrine as their oral decongestant of choice (FDA Category C), while still noting case control studies associate use with fetal gastroschises, especially in first trimester use [343–346]. Similarly, H-1 receptor antagonists should be avoided in first trimester. First generation antihistamines are preferred to second generation due to longevity, but if unable to be tolerated, cetirizine or loratadine (Category B) can be used in third trimester [347, 348].

Third Window Syndrome

Third window syndrome (TWS) is a group of characteristic signs and symptoms affecting hearing and balance related to underlying dehiscence of the otic capsule resulting in a third mobile window. While superior semicircular canal dehiscence (SSCD) is the most common site for a pathological third mobile window, over one dozen sites can be seen with high-resolution temporal bone CT scans, and there are also patients in whom a TWS exists in which no site of dehiscence can be seen (CT- TWS) [64]. Many locations of dehiscence have been identified and reported that lead to an artificial "third mobile window" and resulting phenotype, including cochlea-facial nerve dehiscence, cochlea-internal auditory canal dehiscence, enlarged (wide) vestibular aqueduct, lateral semicircular canal dehiscence, lateral semicircular canal-facial nerve dehiscence, vestibule-middle ear dehiscence, posttraumatic hypermobile stapes footplate, modiolus dehiscence, superior semicircular canal-superior petrosal vein dehiscence, posterior semicircular canal dehiscence, and posterior semicircular canal-jugular bulb dehiscence—all of which can be seen by high-resolution temporal bone CT [66]; likewise, similar symptoms and audiologic exam signs may be seen in conditions such as perilymphatic fistula. A common structural finding in all of these conditions is an otic capsule defect that creates a "third mobile window." As a minority of SSCD and near-SSCD patients may have persistent or recurrent TWS symptoms after surgery, the presence of multiple-sites of dehiscence is an important principle to understand [64–66, 349–351].

Pathophysiology

Due to the numerous sites of dehiscence and labyrinth defects that can cause TWS, no one etiology can be identified. In the case of SSCD and other canal defects, dehiscence may be due to congenital underdevelopment or weakening of the temporal bone followed by an inciting event later in life including high intracranial or middle ear pressures or age-related bony erosion [352]. A hereditary predisposition has been proposed as well due to familial occurrence [353]. Bilateral dehiscence is seen in about 25% of patients, with a predilection for the left side in unilateral SSCD [352]. Canal bony thinning is seen in 1.3% of individuals, and frank dehiscence is estimated in about 0.7% of the population through cadaveric temporal bone examination [354]. Though one study found higher rates of SSCD in women (55%), the authors noted that women aged 26–54 exhibit higher rates of outpatient healthcare utilization compared to men, most disparately among ages 26–54 (the same age range in which SSCD is most commonly diagnosed) [352].

These TWS patients experience sound-induced dizziness (gravitational receptor [otolithic] dysfunction type of vertigo) and autophony (e.g., resonant voice, hearing heartbeat, hearing eyes move or blink, joints moving, chewing, hearing heel strikes, and/or joints popping or moving). They also experience auditory symptoms such as autophony and aural fullness (94%) or tinnitus, improved with Valsalva or supine positioning (50%) [355]. Cognitive dysfunction, migraine headaches, and migraine variants including vestibular migraine, oscillopsia, autonomic dysfunction, and spatial disorientation may be seen as well [65, 66, 350]. On audiologic exam, ipsilateral pseudoconductive hearing loss may be seen in the ear with TWS. Cervical vestibular-evoked myogenic potential (cVEMP) testing can aid diagnosis with findings of abnormally reduced cVEMP response threshold and increased amplitude [64, 65]. In patients with high index of suspicion for SSCD or TWS, high-resolution temporal bone CT without contrast should be used to identify an area of dehiscence. It is important to have the images formatted in the axial, coronal, Pöschl, and Stenvers views and inverted images are particularly well-suited to identifying the site of dehiscence [66].

Treatment

For patients with debilitating symptoms, treatment options consist of surgical elimination of the third window returning to the natural two windows. For the most common etiology, SSCD, this can be accomplished by surgical resurfacing and/or plugging of the superior semicircular canal by a middle cranial fossa or transmastoid approach [356]. This definitive correction generally improves autophony and dizziness symptoms as well as quality of life and shows normalization on audiologic and cVEMP testing [65, 356–358]. Round window reinforcement has also been introduced as a less invasive potential approach for reducing SSCD symptoms [359]. For third windows that cannot be accessed and managed directly because of potential morbidity, such as cochlea-facial nerve dehiscence, round window reinforcement is the management strategy used [66].

Pregnancy

TWS secondary to SSCD has been reported to occur during pregnancy, hypothesized to result from bone demineralization that may occur during pregnancy [360]. Contraction-related Valsalva maneuver during labor has been reported to act as an inciting event for TWS during the peripartum period [361]. Therefore, new-onset gravitational receptor (otolithic) dysfunction type of vertigo during pregnancy or the peripartum period with symptoms consistent with TWS should be appropriately referred to a neurotologist for management.

Patients with history of traumatic brain injury and psychiatric comorbidities such as posttraumatic stress disorder, major depressive disorder, functional neurologic symptom disorder, and somatic symptom disorder (formerly conversion disorder) may have worse surgical outcomes [65].

Conclusion

Otologic and neurologic disorders can commonly occur during pregnancy. While some symptoms and complaints are related to physiologic changes of pregnancy, are transient in nature, and resolve in the postpartum period, a number of otologic and neurotological disorders have increased incidence and morbidity among the pregnant population. Proper recognition and appropriate treatment of otologic and neurotological disorders is incumbent upon all providers seeing pregnant patients in a healthcare setting. In management decision-making, proper consideration must be given to fetal risk, maternal risk, natural course and prognosis of disorder, and patient preferences. The second trimester is the safest time to initiate treatment. Treatment of otologic symptoms among pregnant patients should be co-managed between obstetricians and otologists–neurotologists.

Disclosure The authors have no conflicts of interest to disclose.

References

1. Wu PH, Cheng PW, Young YH. Inner ear disorders in 68 pregnant women: a 20-year experience. Clin Otolaryngol. 2017;42(4):844–6. https://doi.org/10.1111/coa.12693.

2. Shiny Sherlie V, Varghese A. ENT changes of pregnancy and its management. Indian J Otolaryngol Head Neck Surg. 2014;66(Suppl 1):6–9. https://doi.org/10.1007/s12070-011-0376-6.

3. Radtke A, Lempert T, von Brevern M, Feldmann M, Lezius F, Neuhauser H. Prevalence and complications of orthostatic dizziness in the general population. Clin Auton Res. 2011;21(3):161–8. https://doi.org/10.1007/s10286-010-0114-2.

4. Harris JP, Alexander TH. Current-day prevalence of Meniere's syndrome. Audiol Neurootol. 2010;15(5):318–22. https://doi.org/10.1159/000286213.

5. House JW, Doherty JK, Fisher LM, Derebery MJ, Berliner KI. Meniere's disease: prevalence of contralateral ear involvement. Otol Neurotol. 2006;27(3):355–61. https://doi.org/10.1097/00129492-200604000-00011.

6. Havia M, Kentala E. Progression of symptoms of dizziness in Meniere's disease. Arch Otolaryngol Head Neck Surg. 2004;130(4):431–5. https://doi.org/10.1001/archotol.130.4.431.

7. Silverstein H, Smouha E, Jones R. Natural history vs. surgery for Meniere's disease. Otolaryngol Head Neck Surg. 1989;100(1):6–16. https://doi.org/10.1177/019459988910000102.

8. Murofushi T, Tsubota M, Kitao K, Yoshimura E. Simultaneous presentation of definite vestibular migraine and definite Meniere's disease: overlapping syndrome of two diseases. Front Neurol. 2018;9:749. https://doi.org/10.3389/fneur.2018.00749.

9. Foster CA, Breeze RE. Endolymphatic hydrops in Meniere's disease: cause, consequence, or epiphenomenon? Otol Neurotol. 2013;34(7):1210–4. https://doi.org/10.1097/MAO.0b013e31829e83df.

10. Rauch SD, Merchant SN, Thedinger BA. Meniere's syndrome and endolymphatic hydrops. Double-blind temporal bone study. Ann Otol Rhinol Laryngol. 1989;98(11):873–83. https://doi.org/10.1177/000348948909801108.

11. Gurkov R, Flatz W, Louza J, Strupp M, Krause E. In vivo visualization of endolymphatic hydrops in patients with Meniere's disease: correlation with audiovestibular function. Eur Arch Otorhinolaryngol. 2011;268(12):1743–8. https://doi.org/10.1007/s00405-011-1573-3.

12. Luryi AL, Morse E, Michaelides E. Pathophysiology and diagnosis of Meniere's disease. In: Babu S, Schutt CA, Bojrab DI, editors. Diagnosis and treatment of vestibular disorders. Cham: Springer International; 2019. p. 165–88.

13. Nakashima T, Pyykko I, Arroll MA, et al. Meniere's disease. Nat Rev Dis Primers. 2016;2:16028. https://doi.org/10.1038/nrdp.2016.28.

14. Greco A, Gallo A, Fusconi M, Marinelli C, Macri GF, de Vincentiis M. Meniere's disease might be an autoimmune condition? Autoimmun Rev. 2012;11(10):731–8. https://doi.org/10.1016/j.autrev.2012.01.004.

15. Filipo R, Ciciarello F, Attanasio G, et al. Chronic cerebrospinal venous insufficiency in patients with Meniere's disease. Eur Arch Otorhinolaryngol. 2015;272(1):77–82. https://doi.org/10.1007/s00405-013-2841-1.

16. Paparella MM, Mancini F. Vestibular Meniere's disease. Otolaryngol Head Neck Surg. 1985;93(2):148–51. https://doi.org/10.1177/019459988509300203.

17. Ueberfuhr MA, Wiegrebe L, Krause E, Gurkov R, Drexl M. Tinnitus in normal-hearing participants after exposure to intense low-frequency sound and in Meniere's disease patients. Front Neurol. 2016;7:239. https://doi.org/10.3389/fneur.2016.00239.

18. Colebatch JG, Day BL, Bronstein AM, et al. Vestibular hypersensitivity to clicks is characteristic of the Tullio phenomenon. J Neurol Neurosurg Psychiatry. 1998;65(5):670–8. https://doi.org/10.1136/jnnp.65.5.670.

19. Lopez-Escamez JA, Viciana D, Garrido-Fernandez P. Impact of bilaterality and headache on health-related quality of life in Meniere's disease. Ann Otol Rhinol Laryngol. 2009;118(6):409–16. https://doi.org/10.1177/000348940911800603.

20. Ozeki H, Iwasaki S, Murofushi T. Vestibular drop attack secondary to Meniere's disease results from unstable otolithic function. Acta Otolaryngol. 2008;128(8):887–91. https://doi.org/10.1080/00016480701767390.

21. Lopez-Escamez JA, Carey J, Chung WH, et al. Diagnostic criteria for Meniere's disease according to the classification Committee of the Barany Society. HNO. 2017;65(11):887–93. https://doi.org/10.1007/s00106-017-0387-z.

22. Kim CH, Shin JE, Kim TS, Shim BS, Park HJ. Two-dimensional analysis of head-shaking nystagmus in patients with Meniere's disease. J Vestib Res. 2013;23(2):95–100. https://doi.org/10.3233/VES-130478.

23. Lee SU, Kim HJ, Koo JW, Kim JS. Comparison of caloric and head-impulse tests during the attacks of Meniere's disease. Laryngoscope. 2017;127(3):702–8. https://doi.org/10.1002/lary.26103.

24. Kim HH, Kumar A, Battista RA, Wiet RJ. Electrocochleography in patients with Meniere's disease. Am J Otolaryngol. 2005;26(2):128–31. https://doi.org/10.1016/j.amjoto.2004.11.005.

25. Schick B, Brors D, Koch O, Schafers M, Kahle G. Magnetic resonance imaging in patients with sudden hearing loss, tinnitus and vertigo. Otol Neurotol. 2001;22(6):808–12. https://doi.org/10.1097/00129492-200111000-00016.

26. Ito T, Inui H, Miyasaka T, et al. Three-dimensional magnetic resonance imaging reveals the relationship between the control of vertigo and decreases in endolymphatic hydrops after endolymphatic sac drainage with steroids for Meniere's disease. Front Neurol. 2019;10:46. https://doi.org/10.3389/fneur.2019.00046.

27. Cass SP, Machala MC, Ambrose EC. Medical management of Meniere's disease. In: Babu S, Schutt CA, Bojrab DI, editors. Diagnosis and treatment of vestibular disorders. Cham: Springer International; 2019. p. 189–98.

28. Crowson MG, Patki A, Tucci DL. A systematic review of diuretics in the medical management of Meniere's disease. Otolaryngol Head Neck Surg. 2016;154(5):824–34. https://doi.org/10.1177/0194599816630733.

29. Adrion C, Fischer CS, Wagner J, et al. Efficacy and safety of betahistine treatment in patients with Meniere's disease: primary results of a long term, multicentre, double blind, randomised, placebo controlled, dose defining trial (BEMED trial). BMJ. 2016;352:h6816. https://doi.org/10.1136/bmj.h6816.

30. Morales-Luckie E, Cornejo-Suarez A, Zaragoza-Contreras MA, Gonzalez-Perez O. Oral administration of prednisone to control refractory vertigo in Meniere's disease: a pilot study. Otol Neurotol. 2005;26(5):1022–6. https://doi.org/10.1097/01.mao.0000185057.81962.51.

31. Fisher LM, Derebery MJ, Friedman RA. Oral steroid treatment for hearing improvement in Meniere's disease and endolymphatic hydrops. Otol Neurotol. 2012;33(9):1685–91. https://doi.org/10.1097/MAO.0b013e31826dba83.

32. Neff BA, Staab JP, Eggers SD, et al. Auditory and vestibular symptoms and chronic subjective dizziness in patients with Meniere's disease, vestibular migraine, and Meniere's disease with concomitant vestibular migraine. Otol Neurotol. 2012;33(7):1235–44. https://doi.org/10.1097/MAO.0b013e31825d644a.

33. Viscomi GJ, Bojrab DI. Use of electrocochleography to monitor antigenic challenge in Meniere's disease. Otolaryngol Head Neck Surg. 1992;107(6 Pt 1):733–7. https://doi.org/10.1177/019459988910700604.1.

34. Derebery MJ. Allergic management of Meniere's disease: an outcome study. Otolaryngol Head Neck Surg. 2000;122(2):174–82. https://doi.org/10.1016/S0194-5998(00)70235-X.

35. Keles E, Godekmerdan A, Kalidag T, et al. Meniere's disease and allergy: allergens and cytokines. J Laryngol Otol. 2004;118(9):688–93. https://doi.org/10.1258/0022215042244822.

36. Hall CD, Herdman SJ, Whitney SL, et al. Vestibular rehabilitation for peripheral vestibular hypofunction: an evidence-based clinical practice guideline: from the American Physical Therapy Association Neurology Section. J Neurol Phys Ther. 2016;40(2):124–55. https://doi.org/10.1097/NPT.0000000000000120.

37. Arif M, Sadlier M, Rajenderkumar D, James J, Tahir T. A randomised controlled study of mindfulness meditation versus relaxation therapy in the management of tinnitus. J Laryngol Otol. 2017;131(6):501–7. https://doi.org/10.1017/S002221511700069X.

38. Jackson NM, LaRouere MJ. Surgical treatment of Meniere's disease. In: Babu S, Schutt CA, Bojrab

DI, editors. Diagnosis and treatment of vestibular disorders. Cham: Springer International; 2019. p. 199–213.

39. Wackym PA, Friberg U, Bagger-Sjoback D, Linthicum FH Jr, Friedmann I, Rask-Andersen H. Human endolymphatic sac: possible mechanisms of pressure regulation. J Laryngol Otol. 1987;101(8):768–79. https://doi.org/10.1017/s0022215100102713.

40. Wackym PA, Linthicum FH Jr, Ward PH, House WF, Micevych PE, Bagger-Sjoback D. Re-evaluation of the role of the human endolymphatic sac in Meniere's disease. Otolaryngol Head Neck Surg. 1990;102(6):732–44. https://doi.org/10.1177/019459989010200618.

41. Wackym PA. Histopathologic findings in Meniere's disease. Otolaryngol Head Neck Surg. 1995;112(1):90–100. https://doi.org/10.1016/S0194-59989570307-1.

42. Sood AJ, Lambert PR, Nguyen SA, Meyer TA. Endolymphatic sac surgery for Menier's disease: a systematic review and meta-analysis. Otol Neurotol. 2014;35(6):1033–45. https://doi.org/10.1097/MAO.0000000000000324.

43. Kato BM, LaRouere MJ, Bojrab DI, Michaelides EM. Evaluating quality of life after endolymphatic sac surgery: the Meniere's disease outcomes questionnaire. Otol Neurotol. 2004;25(3):339–44. https://doi.org/10.1097/00129492-200405000-00023.

44. Ozturk K, Ata N. Intratympanic mixture gentamicin and dexamethasone versus dexamethasone for unilateral Meniere's disease. Am J Otolaryngol. 2019;40(5):711–4. https://doi.org/10.1016/j.amjoto.2019.06.008.

45. Minor LB. Intratympanic gentamicin for control of vertigo in Meniere's disease: vestibular signs that specify completion of therapy. Am J Otol. 1999;20(2):209–19. https://www.ncbi.nlm.nih.gov/pubmed/10100525.

46. Nedzelski JM, Chiong CM, Fradet G, Schessel DA, Bryce GE, Pfleiderer AG. Intratympanic gentamicin instillation as treatment of unilateral Meniere's disease: update of an ongoing study. Am J Otol. 1993;14(3):278–82. https://www.ncbi.nlm.nih.gov/pubmed/8372926.

47. Kemink JL, Telian SA, Graham MD, Joynt L. Transmastoid labyrinthectomy: reliable surgical management of vertigo. Otolaryngol Head Neck Surg. 1989;101(1):5–10. https://doi.org/10.1177/019459988910100102.

48. Graham MD, Kemink JL. Transmastoid labyrinthectomy: surgical management of vertigo in the nonserviceable hearing ear. A five-year experience. Am J Otol. 1984;5(4):295–9. https://www.ncbi.nlm.nih.gov/pubmed/6720881.

49. Swain S, Pattnaik T, Mohanty J. Otological and rhinological manifestations in pregnancy: our experiences at a tertiary care teaching hospital of East India. Int J Health Allied Sci. 2020;9(2):159–63. (Original Article). https://doi.org/10.4103/ijhas.IJHAS_87_19.

50. Schmidt PM, Flores Fda T, Rossi AG, Silveira AF. Hearing and vestibular complaints during pregnancy. Braz J Otorhinolaryngol. 2010;76(1):29–33. https://www.ncbi.nlm.nih.gov/pubmed/20339686; https://pdf.sciencedirectassets.com/306588/1-s2.0-S1808869415X70546/1-s2.0-S1808869415313501/main.pdf.

51. Swain SK, Nayak S, Ravan JR, Sahu MC. Tinnitus and its current treatment—still an enigma in medicine. J Formos Med Assoc. 2016;115(3):139–44. https://doi.org/10.1016/j.jfma.2015.11.011.

52. Shapiro JL, Yudin MH, Ray JG. Bell's palsy and tinnitus during pregnancy: predictors of pre-eclampsia? Three cases and a detailed review of the literature. Acta Otolaryngol. 1999;119(6):647–51. https://doi.org/10.1080/00016489950180577.

53. Mukhophadhyay S, Biswas S, Vindla S. Severe tinnitus in pregnancy, necessitating caesarean delivery. J Obstet Gynaecol. 2007;27(1):81–2. https://doi.org/10.1080/01443610601062689.

54. Uchide K, Suzuki N, Takiguchi T, Terada S, Inoue M. The possible effect of pregnancy on Meniere's disease. ORL J Otorhinolaryngol Relat Spec. 1997;59(5):292–5. https://doi.org/10.1159/000276956.

55. Stevens MN, Hullar TE. Improvement in sensorineural hearing loss during pregnancy. Ann Otol Rhinol Laryngol. 2014;123(9):614–8. https://doi.org/10.1177/0003489414525590.

56. Andrews JC, Honrubia V. Premenstrual exacerbation of Meniere's disease revisited. Otolaryngol Clin North Am. 2010;43(5):1029–40. https://doi.org/10.1016/j.otc.2010.05.012.

57. Morse GG, House JW. Changes in Meniere's disease responses as a function of the menstrual cycle. Nurs Res. 2001;50(5):286–92. https://doi.org/10.1097/00006199-200109000-00006.

58. Holt GR, Mabry RL. ENT medications in pregnancy. Otolaryngol Head Neck Surg. 1983;91(3):338–41. https://doi.org/10.1177/019459988309100330.

59. Huynh-Do U, Frey FJ. Potential dangers of diuretics. Ther Umsch. 2000;57(6):408–11. https://doi.org/10.1024/0040-5930.57.6.408.

60. Vlastarakos PV, Nikolopoulos TP, Manolopoulos L, Ferekidis E, Kreatsas G. Treating common ear problems in pregnancy: what is safe? Eur Arch Otorhinolaryngol. 2008;265(2):139–45. https://doi.org/10.1007/s00405-007-0534-3.

61. Lempert T, Neuhauser H. Epidemiology of vertigo, migraine and vestibular migraine. J Neurol. 2009;256(3):333–8. https://doi.org/10.1007/s00415-009-0149-2.

62. Oh AK, Lee H, Jen JC, Corona S, Jacobson KM, Baloh RW. Familial benign recurrent vertigo. Am J Med Genet. 2001;100(4):287–91. https://doi.org/10.1002/ajmg.1294.

63. Baloh RW, Foster CA, Yue Q, Nelson SF. Familial migraine with vertigo and essential tremor.

Neurology. 1996;46(2):458–60. https://doi.org/10.1212/wnl.46.2.458.

64. Wackym PA, Wood SJ, Siker DA, Carter DM. Otic capsule dehiscence syndrome: superior semicircular canal dehiscence syndrome with no radiographically visible dehiscence. Ear Nose Throat J. 2015;94(8):E8–E24. https://doi.org/10.1177/014556131509400802.

65. Wackym PA, Balaban CD, Mackay HT, et al. Longitudinal cognitive and neurobehavioral functional outcomes before and after repairing Otic capsule dehiscence. Otol Neurotol. 2016;37(1):70–82. https://doi.org/10.1097/MAO.0000000000000928.

66. Wackym PA, Balaban CD, Zhang P, Siker DA, Hundal JS. Third window syndrome: surgical management of cochlea-facial nerve dehiscence. Front Neurol. 2019;10:1281. https://doi.org/10.3389/fneur.2019.01281.

67. Bayazit Y, Yilmaz M, Mumbuc S, Kanlikama M. Assessment of migraine-related cochleovestibular symptoms. Rev Laryngol Otol Rhinol (Bord). 2001;122(2):85–8. https://www.ncbi.nlm.nih.gov/pubmed/11715266.

68. Kuritzky A, Ziegler DK, Hassanein R. Vertigo, motion sickness and migraine. Headache. 1981;21(5):227–31. https://doi.org/10.1111/j.1526-4610.1981.hed2105227.x.

69. Selby G, Lance JW. Observations on 500 cases of migraine and allied vascular headache. J Neurol Neurosurg Psychiatry. 1960;23:23–32. https://doi.org/10.1136/jnnp.23.1.23.

70. Johnson GD. Medical management of migraine-related dizziness and vertigo. Laryngoscope. 1998;108(1 Pt 2):1–28. https://doi.org/10.1097/00005537-199801001-00001.

71. Kayan A, Hood JD. Neuro-otological manifestations of migraine. Brain. 1984;107(Pt 4):1123–42. https://doi.org/10.1093/brain/107.4.1123.

72. Murdin L, Chamberlain F, Cheema S, et al. Motion sickness in migraine and vestibular disorders. J Neurol Neurosurg Psychiatry. 2015;86(5):585–7. https://doi.org/10.1136/jnnp-2014-308331.

73. Drummond PD. Triggers of motion sickness in migraine sufferers. Headache. 2005;45(6):653–6. https://doi.org/10.1111/j.1526-4610.2005.05132.x.

74. Furman JM, Marcus DA, Balaban CD. Migrainous vertigo: development of a pathogenetic model and structured diagnostic interview. Curr Opin Neurol. 2003;16(1):5–13. https://doi.org/10.1097/01.wco.0000053582.70044.e2.

75. Radtke A, von Brevern M, Neuhauser H, Hottenrott T, Lempert T. Vestibular migraine: long-term follow-up of clinical symptoms and vestibulo-cochlear findings. Neurology. 2012;79(15):1607–14. https://doi.org/10.1212/WNL.0b013e31826e264f.

76. Dieterich M, Brandt T. Episodic vertigo related to migraine (90 cases): vestibular migraine? J Neurol. 1999;246(10):883–92. https://doi.org/10.1007/s004150050478.

77. Wackym PA. Ultrastructural organization of calcitonin gene-related peptide immunoreactive efferent axons and terminals in the vestibular periphery. Am J Otol. 1993;14(1):41–50. https://www.ncbi.nlm.nih.gov/pubmed/8424475.

78. Jen JC, Baloh RW. Familial episodic ataxia: a model for migrainous vertigo. Ann N Y Acad Sci. 2009;1164:252–6. https://doi.org/10.1111/j.1749-6632.2008.03723.x.

79. Jen J, Kim GW, Baloh RW. Clinical spectrum of episodic ataxia type 2. Neurology. 2004;62(1):17–22. https://doi.org/10.1212/01.wnl.0000101675.61074.50.

80. Radtke A, Lempert T, Gresty MA, Brookes GB, Bronstein AM, Neuhauser H. Migraine and Meniere's disease: is there a link? Neurology. 2002;59(11):1700–4. https://doi.org/10.1212/01.wnl.0000036903.22461.39.

81. Harno H, Hirvonen T, Kaunisto MA, et al. Subclinical vestibulocerebellar dysfunction in migraine with and without aura. Neurology. 2003;61(12):1748–52. https://doi.org/10.1212/01.wnl.0000098882.82690.65.

82. Cutrer FM, Baloh RW. Migraine-associated dizziness. Headache. 1992;32(6):300–4. https://doi.org/10.1111/j.1526-4610.1992.hed3206300.x.

83. Headache Classification Committee of the International Headache Society (IHS) the International Classification of Headache Disorders, 3rd edition. Cephalalgia. 2018;38(1):1–211. https://doi.org/10.1177/0333102417738202.

84. Maldonado Fernández M, Birdi JS, Irving GJ, Murdin L, Kivekäs I, Strupp M. Pharmacological agents for the prevention of vestibular migraine. Cochrane Database Syst Rev. 2015;(6):CD010600. https://doi.org/10.1002/14651858.CD010600.pub2.

85. Strupp M, Dieterich M, Brandt T. The treatment and natural course of peripheral and central vertigo. Dtsch Arztebl Int. 2013;110(29–30):505–15; quiz 515–6. https://doi.org/10.3238/arztebl.2013.0505.

86. Seemungal B, Kaski D, Lopez-Escamez JA. Early diagnosis and management of acute vertigo from vestibular migraine and Meniere's disease. Neurol Clin. 2015;33(3):619–28, ix. https://doi.org/10.1016/j.ncl.2015.04.008.

87. Bikhazi P, Jackson C, Ruckenstein MJ. Efficacy of antimigrainous therapy in the treatment of migraine-associated dizziness. Am J Otol. 1997;18(3):350–4. https://www.ncbi.nlm.nih.gov/pubmed/9149830.

88. Furman JM, Marcus DA, Balaban CD. Rizatriptan reduces vestibular-induced motion sickness in migraineurs. J Headache Pain. 2011;12(1):81–8. https://doi.org/10.1007/s10194-010-0250-z.

89. Neuhauser H, Radtke A, von Brevern M, Lempert T. Zolmitriptan for treatment of migrainous vertigo: a pilot randomized placebo-controlled trial. Neurology. 2003;60(5):882–3. https://doi.org/10.1212/01.wnl.0000049476.40047.a3.

90. Cassano D, Pizza V, Busillo V. P074. Almotriptan in the acute treatment of vestibular migraine: a retrospective study. J Headache Pain. 2015;16(Suppl 1):A114. https://doi.org/10.1186/1129-2377-16-S1-A114.

91. Prakash S, Chavda BV, Mandalia H, Dhawan R, Padmanabhan D. Headaches related to triptans therapy in patients of migrainous vertigo. J Headache Pain. 2008;9(3):185–8. https://doi.org/10.1007/s10194-008-0035-9.

92. Prakash S, Shah ND. Migrainous vertigo responsive to intravenous methylprednisolone: case reports. Headache. 2009;49(8):1235–9. https://doi.org/10.1111/j.1526-4610.2009.01474.x.

93. Harker LA, Rassekh C. Migraine equivalent as a cause of episodic vertigo. Laryngoscope. 1988;98(2):160–4. https://doi.org/10.1288/00005537-198802000-00008.

94. Salviz M, Yuce T, Acar H, Karatas A, Acikalin RM. Propranolol and venlafaxine for vestibular migraine prophylaxis: a randomized controlled trial. Laryngoscope. 2016;126(1):169–74. https://doi.org/10.1002/lary.25445.

95. Reploeg MD, Goebel JA. Migraine-associated dizziness: patient characteristics and management options. Otol Neurotol. 2002;23(3):364–71. https://doi.org/10.1097/00129492-200205000-00024.

96. Maione A. Migraine-related vertigo: diagnostic criteria and prophylactic treatment. Laryngoscope. 2006;116(10):1782–6. https://doi.org/10.1097/01.mlg.0000231302.77922.c5.

97. Linde M, Mulleners WM, Chronicle EP, McCrory DC. Antiepileptics other than gabapentin, pregabalin, topiramate, and valproate for the prophylaxis of episodic migraine in adults. Cochrane Database Syst Rev. 2013;2013(6):CD010608. https://doi.org/10.1002/14651858.CD010608.

98. Brodsky JR, Cusick BA, Zhou G. Evaluation and management of vestibular migraine in children: experience from a pediatric vestibular clinic. Eur J Paediatr Neurol. 2016;20(1):85–92. https://doi.org/10.1016/j.ejpn.2015.09.011.

99. Gode S, Celebisoy N, Kirazli T, et al. Clinical assessment of topiramate therapy in patients with migrainous vertigo. Headache. 2010;50(1):77–84. https://doi.org/10.1111/j.1526-4610.2009.01496.x.

100. Bisdorff AR. Treatment of migraine related vertigo with lamotrigine an observational study. Bull Soc Sci Med Grand Duche Luxemb. 2004;2:103–8. https://www.ncbi.nlm.nih.gov/pubmed/15641316.

101. Salmito MC, Duarte JA, Morganti LOG, et al. Prophylactic treatment of vestibular migraine. Braz J Otorhinolaryngol. 2017;83(4):404–10. https://doi.org/10.1016/j.bjorl.2016.04.022.

102. Jackson JL, Cogbill E, Santana-Davila R, et al. A comparative effectiveness meta-analysis of drugs for the prophylaxis of migraine headache. PloS One. 2015;10(7):e0130733. https://doi.org/10.1371/journal.pone.0130733.

103. Lepcha A, Amalanathan S, Augustine AM, Tyagi AK, Balraj A. Flunarizine in the prophylaxis of migrainous vertigo: a randomized controlled trial. Eur Arch Otorhinolaryngol. 2014;271(11):2931–6. https://doi.org/10.1007/s00405-013-2786-4.

104. Taghdiri F, Togha M, Razeghi Jahromi S, Refaeian F. Cinnarizine for the prophylaxis of migraine associated vertigo: a retrospective study. SpringerPlus. 2014;3:231. https://doi.org/10.1186/2193-1801-3-231.

105. Whitney SL, Wrisley DM, Brown KE, Furman JM. Physical therapy for migraine-related vestibulopathy and vestibular dysfunction with history of migraine. Laryngoscope. 2000;110(9):1528–34. https://doi.org/10.1097/00005537-200009000-00022.

106. Kinne BL, Baker BJ, Chesser BT. The use of vestibular rehabilitation for individuals with migraines: a systematic review. Otolaryngology. 2017;7(6):334. https://doi.org/10.4172/2161-119X.1000334.

107. Schettino A, Navaratnam D. Vestibular migraine. In: Babu S, Schutt CA, Bojrab DI, editors. Diagnosis and treatment of vestibular disorders. Cham: Springer International; 2019. p. 255–76.

108. Formeister EJ, Rizk HG, Kohn MA, Sharon JD. The epidemiology of vestibular migraine: a population-based survey study. Otol Neurotol. 2018;39(8):1037–44. https://doi.org/10.1097/MAO.0000000000001900.

109. Brodsky J, Kaur K, Shoshany T, Lipson S, Zhou G. Benign paroxysmal migraine variants of infancy and childhood: transitions and clinical features. Eur J Paediatr Neurol. 2018;22(4):667–73. https://doi.org/10.1016/j.ejpn.2018.03.008.

110. Neuhauser HK, Radtke A, von Brevern M, et al. Migrainous vertigo: prevalence and impact on quality of life. Neurology. 2006;67(6):1028–33. https://doi.org/10.1212/01.wnl.0000237539.09942.06.

111. Neuhauser H, Leopold M, von Brevern M, Arnold G, Lempert T. The interrelations of migraine, vertigo, and migrainous vertigo. Neurology. 2001;56(4):436–41. https://doi.org/10.1212/wnl.56.4.436.

112. Yin M, Ishikawa K, Wong WH, Shibata Y. A clinical epidemiological study in 2169 patients with vertigo. Auris Nasus Larynx. 2009;36(1):30–5. https://doi.org/10.1016/j.anl.2008.03.006.

113. Weisleder P, Fife TD. Dizziness and headache: a common association in children and adolescents. J Child Neurol. 2001;16(10):727–30. https://doi.org/10.1177/088307380101601004.

114. Riina N, Ilmari P, Kentala E. Vertigo and imbalance in children: a retrospective study in a Helsinki university otorhinolaryngology clinic. Arch Otolaryngol Head Neck Surg. 2005;131(11):996–1000. https://doi.org/10.1001/archotol.131.11.996.

115. Choung YH, Park K, Moon SK, Kim CH, Ryu SJ. Various causes and clinical characteristics in vertigo in children with normal eardrums. Int J Pediatr Otorhinolaryngol. 2003;67(8):889–94. https://doi.org/10.1016/s0165-5876(03)00136-8.

116. Cass SP, Furman JM, Ankerstjerne K, Balaban C, Yetiser S, Aydogan B. Migraine-related vestibulopathy. Ann Otol Rhinol Laryngol. 1997;106(3):182–9. https://doi.org/10.1177/000348949710600302.

117. Frederick IO, Qiu C, Enquobahrie DA, et al. Lifetime prevalence and correlates of migraine among women in a pacific northwest pregnancy cohort study. Headache. 2014;54(4):675–85. https://doi.org/10.1111/head.12206.

118. Chen J, Chang H, Chen D. Vestibular migraine in a female with unexpected pregnancy. Arch Neurosci. 2016;3(1):e22924. (Case Report) (In en). https://doi.org/10.5812/archneurosci.22924.

119. Park JH, Viirre E. Vestibular migraine may be an important cause of dizziness/vertigo in perimenopausal period. Med Hypotheses. 2010;75(5):409–14. https://doi.org/10.1016/j.mehy.2009.04.054.

120. Silberstein SD. Migraine and pregnancy. Neurol Clin. 1997;15(1):209–31. https://doi.org/10.1016/s0733-8619(05)70305-4.

121. Wells RE, Turner DP, Lee M, Bishop L, Strauss L. Managing migraine during pregnancy and lactation. Curr Neurol Neurosci Rep. 2016;16(4):40. https://doi.org/10.1007/s11910-016-0634-9.

122. Flake ZA, Scalley RD, Bailey AG. Practical selection of antiemetics. Am Fam Physician. 2004;69(5):1169–74. https://www.ncbi.nlm.nih.gov/pubmed/15023018.

123. Matthews A, Dowswell T, Haas DM, Doyle M, O'Mathuna DP. Interventions for nausea and vomiting in early pregnancy. Cochrane Database Syst Rev. 2010;(9):CD007575. https://doi.org/10.1002/14651858.CD007575.pub2.

124. Jewell D, Young G. Interventions for nausea and vomiting in early pregnancy. Cochrane Database Syst Rev. 2003;(4):CD000145. https://doi.org/10.1002/14651858.CD000145.

125. Robbins MS, Farmakidis C, Dayal AK, Lipton RB. Acute headache diagnosis in pregnant women: a hospital-based study. Neurology. 2015;85(12):1024–30. https://doi.org/10.1212/WNL.0000000000001954.

126. Eckhardt-Henn A, Best C, Bense S, et al. Psychiatric comorbidity in different organic vertigo syndromes. J Neurol. 2008;255(3):420–8. https://doi.org/10.1007/s00415-008-0697-x.

127. Fawcett EJ, Fairbrother N, Cox ML, White IR, Fawcett JM. The prevalence of anxiety disorders during pregnancy and the postpartum period: a multivariate Bayesian meta-analysis. J Clin Psychiatry. 2019;80(4):18r12527. https://doi.org/10.4088/JCP.18r12527.

128. Ornoy A, Koren G. SSRIs and SNRIs (SRI) in pregnancy: effects on the course of pregnancy and the offspring: how far are we from having all the answers? Int J Mol Sci. 2019;20(10):2370. https://doi.org/10.3390/ijms20102370.

129. Bisdorff AR. Management of vestibular migraine. Ther Adv Neurol Disord. 2011;4(3):183–91. https://doi.org/10.1177/1756285611401647.

130. Ealy M, Smith RJH. Otosclerosis. Adv Otorhinolaryngol. 2011;70:122–9. https://doi.org/10.1159/000322488.

131. Rudic M, Keogh I, Wagner R, et al. The pathophysiology of otosclerosis: review of current research. Hear Res. 2015;330(Pt A):51–6. https://doi.org/10.1016/j.heares.2015.07.014.

132. Thomas JP, Minovi A, Dazert S. Current aspects of etiology, diagnosis and therapy of otosclerosis. Otolaryngol Pol. 2011;65(3):162–70. https://doi.org/10.1016/S0030-6657(11)70670-9.

133. Babcock TA, Liu XZ. Otosclerosis: from genetics to molecular biology. Otolaryngol Clin North Am. 2018;51(2):305–18. https://doi.org/10.1016/j.otc.2017.11.002.

134. Batson L, Rizzolo D. Otosclerosis: an update on diagnosis and treatment. JAAPA. 2017;30(2):17–22. https://doi.org/10.1097/01.JAA.0000511784.21936.1b.

135. Crompton M, Cadge BA, Ziff JL, et al. The epidemiology of Otosclerosis in a British cohort. Otol Neurotol. 2019;40(1):22–30. https://doi.org/10.1097/MAO.0000000000002047.

136. Lippy WH, Berenholz LP. Pearls on otosclerosis and stapedectomy. Ear Nose Throat J. 2008;87(6):326–8. https://www.ncbi.nlm.nih.gov/pubmed/18561115.

137. Vincent R, Sperling NM, Oates J, Jindal M. Surgical findings and long-term hearing results in 3,050 stapedotomies for primary otosclerosis: a prospective study with the otology-neurotology database. Otol Neurotol. 2006;27(8 Suppl 2):S25–47. https://doi.org/10.1097/01.mao.0000235311.80066.df.

138. Meyer TA, Lambert PR. Primary and revision stapedectomy in elderly patients. Curr Opin Otolaryngol Head Neck Surg. 2004;12(5):387–92. https://www.ncbi.nlm.nih.gov/pubmed/15377949.

139. Redfors YD, Moller C. Otosclerosis: thirty-year follow-up after surgery. Ann Otol Rhinol Laryngol. 2011;120(9):608–14. https://doi.org/10.1177/000348941112000909.

140. Venail F, Lavieille JP, Meller R, Deveze A, Tardivet L, Magnan J. New perspectives for middle ear implants: first results in otosclerosis with mixed hearing loss. Laryngoscope. 2007;117(3):552–5. https://doi.org/10.1097/MLG.0b013e31802dfc59.

141. van Loon MC, Merkus P, Smit CF, Smits C, Witte BI, Hensen EF. Stapedotomy in cochlear implant candidates with far advanced otosclerosis: a systematic review of the literature and meta-analysis. Otol Neurotol. 2014;35(10):1707–14. https://doi.org/10.1097/MAO.0000000000000637.

142. Lenarz T, Zwartenkot JW, Stieger C, et al. Multicenter study with a direct acoustic cochlear implant. Otol Neurotol. 2013;34(7):1215–25. https://doi.org/10.1097/MAO.0b013e318298aa76.

143. Cruise AS, Singh A, Quiney RE. Sodium fluoride in otosclerosis treatment: review. J Laryngol Otol. 2010;124(6):583–6. https://doi.org/10.1017/S0022215110000241.

144. Liktor B, Szekanecz Z, Batta TJ, Sziklai I, Karosi T. Perspectives of pharmacological treatment in otosclerosis. Eur Arch Otorhinolaryngol. 2013;270(3):793–804. https://doi.org/10.1007/s00405-012-2126-0.

145. Podoshin L, Gertner R, Fradis M, et al. Oral contraceptive pills and clinical otosclerosis. Int J Gynaecol Obstet. 1978;15(6):554–5. https://doi.org/10.1002/j.1879-3479.1977.tb00755.x.

146. Gristwood RE, Venables WN. Pregnancy and otosclerosis. Clin Otolaryngol Allied Sci. 1983;8(3):205–10. https://doi.org/10.1111/j.1365-2273.1983.tb01428.x.

147. Vessey M, Painter R. Oral contraception and ear disease: findings in a large cohort study. Contraception. 2001;63(2):61–3. https://doi.org/10.1016/s0010-7824(01)00176-7.

148. Lippy WH, Berenholz LP, Schuring AG, Burkey JM. Does pregnancy affect otosclerosis? Laryngoscope. 2005;115(10):1833–6. https://doi.org/10.1097/01.MLG.0000187573.99335.85.

149. Kameda T, Mano H, Yuasa T, et al. Estrogen inhibits bone resorption by directly inducing apoptosis of the bone-resorbing osteoclasts. J Exp Med. 1997;186(4):489–95. https://doi.org/10.1084/jem.186.4.489.

150. Pacifici R. Estrogen, cytokines, and pathogenesis of postmenopausal osteoporosis. J Bone Miner Res. 1996;11(8):1043–51. https://doi.org/10.1002/jbmr.5650110802.

151. Markou K, Goudakos J. An overview of the etiology of otosclerosis. Eur Arch Otorhinolaryngol. 2009;266(1):25–35. https://doi.org/10.1007/s00405-008-0790-x.

152. McKenna MJ, Kristiansen AG. Molecular biology of otosclerosis. Adv Otorhinolaryngol. 2007;65:68–74. https://doi.org/10.1159/000098674.

153. Imauchi Y, Laine P, Sterkers O, Ferrary E, Bozorg GA. Effect of 17 beta-estradiol on diastrophic dysplasia sulfate transporter activity in otosclerotic bone cell cultures and SaOS-2 cells. Acta Otolaryngol. 2004;124(8):890–5. https://doi.org/10.1080/00016480310017081.

154. Qian ZJ, Alyono JC. Effects of pregnancy on Otosclerosis. Otolaryngol Head Neck Surg. 2020;162:544–7. https://doi.org/10.1177/0194599820907093.

155. Morrison AW. Genetic factors in otosclerosis. Ann R Coll Surg Engl. 1967;41(2):202–37. https://www.ncbi.nlm.nih.gov/pubmed/5298472; https://www.ncbi.nlm.nih.gov/pmc/articles/PMC2311999/pdf/annrcse00242-0022.pdf.

156. Larsson A. Otosclerosis. A genetic and clinical study. Acta Otolaryngol Suppl. 1960;154:1–86. https://www.ncbi.nlm.nih.gov/pubmed/14414297.

157. Fisher JL, Pettersson D, Palmisano S, et al. Loud noise exposure and acoustic neuroma. Am J Epidemiol. 2014;180(1):58–67. https://doi.org/10.1093/aje/kwu081.

158. Lin D, Hegarty JL, Fischbein NJ, Jackler RK. The prevalence of "incidental" acoustic neuroma. Arch Otolaryngol Head Neck Surg. 2005;131(3):241–4. https://doi.org/10.1001/archotol.131.3.241.

159. Propp JM, McCarthy BJ, Davis FG, Preston-Martin S. Descriptive epidemiology of vestibular schwannomas. Neuro Oncol. 2006;8(1):1–11. https://doi.org/10.1215/S1522851704001097.

160. Kasantikul V, Netsky MG, Glasscock ME 3rd, Hays JW. Acoustic neurilemmoma. Clinicoanatomical study of 103 patients. J Neurosurg. 1980;52(1):28–35. https://doi.org/10.3171/jns.1980.52.1.0028.

161. Babu R, Sharma R, Bagley JH, Hatef J, Friedman AH, Adamson C. Vestibular schwannomas in the modern era: epidemiology, treatment trends, and disparities in management. J Neurosurg. 2013;119(1):121–30. https://doi.org/10.3171/2013.1.JNS121370.

162. Matthies C, Samii M. Management of 1000 vestibular schwannomas (acoustic neuromas): clinical presentation. Neurosurgery. 1997;40(1):1–9; discussion 9–10. https://doi.org/10.1097/00006123-199701000-00001.

163. Harun A, Agrawal Y, Tan M, Niparko JK, Francis HW. Sex and age associations with vestibular schwannoma size and presenting symptoms. Otol Neurotol. 2012;33(9):1604–10. https://doi.org/10.1097/MAO.0b013e31826dba9e.

164. Montgomery BK, Alimchandani M, Mehta GU, et al. Tumors displaying hybrid schwannoma and neurofibroma features in patients with neurofibromatosis type 2. Clin Neuropathol. 2016;35(2):78–83. https://doi.org/10.5414/NP300895.

165. Schneider AB, Ron E, Lubin J, et al. Acoustic neuromas following childhood radiation treatment for benign conditions of the head and neck. Neuro Oncol. 2008;10(1):73–8. https://doi.org/10.1215/15228517-2007-047.

166. Edwards CG, Schwartzbaum JA, Lonn S, Ahlbom A, Feychting M. Exposure to loud noise and risk of acoustic neuroma. Am J Epidemiol. 2006;163(4):327–33. https://doi.org/10.1093/aje/kwj044.

167. Preston-Martin S, Thomas DC, Wright WE, Henderson BE. Noise trauma in the aetiology of acoustic neuromas in men in Los Angeles County, 1978-1985. Br J Cancer. 1989;59(5):783–6. https://doi.org/10.1038/bjc.1989.163.

168. Schlehofer B, Schlaefer K, Blettner M, et al. Environmental risk factors for sporadic acoustic neuroma (Interphone Study Group, Germany). Eur J Cancer. 2007;43(11):1741–7. https://doi.org/10.1016/j.ejca.2007.05.008.

169. Cao Z, Zhao F, Mulugeta H. Noise exposure as a risk factor for acoustic neuroma: a systematic review and meta-analysis. Int J Audiol. 2019;58(9):525–32. https://doi.org/10.1080/14992027.2019.1602289.

170. Khurana VG, Teo C, Kundi M, Hardell L, Carlberg M. Cell phones and brain tumors: a review including the long-term epidemiologic data. Surg Neurol.

2009;72(3):205–14; discussion 214–5. https://doi.org/10.1016/j.surneu.2009.01.019.

171. Chen M, Fan Z, Zheng X, Cao F, Wang L. Risk factors of acoustic neuroma: systematic review and meta-analysis. Yonsei Med J. 2016;57(3):776–83. https://doi.org/10.3349/ymj.2016.57.3.776.

172. Kim SH, Lee SH, Choi SK, Lim YJ, Na SY, Yeo SG. Audiologic evaluation of vestibular schwannoma and other cerebellopontine angle tumors. Acta Otolaryngol. 2016;136(2):149–53. https://doi.org/10.3109/00016489.2015.1100326.

173. Koors PD, Thacker LR, Coelho DH. ABR in the diagnosis of vestibular schwannomas: a meta-analysis. Am J Otolaryngol. 2013;34(3):195–204. https://doi.org/10.1016/j.amjoto.2012.11.011.

174. Salem N, Galal A, Mastronardi V, Talaat M, Sobhy O, Sanna M. Audiological evaluation of vestibular schwannoma patients with normal hearing. Audiol Neurootol. 2019;24(3):117–26. https://doi.org/10.1159/000500660.

175. Waterval J, Kania R, Somers T. EAONO position statement on vestibular schwannoma: imaging assessment. What are the indications for performing a screening MRI scan for a potential vestibular schwannoma? J Int Adv Otol. 2018;14(1):95–9. https://doi.org/10.5152/iao.2018.5364.

176. Fortnum H, O'Neill C, Taylor R, et al. The role of magnetic resonance imaging in the identification of suspected acoustic neuroma: a systematic review of clinical and cost effectiveness and natural history. Health Technol Assess. 2009;13(18):iii–iv, ix-xi, 1–154. https://doi.org/10.3310/hta13180.

177. Matthies C, Samii M, Krebs S. Management of vestibular schwannomas (acoustic neuromas): radiological features in 202 cases--their value for diagnosis and their predictive importance. Neurosurgery. 1997;40(3):469–81; discussion 481–2. https://doi.org/10.1097/00006123-199703000-00009.

178. Goldbrunner R, Weller M, Regis J, et al. EANO guideline on the diagnosis and treatment of vestibular schwannoma. Neuro Oncol. 2020;22(1):31–45. https://doi.org/10.1093/neuonc/noz153.

179. Raheja A, Bowers CA, MacDonald JD, et al. Middle fossa approach for vestibular schwannoma: good hearing and facial nerve outcomes with low morbidity. World Neurosurg. 2016;92:37–46. https://doi.org/10.1016/j.wneu.2016.04.085.

180. Lanman TH, Brackmann DE, Hitselberger WE, Subin B. Report of 190 consecutive cases of large acoustic tumors (vestibular schwannoma) removed via the translabyrinthine approach. J Neurosurg. 1999;90(4):617–23. https://doi.org/10.3171/jns.1999.90.4.0617.

181. Samii M, Matthies C. Management of 1000 vestibular schwannomas (acoustic neuromas): surgical management and results with an emphasis on complications and how to avoid them. Neurosurgery. 1997;40(1):11–21; discussion 21–3. https://doi.org/10.1097/00006123-199701000-00002.

182. Darrouzet V, Martel J, Enee V, Bebear JP, Guerin J. Vestibular schwannoma surgery outcomes: our multidisciplinary experience in 400 cases over 17 years. Laryngoscope. 2004;114(4):681–8. https://doi.org/10.1097/00005537-200404000-00016.

183. Nakatomi H, Jacob JT, Carlson ML, et al. Long-term risk of recurrence and regrowth after gross-total and subtotal resection of sporadic vestibular schwannoma. J Neurosurg. 2017;133:1–7. https://doi.org/10.3171/2016.11.JNS16498.

184. Ahmad RA, Sivalingam S, Topsakal V, Russo A, Taibah A, Sanna M. Rate of recurrent vestibular schwannoma after total removal via different surgical approaches. Ann Otol Rhinol Laryngol. 2012;121(3):156–61. https://doi.org/10.1177/000348941212100303.

185. Sughrue ME, Yang I, Aranda D, et al. Beyond audiofacial morbidity after vestibular schwannoma surgery. J Neurosurg. 2011;114(2):367–74. https://doi.org/10.3171/2009.10.JNS091203.

186. Schankin CJ, Gall C, Straube A. Headache syndromes after acoustic neuroma surgery and their implications for quality of life. Cephalalgia. 2009;29(7):760–71. https://doi.org/10.1111/j.1468-2982.2008.01790.x.

187. Sylvester MJ, Shastri DN, Patel VM, et al. Outcomes of vestibular schwannoma surgery among the elderly. Otolaryngol Head Neck Surg. 2017;156(1):166–72. https://doi.org/10.1177/0194599816677522.

188. Barker FG 2nd, Carter BS, Ojemann RG, Jyung RW, Poe DS, McKenna MJ. Surgical excision of acoustic neuroma: patient outcome and provider caseload. Laryngoscope. 2003;113(8):1332–43. https://doi.org/10.1097/00005537-200308000-00013.

189. Murphy ES, Suh JH. Radiotherapy for vestibular schwannomas: a critical review. Int J Radiat Oncol Biol Phys. 2011;79(4):985–97. https://doi.org/10.1016/j.ijrobp.2010.10.010.

190. Niu NN, Niemierko A, Larvie M, et al. Pretreatment growth rate predicts radiation response in vestibular schwannomas. Int J Radiat Oncol Biol Phys. 2014;89(1):113–9. https://doi.org/10.1016/j.ijrobp.2014.01.038.

191. Pollock BE. Management of vestibular schwannomas that enlarge after stereotactic radiosurgery: treatment recommendations based on a 15 year experience. Neurosurgery. 2006;58(2):241–8; discussion 241–8. https://doi.org/10.1227/01.NEU.0000194833.66593.8B.

192. Hasegawa T, Kida Y, Kato T, Iizuka H, Kuramitsu S, Yamamoto T. Long-term safety and efficacy of stereotactic radiosurgery for vestibular schwannomas: evaluation of 440 patients more than 10 years after treatment with gamma knife surgery. J Neurosurg. 2013;118(3):557–65. https://doi.org/10.3171/2012.10.JNS12523.

193. Pollock BE, Link MJ, Stafford SL, Parney IF, Garces YI, Foote RL. The risk of radiation-induced tumors or malignant transformation after single-fraction intracranial radiosurgery: results based

on a 25-year experience. Int J Radiat Oncol Biol Phys. 2017;97(5):919–23. https://doi.org/10.1016/j.ijrobp.2017.01.004.

194. Patel MA, Marciscano AE, Hu C, et al. Long-term treatment response and patient outcomes for vestibular schwannoma patients treated with Hypofractionated stereotactic radiotherapy. Front Oncol. 2017;7:200. https://doi.org/10.3389/fonc.2017.00200.

195. Combs SE, Welzel T, Schulz-Ertner D, Huber PE, Debus J. Differences in clinical results after LINAC-based single-dose radiosurgery versus fractionated stereotactic radiotherapy for patients with vestibular schwannomas. Int J Radiat Oncol Biol Phys. 2010;76(1):193–200. https://doi.org/10.1016/j.ijrobp.2009.01.064.

196. Barnes CJ, Bush DA, Grove RI, Loredo LN, Slater JD. Fractionated proton beam therapy for acoustic neuromas: tumor control and hearing preservation. Int J Part Ther. 2018;4(4):28–36. https://doi.org/10.14338/IJPT-14-00014.1.

197. Wackym PA, Runge-Samuelson CL, Nash JJ, et al. Gamma knife surgery of vestibular schwannomas: volumetric dosimetry correlations to hearing loss suggest stria vascularis devascularization as the mechanism of early hearing loss. Otol Neurotol. 2010;31(9):1480–7. https://doi.org/10.1097/MAO.0b013e3181f7d7d4.

198. Wackym PA, Hannley MT, Runge-Samuelson CL, Jensen J, Zhu YR. Gamma knife surgery of vestibular schwannomas: longitudinal changes in vestibular function and measurement of the dizziness handicap inventory. J Neurosurg. 2008;109(Suppl):137–43. https://doi.org/10.3171/JNS/2008/109/12/S21.

199. Smouha EE, Yoo M, Mohr K, Davis RP. Conservative management of acoustic neuroma: a meta-analysis and proposed treatment algorithm. Laryngoscope. 2005;115(3):450–4. https://doi.org/10.1097/00005537-200503000-00011.

200. Bakkouri WE, Kania RE, Guichard JP, Lot G, Herman P, Huy PT. Conservative management of 386 cases of unilateral vestibular schwannoma: tumor growth and consequences for treatment. J Neurosurg. 2009;110(4):662–9. https://doi.org/10.3171/2007.5.16836.

201. Sughrue ME, Yang I, Aranda D, et al. The natural history of untreated sporadic vestibular schwannomas: a comprehensive review of hearing outcomes. J Neurosurg. 2010;112(1):163–7. https://doi.org/10.3171/2009.4.JNS08895.

202. Akpinar B, Mousavi SH, McDowell MM, et al. Early radiosurgery improves hearing preservation in vestibular schwannoma patients with Normal hearing at the time of diagnosis. Int J Radiat Oncol Biol Phys. 2016;95(2):729–34. https://doi.org/10.1016/j.ijrobp.2016.01.019.

203. Kumar P, Joshna BM, Nair SS. A clinical study of otorhinolaryngological symptoms in pregnancy. Orissa J Otolaryngol Head Neck Surg. 2019:62–5. https://doi.org/10.21176/ojolhns.2019.13.2.4.

204. Figueiro-Filho EA, Horgan RP, Muhanna N, Parrish J, Irish JC, Maxwell CV. Obstetrical outcomes of head and neck (nonthyroid) cancers: a 27-year retrospective series and literature review. AJP Rep. 2019;9(1):e15–22. https://doi.org/10.1055/s-0039-1677876.

205. Shah KJ, Chamoun RB. Large vestibular schwannomas presenting during pregnancy: management strategies. J Neurol Surg B Skull Base. 2014;75(3):214–20. https://doi.org/10.1055/s-0034-1370784.

206. Xie S, Wu X. Clinical management and progress in sudden sensorineural hearing loss during pregnancy. J Int Med Res. 2019;48:300060519870718. https://doi.org/10.1177/0300060519870718.

207. Allen J, Eldridge R, Koerber T. Acoustic neuroma in the last months of pregnancy. Am J Obstet Gynecol. 1974;119(4):516–20. https://doi.org/10.1016/0002-9378(74)90212-9.

208. Kachhara R, Devi CG, Nair S, Bhattacharya RN, Radhakrishnan VV. Acoustic neurinomas during pregnancy: report of two cases and review of literature. Acta Neurochir. 2001;143(6):587–91. https://doi.org/10.1007/s007010170063.

209. Gaughan RK, Harner SG. Acoustic neuroma and pregnancy. Am J Otol. 1993;14(1):88–91. https://www.ncbi.nlm.nih.gov/pubmed/8424484.

210. Misra BK, Rout D, Bhiladvala DB, Radhakrishnan V. Spontaneous haemorrhage in acoustic neurinomas. Br J Neurosurg. 1995;9(2):219–21. https://doi.org/10.1080/02688699550041593.

211. Stidham KR, Roberson JB Jr. Effects of estrogen and tamoxifen on growth of human vestibular schwannomas in the nude mouse. Otolaryngol Head Neck Surg. 1999;120(2):262–4. https://doi.org/10.1016/S0194-5998(99)70416-X.

212. Doyle KJ, Luxford WM. Acoustic neuroma in pregnancy. Am J Otol. 1994;15(1):111–3. https://www.ncbi.nlm.nih.gov/pubmed/8109621.

213. Kasantikul V, Brown WJ. Estrogen receptors in acoustic neurilemmomas. Surg Neurol. 1981;15(2):105–9. https://doi.org/10.1016/0090-3019(81)90023-9.

214. Brown CM, Ahmad ZK, Ryan AF, Doherty JK. Estrogen receptor expression in sporadic vestibular schwannomas. Otol Neurotol. 2011;32(1):158–62. https://doi.org/10.1097/MAO.0b013e3181feb92a.

215. Sagers JE, Brown AS, Vasilijic S, et al. Computational repositioning and preclinical validation of mifepristone for human vestibular schwannoma. Sci Rep. 2018;8(1):5437. https://doi.org/10.1038/s41598-018-23609-7.

216. Kal HB, Struikmans H. Radiotherapy during pregnancy: fact and fiction. Lancet Oncol. 2005;6(5):328–33. https://doi.org/10.1016/S1470-2045(05)70169-8.

217. Akella SS, Mattson JN, Moreira NN. Vestibular schwannoma growth during pregnancy: case report of neurofibromatosis type 2 in pregnancy. Proc Obstet Gynecol. 2019;9(1):1–9. https://doi.org/10.17077/2154-4751.1409.

218. Magliulo G, Ronzoni R, Petti R, Marcotullio D, Marini M. Acoustic neuroma in the pregnant patient. Eur Arch Otorhinolaryngol. 1995;252(2):123–4. https://doi.org/10.1007/BF00168034.

219. Tschudi DC, Linder TE, Fisch U. Conservative management of unilateral acoustic neuromas. Am J Otol. 2000;21(5):722–8. https://www.ncbi.nlm.nih.gov/pubmed/10993466.

220. Beni-Adani L, Pomeranz S, Flores I, Shoshan Y, Ginosar Y, Ben-Shachar I. Huge acoustic neurinomas presenting in the late stage of pregnancy. Treatment options and review of literature. Acta Obstet Gynecol Scand. 2001;80(2):179–84. https://www.ncbi.nlm.nih.gov/pubmed/11167216.

221. Esmaeilzadeh M, Uksul N, Hong B, et al. Intracranial emergencies during pregnancy requiring urgent neurosurgical treatment. Clin Neurol Neurosurg. 2020;195:105905. https://doi.org/10.1016/j.clineuro.2020.105905.

222. Priddy BH, Otto BA, Carrau RL, Prevedello DM. Management of skull base tumors in the obstetric population: a case series. World Neurosurg. 2018;113:e373–82. https://doi.org/10.1016/j.wneu.2018.02.038.

223. Thacker JG, Wallace EM, Whittle IR, Calder AA. Successful excision of a giant acoustic neuroma in the third trimester of pregnancy. Scott Med J. 1995;40(4):117–8. https://doi.org/10.1177/003693309504000405.

224. De Diego-Sastre JI, Prim-Espada MP, Fernandez-Garcia F. The epidemiology of Bell's palsy. Rev Neurol. 2005;41(5):287–90. https://www.ncbi.nlm.nih.gov/pubmed/16138286.

225. Hilsinger RL Jr, Adour KK, Doty HE. Idiopathic facial paralysis, pregnancy, and the menstrual cycle. Ann Otol Rhinol Laryngol. 1975;84(4 Pt 1):433–42. https://doi.org/10.1177/000348947508400402.

226. Hussain A, Nduka C, Moth P, Malhotra R. Bell's facial nerve palsy in pregnancy: a clinical review. J Obstet Gynaecol. 2017;37(4):409–15. https://doi.org/10.1080/01443615.2016.1256973.

227. Riga M, Kefalidis G, Danielides V. The role of diabetes mellitus in the clinical presentation and prognosis of bell palsy. J Am Board Fam Med. 2012;25(6):819–26. https://doi.org/10.3122/jabfm.2012.06.120084.

228. Pecket P, Schattner A. Concurrent Bell's palsy and diabetes mellitus: a diabetic mononeuropathy? J Neurol Neurosurg Psychiatry. 1982;45(7):652–5. https://doi.org/10.1136/jnnp.45.7.652.

229. Adour KK, Byl FM, Hilsinger RL Jr, Kahn ZM, Sheldon MI. The true nature of Bell's palsy: analysis of 1,000 consecutive patients. Laryngoscope. 1978;88(5):787–801. https://doi.org/10.1002/lary.1978.88.5.787.

230. Fu L, Bundy C, Sadiq SA. Psychological distress in people with disfigurement from facial palsy. Eye (Lond). 2011;25(10):1322–6. https://doi.org/10.1038/eye.2011.158.

231. Benatar M, Edlow J. The spectrum of cranial neuropathy in patients with Bell's palsy. Arch Intern Med. 2004;164(21):2383–5. https://doi.org/10.1001/archinte.164.21.2383.

232. Peitersen E. Bell's palsy: the spontaneous course of 2,500 peripheral facial nerve palsies of different etiologies. Acta Otolaryngol Suppl. 2002;549:4–30. https://www.ncbi.nlm.nih.gov/pubmed/12482166.

233. Murakami S, Sugita T, Hirata Y, Yanagihara N, Desaki J. Histopathology of facial nerve neuritis caused by herpes simplex virus infection in mice. Eur Arch Otorhinolaryngol. 1994:S487–8. https://doi.org/10.1007/978-3-642-85090-5_192.

234. Liston SL, Kleid MS. Histopathology of Bell's palsy. Laryngoscope. 1989;99(1):23–6. https://doi.org/10.1288/00005537-198901000-00006.

235. Murakami S, Mizobuchi M, Nakashiro Y, Doi T, Hato N, Yanagihara N. Bell palsy and herpes simplex virus: identification of viral DNA in endoneurial fluid and muscle. Ann Intern Med. 1996;124(1 Pt 1):27–30. https://doi.org/10.7326/0003-4819-124-1_part_1-199601010-00005.

236. Carreno M, Ona M, Melon S, Llorente JL, Diaz JJ, Suarez C. Amplification of herpes simplex virus type 1 DNA in human geniculate ganglia from formalin-fixed, nonembedded temporal bones. Otolaryngol Head Neck Surg. 2000;123(4):508–11. https://doi.org/10.1067/mhn.2000.107886.

237. Burgess RC, Michaels L, Bale JF Jr, Smith RJ. Polymerase chain reaction amplification of herpes simplex viral DNA from the geniculate ganglion of a patient with Bell's palsy. Ann Otol Rhinol Laryngol. 1994;103(10):775–9. https://doi.org/10.1177/000348949410301006.

238. Takasu T, Furuta Y, Sato KC, Fukuda S, Inuyama Y, Nagashima K. Detection of latent herpes simplex virus DNA and RNA in human geniculate ganglia by the polymerase chain reaction. Acta Otolaryngol. 1992;112(6):1004–11. https://doi.org/10.3109/00016489209137502.

239. Morgan M, Nathwani D. Facial palsy and infection: the unfolding story. Clin Infect Dis. 1992;14(1):263–71. https://doi.org/10.1093/clinids/14.1.263.

240. Wackym PA, Popper P, Kerner MM, Grody WW. Varicella-zoster DNA in temporal bones of patients with Ramsay Hunt syndrome. Lancet. 1993;342(8886–8887):1555. https://doi.org/10.1016/s0140-6736(05)80126-6.

241. Wackym PA. Molecular temporal bone pathology: II. Ramsay Hunt syndrome (herpes zoster oticus). Laryngoscope. 1997;107(9):1165–75. https://doi.org/10.1097/00005537-199709000-00003.

242. Zhang W, Xu L, Luo T, Wu F, Zhao B, Li X. The etiology of Bell's palsy: a review. J Neurol. 2019;267:1896. https://doi.org/10.1007/s00415-019-09282-4.

243. Mutsch M, Zhou W, Rhodes P, et al. Use of the inactivated intranasal influenza vaccine and the risk of Bell's palsy in Switzerland. N Engl J Med. 2004;350(9):896–903. https://doi.org/10.1056/NEJMoa030595.

244. Clement WA, White A. Idiopathic familial facial nerve paralysis. J Laryngol Otol. 2000;114(2):132–4. https://doi.org/10.1258/0022215001904879.

245. Kanoh N, Nomura J, Satomi F. Nocturnal onset and development of Bell's palsy. Laryngoscope. 2005;115(1):99–100. https://doi.org/10.1097/01.mlg.0000150700.46377.96.

246. Sax TW, Rosenbaum RB. Neuromuscular disorders in pregnancy. Muscle Nerve. 2006;34(5):559–71. https://doi.org/10.1002/mus.20661.

247. Heckmann JG, Urban PP, Pitz S, Guntinas-Lichius O, Gagyor I. The diagnosis and treatment of idiopathic facial paresis (Bell's palsy). Dtsch Arztebl Int. 2019;116(41):692–702. https://doi.org/10.3238/arztebl.2019.0692.

248. Su BM, Kuan EC, St John MA. What is the role of imaging in the evaluation of the patient presenting with unilateral facial paralysis? Laryngoscope. 2018;128(2):297–8. https://doi.org/10.1002/lary.26825.

249. House JW, Brackmann DE. Facial nerve grading system. Otolaryngol Head Neck Surg. 1985;93(2):146–7. https://doi.org/10.1177/019459988509300202.

250. Gronseth GS, Paduga R, American Academy of N. Evidence-based guideline update: steroids and antivirals for bell palsy: report of the guideline development Subcommittee of the American Academy of Neurology. Neurology. 2012;79(22):2209–13. https://doi.org/10.1212/WNL.0b013e318275978c.

251. de Almeida JR, Guyatt GH, Sud S, et al. Management of Bell palsy: clinical practice guideline. CMAJ. 2014;186(12):917–22. https://doi.org/10.1503/cmaj.131801.

252. Madhok VB, Gagyor I, Daly F, et al. Corticosteroids for Bell's palsy (idiopathic facial paralysis). Cochrane Database Syst Rev. 2016;7:CD001942. https://doi.org/10.1002/14651858.CD001942.pub5.

253. Sullivan FM, Swan IR, Donnan PT, et al. Early treatment with prednisolone or acyclovir in Bell's palsy. N Engl J Med. 2007;357(16):1598–607. https://doi.org/10.1056/NEJMoa072006.

254. Engstrom M, Berg T, Stjernquist-Desatnik A, et al. Prednisolone and valaciclovir in Bell's palsy: a randomised, double-blind, placebo-controlled, multicentre trial. Lancet Neurol. 2008;7(11):993–1000. https://doi.org/10.1016/S1474-4422(08)70221-7.

255. de Almeida JR, Al Khabori M, Guyatt GH, et al. Combined corticosteroid and antiviral treatment for bell palsy: a systematic review and meta-analysis. JAMA. 2009;302(9):985–93. https://doi.org/10.1001/jama.2009.1243.

256. Quant EC, Jeste SS, Muni RH, Cape AV, Bhussar MK, Peleg AY. The benefits of steroids versus steroids plus antivirals for treatment of Bell's palsy: a meta-analysis. BMJ. 2009;339:b3354. https://doi.org/10.1136/bmj.b3354.

257. Turgeon RD, Wilby KJ, Ensom MH. Antiviral treatment of Bell's palsy based on baseline severity: a systematic review and meta-analysis. Am J Med. 2015;128(6):617–28. https://doi.org/10.1016/j.amjmed.2014.11.033.

258. Gagyor I, Madhok VB, Daly F, Sullivan F. Antiviral treatment for Bell's palsy (idiopathic facial paralysis). Cochrane Database Syst Rev. 2019;9:CD001869. https://doi.org/10.1002/14651858.CD001869.pub9.

259. Birgfeld C, Neligan P. Surgical approaches to facial nerve deficits. Skull Base. 2011;21(3):177–84. https://doi.org/10.1055/s-0031-1275252.

260. Teixeira LJ, Valbuza JS, Prado GF. Physical therapy for Bell's palsy (idiopathic facial paralysis). Cochrane Database Syst Rev. 2011;(12):CD006283. https://doi.org/10.1002/14651858.CD006283.pub3.

261. Nicastri M, Mancini P, De Seta D, et al. Efficacy of early physical therapy in severe Bell's palsy: a randomized controlled trial. Neurorehabil Neural Repair. 2013;27(6):542–51. https://doi.org/10.1177/1545968313481280.

262. Andresen NS, Sun DQ, Hansen MR. Facial nerve decompression. Curr Opin Otolaryngol Head Neck Surg. 2018;26(5):280–5. https://doi.org/10.1097/MOO.0000000000000478.

263. Lee SY, Seong J, Kim YH. Clinical implication of facial nerve decompression in complete Bell's palsy: a systematic review and meta-analysis. Clin Exp Otorhinolaryngol. 2019;12(4):348–59. https://doi.org/10.21053/ceo.2019.00535.

264. Peitersen E. The natural history of Bell's palsy. Am J Otol. 1982;4(2):107–11. https://www.ncbi.nlm.nih.gov/pubmed/7148998.

265. Jabor MA, Gianoli G. Management of Bell's palsy. J La State Med Soc. 1996;148(7):279–83. https://www.ncbi.nlm.nih.gov/pubmed/8816019.

266. Cirpaciu D, Goanta CM, Cirpaciu MD. Recurrences of Bell's palsy. J Med Life. 2014;7:68–77. https://www.ncbi.nlm.nih.gov/pubmed/25870699.

267. Reece EA, Leguizamon G, Wiznitzer A. Gestational diabetes: the need for a common ground. Lancet. 2009;373(9677):1789–97. https://doi.org/10.1016/S0140-6736(09)60515-8.

268. Naib ZM, Nahmias AJ, Josey WE, Zaki SA. Relation of cytohistopathology of genital herpesvirus infection to cervical anaplasia. Cancer Res. 1973;33(6):1452–63. https://www.ncbi.nlm.nih.gov/pubmed/4352382.

269. McGregor JA, Guberman A, Amer J, Goodlin R. Idiopathic facial nerve paralysis (Bell's palsy) in late pregnancy and the early puerperium. Obstet Gynecol. 1987;69(3 Pt 2):435–8. https://www.ncbi.nlm.nih.gov/pubmed/3808518.

270. Shmorgun D, Chan WS, Ray JG. Association between Bells palsy in pregnancy and pre-eclampsia.

QJM. 2002;95(6):359–62. https://doi.org/10.1093/qjmed/95.6.359.

271. Katz A, Sergienko R, Dior U, Wiznitzer A, Kaplan DM, Sheiner E. Bell's palsy during pregnancy: is it associated with adverse perinatal outcome? Laryngoscope. 2011;121(7):1395–8. https://doi.org/10.1002/lary.21860.

272. Gillman GS, Schaitkin BM, May M, Klein SR. Bell's palsy in pregnancy: a study of recovery outcomes. Otolaryngol Head Neck Surg. 2002;126(1):26–30. https://doi.org/10.1067/mhn.2002.121321.

273. Kunze M, Arndt S, Zimmer A, et al. Idiopathic facial palsy during pregnancy. HNO. 2012;60(2):98–101. https://doi.org/10.1007/s00106-011-2394-9.

274. Sharma K, Sharma S, Chander D. Evaluation of audio-rhinological changes during pregnancy. Indian J Otolaryngol Head Neck Surg. 2011;63(1):74–8. https://doi.org/10.1007/s12070-010-0103-8.

275. Sennaroglu G, Belgin E. Audiological findings in pregnancy. J Laryngol Otol. 2001;115(8):617–21. https://doi.org/10.1258/0022215011908603.

276. Dag EK, Gulumser C, Erbek S. Decrease in middle ear resonance frequency during pregnancy. Audiol Res. 2016;6(1):147. https://doi.org/10.4081/audiores.2016.147.

277. Kwatra D, Kumar S, Singh GB, Biswas R, Upadhyay P. Can pregnancy Lead to changes in hearing threshold? Ear Nose Throat J. 2019;100:145561319871240. https://doi.org/10.1177/0145561319871240.

278. Tsunoda K, Takahashi S, Takanosawa M, Shimoji Y. The influence of pregnancy on sensation of ear problems--ear problems associated with healthy pregnancy. J Laryngol Otol. 1999;113(4):318–20. https://doi.org/10.1017/s0022215100143877.

279. Klemm E, Deutscher A, Mosges R. A present investigation of the epidemiology in idiopathic sudden sensorineural hearing loss. Laryngorhinootologie. 2009;88(8):524–7. https://doi.org/10.1055/s-0028-1128133.

280. Alexander TH, Harris JP. Incidence of sudden sensorineural hearing loss. Otol Neurotol. 2013;34(9):1586–9. https://doi.org/10.1097/MAO.0000000000000222.

281. Yen TT, Lin CH, Shiao JY, Liang KL. Pregnancy is not a risk factor for idiopathic sudden sensorineural hearing loss: a nationwide population-based study. Acta Otolaryngol. 2016;136(5):446–50. https://doi.org/10.3109/00016489.2015.1123292.

282. Hou ZQ, Wang QJ. A new disease: pregnancy-induced sudden sensorineural hearing loss? Acta Otolaryngol. 2011;131(7):779–86. https://doi.org/10.3109/00016489.2011.553630.

283. Fetterman BL, Luxford WM, Saunders JE. Sudden bilateral sensorineural hearing loss. Laryngoscope. 1996;106(11):1347–50. https://doi.org/10.1097/00005537-199611000-00008.

284. Schuknecht HF, Donovan ED. The pathology of idiopathic sudden sensorineural hearing loss. Arch Otorhinolaryngol. 1986;243(1):1–15. https://doi.org/10.1007/BF00457899.

285. Capaccio P, Ottaviani F, Cuccarini V, et al. Genetic and acquired prothrombotic risk factors and sudden hearing loss. Laryngoscope. 2007;117(3):547–51. https://doi.org/10.1097/MLG.0b013e31802f3c6a.

286. Toubi E, Ben-David J, Kessel A, Halas K, Sabo E, Luntz M. Immune-mediated disorders associated with idiopathic sudden sensorineural hearing loss. Ann Otol Rhinol Laryngol. 2004;113(6):445–9. https://doi.org/10.1177/000348940411300605.

287. Goh AY, Hussain SS. Sudden hearing loss and pregnancy: a review. J Laryngol Otol. 2012;126(4):337–9. https://doi.org/10.1017/S0022215112000114.

288. Kenny R, Patil N, Considine N. Sudden (reversible) sensorineural hearing loss in pregnancy. Ir J Med Sci. 2011;180(1):79–84. https://doi.org/10.1007/s11845-010-0525-z.

289. Lee JH, Marcus DC. Estrogen acutely inhibits ion transport by isolated stria vascularis. Hear Res. 2001;158(1–2):123–30. https://doi.org/10.1016/s0378-5955(01)00316-1.

290. Stenberg AE, Wang H, Fish J 3rd, Schrott-Fischer A, Sahlin L, Hultcrantz M. Estrogen receptors in the normal adult and developing human inner ear and in Turner's syndrome. Hear Res. 2001;157(1–2):87–92. https://doi.org/10.1016/s0378-5955(01)00280-5.

291. Carlin A, Alfirevic Z. Physiological changes of pregnancy and monitoring. Best Pract Res Clin Obstet Gynaecol. 2008;22(5):801–23. https://doi.org/10.1016/j.bpobgyn.2008.06.005.

292. Baylan MY, Kuyumcuoglu U, Kale A, Celik Y, Topcu I. Is preeclampsia a new risk factor for cochlear damage and hearing loss? Otol Neurotol. 2010;31(8):1180–3. https://doi.org/10.1097/MAO.0b013e3181edb6eb.

293. Terzi H, Kale A, Hasdemir PS, Selcuk A, Yavuz A, Genc S. Hearing loss: an unknown complication of pre-eclampsia? J Obstet Gynaecol Res. 2015;41(2):188–92. https://doi.org/10.1111/jog.12505.

294. Schreiber BE, Agrup C, Haskard DO, Luxon LM. Sudden sensorineural hearing loss. Lancet. 2010;375(9721):1203–11. https://doi.org/10.1016/S0140-6736(09)62071-7.

295. Yin T, Huang F, Ren J, et al. Bilateral sudden hearing loss following habitual abortion: a case report and review of literature. Int J Clin Exp Med. 2013;6(8):720–3. https://www.ncbi.nlm.nih.gov/pubmed/24040484.

296. Wiles NM, Hunt BJ, Callanan V, Chevretton EB. Sudden sensorineural hearing loss and antiphospholipid syndrome. Haematologica. 2006;91(12 Suppl):ECR46. https://www.ncbi.nlm.nih.gov/pubmed/17194652.

297. Wang YP, Young YH. Experience in the treatment of sudden deafness during pregnancy. Acta Otolaryngol. 2006;126(3):271–6. https://doi.org/10.1080/00016480500388984.

298. Xu M, Jiang Q, Tang H. Sudden sensorineural hearing loss during pregnancy: clinical characteristics, management and outcome. Acta Otolaryngol. 2019;139(1):38–41. https://doi.org/10.1080/00016489.2018.1535192.

299. Fu Y, Jing J, Ren T, Zhao H. Intratympanic dexamethasone for managing pregnant women with sudden hearing loss. J Int Med Res. 2019;47(1):377–82. https://doi.org/10.1177/0300060518802725.

300. Slattery WH, Fisher LM, Iqbal Z, Liu N. Oral steroid regimens for idiopathic sudden sensorineural hearing loss. Otolaryngol Head Neck Surg. 2005;132(1):5–10. https://doi.org/10.1016/j.otohns.2004.09.072.

301. Chandrasekhar SS, Tsai Do BS, Schwartz SR, et al. Clinical practice guideline: sudden hearing loss (update) executive summary. Otolaryngol Head Neck Surg. 2019;161(2):195–210. https://doi.org/10.1177/0194599819859883.

302. Bakhshaee M, Hassanzadeh M, Nourizadeh N, Karimi E, Moghiman T, Shakeri M. Hearing impairment in pregnancy toxemia. Otolaryngol Head Neck Surg. 2008;139(2):298–300. https://doi.org/10.1016/j.otohns.2008.04.016.

303. Gomaa M, Elbadery M, Samy H, Moniem R, Ali H. Hearing impairment in pre-eclampsia. Online. J Otolaryngol. 2016;6(3):135. http://www.jorl.net/otolaryngology/hearing-impairment-in-preeclampsia-5981.html.

304. Atmaja OS, Sudarman K, Surono A. Preeclampsia as a risk factor for damage of the Cochlear outer hair cells function. Adv Otolaryngol. 2016;2016:1798382. https://doi.org/10.1155/2016/1798382.

305. Simen RCM, Vieira AA, Miterhof MEV, de Faria AOP. Correlation between the presence of maternal gestational or pre-gestational pathologies and hearing impairment in the puerperal period. Clin J Obstetr Gynecol. 2019;2:122–6. https://doi.org/10.29328/journal.cjog.1001033.

306. Altuntas EE, Yenicesu AG, Mutlu AE, Muderris S, Cetin M, Cetin A. An evaluation of the effects of hypertension during pregnancy on postpartum hearing as measured by transient-evoked otoacoustic emissions. Acta Otorhinolaryngol Ital. 2012;32(1):31–6. https://www.ncbi.nlm.nih.gov/pubmed/22500064.

307. Han CS, Park JR, Boo SH, et al. Clinical efficacy of initial intratympanic steroid treatment on sudden sensorineural hearing loss with diabetes. Otolaryngol Head Neck Surg. 2009;141(5):572–8. https://doi.org/10.1016/j.otohns.2009.06.084.

308. Suzuki H, Hashida K, Nguyen KH, et al. Efficacy of intratympanic steroid administration on idiopathic sudden sensorineural hearing loss in comparison with hyperbaric oxygen therapy. Laryngoscope. 2012;122(5):1154–7. https://doi.org/10.1002/lary.23245.

309. Rhee TM, Hwang D, Lee JS, Park J, Lee JM. Addition of hyperbaric oxygen therapy vs medical therapy alone for idiopathic sudden sensorineural hearing loss: a systematic review and meta-analysis. JAMA Otolaryngol Head Neck Surg. 2018;144(12):1153–61. https://doi.org/10.1001/jamaoto.2018.2133.

310. Guller S, Kong L, Wozniak R, Lockwood CJ. Reduction of extracellular matrix protein expression in human amnion epithelial cells by glucocorticoids: a potential role in preterm rupture of the fetal membranes. J Clin Endocrinol Metab. 1995;80(7):2244–50. https://doi.org/10.1210/jcem.80.7.7608287.

311. Lockwood CJ, Radunovic N, Nastic D, Petkovic S, Aigner S, Berkowitz GS. Corticotropin-releasing hormone and related pituitary-adrenal axis hormones in fetal and maternal blood during the second half of pregnancy. J Perinat Med. 1996;24(3):243–51. https://doi.org/10.1515/jpme.1996.24.3.243.

312. Canlon B, Erichsen S, Nemlander E, et al. Alterations in the intrauterine environment by glucocorticoids modifies the developmental programme of the auditory system. Eur J Neurosci. 2003;17(10):2035–41. https://doi.org/10.1046/j.1460-9568.2003.02641.x.

313. Ostensen M, Khamashta M, Lockshin M, et al. Anti-inflammatory and immunosuppressive drugs and reproduction. Arthritis Res Ther. 2006;8(3):209. https://doi.org/10.1186/ar1957.

314. Pawlak-Osinska K, Burduk PK, Kopczynski A. Episodes of repeated sudden deafness following pregnancies. Am J Obstet Gynecol. 2009;200(4):e7–9. https://doi.org/10.1016/j.ajog.2008.09.880.

315. Ambro BT, Scheid SC, Pribitkin EA. Prescribing guidelines for ENT medications during pregnancy. Ear Nose Throat J. 2003;82(8):565–8. https://www.ncbi.nlm.nih.gov/pubmed/14503092.

316. Elkharrat D, Raphael JC, Korach JM, et al. Acute carbon monoxide intoxication and hyperbaric oxygen in pregnancy. Intensive Care Med. 1991;17(5):289–92. https://doi.org/10.1007/BF01713940.

317. Van Hoesen KB, Camporesi EM, Moon RE, Hage ML, Piantadosi CA. Should hyperbaric oxygen be used to treat the pregnant patient for acute carbon monoxide poisoning? A case report and literature review. JAMA. 1989;261(7):1039–43. https://doi.org/10.1001/jama.261.7.1039.

318. Huisman JML, Verdam FJ, Stegeman I, de Ru JA. Treatment of Eustachian tube dysfunction with balloon dilation: a systematic review. Laryngoscope. 2018;128(1):237–47. https://doi.org/10.1002/lary.26800.

319. Shan A, Ward BK, Goman AM, et al. Prevalence of Eustachian tube dysfunction in adults in the United States. JAMA Otolaryngol Head Neck Surg. 2019;145:974. https://doi.org/10.1001/jamaoto.2019.1917.

320. Licameli GR. The eustachian tube. Update on anatomy, development, and function. Otolaryngol Clin North Am. 2002;35(4):803–9. https://doi.org/10.1016/s0030-6665(02)00047-6.

321. Schilder AG, Bhutta MF, Butler CC, et al. Eustachian tube dysfunction: consensus statement on definition, types, clinical presentation and diagnosis.

Clin Otolaryngol. 2015;40(5):407–11. https://doi.org/10.1111/coa.12475.

322. Choi SW, Kim J, Lee HM, et al. Prevalence and incidence of clinically significant patulous Eustachian tube: a population-based study using the Korean National Health Insurance Claims Database. Am J Otolaryngol. 2018;39(5):603–8. https://doi.org/10.1016/j.amjoto.2018.07.010.

323. Adil E, Poe D. What is the full range of medical and surgical treatments available for patients with Eustachian tube dysfunction? Curr Opin Otolaryngol Head Neck Surg. 2014;22(1):8–15. https://doi.org/10.1097/MOO.0000000000000020.

324. McCoul ED, Anand VK, Christos PJ. Validating the clinical assessment of eustachian tube dysfunction: the Eustachian tube dysfunction questionnaire (ETDQ-7). Laryngoscope. 2012;122(5):1137–41. https://doi.org/10.1002/lary.23223.

325. Doyle WJ, Swarts JD, Banks J, Casselbrant ML, Mandel EM, Alper CM. Sensitivity and specificity of eustachian tube function tests in adults. JAMA Otolaryngol Head Neck Surg. 2013;139(7):719–27. https://doi.org/10.1001/jamaoto.2013.3559.

326. Chua MLK, Wee JTS, Hui EP, Chan ATC. Nasopharyngeal carcinoma. Lancet. 2016;387(10022):1012–24. https://doi.org/10.1016/S0140-6736(15)00055-0.

327. Ribassin-Majed L, Marguet S, Lee AWM, et al. What is the best treatment of locally advanced nasopharyngeal carcinoma? An individual patient data network meta-analysis. J Clin Oncol. 2017;35(5):498–505. https://doi.org/10.1200/JCO.2016.67.4119.

328. Norman G, Llewellyn A, Harden M, et al. Systematic review of the limited evidence base for treatments of Eustachian tube dysfunction: a health technology assessment. Clin Otolaryngol. 2014;39(1):6–21. https://doi.org/10.1111/coa.12220.

329. McCoul ED, Lucente FE, Anand VK. Evolution of Eustachian tube surgery. Laryngoscope. 2011;121(3):661–6. https://doi.org/10.1002/lary.21453.

330. Wang TC, Lin CD, Shih TC, et al. Comparison of balloon dilation and laser Eustachian Tuboplasty in patients with Eustachian tube dysfunction: a meta-analysis. Otolaryngol Head Neck Surg. 2018;158(4):617–26. https://doi.org/10.1177/0194599817753609.

331. Miller BJ, Jaafar M, Elhassan HA. Laser Eustachian Tuboplasty for Eustachian tube dysfunction: a case series review. Eur Arch Otorhinolaryngol. 2017;274(6):2381–7. https://doi.org/10.1007/s00405-017-4476-0.

332. Poe DS, Grimmer JF, Metson R. Laser eustachian tuboplasty: two-year results. Laryngoscope. 2007;117(2):231–7. https://doi.org/10.1097/01.mlg.0000246227.65877.1f.

333. Siow JK, Tan JL. Indications for Eustachian tube dilation. Curr Opin Otolaryngol Head Neck Surg. 2020;28(1):31–5. https://doi.org/10.1097/MOO.0000000000000601.

334. Rotenberg BW, Busato GM, Agrawal SK. Endoscopic ligation of the patulous eustachian tube as treatment for autophony. Laryngoscope. 2013;123(1):239–43. https://doi.org/10.1002/lary.23635.

335. Dyer RK Jr, McElveen JT Jr. The patulous eustachian tube: management options. Otolaryngol Head Neck Surg. 1991;105(6):832–5. https://doi.org/10.1177/019459989110500610.

336. Vaezeafshar R, Turner JH, Li G, Hwang PH. Endoscopic hydroxyapatite augmentation for patulous Eustachian tube. Laryngoscope. 2014;124(1):62–6. https://doi.org/10.1002/lary.24250.

337. Doherty JK, Slattery WH 3rd. Autologous fat grafting for the refractory patulous eustachian tube. Otolaryngol Head Neck Surg. 2003;128(1):88–91. https://doi.org/10.1067/mhn.2003.34.

338. Reiss M, Reiss G. Patulous eustachian tube-diagnosis and therapy. Wien Med Wochenschr. 2000;150(22):454–6. https://www.ncbi.nlm.nih.gov/pubmed/11191956.

339. Mabry RL. Rhinitis of pregnancy. South Med J. 1986;79(8):965–71. https://doi.org/10.1097/00007611-198608000-00012.

340. Demir UL, Demir BC, Oztosun E, Uyaniklar OO, Ocakoglu G. The effects of pregnancy on nasal physiology. Int Forum Allergy Rhinol. 2015;5(2):162–6. https://doi.org/10.1002/alr.21438.

341. Derkay CS. Eustachian tube and nasal function during pregnancy: a prospective study. Otolaryngol Head Neck Surg. 1988;99(6):558–66. https://doi.org/10.1177/019459988809900604.

342. Plate S, Johnsen NJ, Nodskov Pedersen S, Thomsen KA. The frequency of patulous Eustachian tubes in pregnancy. Clin Otolaryngol Allied Sci. 1979;4(6):393–400. https://doi.org/10.1111/j.1365-2273.1979.tb01771.x.

343. Demoly P, Piette V, Daures JP. Treatment of allergic rhinitis during pregnancy. Drugs. 2003;63(17):1813–20. https://doi.org/10.2165/00003495-200363170-00004.

344. Gilbert-Barness E, Drut RM. Association of sympathomimetic drugs with malformations. Vet Hum Toxicol. 2000;42(3):168–71. https://www.ncbi.nlm.nih.gov/pubmed/10839324.

345. Ugen KE, Scott WJ Jr. Reduction of uterine blood flow by phenylephrine, an alpha-adrenergic agonist, in the day 11 pregnant rat: relationship to potentiation of acetazolamide teratogenesis. Teratology. 1987;36(1):133–41. https://doi.org/10.1002/tera.1420360117.

346. Gastroschisis and pseudoephedrine during pregnancy. Prescrire Int. 2004;13(72):141–3. https://www.ncbi.nlm.nih.gov/pubmed/15532139.

347. Gilbert C, Mazzotta P, Loebstein R, Koren G. Fetal safety of drugs used in the treatment of allergic rhinitis: a critical review. Drug Saf. 2005;28(8):707–19. https://doi.org/10.2165/00002018-200528080-00005.

348. Blaiss MS, Food DA, Acaai A. Management of rhinitis and asthma in pregnancy. Ann Allergy Asthma Immunol. 2003;90(6 Suppl 3):16–22. https://doi.org/10.1016/s1081-1206(10)61655-9.

349. Song Y, Alyono JC, Bartholomew RA, Vaisbuch Y, Corrales CE, Blevins NH. Prevalence of radiographic Cochlear-facial nerve dehiscence. Otol Neurotol. 2018;39(10):1319–25. https://doi.org/10.1097/MAO.0000000000002015.

350. Wackym PA, Mackay-Promitas HT, Demirel S, et al. Comorbidities confounding the outcomes of surgery for third window syndrome: outlier analysis. Laryngosc Investig Otolaryngol. 2017;2(5):225–53. https://doi.org/10.1002/lio2.89.

351. Schart-Moren N, Larsson S, Rask-Andersen H, Li H. Anatomical characteristics of facial nerve and cochlea interaction. Audiol Neurootol. 2017;22(1):41–9. https://doi.org/10.1159/000475876.

352. Karimnejad K, Czerny MS, Lookabaugh S, Lee DJ, Mikulec AA. Gender and laterality in semicircular canal dehiscence syndrome. J Laryngol Otol. 2016;130(8):712–6. https://doi.org/10.1017/S0022215116008185.

353. Mikulec AA, McKenna MJ, Ramsey MJ, et al. Superior semicircular canal dehiscence presenting as conductive hearing loss without vertigo. Otol Neurotol. 2004;25(2):121–9. https://doi.org/10.1097/00129492-200403000-00007.

354. Carey JP, Minor LB, Nager GT. Dehiscence or thinning of bone overlying the superior semicircular canal in a temporal bone survey. Arch Otolaryngol Head Neck Surg. 2000;126(2):137–47. https://doi.org/10.1001/archotol.126.2.137.

355. Zhou G, Gopen Q, Poe DS. Clinical and diagnostic characterization of canal dehiscence syndrome: a great Otologic mimicker. Otol Neurotol. 2007;28(7):920–6. https://doi.org/10.1097/MAO.0b013e31814b25f2.

356. Ward BK, Carey JP, Minor LB. Superior Canal dehiscence syndrome: lessons from the first 20 years. Front Neurol. 2017;8:177. https://doi.org/10.3389/fneur.2017.00177.

357. Crane BT, Lin FR, Minor LB, Carey JP. Improvement in autophony symptoms after superior canal dehiscence repair. Otol Neurotol. 2010;31(1):140–6. https://doi.org/10.1097/mao.0b013e3181bc39ab.

358. Crane BT, Minor LB, Carey JP. Superior canal dehiscence plugging reduces dizziness handicap. Laryngoscope. 2008;118(10):1809–13. https://doi.org/10.1097/MLG.0b013e31817f18fa.

359. Nikkar-Esfahani A, Whelan D, Banerjee A. Occlusion of the round window: a novel way to treat hyperacusis symptoms in superior semicircular canal dehiscence syndrome. J Laryngol Otol. 2013;127(7):705–7. https://doi.org/10.1017/S0022215113001096.

360. Meehan T, Nogueira C, Rajenderkumar D, Shah J, Stephens D, Dyer K. Dehiscence of the posterior and superior semicircular canal presenting in pregnancy. B-ENT. 2013;9(2):165–8. https://www.ncbi.nlm.nih.gov/pubmed/23909125.

361. Ogutha J, Page NC, Hullar TE. Postpartum vertigo and superior semicircular canal dehiscence syndrome. Obstet Gynecol. 2009;114(2 Pt 2):434–6. https://doi.org/10.1097/AOG.0b013e3181ae8da0.

Management of Mental Health Disorders in Pregnancy

Diego Garces Grosse and Rashi Aggarwal

Introduction

The term perinatal mental illness encompasses psychiatric disorders that are prevalent during both pregnancy and the postpartum. The typical associated postpartum timeframe is between 4 weeks and 3 months after delivery, but some authors consider the duration to be up to 1 year after delivery. Mental disorders that predate the pregnancy but relapse during pregnancy or postpartum are also considered perinatal mental illness [1]. What is considered perinatal mental illness ranges from mild anxiety or depression to mania and full-blown psychosis.

The estimated worldwide prevalence rate for mental illness is 10% in pregnant women and 13% in postpartum women [2]. In the USA, there is no significant difference in the 12-month prevalence of mental illness between women who were pregnant in the past year (25.35%), those in the postpartum phase (27.5%), and non-pregnant women of childbearing age (30.1%) except for the increased risk of depressive disorders in postpartum women (9.3%) versus non-pregnant women (8.1%). Pregnancy, per se, is not considered a risk factor for mental illness, nor is it pro-

tective from mental illness as was erroneously believed in the past [3].

One study [4] reported that 10.3% of over 340,000 American women who delivered a child between the years 2006 and 2011 were prescribed a psychotropic medication. The percentage varied from state to state, ranging from 6% to 15%. The most common drugs prescribed were selective serotonin reuptake inhibitors (SSRIs) and benzodiazepines.

Therefore, many questions arise regarding the management of mental illness in pregnant women such as the type of treatment to use, the necessity of medications, and the relative risks of treatment and side effects.

In the sections that follow we discuss the above questions in the context of the major classes of mental illness: depressive disorders, anxiety, bipolar disorder, and psychoses. Depressive disorders include both major depression and the so-called postpartum blues and we discuss both.

Depressive Disorders

Major Depression

Major depressive disorder (MDD) is defined as a period of at least 2 weeks with depressed mood or anhedonia (loss of interest or pleasure in previously pleasurable activities) for the majority of

D. G. Grosse (✉) · R. Aggarwal
Rutgers, New Jersey Medical School,
Newark, NJ, USA
e-mail: diego.garces@rutgers.edu; aggarwra@njms.rutgers.edu

© The Author(s), under exclusive license to Springer Nature Switzerland AG 2023
G. Gupta et al. (eds.), *Neurological Disorders in Pregnancy*,
https://doi.org/10.1007/978-3-031-36490-7_31

Table 31.1 DSM-5 diagnostic criteria for major depressive episode

DSM-5 diagnostic criteria for major depressive episode [5]
At least one of following 2 for at least 2 weeks:
1 Depressed mood most of the time
2 Diminished interest or pleasure in all or almost all activities
Five or more of the following symptoms for at least 2 weeks:
3 Significant weight loss or weight gain. Alternatively, decreased or increased appetite
4 Insomnia or hypersomnia almost every day
5 Psychomotor agitation or retardation nearly every day
6 Fatigue or loss of energy nearly every day
7 Feelings of worthlessness or excessive or inappropriate guilt
8 Diminished ability to think or concentrate
9 Recurrent thoughts of death or suicidal ideation

the time, accompanied by at least five of the following: unintended increase or decrease in appetite or weight, insomnia or hypersomnia, psychomotor agitation or retardation, fatigue or loss of energy, feelings of worthlessness or guilt, difficulty with attention and concentration, and recurrent thoughts of death or suicide [5] (Table 31.1).

Following puberty, the prevalence of MDD in women ranges from 10% to 20%, which is almost twice that of men [6]. The prevalence of depression during pregnancy is around 11% in the first trimester and 8.5% in the second and third trimesters [7]. Many of the depressive episodes that occur during pregnancy represent the first such event in the woman's lifetime [8] and can go undiagnosed more frequently in pregnant women than in non-pregnant women [9].

The pathogenesis of depression remains unknown, as does the degree to which perinatal depression differs from non-perinatal depression [10]. It is suggested that some of the factors that are involved in perinatal depression are genetic inheritance [11], hormonal changes, and social and psychological factors.

The prevalence of suicide in pregnant women is lower than that of the general population of women in the same age group [12]. One study found that the rate of suicide in pregnant women is approximately one quarter (27%) of that of the general population of women in the same age group [13].

Special Considerations Related to Pregnancy

Prenatal maternal depression has been associated with multiple negative obstetrical outcomes during both pregnancy and delivery as well as in developmental problems of the neonate, infant, and child [6, 14]. Table 31.2 lists the major associated risks and potential risks where association with prenatal maternal depression has not been clearly established.

Further, prenatal depression has not been found to be associated with hypertensive disorders during pregnancy, gestational diabetes, or placental abruption [18].

Treatment During Pregnancy

A pregnant patient diagnosed with depression needs to be initially assessed in terms of severity of the depressive episode. Combinations of psychotherapy and pharmacological treatment are often used to varying degrees depending on severity. It is also important to take into account if the patient has been diagnosed with depression, and treated, prior to pregnancy. In these cases, continuation of previous treatment is generally indicated. If a patient has been effectively treated with psychotherapy before, it would be expected to be effective again. The same applies to pharmacologic treatment.

For patients newly diagnosed with mild to moderate episodes, the first recommendation is psychotherapy—most commonly cognitive-behavioral therapy (CBT) and interpersonal therapy [27–29].

Cognitive-Behavioral Therapy (CBT)

As the name implies, CBT consists of two approaches to therapy: a cognitive approach and a behavioral approach. The cognitive portion of CBT aims to modify a patient's dysfunctional thoughts by cognitive restructuring. This involves reframing distorted beliefs (e.g. "I'm a bad person") by challenging them while considering alternative, more benign explanations for those beliefs.

Table 31.2 Major associated risks and potential risks association with prenatal maternal

Associated increased risk	
Spontaneous abortion	Maternal depression during pregnancy appears to be associated with a small increase in risk of spontaneous abortions, with a relative risk of 1.1–1.2 compared to non-depressed women [15, 16]
Bleeding	A small increase in risk of hemorrhage during pregnancy and/or the postpartum period has been observed [17, 18]
Operative delivery	Maternal depression has been observed to be associated with operative deliveries, caesarian sections, or instrumentally assisted deliveries [18] with a relative risk of up to 1.3 compared to non-depressed women [19]
Preterm birth	Several studies have consistently shown an association between maternal depression and preterm birth [18, 20]
Breastfeeding	Maternal depression is associated with a small increased risk of delay in starting breastfeeding [14]
Sudden infant death syndrome	Untreated depression during pregnancy may be associated with sudden infant death syndrome [21]
Sleep problems	Neonates born of depressed mothers show a disturbed and disorganized sleep pattern, with less time in deep sleep [22]
Cognitive functioning	High levels of depressive symptoms during pregnancy are associated with delayed development and decreased cognitive performance in children born to depressed mothers [23]
Depression later in life	Children born to mothers depressed during pregnancy have a greater risk of suffering from depression through childhood and adolescence [24]
Association not clearly established	
Teratogenicity	It is unclear if there is an increased risk for teratogenicity with maternal depression because the evidence is conflicting [25, 26]
Stillbirth	As with teratogenicity, conflicting evidence makes it difficult to clarify if there is a real association between maternal depression and risk for stillbirths [25, 26]

The behavioral part of CBT aims to modify problematic behaviors that result from distorted beliefs, depressive symptoms, and multiple stimuli. It does this by different techniques like problem solving, behavioral activation, breathing exercises, physical exercise, and muscle relaxation. The use of CBT has proven effective in the general population of patients with depression [30] and also in patients with antenatal depression [31].

Interpersonal Psychotherapy

Interpersonal psychotherapy during pregnancy mainly focuses on role transitions (becoming a mother) and role disputes (conflicts with others who have different expectations in the relationship). Studies have found that interpersonal psychotherapy is effective for treating perinatal depression [32]

Medications

In some cases of mild to moderate depression, antidepressant medication may be a reasonable option given the following considerations [33]:

- Psychotherapy is not available, or the patient does not accept it.
- Patient prefers pharmacotherapy (has received previous treatment and responded well).
- Patient has a history of severe depression, and thus, mild depression could progress to severe.

In such cases, three classes of drugs are considered: SSRIs, SNRIs, and bupropion.

SSRIs

Selective serotonin reuptake inhibitors (SSRIs) are the most studied class of antidepressants in pregnancy. In a study [34] with more than 64,000 pregnant women who were prescribed antidepressants in the first trimester, 72% were prescribed SSRIs. The most commonly prescribed and studied SSRIs are fluoxetine and sertraline. Less commonly studied are citalopram, escitalopram, fluvoxamine, and paroxetine. Of these, paroxetine is considered the riskiest.

Most of the studies suggest that the use of SSRIs during pregnancy is not associated with malformations or birth defects [18, 35, 36]. There are a few studies that have found a small potential increase in cardiovascular defects [37], most specifically with paroxetine [38]. The use of SSRIs during pregnancy has not been associated with perinatal death [39] nor with spontaneous abortions [40].

Pertaining to maternal health, the relative risk of postpartum hemorrhage is doubled when taking SSRIs as shown in a study where 18% of women taking SSRIs had postpartum hemorrhage compared to 9% of those who were not exposed [41]. Also, in women who did have postpartum hemorrhage, the average amount of blood lost was greater in those taking SSRIs [41].

A small association has also been found between women taking SSRIs and preterm delivery [42]. A study found that, on average, women taking SSRIs deliver 3 days earlier than women not exposed to SSRIs [40].

It is unclear if exposure to SSRIs during pregnancy is associated with low birth weight. Some evidence suggests that the relative risk for low birth weight is 1.5 in neonates born to mothers exposed to SSRIs during pregnancy [43]. A meta-analysis found that, on average, neonates born to mothers exposed to SSRIs weigh 74 g less than those born to non-exposed mothers. However, the difference is not considered clinically significant [40].

There is conflicting evidence about the rates of preeclampsia in women being treated with SSRIs. Some studies have found an increase [44], some no change [18], and some a decrease [45].

SNRIs

In addition to SSRIs, another class of medications often used for the treatment of depressive episodes is serotonin and norepinephrine reuptake inhibitors (SNRIs). These are far less commonly prescribed than SSRIs and consequently, much less studied. The most studied among the SNRIs are duloxetine and venlafaxine. There is very little evidence for the use of other SNRIs like milnacipran, levomilnacipran, and desvenlafaxine [46].

SNRIs are not considered teratogenic and they have not been associated with malformations [35]. Neonates born to mothers taking SNRIs during pregnancy have not shown to have an increased risk of congenital cardiac defects [34].

Several studies suggest that SNRIs are associated with postpartum hemorrhage [47]. More specifically, a study found that women who were treated with venlafaxine during the last 30 days of pregnancy have a higher risk of postpartum hemorrhage (11%) than those who were not exposed (7%) [48].

It is not clear if SNRIs are associated with spontaneous abortions. For example, there are conflicting results regarding duloxetine; one study showed a relative risk of 3 [49], while the Eli Lilly pharmacovigilance system reports an incidence equal to that of general population [50]. Results for venlafaxine have been also conflicting; however, the evidence suggests that it is not likely to be associated with spontaneous abortions [51, 52].

There is also conflicting evidence about the association of SNRIs with hypertensive disorders in pregnancy. Some studies suggest that venlafaxine results in a mild increase in the risk of preeclampsia [53]. Duloxetine, however, was not found to increase the risk for preeclampsia [54].

Bupropion

Bupropion is yet another therapeutic agent commonly used for treating depression. It belongs to the class of norepinephrine and dopamine reuptake inhibitors (NDRIs).

Bupropion is generally considered low risk for teratogenicity [29, 34, 35]. The "Bupropion Pregnancy Registry" study found that there is no significant increase in the risk of birth defects as a result of the use of bupropion during pregnancy [55]. A few studies have found an association with the increase in risk of cardiac defects in newborns whose mothers were exposed to bupropion during pregnancy; this risk is considered to be 2–3 times that of the general population, however the absolute risk is considered small with 2.1–2.8 cases per 1000 births [56].

There is evidence that the use of bupropion may be associated with spontaneous abortions with a relative risk of 3 compared to women who were not exposed to it [57].

Bupropion does not appear to be associated with increased risk of hypertensive disorders during pregnancy [53], postpartum hemorrhage [58], low birth weight [59], or preterm birth. In fact, one study found that women who received bupropion during pregnancy have a lower likelihood of having a preterm delivery [60].

Recommended Treatment

Overall, the recommend course of action is to identify patients who may be showing symptoms of depression as described in Table 31.1. Mild to moderate cases may receive initial treatment with psychotherapy alone, while more severe cases, or patients who have had severe episodes in the past, or patients not amenable to receive psychotherapy should be started on SSRIs as the first line of pharmacological management. Patients who have responded to medications other than SSRIs in the past may be started on that same medication. Patients who continue to worsen or do not show improvement may need inpatient psychiatric treatment.

Postpartum Blues

Postpartum blues, belonging to the cluster of postpartum mood disturbances, is a transient condition that presents with several mild depressive symptoms that develop in nearly 50% of women who have given birth within a week of delivery [61]. The symptoms include a depressed mood, crying, irritability, anxiety, insomnia, exhaustion, and decreased concentration. It is considered nonpathological subclinical depression. Nonetheless, it is important that it be recognized because women who go through postpartum blues are nearly 4 times as likely to develop post-

partum depression and anxiety disorders than women who do not [62].

Though the etiology is still unknown, studies suggest that postpartum blues result from a decrease in estrogen levels during the days following delivery, which in turn results in an elevation of monoamine oxidase-A (MAO-A) [63] and decreased serotonergic activity [64].

Postpartum blues usually does not require specific treatment as it resolves spontaneously over 2 weeks. Management is generally conservative, with watchful waiting, and frequent support and reassurance.

Patient should be referred for treatment if symptoms do not improve or worsen over 2 weeks or if there is suicidal ideation or risk for suicidality. In this case, the patient is likely to have developed postpartum depression and needs treatment.

Anxiety

Anxiety is the second most common psychiatric disorder during pregnancy and in the postpartum period [65], with a prevalence ranging between 15% and 22% [66].

Pregnancy by itself is a stressful period with the many physiological and social changes it brings and the potential challenges it introduces. These stressors can result in higher anxiety levels in pregnant and postpartum women. Given that pregnancy comes with physical changes, it may be difficult to differentiate between the physical symptoms and unspecific complaints such as fatigue, loss of energy or appetite, and sleep changes that arise from pregnancy and those arising from anxiety. It is as a result of this that anxiety often goes undiagnosed [67, 68].

Special Considerations Related to Pregnancy

A meta-analysis of 29 studies concluded that maternal prenatal anxiety is significantly associated with preterm birth (OR of 1.54 versus controls) and low birth weight (OR of 1.8 versus controls) with an average of 143 g below controls for babies with diagnosed mothers and 55 g below controls for babies with symptomatic undiagnosed mothers [69].

Anxiety has not been shown to be associated with lower Apgar scores or preeclampsia. Anxiety has also not been shown to be associated with incidence of instrumental or operative delivery [70].

Treatment During Pregnancy

Family support and relaxation techniques are usually the first step in managing anxiety during pregnancy [71]. Psychotherapeutic techniques like cognitive-behavioral and interpersonal therapy are also effective methods in treating anxiety [72]. Their use during pregnancy is discussed in the depressive disorder section above. It is when support and psychotherapeutic approaches do not appear to improve a patient's condition or when symptoms are becoming too distressing that medication is indicated.

Medications

The most commonly used classes of medication for the treatment of anxiety in pregnant women are SSRIs, benzodiazepines, gabapentin, and antihistamines.

SSRIs

SSRIs are commonly used to treat moderate to severe anxiety disorders. Considerations for their use during pregnancy are discussed above in the depressive disorder section.

Benzodiazepines

Benzodiazepines are commonly used to treat severe anxiety (as in panic disorder or GAD) in the general population. They can also be used to manage severe anxiety during pregnancy. Benzodiazepines with shorter half-lives are gen-

erally preferred. Benzodiazepines do, however, appear to be associated with an increased risk for spontaneous abortions as evidenced by a meta-analysis with an OR of 2 [73].

It is unclear if benzodiazepines are teratogenic as conflicting results have supported both association and non-association [74]. If a real association does exist, the effect is considered small [75]. For example, benzodiazepines have been associated with an increased risk for oral clefts (lip, palate, or both) [75]. However, the increased risk is considered small because only about 6 in 10,000 births in the general population result in these birth defects and benzodiazepines raise that risk to 11 in 10,000 births. Even though the increase is almost double, the absolute numbers remain small [74].

Benzodiazepines may be associated with preterm birth with greater likelihood stemming from earlier exposure, i.e. in the first trimester [76]. There does not appear to be any correlation between exposure to benzodiazepines during pregnancy and low birth weight [73].

Notably, studies have found some postnatal effects in neonates when exposure to benzodiazepine was close to delivery. Symptoms include low Apgar scores, apnea/hypopnea, lethargy, tremors, hypotonia, irritability, and poor feeding [75, 76]. Neonates may experience withdrawal symptoms, such as hypoventilation, irritability, hypertonicity, and a syndrome that includes hypotonia, lethargy, and sucking difficulties, soon after delivery if exposure was long and symptoms may persist for up to 3 months [76]. There does not appear to be any correlation between exposure to benzodiazepines during pregnancy and neurocognitive or behavioral development in babies [77].

Gabapentin

Gabapentin is a GABA analogue drug with an inhibitory neurotransmission effect traditionally used as an antiepileptic. It is also often used to treat anxiety and insomnia. No associations have been found between gabapentin treatment during pregnancy and birth defects, abortions, or stillbirths [78]. However, although considered safe, it does present an overall increase in the risk for preterm birth (10.5% vs 3.9%) and low birth weight (10.5 vs. 4.4%) [78]. It should be noted that maternal gabapentin in the third trimester significantly increases the risk for need of neonatal ICU after delivery [78].

Buspirone

Buspirone is another commonly used anxiolytic proven to decrease symptoms of anxiety, comparable to benzodiazepines over long term use with lower frequency of side effects [79]. Over the short term, benzodiazepines have a quicker onset on decreasing anxiety symptoms. Although animal models have shown no association of buspirone with negative outcomes of pregnancy, there are no studies to support that the same applies in human subjects. Interestingly enough, rat models have shown that maternal buspirone may have a protective factor against stress in infant and adult rats [80, 81].

Antihistamines

Some antihistamines, specifically hydroxyzine and diphenhydramine, can be used for the treatment of anxiety. Of these, hydroxyzine is the preferred course for treatment of anxiety during pregnancy. It is often considered equivalent to buspirone in efficacy [82]. The sedating effects of antihistamines can also help with insomnia associated with anxiety [82]. The above being said, there are few studies on the use of antihistamines for anxiety during pregnancy given that they are contraindicated in all three trimesters [83, 84]. Hydroxyzine and diphenhydramine have been associated with orofacial clefts in the neonate if taken during the first trimester [85]. Several other antihistamines have been reported to increase the risk of spontaneous abortions and preterm births, although the evidence has been conflicting [86]. A case report suggested that the use of hydroxyzine during the third trimester may be associated with neonatal seizures [87].

Antihistamines are sometimes used for the prevention and management of extra-pyramidal symptoms (EPS) secondary to antipsychotic use. Anticholinergics like benztropine and trihexyphenidyl are more commonly used for EPS in the general population; however, their risk of teratogenicity is greater than that of antihistamines [88]. Therefore, the antihistamine diphenhydramine with its lower risk of teratogenicity is considered the treatment of choice for secondary EPS in pregnant women. Note that given the associated risks of malformation and the unclear risk of preterm birth [86, 88], the dose should be the lowest possible that is still effective and the duration of treatment the shortest possible.

Recommended Treatment

As with depression, the recommended course of action is relaxation techniques and family support. If those do not prove adequate, mild and moderate cases of anxiety should be treated with psychotherapeutic approaches like CTB and interpersonal therapy. Treatment can be escalated from there if symptoms progress.

In more severe cases, the clinician should weigh the risk of treatment versus the risk of non-treatment. SSRIs are considered mostly safe and effective, but they typically take longer to result in clinical improvement compared to other medications [34]. In cases of severe anxiety or agitation or when clinical improvement is required in a shorter period, benzodiazepines can be used with the lowest effective dose and for the shortest period possible [73].

Bipolar Disorder

Bipolar disorder is a mood disorder characterized by the presence of depressive episodes and manic or hypomanic episodes. To diagnose a patient with bipolar disorder, there must be at least one manic episode or one hypomanic episode and one depressive episode [5].

Manic episodes are defined as a period of abnormally and persistently elevated, expansive, or irritable mood along with increased energy for a least 1 week. They must be accompanied by at least three of the following: inflated self-esteem or grandiosity; decreased need for sleep; talkativeness or pressured speech; flight of ideas; distractibility; increased activity levels or psychomotor agitation; and/or excessive involvement in activities with potential for negative outcomes (buying sprees, sexual indiscretion, foolish investments). A hypomanic episode constitutes the same symptoms, albeit milder and for at least 4 days [5] (Table 31.3).

The prevalence of bipolar disorder in the USA is about 0.6%. The prevalence around the world ranges from 0.0% to 0.6% and affects males more than females in a ratio of 1.1:1 [5].

Bipolar disorder in women usually begins during the onset of reproductive age and after the first episode most patients are at risk for recurrent episodes. Euthymic (i.e. controlled patients without symptoms of mania or depression) bipolar patients usually receive maintenance therapy to prevent new episodes [75].

It is not known if pregnancy has an effect on mood episodes as there is conflicting evidence stating that some patients may have decreased risk of mood episodes during pregnancy, whereas in other patients the course of illness may worsen or remain unchanged during pregnancy [89].

The risk of recurrence of mood episodes appears to be highest in the first trimester. A study that included 63 patients who had mood episodes during the course of their pregnancy found that 66.6% of the patients had mood episodes in the first trimester, 28.3% in the second trimester, and 9.5% in the third trimester [89].

Special Considerations Related to Pregnancy

Women who experience mood episodes (manic, hypomanic, or depressive) during pregnancy may be affected negatively by these episodes, resulting in potential harm to themselves and/or the fetus. The recognized risks are:

- Manic/hypomanic episodes: Impulsive and risky behavior, substance abuse, malnutrition, poor adherence to prenatal care, disrupted family functioning.
- Depressive episodes: Suicidal behavior, poor self-care, poor adherence to prenatal care, malnutrition resulting in low birth weight, diminished mother-infant bonding, and the obstetric and developmental outcomes described in depression section.

For patients already on medication (prior to the onset of pregnancy or during pregnancy), there are significant risks of discontinuing medication during pregnancy [90]. These include:

- Increased recurrence of episodes during pregnancy
- Abrupt discontinuation may precipitate a mood episode.
- More difficulty in treating recurrent episodes during pregnancy
- Possible exposure of the fetus to more medications, or higher doses of medication
- Higher risk of postpartum recurrences

Table 31.3 DSM-5 diagnostic criteria for manic episode

DSM-5 diagnostic criteria for manic Episode [5]
A period of abnormally elevated, expansive, or irritable mood and increased activity or energy for at least 1 week, accompanied by three or more of the following:
1 Inflated self-esteem or grandiosity
2 Decreased need for sleep
3 More talkativeness than usual
4 Flight of ideas or racing thoughts
5 Distractibility
6 Increased goal-directed activity
7 Excessive involvement in activities with potential for negative consequences
Note: The mood disturbance has to be severe enough to impair social or occupational functioning.

Treatment During Pregnancy

Maintenance treatment during pregnancy prevents the recurrence of mood episodes. A study that included euthymic pregnant patients found a recurrence rate of 37% in those who were on maintenance medication versus 86% in those who were not [89].

The current recommendation for bipolar patients who want to conceive is to wait until a period of clinical stability of at least 6–12 months [91]. A study found that a shorter period of clinical stability between the last mood episode and pregnancy is correlated with an increased risk of mood episodes and recurrences during pregnancy [89].

Pharmacotherapy

For most patients with an established diagnosis, continued treatment is recommended. Some pregnant women may develop a new onset of mild mood episodes during pregnancy that can self-limit such as minor depressive episodes or some episodes of hypomania. These cases may not require medication. Pharmacotherapy is indicated if more severe symptoms arise, such as suicidal or homicidal ideations or behavior, psychosis, poor judgment, or involvement in activities that may pose risk for harm to patient or others, social or occupational impairment, or aggression [10].

Antipsychotics

Antipsychotics are commonly the first line of treatment in episodes of acute mania. Haloperidol is usually the first choice given its efficacy and safety in pregnancy [92]. Nonetheless, a study of prevalence of antipsychotic use during pregnancy between 2001 and 2007 found that second-generation antipsychotics are used more often (0.7%) than first-generation antipsychotics (0.1%) [93]. In episodes of bipolar depression, quetiapine, of all antipsychotics, has proven greater efficacy [94]. Most of the studies have found that there is no increased risk of malformations with prenatal exposure to first- and second-generation antipsychotics [95, 96], with the exception of one study that found that risperidone showed a small increase in risk for overall malformations of 1.2 when compared to unexposed newborns [97].

Postnatal effects have been observed in neonates born to mothers taking antipsychotics during the third trimester. The effects may be a consequence of neonatal toxicity and/or withdrawal from the antipsychotics [75]. Symptoms of these effects in neonates may include: increased or decreased muscle tone, hyperreflexia, tremors, irritability, crying, or restlessness. The frequency of incidence is low and symptoms are more likely to occur with first-generation antipsychotics and risperidone than with second-generation antipsychotics [96]. Symptoms are usually self-limited, subside within hours to days, and usually do not require specific treatment [96].

An association with birth weight is unclear for both first- and second-generation antipsychotics. For first generation, there is conflictive evidence showing no association with abnormal birth weight [98], while others suggest that, on average, newborns exposed in-utero have a decreased birth weight than those who were not exposed [99]. Similarly, for second generation, conflicting results have shown association with both higher [99] and lower [100] birth weights.

Lithium

Lithium is the third element in the periodic table and in the 1950s its salts became the first medication dedicated to treating bipolar disorder. [101] Since then, lithium has remained one of the main medications for treating bipolar disorder because of its high efficacy, especially in acute mania. There is evidence that shows that it also helps decrease suicidality [102].

While lithium's mechanism of action is still unknown, several hypotheses suggest that it works by the stimulation of inhibitory neurotransmission and the inhibition of excitatory neurotransmission [103].

Unfortunately, lithium is largely associated with congenital defects and malformations [104]. The most commonly associated conditions appear to be cardiac defects, mainly Ebstein's anomaly (abnormal tricuspid valve and right ventricle), right ventricle obstruction defects, coarctation of the aorta, and mitral atresia [75, 105].

It is unclear if the use of lithium is associated with spontaneous abortions. One study found similar frequencies of spontaneous abortions and stillbirths with controls [106]. However, a second study found that women exposed to lithium during the first trimester had a higher risk (16%) for spontaneous abortions than non-exposed women (6%) [104].

The use of lithium during pregnancy appears to be associated with preterm birth. A prospective study found that women who received lithium during the first trimester had a greater rate of preterm delivery (14%) than women who were treated with non-teratogenic substances (6%) [104]. Birth weight appears to increase upon in-utero exposure to lithium but the increase has not been found to be significant [106].

The use of lithium during the second and third trimesters is associated with neonatal complications such as cardiomegaly, GI bleeding, thyroid problems, hepatomegaly, and nephrogenic diabetes insipidus [107, 108].

Newborns exposed to lithium near delivery may experience lithium toxicity characterized by low Apgar scores, apnea/hypopnea, bradycardia/tachycardia, arrhythmias, lethargy, hypotonia, poor reflexes, twitching, and seizures. Lithium toxicity is more commonly seen in newborns with higher serum lithium levels [107, 108].

Antiepileptics

Antiepileptic drugs (AEDs) are generally used as mood stabilizers for maintenance treatment of bipolar disorder [109]. The AEDs typically prescribed for mood stabilization are valproic acid, lamotrigine, carbamazepine, and oxcarbazepine. It is recommended that female bipolar patients begin counseling before starting maintenance therapy because AEDs have a high risk for teratogenicity. Thus, they are usually not recommended for women of childbearing age and are usually given in conjunction with contraceptive methods [95]. Of the AEDs, lamotrigine is preferred for maintenance during pregnancy [110]. In such cases, it is recommended to start lamotrigine before pregnancy because initiating it during pregnancy may be complicated by the need for a slow titration and the difficulty in achieving therapeutic levels.

Recommended Treatment

Mania or Hypomania

In cases of acute mania, the general recommendation is first-generation antipsychotics; namely, haloperidol, given its efficacy and safety [92]. Alternative first-generation antipsychotics include fluphenazine, chlorpromazine, and perphenazine. Approximately 50% of the patients are expected to respond to the treatment by first-generation antipsychotics [111]. The efficacy of haloperidol is comparable to that of risperidone and olanzapine and appears to be superior to that of quetiapine and lithium [92].

Bipolar Depression

In cases of bipolar depression, quetiapine appears to have comparable efficacy with lamotrigine [112], in addition to the advantage of easier titration and shorter time of response. For patients who fail to respond to quetiapine and lamotrigine, a combination of fluoxetine and olanzapine [113] appears to be comparable to the combination of lamotrigine and lithium; however, the former is preferred given the potential teratogenicity of lithium.

Psychoses

Psychotic disorders are defined in DSM-5 by five main symptoms, which are delusions, hallucinations, disorganized thinking or speech, disorganized or abnormal motor behavior, and negative symptoms [5]. The prevalence of organic psychotic disorders is usually under 1%, although medication-induced psychoses and psychoses secondary to medical conditions can go as high as 25% in the USA [5]. Although psychosis is the most recognized symptom of disorders like schizophrenia and schizoaffective disorders, many other psychiatric disorders like severe depression and mania can present with psychotic symptoms.

DSM-5 defines peripartum psychosis and postpartum psychosis separately. Peripartum psychosis refers to onset from time of delivery to 4 weeks following, while postpartum psychosis refers to onset after 4 weeks [5]. Postpartum psychosis is often seen in bipolar patients but can also occur in women with depressive disorder, schizophrenia, or schizoaffective disorder. Postpartum psychosis is considered a psychiatric emergency because of an associated risk of infanticide.

Special Considerations Related to Pregnancy

It is recommended that women with psychotic disorders strive for clinical stability before attempting to get pregnant. The risks associated with psychosis during pregnancy are similar to the risks associated with the disorders discussed above. They include suicidal ideation or behavior, disorganized thought or behavior, overall risky behavior that poses a threat to the patient and the fetus. All of these behaviors warrant emergent treatment.

Recommended Treatment

Women who are not already under treatment and develop psychosis during pregnancy require emergent treatment to prevent harm to self and possible negative outcomes of pregnancy. Treatment is usually started with antipsychotics as described above in the bipolar disorders section. The risks and recommendations associated with antipsychotics during pregnancy are discussed in the prior section.

For women who are already on antipsychotic treatment and develop psychosis during pregnancy, it is recommended that the dosage of the antipsychotic be increased and titrated to the maximum therapeutically tolerated dose before starting a second drug in order to prevent exposure of the fetus to multiple drugs. Although first- and second-generation antipsychotics are generally considered safe during pregnancy, it is preferred to minimize multiple drug exposure. If poor or no response is noted, then other medications can be added in a step-by-step approach. Electroconvulsive therapy, while used less often nowadays, is also a relatively safe option for treatment of acute psychotic episodes.

While anxiety and mild to moderate depressive disorders may be managed by general practitioners, it is important to note that more severe cases and conditions like bipolar disorder and psychotic disorders should ideally be managed by a psychiatrist.

Conclusion

Mental illnesses have a significant prevalence during pregnancy and the postpartum period. Pregnancy, per se, is not considered to be a risk factor or protective factor for mental illness. Mental illnesses can be present before and continue through pregnancy, as well as they can newly develop during the course of pregnancy. The treatment of mental illnesses during pregnancy should focus on resolving the symptoms of the pregnant woman while minimizing the potential risks to the fetus. Milder forms of depression and anxiety can often be treated with and respond well to psychotherapeutic interventions and family support. More severe cases, or patients who have presented severe forms prior to pregnancy often require medication to control symptoms. Women presenting with psychosis or mania during require emergent intervention and medication to control symptoms. While several interventions can be initiated by a primary care physician, an emergency medicine doctor, or an obstetrician, consultation to a psychiatrist to manage psychotropic medications remains the standard of care. Better medical care is provided when a psychiatrist is involved in the multidisciplinary team.

Risks of Different Medications

Table 31.4 lists the common complications with the different medications discussed in the sections above.

Table 31.4 Risks of different medications

	Risk of complications						
	Teratogenicity	Stillbirth	Preterm birth	Spontaneous abortion	Low birth weight	Bleeding	Preeclampsia
Antidepressants and anxiolytics							
SSRIs	No association [18, 35, 36] Except paroxetine [38]	No association [39]	Small increase [42]	No association [40]	Unclear [43]	Double [41]	Unclear [18, 44, 45]
SNRIs	No association [34, 35]	No association [34, 35]	No evidence	Unclear [49–52]	No evidence	Increase [47, 48]	Small increase (venlafaxine) [53]
Bupropion	Small risk [29, 34, 35]	No association [59]	No association [59] Protective [60]	Increase [57]	No association [59]	No association [58]	No association [53]
Benzodiazepines	Orofacial clefts [75]	Unclear	Increase [76]	Increase [73]	No association [73]	Unclear	Unclear
Gabapentin	No association [78]	No association [78]	Small increase [78]	No association [78]	Small increase [78]	Unclear	Unclear
Buspirone	No evidence	No evidence	No evidence	No evidence	No evidence	No evidence	No evidence
Antihistamines	Orofacial clefts [85]	Unclear	Unclear [86, 88]	Unclear	No evidence	No evidence	No evidence
Antipsychotics							
First generation	No association [95, 96]	No association [96]	No association [96]	No association [96]	Unclear [98, 99]	No association [96]	No association [96]
Second generation	Small increase (only risperidone) [97]	No association [92]	No association [96]	No association [96]	Unclear [99, 100]	No association [96]	No association [96]
Mood stabilizers							
Lithium	Cardiac defects [104]	Unclear	Small increase [104]	Unclear [106]	Protective [106]	Unclear	Unclear
Antiepileptics	High increase [95]	Unclear	Increase [95]	Unclear	Increase [95]	Unclear	Unclear

References

1. O'Hara MW, Wisner KL. Perinatal mental illness: definition, description and aetiology. Best Pract Res Clin Obstet Gynaecol. 2014;28(1):3–12. https://doi.org/10.1016/j.bpobgyn.2013.09.002.
2. Creeley CE, Denton LK. Use of prescribed Psychotropics during pregnancy: a systematic review of pregnancy, neonatal, and childhood outcomes. Brain Sci. 2019;9(9):235. https://doi.org/10.3390/brainsci9090235.
3. Vesga-Lopez O, Blanco C, Keyes K, Olfson M, Grant BF, Hasin DS. Psychiatric disorders in pregnant and postpartum women in the United States. Arch Gen Psychiatry. 2008;65(7):805–15. https://doi.org/10.1001/archpsyc.65.7.805.
4. Hanley GE, Mintzes B. Patterns of psychotropic medicine use in pregnancy in the United States from 2006 to 2011 among women with private insurance. BMC Pregnancy Childbirth. 2014;14:242. https://doi.org/10.1186/1471-2393-14-242.
5. American Psychiatric Association. Diagnostic and statistical manual of mental disorders. Fifth ed. Washington, DC: American Psychiatric Association; 2013. https://doi.org/10.1176/appi.books.9780890425596.
6. Pearlstein T. Depression during pregnancy. Best Pract Res Clin Obstet Gynaecol. 2015;29(5):754–64. https://doi.org/10.1016/j.bpobgyn.2015.04.004.
7. Gavin N, Gaynes B, Lohr K, Meltzer-Brody S, Gartlehner G, Swinson T. Perinatal depression: a systematic review of prevalence and incidence. Obstet Gynecol. 2005;106:1071–83. https://doi.org/10.1097/01.AOG.0000183597.31630.db.
8. Patton GC, Romaniuk H, Spry E, et al. Prediction of perinatal depression from adolescence and before conception (VIHCS): 20-year prospective cohort study. Lancet. 2015;386(9996):875–83. https://doi.org/10.1016/S0140-6736(14)62248-0.
9. Ko JY, Farr SL, Dietz PM, Robbins CL, Depression and Treatment Among U.S. Pregnant and nonpregnant women of reproductive age, 2005–2009. J Women's Health. 2012;21(8):830–6. https://doi.org/10.1089/jwh.2011.3466.
10. Yonkers KA, Vigod S, Ross LE. Diagnosis, pathophysiology, and management of mood disorders in pregnant and postpartum women. Obstet Gynecol. 2011;117(4):961–77. https://doi.org/10.1097/AOG.0b013e31821187a7.
11. Viktorin A, Meltzer-Brody S, Kuja-Halkola R, et al. Heritability of perinatal depression and genetic overlap with nonperinatal depression. Am J Psychiatry. 2015;173(2):158–65. https://doi.org/10.1176/appi.ajp.2015.15010085.
12. Fuhr DC, Calvert C, Ronsmans C, et al. Contribution of suicide and injuries to pregnancy-related mortality in low-income and middle-income countries: a systematic review and meta-analysis. Lancet Psychiatry. 2014;1(3):213–25. https://doi.org/10.1016/S2215-0366(14)70282-2.
13. Samandari G, Martin SL, Kupper LL, Schiro S, Norwood T, Avery M. Are pregnant and postpartum women: at increased risk for violent death? Suicide and homicide findings from North Carolina. Matern Child Health J. 2011;15(5):660–9. https://doi.org/10.1007/s10995-010-0623-6.
14. Grigoriadis S, VonderPorten EH, Mamisashvili L, et al. The impact of maternal depression during pregnancy on perinatal outcomes: a systematic review and meta-analysis. J Clin Psychiatry. 2013;74(4):e321–41. https://doi.org/10.4088/JCP.12r07968.
15. Almeida ND, Basso O, Abrahamowicz M, Gagnon R, Tamblyn R. Risk of miscarriage in women receiving antidepressants in early pregnancy, correcting for induced abortions. Epidemiology. 2016;27(4):538–46. https://doi.org/10.1097/EDE.0000000000000484.
16. Johansen RLR, Mortensen LH, Andersen AMN, Hansen AV, Strandberg-Larsen K. Maternal use of selective serotonin reuptake inhibitors and risk of miscarriage—assessing potential biases. Paediatr Perinat Epidemiol. 2015;29(1):72–81. https://doi.org/10.1111/ppe.12160.
17. Lupattelli A, Spigset O, Koren G, Nordeng H. Risk of vaginal bleeding and postpartum hemorrhage after use of antidepressants in pregnancy: a study from the Norwegian mother and child cohort study. J Clin Psychopharmacol. 2014;34(1):143–8. https://doi.org/10.1097/JCP.0000000000000036.
18. Malm H, Sourander A, Gissler M, et al. Pregnancy complications following prenatal exposure to SSRIs or maternal psychiatric disorders: results from population-based National register data. Am J Psychiatry. 2015;172(12):1224–32. https://doi.org/10.1176/appi.ajp.2015.14121575.
19. Hu R, Li Y, Zhang Z, Yan W. Antenatal depressive symptoms and the risk of preeclampsia or operative deliveries: a meta-analysis. PLoS One. 2015;10(3):e0119018. https://doi.org/10.1371/journal.pone.0119018.
20. Oberlander TF, Warburton W, Misri S, Aghajanian J, Hertzman C. Neonatal outcomes after prenatal exposure to selective serotonin reuptake inhibitor antidepressants and maternal depression using population-based linked health data. Arch Gen Psychiatry. 2006;63(8):898–906. https://doi.org/10.1001/archpsyc.63.8.898.
21. Howard LM, Kirkwood G, Latinovic R. Sudden infant death syndrome and maternal depression. J Clin Psychiatry. 2007;68(8):1279–83. https://doi.org/10.4088/jcp.v68n0816.
22. Field T, Diego M, Hernandez-Reif M, Figueiredo B, Schanberg S, Kuhn C. Sleep disturbances in depressed pregnant women and their newborns. Infant Behav Dev. 2007;30(1):127–33. https://doi.org/10.1016/j.infbeh.2006.08.002.
23. Koutra K, Chatzi L, Bagkeris M, Vassilaki M, Bitsios P, Kogevinas M. Antenatal and postnatal maternal

mental health as determinants of infant neurodevelopment at 18 months of age in a mother-child cohort (Rhea study) in Crete, Greece. Soc Psychiatry Psychiatr Epidemiol. 2013;48(8):1335–45. https://doi.org/10.1007/s00127-012-0636-0.

24. Stein A, Pearson RM, Goodman SH, et al. Effects of perinatal mental disorders on the fetus and child. Lancet. 2014;384(9956):1800–19. https://doi.org/10.1016/S0140-6736(14)61277-0.

25. Räisänen S, Lehto SM, Nielsen HS, Gissler M, Kramer MR, Heinonen S. Risk factors for and perinatal outcomes of major depression during pregnancy: a population-based analysis during 2002-2010 in Finland. BMJ Open. 2014;4(11):e004883. https://doi.org/10.1136/bmjopen-2014-004883.

26. Mei-Dan E, Ray JG, Vigod SN. Perinatal outcomes among women with bipolar disorder: a population-based cohort study. Am J Obstet Gynecol. 2015;212(3):367.e1–8. https://doi.org/10.1016/j.ajog.2014.10.020.

27. Stuart S, Koleva H. Psychological treatments for perinatal depression. Best Pract Res Clin Obstet Gynaecol. 2014;28(1):61–70. https://doi.org/10.1016/j.bpobgyn.2013.09.004.

28. Meltzer-Brody S, Jones I. Optimizing the treatment of mood disorders in the perinatal period. Dialogues Clin Neurosci. 2015;17(2):207–18.

29. Yonkers KA, Wisner KL, Stewart DE, et al. The management of depression during pregnancy: a report from the American Psychiatric Association and the American College of Obstetricians and Gynecologists. Gen Hosp Psychiatry. 2009;31(5):403–13. https://doi.org/10.1016/j.genhosppsych.2009.04.003.

30. Cuijpers P, Berking M, Andersson G, Quigley L, Kleiboer A, Dobson KS. A meta-analysis of cognitive-behavioural therapy for adult depression, alone and in comparison with other treatments. Can J Psychiatry. 2013;58(7):376–85. https://doi.org/10.1177/070674371305800702.

31. Sockol LE. A systematic review of the efficacy of cognitive behavioral therapy for treating and preventing perinatal depression. J Affect Disord. 2015;177:7–21. https://doi.org/10.1016/j.jad.2015.01.052.

32. Claridge AM. Efficacy of systemically oriented psychotherapies in the treatment of perinatal depression: a meta-analysis. Arch Womens Ment Health. 2014;17(1):3–15. https://doi.org/10.1007/s00737-013-0391-6.

33. Chaudron LH. Complex challenges in treating depression during pregnancy. Am J Psychiatry. 2013;170(1):12–20. https://doi.org/10.1176/appi.ajp.2012.12040440.

34. Huybrechts KF, Palmsten K, Avorn J, et al. Antidepressant use in pregnancy and the risk of cardiac defects. N Engl J Med. 2014;370(25):2397–407. https://doi.org/10.1056/NEJMoa1312828.

35. Byatt N, Deligiannidis KM, Freeman MP. Antidepressant use in pregnancy: a critical review focused on risks and controversies. Acta Psychiatr Scand. 2013;127(2):94–114. https://doi.org/10.1111/acps.12042.

36. Kulin NA, Pastuszak A, Sage SR, et al. Pregnancy outcome following maternal use of the new selective serotonin reuptake inhibitors: a prospective controlled multicenter study. JAMA. 1998;279(8):609–10. https://doi.org/10.1001/jama.279.8.609.

37. Alwan S, Reefhuis J, Rasmussen SA, Olney RS, Friedman JM, National Birth Defects Prevention Study. Use of selective serotonin-reuptake inhibitors in pregnancy and the risk of birth defects. N Engl J Med. 2007;356(26):2684–92. https://doi.org/10.1056/NEJMoa066584.

38. Grigoriadis S, VonderPorten EH, Mamisashvili L, et al. Antidepressant exposure during pregnancy and congenital malformations: is there an association? A systematic review and meta-analysis of the best evidence. J Clin Psychiatry. 2013;74(4):e293–308. https://doi.org/10.4088/JCP.12r07966.

39. Jimenez-Solem E, Andersen JT, Petersen M, et al. SSRI use during pregnancy and risk of stillbirth and neonatal mortality. Am J Psychiatry. 2013;170(3):299–304. https://doi.org/10.1176/appi.ajp.2012.11081251.

40. Ross LE, Grigoriadis S, Mamisashvili L, et al. Selected pregnancy and delivery outcomes after exposure to antidepressant medication: a systematic review and meta-analysis. JAMA Psychiat. 2013;70(4):436–43. https://doi.org/10.1001/jamapsychiatry.2013.684.

41. Lindqvist PG, Nasiell J, Gustafsson LL, Nordstrom L. Selective serotonin reuptake inhibitor use during pregnancy increases the risk of postpartum hemorrhage and anemia: a hospital-based cohort study. J Thromb Haemost. 2014;12(12):1986–92. https://doi.org/10.1111/jth.12757.

42. Yang A, Ciolino JD, Pinheiro E, Rasmussen-Torvik LJ, Sit DKY, Wisner KL. Neonatal discontinuation syndrome in serotonergic antidepressant-exposed neonates. J Clin Psychiatry. 2017;78(5):605–11. https://doi.org/10.4088/JCP.16m11044.

43. Huang H, Coleman S, Bridge JA, Yonkers K, Katon W. A meta-analysis of the relationship between antidepressant use in pregnancy and the risk of preterm birth and low birth weight. Gen Hosp Psychiatry. 2014;36(1):13–8. https://doi.org/10.1016/j.genhosppsych.2013.08.002.

44. Palmsten K, Setoguchi S, Margulis AV, Patrick AR, Hernández-Díaz S. Elevated risk of preeclampsia in pregnant women with depression: depression or antidepressants? Am J Epidemiol. 2012;175(10):988–97. https://doi.org/10.1093/aje/kwr394.

45. Palmsten K, Huybrechts KF, Michels KB, et al. Antidepressant use and risk for preeclampsia. Epidemiology. 2013;24(5):682–91. https://doi.org/10.1097/EDE.0b013e31829e0aaa.

46. Bérard A, Zhao JP, Sheehy O. Antidepressant use during pregnancy and the risk of major congenital

malformations in a cohort of depressed pregnant women: an updated analysis of the Quebec pregnancy cohort. BMJ Open. 2017;7(1):e013372. https://doi.org/10.1136/bmjopen-2016-013372.

47. Jiang HY, Xu LL, Li YC, Deng M, Peng CT, Ruan B. Antidepressant use during pregnancy and risk of postpartum hemorrhage: a systematic review and meta-analysis. J Psychiatr Res. 2016;83:160–7. https://doi.org/10.1016/j.jpsychires.2016.09.001.

48. Hanley GE, Smolina K, Mintzes B, Oberlander TF, Morgan SG. Postpartum hemorrhage and use of serotonin reuptake inhibitor antidepressants in pregnancy. Obstet Gynecol. 2016;127(3):553–61. https://doi.org/10.1097/AOG.0000000000001200.

49. Kjaersgaard MIS, Parner ET, Vestergaard M, et al. Prenatal antidepressant exposure and risk of spontaneous abortion—a population-based study. PLoS One. 2013;8(8):e72095. https://doi.org/10.1371/journal.pone.0072095.

50. Hoog SL, Cheng Y, Elpers J, Dowsett SA. Duloxetine and pregnancy outcomes: safety surveillance findings. Int J Med Sci. 2013;10(4):413–9. https://doi.org/10.7150/ijms.5213.

51. Einarson A, Fatoye B, Sarkar M, et al. Pregnancy outcome following gestational exposure to venlafaxine: a multicenter prospective controlled study. Am J Psychiatry. 2001;158(10):1728–30. https://doi.org/10.1176/appi.ajp.158.10.1728.

52. Richardson JL, Martin F, Dunstan H, et al. Pregnancy outcomes following maternal venlafaxine use: a prospective observational comparative cohort study. Reprod Toxicol. 2019;84:108–13. https://doi.org/10.1016/j.reprotox.2019.01.003.

53. Newport DJ, Hostetter AL, Juul SH, Porterfield SM, Knight BT, Stowe ZN. Prenatal psychostimulant and antidepressant exposure and risk of hypertensive disorders of pregnancy. J Clin Psychiatry. 2016;77(11):1538–45. https://doi.org/10.4088/JCP.15m10506.

54. Huybrechts KF, Bateman BT, Pawar A, et al. Maternal and fetal outcomes following exposure to duloxetine in pregnancy: cohort study. BMJ. 2020;368:m237. https://doi.org/10.1136/bmj.m237.

55. GlaxoSmithKline Pregnancy Registries » Bupropion. https://pregnancyregistry.gsk.com/bupropion.html. Accessed 29 May 2020.

56. Hendrick V, Suri R, Gitlin MJ, Ortiz-Portillo E. Bupropion use during pregnancy: a systematic review. Prim Care Companion CNS Disord. 2017;19(5):17r02160. https://doi.org/10.4088/PCC.17r02160.

57. Chun-Fai-Chan B, Koren G, Fayez I, et al. Pregnancy outcome of women exposed to bupropion during pregnancy: a prospective comparative study. Am J Obstet Gynecol. 2005;192(3):932–6. https://doi.org/10.1016/j.ajog.2004.09.027.

58. Palmsten K, Hernández-Díaz S, Huybrechts KF, et al. Use of antidepressants near delivery and risk of postpartum hemorrhage: cohort study of low income women in the United States. BMJ. 2013;347:f4877. https://doi.org/10.1136/bmj.f4877.

59. Nanovskaya TN, Oncken C, Fokina VM, et al. Bupropion sustained release for pregnant smokers: a randomized, placebo-controlled trial. Am J Obstet Gynecol. 2017;216(4):420.e1–9. https://doi.org/10.1016/j.ajog.2016.11.1036.

60. Bérard A, Zhao JP, Sheehy O. Success of smoking cessation interventions during pregnancy. Am J Obstet Gynecol. 2016;215(5):611.e1–8. https://doi.org/10.1016/j.ajog.2016.06.059.

61. Howard LM, Molyneaux E, Dennis CL, Rochat T, Stein A, Milgrom J. Non-psychotic mental disorders in the perinatal period. Lancet. 2014;384(9956):1775–88. https://doi.org/10.1016/S0140-6736(14)61276-9.

62. Reck C, Stehle E, Reinig K, Mundt C. Maternity blues as a predictor of DSM-IV depression and anxiety disorders in the first three months postpartum. J Affect Disord. 2009;113(1–2):77–87. https://doi.org/10.1016/j.jad.2008.05.003.

63. Sacher J, Wilson AA, Houle S, et al. Elevated brain monoamine oxidase a binding in the early postpartum period. Arch Gen Psychiatry. 2010;67(5):468–74. https://doi.org/10.1001/archgenpsychiatry.2010.32.

64. Doornbos B, Fekkes D, Tanke MAC, de Jonge P, Korf J. Sequential serotonin and noradrenalin associated processes involved in postpartum blues. Prog Neuro-Psychopharmacol Biol Psychiatry. 2008;32(5):1320–5. https://doi.org/10.1016/j.pnpbp.2008.04.010.

65. Alipour Z, Lamyian M, Hajizadeh E. Anxiety and fear of childbirth as predictors of postnatal depression in nulliparous women. Women Birth. 2012;25(3):e37–43. https://doi.org/10.1016/j.wombi.2011.09.002.

66. Dennis CL, Falah-Hassani K, Shiri R. Prevalence of antenatal and postnatal anxiety: systematic review and meta-analysis. Br J Psychiatry. 2017;210(5):315–23. https://doi.org/10.1192/bjp.bp.116.187179.

67. Posternak MA, Zimmerman M. Symptoms of atypical depression. Psychiatry Res. 2001;104(2):175–81. https://doi.org/10.1016/s0165-1781(01)00301-8.

68. Marchesi C, Bertoni S, Maggini C. Major and minor depression in pregnancy. Obstet Gynecol. 2009;113(6):1292–8. https://doi.org/10.1097/AOG.0b013e3181a45e90.

69. Grigoriadis S, Graves L, Peer M, et al. Maternal anxiety during pregnancy and the association with adverse perinatal outcomes: systematic review and meta-analysis. J Clin Psychiatry. 2018;79(5):17r12011. https://doi.org/10.4088/JCP.17r12011.

70. Shahhosseini Z, Pourasghar M, Khalilian A, Salehi F. A review of the effects of anxiety during pregnancy on children's health. Mater Sociomed. 2015;27(3):200–2. https://doi.org/10.5455/msm.2015.27.200-202.

71. Glazier RH, Elgar FJ, Goel V, Holzapfel S. Stress, social support, and emotional distress in a com-

munity sample of pregnant women. J Psychosom Obstet Gynaecol. 2004;25(3–4):247–55. https://doi.org/10.1080/01674820400024406.

72. van Ravesteyn LM, Lambregtse-van den Berg MP, Hoogendijk WJG, Kamperman AM. Interventions to treat mental disorders during pregnancy: a systematic review and multiple treatment meta-analysis. PLoS One. 2017;12(3):e0173397. https://doi.org/10.1371/journal.pone.0173397.

73. Overview | Antenatal and postnatal mental health: clinical management and service guidance | Guidance | NICE. https://www.nice.org.uk/guidance/cg192. Accessed 31 May 2020.

74. Dolovich LR, Addis A, Vaillancourt JM, Power JD, Koren G, Einarson TR. Benzodiazepine use in pregnancy and major malformations or oral cleft: meta-analysis of cohort and case-control studies. BMJ. 1998;317(7162):839–43. https://doi.org/10.1136/bmj.317.7162.839.

75. Yonkers KA, Wisner KL, Stowe Z, et al. Management of bipolar disorder during pregnancy and the postpartum period. Am J Psychiatry. 2004;161(4):608–20. https://doi.org/10.1176/appi.ajp.161.4.608.

76. Wikner BN, Stiller CO, Bergman U, Asker C, Källén B. Use of benzodiazepines and benzodiazepine receptor agonists during pregnancy: neonatal outcome and congenital malformations. Pharmacoepidemiol Drug Saf. 2007;16(11):1203–10. https://doi.org/10.1002/pds.1457.

77. Hartz SC, Heinonen OP, Shapiro S, Siskind V, Slone D. Antenatal exposure to meprobamate and chlordiazepoxide in relation to malformations, mental development, and childhood mortality. N Engl J Med. 1975;292(14):726–8. https://doi.org/10.1056/NEJM197504032921405.

78. Fujii H, Goel A, Bernard N, et al. Pregnancy outcomes following gabapentin use: results of a prospective comparative cohort study. Neurology. 2013;80(17):1565–70. https://doi.org/10.1212/WNL.0b013e31828f18c1.

79. Chessick CA, Allen MH, Thase M, et al. Azapirones for generalized anxiety disorder. Cochrane Database Syst Rev. 2006;(3):CD006115. https://doi.org/10.1002/14651858.CD006115.

80. Butkevich IP, Mikhailenko VA, Vershinina EA, Otellin VA, Aloisi AM. Buspirone before prenatal stress protects against adverse effects of stress on emotional and inflammatory pain-related behaviors in infant rats: age and sex differences. Brain Res. 2011;1419:76–84. https://doi.org/10.1016/j.brainres.2011.08.068.

81. Butkevich I, Mikhailenko V, Vershinina E, Semionov P, Makukhina G, Otellin V. Maternal buspirone protects against the adverse effects of in utero stress on emotional and pain-related behaviors in offspring. Physiol Behav. 2011;102(2):137–42. https://doi.org/10.1016/j.physbeh.2010.10.023.

82. Guaiana G, Barbui C, Cipriani A. Hydroxyzine for generalised anxiety disorder. Cochrane Database Syst Rev. 2010;(12):CD006815. https://doi.org/10.1002/14651858.CD006815.pub2.

83. Meadows M. Pregnancy and the drug dilemma. FDA Consumer Magazine. Published online. 2001.

84. Lis-Swiety AD, Brzezińska-Wcisło LA. The safety of the antihistamines in dermatoses of pregnancy. Wiad Lek. 2006;59(1–2):89–91.

85. Aselton P, Jick H, Milunsky A, Hunter JR, Stergachis A. First-trimester drug use and congenital disorders. Obstet Gynecol. 1985;65(4):451–5.

86. Aldridge TD, Hartmann KE, Michels KA, Velez Edwards DR. First-trimester antihistamine exposure and risk of spontaneous abortion or preterm birth. Pharmacoepidemiol Drug Saf. 2014;23(10):1043–50. https://doi.org/10.1002/pds.3637.

87. Serreau R, Komiha M, Blanc F, Guillot F, Jacqz-Aigrain E. Neonatal seizures associated with maternal hydroxyzine hydrochloride in late pregnancy. Reprod Toxicol. 2005;20(4):573–4. https://doi.org/10.1016/j.reprotox.2005.03.005.

88. Altshuler LL, Cohen L, Szuba MP, Burt VK, Gitlin M, Mintz J. Pharmacologic management of psychiatric illness during pregnancy: dilemmas and guidelines. Am J Psychiatry. 1996;153(5):592–606. https://doi.org/10.1176/ajp.153.5.592.

89. Viguera AC, Whitfield T, Baldessarini RJ, et al. Risk of recurrence in women with bipolar disorder during pregnancy: prospective study of mood stabilizer discontinuation. Am J Psychiatry. 2007;164(12):1817–24; quiz 1923. https://doi.org/10.1176/appi.ajp.2007.06101639.

90. Wesseloo R, Kamperman AM, Munk-Olsen T, Pop VJM, Kushner SA, Bergink V. Risk of postpartum relapse in bipolar disorder and postpartum psychosis: a systematic review and meta-analysis. Am J Psychiatry. 2015;173(2):117–27. https://doi.org/10.1176/appi.ajp.2015.15010124.

91. Burt VK, Bernstein C, Rosenstein WS, Altshuler LL. Bipolar disorder and pregnancy: maintaining psychiatric stability in the real world of obstetric and psychiatric complications. Am J Psychiatry. 2010;167(8):892–7. https://doi.org/10.1176/appi.ajp.2009.09081248.

92. Cipriani A, Barbui C, Salanti G, et al. Comparative efficacy and acceptability of antimanic drugs in acute mania: a multiple-treatments meta-analysis. Lancet. 2011;378(9799):1306–15. https://doi.org/10.1016/S0140-6736(11)60873-8.

93. Toh S, Li Q, Cheetham TC, et al. Prevalence and trends in the use of antipsychotic medications during pregnancy in the U.S., 2001-2007: a population-based study of 585,615 deliveries. Arch Women's Ment Health. 2013;16(2):149–57. https://doi.org/10.1007/s00737-013-0330-6.

94. Young AH, McElroy SL, Bauer M, et al. A double-blind, placebo-controlled study of quetiapine and lithium monotherapy in adults in the acute phase of bipolar depression (EMBOLDEN I). J Clin Psychiatry. 2010;71(2):150–62. https://doi.org/10.4088/JCP.08m04995gre.

95. Jones I, Chandra PS, Dazzan P, Howard LM. Bipolar disorder, affective psychosis, and schizophrenia in pregnancy and the post-partum period. Lancet. 2014;384(9956):1789–99. https://doi.org/10.1016/S0140-6736(14)61278-2.

96. Einarson A, Boskovic R. Use and safety of antipsychotic drugs during pregnancy. J Psychiatr Pract. 2009;15(3):183–92. https://doi.org/10.1097/01.pra.0000351878.45260.94.

97. Huybrechts KF, Hernández-Díaz S, Patorno E, et al. Antipsychotic use in pregnancy and the risk for congenital malformations. JAMA Psychiat. 2016;73(9):938–46. https://doi.org/10.1001/jamapsychiatry.2016.1520.

98. Habermann F, Fritzsche J, Fuhlbrück F, et al. Atypical antipsychotic drugs and pregnancy outcome: a prospective, cohort study. J Clin Psychopharmacol. 2013;33(4):453–62. https://doi.org/10.1097/JCP.0b013e318295fe12.

99. Newham JJ, Thomas SH, MacRitchie K, McElhatton PR, McAllister-Williams RH. Birth weight of infants after maternal exposure to typical and atypical antipsychotics: prospective comparison study. Br J Psychiatry J Ment Sci. 2008;192(5):333–7. https://doi.org/10.1192/bjp.bp.107.041541.

100. Newport DJ, Calamaras MR, DeVane CL, et al. Atypical antipsychotic administration during late pregnancy: placental passage and obstetrical outcomes. Am J Psychiatry. 2007;164(8):1214–20. https://doi.org/10.1176/appi.ajp.2007.06111886.

101. Cade JFJ. Lithium salts in the treatment of psychotic excitement. Med J Aust. 1949;2(10):349–52. https://doi.org/10.1080/j.1440-1614.1999.06241.x.

102. Malhi GS, Gessler D, Outhred T. The use of lithium for the treatment of bipolar disorder: recommendations from clinical practice guidelines. J Affect Disord. 2017;217:266–80. https://doi.org/10.1016/j.jad.2017.03.052.

103. Malhi GS, Outhred T. Therapeutic mechanisms of lithium in bipolar disorder: recent advances and current understanding. CNS Drugs. 2016;30(10):931–49. https://doi.org/10.1007/s40263-016-0380-1.

104. Diav-Citrin O, Shechtman S, Tahover E, et al. Pregnancy outcome following in utero exposure to lithium: a prospective, comparative, observational study. Am J Psychiatry. 2014;171(7):785–94. https://doi.org/10.1176/appi.ajp.2014.12111402.

105. Weinstein MR, Goldfield M. Cardiovascular malformations with lithium use during pregnancy. Am J Psychiatry. 1975;132(5):529–31. https://doi.org/10.1176/ajp.132.5.529.

106. Jacobson SJ, Jones K, Johnson K, et al. Prospective multicentre study of pregnancy outcome after lithium exposure during first trimester. Lancet. 1992;339(8792):530–3. https://doi.org/10.1016/0140-6736(92)90346-5.

107. Menon SJ. Psychotropic medication during pregnancy and lactation. Arch Gynecol Obstet. 2008;277(1):1–13. https://doi.org/10.1007/s00404-007-0433-2.

108. Iqbal MM, Gundlapalli SP, Ryan WG, Ryals T, Passman TE. Effects of antimanic mood-stabilizing drugs on fetuses, neonates, and nursing infants. South Med J. 2001;94(3):304–22.

109. Ostacher MJ, Tandon R, Suppes T. Florida best practice psychotherapeutic medication guidelines for adults with bipolar disorder: a novel, practical, patient-centered guide for clinicians. J Clin Psychiatry. 2016;77(7):920–6. https://doi.org/10.4088/JCP.15cs09841.

110. Tomson T, Battino D, Bonizzoni E, et al. Dose-dependent risk of malformations with antiepileptic drugs: an analysis of data from the EURAP epilepsy and pregnancy registry. Lancet Neurol. 2011;10(7):609–17. https://doi.org/10.1016/S1474-4422(11)70107-7.

111. Smith LA, Cornelius V, Warnock A, Tacchi MJ, Taylor D. Pharmacological interventions for acute bipolar mania: a systematic review of randomized placebo-controlled trials. Bipolar Disord. 2007;9(6):551–60. https://doi.org/10.1111/j.1399-5618.2007.00468.x.

112. Sharma V. Management of bipolar II disorder during pregnancy and the postpartum period—Motherisk update 2008. Can J Clin Pharmacol. 2009;16(1):e33–41.

113. Brown EB, McElroy SL, Keck PE, et al. A 7-week, randomized, double-blind trial of olanzapine/fluoxetine combination versus lamotrigine in the treatment of bipolar I depression. J Clin Psychiatry. 2006;67(7):1025–33. https://doi.org/10.4088/jcp.v67n0703.

Part VI

Neoplastic, Congenital, and Other Neurosurgical Disorders in Pregnancy

Management of Brain Tumors in Pregnancy

Oliver Y. Tang and James K. Liu

Brain Tumors in the Pregnant Patient

Overview and Incidence

The management of brain tumors is a multidisciplinary process that requires the concerted efforts of multiple specialties including neurology, neurosurgery, oncology, radiation oncology, and palliative care. However, the treatment of brain tumors during pregnancy is an even greater interdisciplinary challenge that necessitates the insights of additional specialties such as high-risk obstetrics and neonatal medicine. There are no recommendations or consensus guidelines surrounding the care of brain tumors during pregnancy, due to the rarity of this clinical entity. The purpose of this chapter is to summarize the incidence, pathophysiology, diagnostic process, natural history, and treatment of brain tumors in the pregnant patient.

The incidence of central nervous system (CNS) tumors has a slight female predominance (57.9%) [1]. Among female patients, brain tumors have an incidence of approximately 5.2 new cases per 100,000, falling outside of top 10, but are responsible for 3.5 deaths per 100,000, serving as the fifth leading cause of cancer death in women 20–39 years of age [2, 3]. CNS neoplasms in pregnancy are a rare clinical phenomenon. In one consecutive series of 126,413 pregnant patients from 1983 to 1995 in Spain, only 7 patients were found to have brain tumors [4]. Among 5 hospitals in Southern California from 1978 to 1998, brain tumors were diagnosed in 32 out of every 100,000 pregnancies [5]. Another nationwide study from former East Germany from 1961 to 1979 observed a rate of 3.6 brain tumors per million pregnancies [6]. Finally, analysis of nationwide United States (US) administrative data from 1988 to 2009 quantified a rate of 816 pregnant patients with brain tumors out of 19,750,702, or a rate of 4 per 100,000 [7]. In the same study, pregnant patients with brain tumors were 143 times more likely to die during hospitalization compared to counterparts without a brain tumor. Moreover, with improvements in brain tumor treatment, there has been an increase in patients with brain tumors,

O. Y. Tang
Department of Neurosurgery, University of Pittsburgh Medical Center, Pittsburgh, PA, USA

Department of Neurosurgery, Rhode Island Hospital, Providence, RI, USA
e-mail: tango@upmc.edu

J. K. Liu (✉)
Department of Neurological Surgery, New Jersey Medical School, Newark, NJ, USA

Department of Otolaryngology-Head and Neck Surgery, New Jersey Medical School, Newark, NJ, USA

Saint Barnabas Medical Center, RWJ Barnabas Health, Livingston, NJ, USA
e-mail: james.liu.md@rutgers.edu

especially in sustained periods of disease control, considering pregnancy [8]. For example, in one review of 27 studies, one-third of pregnant patients with a brain tumor had a known diagnosis before pregnancy [9].

Some studies have posited that the rate of brain tumors during pregnancy is lower than would be expected based on incidence rates in women of reproductive age in general [6]. There are several hypotheses that have been advanced to explained this. First, certain brain tumors like pituitary adenomas may cause CNS dysfunction with downstream effects on fertility, such as decreased libido or ovulatory dysfunction [6]. Second, some studies have hypothesized that pregnant patients with subclinical and yet undiagnosed tumors may have higher rates of early pregnancy loss [10]. Third, older case series may have likely underestimated brain tumor prevalence as they preceded recent advances in imaging and the modern magnetic resonance imaging (MRI) era.

Several studies have corroborated that there does not seem to be a significant change in the distribution of brain tumor subtypes in pregnant patients compared to nonpregnant patients [3, 10, 11]. Across several case series, the four most common pathologies are glioma, meningioma, vestibular schwannoma, and pituitary tumors. Several studies have also suggested that different brain tumor subtypes may have distinct patterns in which they most commonly present during pregnancy, such as gliomas in the first trimester, compared to meningioma and vascular tumors in the third trimester [10–12].

Presenting Symptoms

Like in nonpregnant patients, brain tumors in pregnant patients may often present with nonspecific symptoms like headache, altered mental status, and vomiting. In an estimated 36–90% of all brain tumors, headache is the initial presenting concern [13]. While new-onset headaches in pregnancy may be due to more benign etiologies like the intravascular volume expansion or the exacerbation of an existing primary headache,

warning signs that clinicians should be mindful of in pregnancy include signs of elevated intracranial pressure (ICP), such as headaches with a positional nature, that are worse in the morning, gradual in onset, or unremitting or increasing in frequency [11]. While vomiting due to a brain tumor may be attributed to hyperemesis gravidarum, the latter commonly remits by the end of the first trimester, and patient vomiting continued into the second and third trimester may warrant suspicion of an intracranial neoplasm.

Other possible presenting symptoms include focal neurologic deficits, cranial nerve palsies, visual changes, and seizures [4]. An estimated 30–50% of brain tumors during pregnancy initially present with seizures, with another 10–30% developing seizures later in disease progression [14]. For new-onset seizures in pregnancy, a differential diagnosis to consider is eclampsia. Focal seizures suggestive of an intracranial mass and onset of seizures before 20 weeks can help differentiate seizures induced by a neoplasm from eclamptic seizures, which are more likely to be generalized. In addition, non-eclamptic patients would lack characteristic disease features like hypertension and proteinuria. Another possible acute presentation for brain tumors during pregnancy is intracranial hemorrhage [4, 15]. In summation, due to other notable pregnancy-related differential diagnoses including hyperemesis gravidarum or eclampsia, a useful rule of thumb is that pregnant patients with focal, prolonged, worsening, or unremitting neurologic sequelae should receive a neurology evaluation and imaging for potential intracranial pathology.

Diagnostic Workup

In the setting of pregnancy, the MRI is advantageous to computed tomography (CT) due to having higher sensitivity and soft tissue resolution as well as not requiring ionizing radiation [16]. Nevertheless, because earlier studies have established that CT radiation is safe in pregnancy with abdominal lead shielding, especially after the first trimester, the lack of an MRI at an institution should not serve as an absolute contraindication for a pregnant patient to receive intracranial imaging and CT imaging may be a viable option for centers that lack MRI capabilities [11, 17].

The use of contrast for the imaging evaluation of a brain tumor in pregnant patients is an area of controversy. While iodinated CT contrast is a physiologically inert substance that poses minimal risk to the developing fetus [4], there is evidence that this increases the risk of congenital hypothyroidism, which necessitates postpartum monitoring accordingly [18]. Additionally, although gadolinium-based contrast used for MRI has been shown to cross the placenta, no study has established link between this contrast and birth defects [19–21]. Nevertheless, due to remaining uncertainty regarding the fetal impact of imaging contrast, the American College of Obstetricians and Gynecologists (ACOG) and other studies have recommended withholding imaging contrast unless there is an absolute clinical indication [8, 16].

Beyond imaging, other noninvasive tests for evaluating the presence of an intracranial mass include a comprehensive neurologic exam, visual field testing, a fundoscopic exam to assess for papilledema, and in the case of functional pituitary tumors, serum screening for elevated hormones.

Natural History of Brain Tumors During Pregnancy

Physiologic Changes in Pregnancy Promoting Tumor Progression

There are several physiologic changes in the pregnant patient that may contribute to the potential progression of intracranial tumors during pregnancy (Fig. 32.1). First, during pregnancy, there is an increase in estrogen and progesterone concentrations by approximately eightfold and fourfold, respectively [22]. These changes in hormonal concentrations may interact with receptors on tumor cells that may promote neoplastic proliferation and growth. Moreover, estrogen induces hypertrophy of the pituitary gland, particularly lactotrophs. Second, there is a 50%

increase in intravascular fluid volume during pregnancy, secondary to increased fluid retention and cardiac output as well as decreased systemic vascular resistance [23]. Third, processes like placental implantation also increase systemic concentrations of angiogenic factors, such as placental growth factor (PGF) and vascular endothelial growth factor (VEGF) [24]. Fourth, the mass effect of the gravid uterus, especially in the third trimester, decreases ventricular compliance due to increasing intraabdominal pressure, which increases the severity of symptoms caused by elevated ICP [12]. Intraoperatively, the gravid uterus may also affect factors like patient respiration and positioning during procedures. Fifth, pregnancy promotes a state of immune tolerance, which may impact immune surveillance of maternal neoplasms [25, 26]. While these mechanisms have been hypothesized to promote the progression and symptomatology of brain tumors across all subtypes, the relative level of evidence and contributing impact for each mechanism may vary between different subtypes, as elaborated in the subsequent sections.

Glioma

Gliomas are the most common primary intra-axial brain tumor in adults and make up 28.8% of all primary CNS tumors [1]. The most aggressive form, glioblastoma multiforme (GBM), accounts for 47.1% of malignant CNS tumors alone [1]. While the 5-year survival rate for low-grade gliomas (LGGs) ranges from 50.1 to 81.3%, GBM has a 5-year survival rate of just 5.5% [1]. Several studies have posited that pregnancy is not a risk factor for the initial pathogenesis of gliomas but does worsen existing and previously undetected neoplasms. Glial cells are known to express hormonal receptors and progesterone has been demonstrated to enhance astrocytic cell growth in vitro [27–29]. Higher expression of progesterone receptors has also been observed in GBM, in comparison to LGGs [30]. Moreover, increased systemic concentration of angiogenic factors like PGF and VEGF may also potentiate tumor growth. Finally, increased intravascular volume

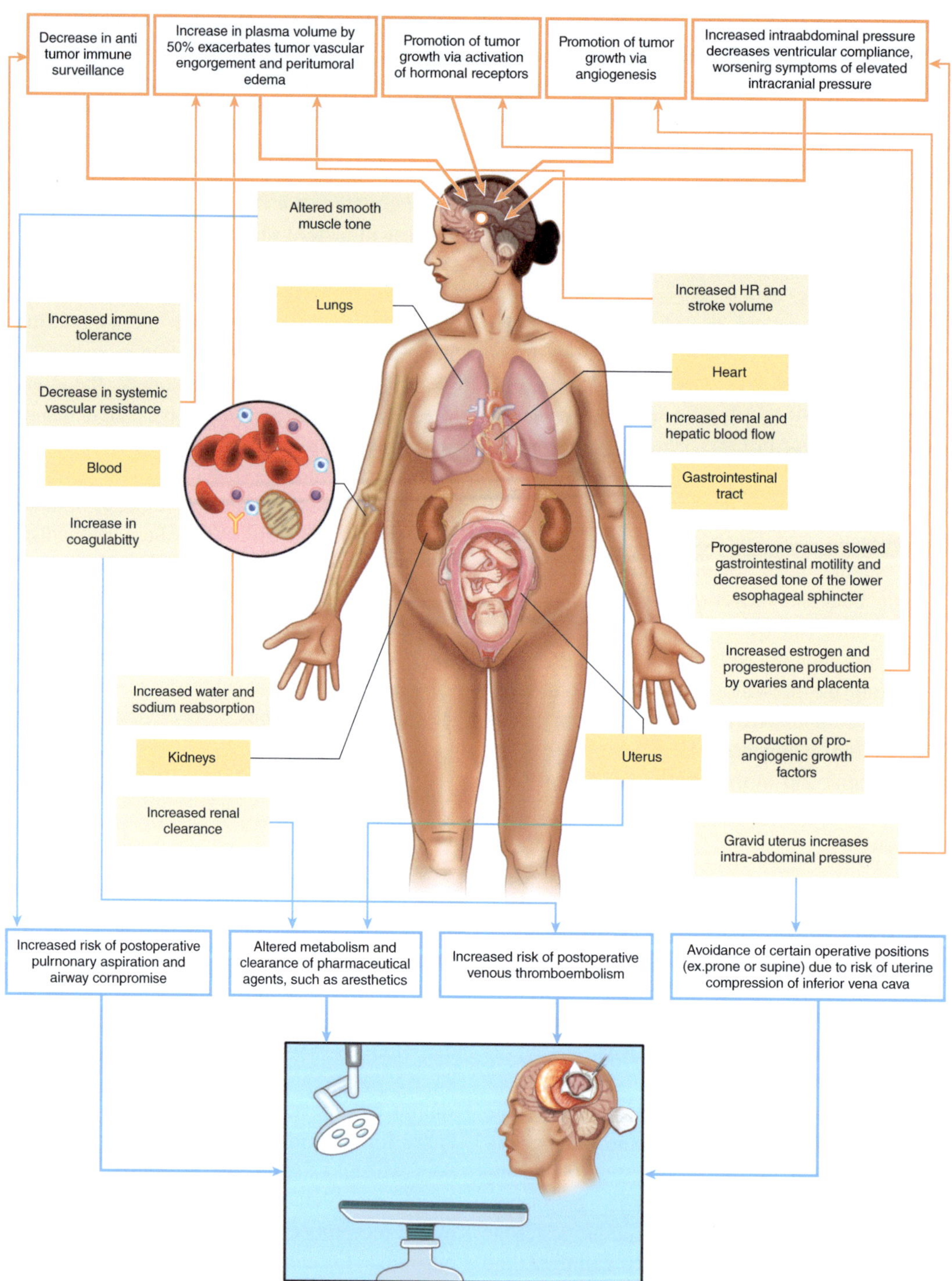

Fig. 32.1 Summary of physiologic changes during pregnancy impacting brain tumor progression and operative management. Summary of pertinent physiologic changes during pregnancy across 6 organ systems (heart, lungs, gastrointestinal tract, kidneys, peripheral circulation, and uterus). Changes impacting tumor progression and operative management are denoted by red and blue boxes and arrows, respectively

may exacerbate peritumoral and vasogenic edema associated with glioma. As a result of these physiologic changes resolving with delivery, the symptomatic burden of gliomas may decrease in the postpartum period. For example, in one case series, 57.2% of pregnant women with seizures due to glioma experienced symptomatic resolution following delivery [31]. Accordingly, patients with gliomas may exhibit a pattern of symptom onset during pregnancy, postpartum remission, and relapse with subsequent pregnancies.

However, these changes likely do not apply uniformly across tumor subtypes. Low-grade tumors, such as oligodendroglioma and astrocytoma, are slow-growing and may often be observed in the absence of progression during pregnancy [32]. For example, in one single-institution case series, there was a 0% progression rate observed among grade I gliomas but a 44% progression rate observed among grade II–III gliomas [8]. High-grade gliomas, such as GBM and anaplastic astrocytoma, may exhibit high growth velocities that may necessitate a planned C-section for early delivery or neurosurgical intervention. Nevertheless, even among LGGs, higher radiological growth rates have been observed during pregnancy, compared to the prepartum and postpartum periods [28]. In another multi-institutional case series of 50 pregnant patients with glioma, 87% of tumors exhibited increased growth rates during pregnancy and 38% experienced clinical deterioration [31]. Accordingly, even if a LGG is indolent throughout the course of a patient's pregnancy, resection of the tumor should be considered if the patient desires subsequent pregnancy, due to the risk of tumor exacerbation.

Meningioma

Meningiomas represent 36.8% of all primary CNS tumors as well as 53% of all benign CNS tumors, with a 5-year survival rate of 86.7% [1]. A 1929 report by Cushing and Eisenhardt of an expanding parasellar meningioma that caused rapid progression of visual impairment during pregnancy, which resolved postpartum and recurred in a subsequent pregnancy, represents the earliest known clinical observation of brain tumors worsening symptomatically during pregnancy [33]. Earlier research into hormonal influences on intracranial tumor growth have most commonly focused on meningioma. 70–90% of meningiomas have been found to have progesterone receptors and 33–38% have been found to have estrogen receptors [32, 34, 35]. Moreover, meningiomas are twice as common in women, with the greatest disparity found during reproductive years, and have been associated with higher rates of other hormone-dependent tumors, including breast cancer [14, 36]. Nevertheless, earlier research into hormone modulation, such as progesterone blockade, has failed to control tumor growth, suggesting a multifactorial cause of tumor progression during progression [37].

Several studies have demonstrated that meningiomas exhibit a similar pattern of growth as gliomas, with an increase in tumor progression during pregnancy that peaks during the third trimester as well as symptoms that often resolve with the end of pregnancy but may recur during a subsequent one [10–12]. Nevertheless, other studies have suggested that even in the immediate postpartum period, highly vascular neoplasms like meningiomas may experience a rapid exacerbation, due to a postpartum fluid shift from extravascular to intravascular, which may rapidly increase mass effect shortly after delivery [3]. As a result, pregnant patients with meningiomas warrant close postpartum monitoring.

Vestibular Schwannoma

8.4% of primary CNS tumors are classified as cranial or spine nerve tumors, of which over 95% are vestibular schwannoma [1]. These benign neoplasms of the myelin sheath have a 93.1% 5-year survival rate [1]. Due to most commonly affecting the vestibulocochlear nerve (CN VIII), the mass effect of vestibular schwannomas most often presents as hearing impairment, tinnitus, vertigo, or facial nerve palsy due to compression in the cerebellopontine angle. Because 50–100%

of vestibular schwannomas have been found to express the estrogen receptor, these tumors have also been documented to grow during pregnancy, with the highest rate in the last months of pregnancy [3, 38]. Nevertheless, an increase in estrogen alone has not been found to promote vestibular schwannoma growth, suggesting that other factors beyond the hormonal milieu of pregnancy drive this change. An increase in engorgement of the tumor's vascular bed has been posited as another cause [3]. In one case series of 36 vestibular schwannomas in pregnant patients, 6 exhibited growth over the course of pregnancy [38].

Pituitary Adenoma

Pituitary adenomas make up 16.2% of primary CNS tumors and are benign neoplasms with a 96.6% 5-year survival rate. Pituitary adenomas may either be nonfunctional (nonsecreting) or functional, with further classification based on the predominant hormone secreted by the neoplasm. While prolactinomas are the most common subtype of pituitary adenomas overall, diagnoses based on serum measurements are confounded by prolactin levels increasing up to tenfold during pregnancy. Pituitary adenomas may also be classified by size as microadenomas (diameter < 1 cm) or macroadenomas (diameter > 1 cm). 5–25% of pituitary adenomas have been documented to enlarge during pregnancy [39]. A significant driver for this growth is physiologic growth of the pituitary gland, due to higher estrogen stimulating lactotroph hyperplasia and hypertrophy [39–41]. The growth of pituitary adenomas may be influenced by the prepartum size of the neoplasm. While under 5% of microadenomas have been observed to grow [41–43], one case series of macroadenomas demonstrated that 35% grew during pregnancy [40]. Due to the proximity of the optic chiasm to the sellar region, sudden pituitary adenoma growth may present as new-onset visual symptoms, such as bitemporal hemianopsia [39–41]. A tumor that suddenly outgrows its blood supply may also result in pituitary apoplexy, which may present as a sudden onset of headache, altered consciousness, nausea and vomiting, and meningeal irritation [44]. Hormonal secretion by other forms of functional pituitary adenomas may also increase the risk of gestational conditions in the mother, such as gestational diabetes (growth hormone) or gestational hypertension (adrenocorticotropic hormone [ACTH]) [41]. Prolactinomas are not a contraindication to breastfeeding, as this has not been shown to increase postpartum growth [42]. Accordingly, in one case series of prolactinomas in the postpartum period, over 60% of tumors were found to recede in size [45].

Given the increased propensity of macroadenomas to grow and become symptomatic during pregnancy, studies have advocated observation as the first-line approach for microadenomas or asymptomatic macroadenomas, whereas symptomatic macroadenomas should be treated by medical management if available, such as a dopamine agonist for prolactinoma, followed by surgery if treatment is refractory [11]. Due to the predilection of macroadenomas in general to grow during pregnancy, a clinical evaluation including visual field assessment should be performed at least every 1–2 months.

Vascular Tumors

Vascular tumors, such as hemangioblastomas, make up approximately 1.6% of all primary CNS tumors and have a 93.6% 5-year survival rate [1]. Like gliomas, vascular tumors may experience growth during pregnancy due to a systemic increase in pro-angiogenic factors, such as PGF and VEGF, and engorgement of the tumor's vascular bed [46]. However, different case series have varied on whether hemangioblastomas exhibit a significantly increased growth velocity during pregnancy [47, 48]. In a patient with several hemangioblastomas, an important diagnosis to consider is Von Hippel-Landau syndrome due to the possibility of a concurrent pheochromocytoma, which carries the risk of hemodynamic lability, especially during potential medical or surgical interventions [49].

Other Primary Brain Tumors

Beyond what has been discussed above, a wide range of intracranial neoplasms have been documented among pregnant patients, including, but not limited to, colloid cysts [11], craniopharyngioma [50], pineal tumors [51], medulloblastoma [52], CNS lymphoma [25], paraganglioma [53], and chordoma [54].

Brain Metastasis

The incidence of overall cancer in pregnant patients has been rising, with one nationwide Dutch registry documenting a rise from 5.4% to 8.3% from 1977 to 2006 [55]. A malignancy of any other organ in the body may serve as a source of metastasis to the brain, and intracranial metastases are estimated to comprise over half of all intracranial tumors [56]. While no study has demonstrated an increased susceptibility for metastasis to the brain during pregnancy, earlier case reports have documented pregnant patients found to have brain metastases from sources including lung cancer [57], breast cancer [58], and melanoma [59]. Brain metastases may progress rapidly and require treatment during pregnancy, as the median survival of untreated metastases has been estimated to be 1–3 months [14, 60, 61].

Another notable source of brain metastasis in the setting of pregnancy is choriocarcinoma, a malignancy of trophoblasts, most commonly from the placenta. While choriocarcinomas are rarely associated with the index pregnancy and are most commonly found after hydatidiform moles or spontaneous abortion [17], there have been reported cases of choriocarcinomas arising during normal gestation and metastasizing to the brain [62]. Following a normal term pregnancy, hydatidiform mole, or spontaneous abortion, choriocarcinomas should be suspected in patients with continued vaginal bleeding, persistently high human chorionic gonadotropin (hCG) levels, and signs of lung or brain metastasis. Due to 20% of choriocarcinomas having metastasized to the brain by time of diagnosis, the diagnosis of choriocarcinoma necessitates an intracranial MRI to evaluate for metastasis [11]. Despite the predilection of these malignancies to metastasize to the brain, neurosurgical intervention is often not needed, as an 83% 5-year survival rate has been documented with chemoradiation alone [63].

Treatment of Brain Tumors During Pregnancy

General Principles

There are two overarching principles that are helpful in guiding the management of brain tumors—as well as any other life-threatening condition—during pregnancy. First, treatment planning should be tailored toward the best possible treatment option for the patient if they were nonpregnant, then subsequently modified based on fetal risks [11]. For example, pregnancy should not be viewed as an absolute contraindication to nonobstetric surgery, but rather a physiologic state with additional considerations that need to be planned around. Second, as expounded by the ACOGs guidelines on "Ethical decision making in obstetrics and gynecology," while the interests of the fetus are generally aligned with those of the pregnant patient, in the event that these interests are in conflict, the fetus' best interests should be considered but respect for a pregnant patient's autonomy and bodily integrity should prevail [64]. In the diametric cases of a pregnant patient who requests a more aggressive treatment regimen that may carry risks to the fetus or a pregnant patient who requests a conservative approach for a tumor that carries a high risk for impairing fetal health, the decision making and autonomy of the patient in both cases should be respected and used to guide treatment selection.

Medical Management

Corticosteroids have been a mainstay for the treatment of brain neoplasms due to alleviating peritumoral edema and, in certain neoplasms, may be used to achieve symptomatic relief to delay surgery and adjuvant therapy until after delivery [4, 65]. Corticosteroids have been found to be safe for use during pregnancy and are also the first-line treatment for accelerating fetal lung maturity in anticipation of a preterm birth, which may have additional utility for patients with a planned cesarean delivery (C-section) due to symptomatic burden from a brain tumor [4]. However, there is evidence connecting maternal corticosteroid use to a higher risk of neonatal adrenal suppression, and long-term use throughout gestation may warrant careful neonatal monitoring for this condition [4].

Antiepileptic drugs (AEDs) are an additional component of treatment for pregnant patients with seizures due to their intracranial neoplasm. Despite the documented teratogenicity of AEDs, the presence of seizures in pregnancy necessitates treatment due to the risk of seizures to the fetus outweighing the risk of teratogenicity [66, 67]. In order to reduce the risk of teratogenicity while preventing the onset of additional seizures, the lowest effective dose should be used. In contrast, AEDs are not indicated as prophylaxis for patients with a brain tumor who have had no lifetime history of seizures. While AEDs have a variable risk profile, several studies have identified levetiracetam or lamotrigine monotherapy as safe options during pregnancy [66, 68]. In contrast, one network meta-analysis identified significantly higher odds for major fetal malformations after maternal use of ethosuximide, valproate, topiramate, phenobarbital, carbamazepine, and phenytoin [69]. While phenytoin is a first-line agent for tonic-clonic seizures in nonpregnant patients, it has been associated with an 11% rate of congenital malformations, such as fetal hydantoin syndrome and cardiac defects [70]. Due to the increased risk of neural tube defects with maternal AED use, folic acid supplementation should also be continued throughout the duration of pregnancy. Management of seizures and considerations for AED use during pregnancy are discussed in detail in Chap. 28.

For glioblastoma, potentially the most aggressive brain malignancy that may affect a pregnant patient, the standard of care in nonpregnant patients is the Stupp protocol, consisting of maximal safe surgical resection, followed by concomitant radiotherapy and chemotherapy, followed by maintenance chemotherapy for 6–12 months [71]. While radiotherapy risks fetal harms such as congenital defects and childhood malignancy, brain radiation may be used to treat intracranial neoplasms if indicated, especially when paired with risk mitigation measures like performance past the first trimester, dose limitation, abdominal lead shielding, and maternal positional changes [11, 72, 73]. Stereotactic radiosurgery has also been demonstrated to be a safe, surgery-sparing treatment modality for other intracranial neoplasms, such as vestibular schwannoma and meningioma, that become symptomatic during pregnancy [11, 72, 73].

There is limited literature on the impact of systemic chemotherapy for brain neoplasms like temozolomide (alkylating agent) or bevacizumab (anti-VEGF agent) on fetal development. While case reports have documented the successful use of systemic chemotherapy without congenital malformations at birth, other studies have advocated for systemic chemotherapy to be deferred whenever possible to after delivery because of the limited knowledge on the potential teratogenicity of these agents [3, 74]. For example, bevacizumab currently does not have an assigned pregnancy risk category from the FDA due to insufficient evidence, and temozolomide is a category D drug, indicating positive evidence of fetal risk but a possibility of benefit in specific scenarios, such as life-threatening situations. Most sources also consider chemotherapy an absolute contraindication to breastfeeding. There is some evidence that there is no loss in efficacy of delaying chemotherapy until weeks after delivery, even if it is not administered concurrently with radiotherapy [3]. Moreover, a potential alternative to systemic chemotherapy may be the administration of implantable local chemotherapy, such as lomustine wafers, which have been found to have virtually undetectable levels in the systemic circulation [3].

The most recent US Food and Drug Administration (FDA)-approved treatment for glioma is tumor-treating fields (TTFs), which deliver low-intensity alternating electric fields through scalp transducer arrays to disrupt tumor mitosis [71]. However, the safety of TTFs has not been studied in pregnancy and the manufacturer currently recommends against the use of TTFs in pregnant patients or patients planning a future pregnancy [14].

Finally, several medical agents may be used for pituitary adenomas, including bromocriptine and cabergoline (prolactinoma), somatostatin analogs (growth hormone-secreting adenoma), and metyrapone and ketoconazole (ACTH-secreting adenoma). For prolactinoma, earlier research has determined that dopamine agonists like bromocriptine and cabergoline both have good safety profiles during pregnancy, but should be used with caution [11, 75–78]. Some studies have preferred the use of bromocriptine, due to it having a shorter half-life and more reported data in the literature [11, 76]. However, other sources have argued that due to the unverified fetal impact of the aforementioned therapies for pituitary adenoma, all prepartum medical management should be stopped with the onset of pregnancy and only resumed in the setting of tumor growth [42].

Neurosurgical Management

Neurosurgical intervention should be considered for brain tumors that are aggressive high-grade malignancies, refractory to medical treatment, or are life-threatening, due to factors like impending herniation, significant mass effect, or unremitting seizures. The ACOG recommends that indicated nonobstetric operations, such as for a neoplasm with high risk of herniation, should be performed regardless of trimester of pregnancy [9, 14, 79]. However, for nonemergent brain tumors that may be resected by a scheduled procedure, several studies have identified the second trimester as the safest period to perform an operation, due to having the lowest risk of inducing preterm labor and intraoperative hemorrhage [9, 14, 79]. For patients in the third trimester, others have recommended delaying surgery until after 28–30 weeks of gestation when fetal survival is 90%, in comparison to 50–70% at 26–27 weeks [80].

Beyond the normal risks of surgery for a nonpregnant patient, nonobstetric operations like neurosurgery carry additional risks in pregnant patients (Fig. 32.1). First, while the ACOG has stated that no currently used anesthetic agents have been shown to have teratogenic effect in humans [79], factors like the changed bioavailability and clearance of agents due to pregnancy-related physiologic changes necessitate the consultation of a neuroanesthesiologist for any potential procedure [25]. Noxious stimulation from perioperative preparation of patients for neurosurgery, such as head pinning and scalp incision, may also elicit hypertensive responses that warrant management with analgesics, such as a short-acting opioid like remifentanil [81]. Second, the use of other medications like vasopressors may jeopardize placental blood flow and in this setting, several studies have recommended the use of epinephrine as the first-line agent [12, 82]. Third, due to the gravid uterus, certain surgical positions, including supine and prone positioning, should be avoided if possible due to the risk of maternal hypotension via inferior vena cava compression [25, 83]. Alternative positions, such as sitting or left lateral decubitus positioning, should be used. Fourth, due to progesterone-mediated relaxation of smooth muscle in the gastrointestinal and respiratory tracts, pregnant patients have a higher risk of postoperative pulmonary aspiration and airway compromise [12, 82]. The hypercoagulable state of pregnancy also increases the postoperative risk of a venous thromboembolism [25, 83]. Finally, 9% of operations in general have been associated with preterm labor [84]. Given these risks, the planning of a neurosurgical operation requires close cooperation with disciplines including maternal-fetal medicine providers, fetal monitoring, and obstetrics, especially in anticipation for the performance of an emergency C-section if needed. Anesthetic, analgesic, and perioperative considerations are discussed in Chaps. 3 and 4.

Despite the aforementioned challenges, neurosurgical procedures have been shown to have acceptable safety with careful planning. Several case series have reported tumor resection with no fetal or maternal morbidity or mortality [12]. A nationwide analysis of pregnant US patients with brain tumors found that 33% of hospitalized patients received neurosurgical intervention and that the performance of a procedure was not associated with pregnancy-related complications [7]. Finally, while tumors present in eloquent or deep cerebral cortex have traditionally been managed by biopsy followed by stereotactic radiosurgery [12], a notable advance in neurosurgical intervention in pregnant patients has been the increased utilization of awake craniotomies for maximal safe surgical resections of neoplasms in eloquent brain areas. Several studies have documented acceptable safety and outcomes for these awake procedures [25, 85, 86].

Beyond the resection of brain tumors, another important role for neurosurgeons is the management of elevated ICP. Possible therapeutic modalities include hyperventilation, mannitol, and a CSF diversion procedure, such as placement of a ventriculoperitoneal (VP) shunt [12]. While mannitol is safe to use in pregnancy, it should be used with caution due to excess levels causing electrolyte abnormalities, dehydration, and disturbances in plasma osmolality [25, 83]. Moreover, during placement of a VP shunt in pregnant patients, careful attention should be paid to gentle insertion into the abdominal cavity to avoid uterine trauma or induction of preterm labor [87]. Laparoscopic-assisted placement of the distal peritoneal catheter has been shown to improve postprocedural recovery and reduce distal shunt obstruction rates [88], but the safety and efficacy of this technique have yet to be studied in pregnancy.

tumors, due to vaginal delivery increasing ICP by an average of 53 mmHg in the first stage of labor and 70 mmHg in the second stage [9, 11, 89]. This risk is especially elevated in nulliparous moms. A brain tumor resection and C-section may be performed under the same general anesthesia to minimize the risk of herniation and adverse effects of anesthetics [5, 9]. Moreover, epidural anesthesia should also be used with caution, due to the risk of a CSF leak promoting herniation. Finally, maternal blood pressure should be carefully controlled in both directions. While overcorrection of hypertension risks placental insufficiency, overcorrection of hypotension may exacerbate elevated ICP.

In several studies, the performance of elective abortion in an earlier stage of pregnancy has also been discussed as an option for patients [8, 11, 12, 82, 90]. This treatment option may be particularly indicated for patients with a neoplasm necessitating radiotherapy or systemic chemotherapy.

Finally, the American Society of Clinical Oncology emphasizes the importance of fertility counseling for future pregnancies in pregnant patients, such as treatment plans before a subsequent pregnancy and patient education on the impact of treatment on future fertility [91]. In one single-center study, 73% of pregnant patients with primary brain tumors readily accepted fertility counseling [92]. The use of assisted reproductive technology should be approached with caution because hormonal stimulation may exacerbate tumor growth and dedifferentiation [9, 93].

Obstetric Management

Brain tumors also raise several important concerns in the management of the patient's pregnancy. In one nationwide US cohort, the presence of a brain tumor during pregnancy was associated with a threefold increased rate of preterm labor and fetal intrauterine growth restriction as well as a sixfold increased rate of C-section [7]. Several studies have argued for the use of C-sections over vaginal delivery in pregnant patients with brain

Controversies in the Management of Brain Tumors During Pregnancy

Table 32.1 summarizes several of the existing controversies and areas for further research in the management of brain tumors in pregnancy. Due to the rarity of these cases, an important next step in this area of study is the development of prospective national or multinational registries to track peripartum and long-term maternal and fetal outcomes.

Table 32.1 Existing areas of controversy in the management of brain tumors in pregnancy

Clinical question	Solutions to address area of controversy
What is the safety of imaging contrast (iodinated or gadolinium) use in pregnancy?	Long-term follow-up of fetal outcomes for pregnancies where imaging contrast was administered Development of consensus guidelines (akin to American College of Radiology Appropriateness Criteria) on situations where contrast use is indicated
What is the relative contribution of different explanations for brain tumor growth and progression during pregnancy?	Increased in vitro work profiling the relation of tumor cells to compounds released in pregnancy, such as estrogen, progesterone, and angiogenic factors Large prospective registries with histopathologic and clinical data as well as sufficient sample size to analyze pregnancy-related factors predictive of tumor progression and growth velocity
What is the safety and long-term impact of systemic chemotherapy during pregnancy?	Long-term follow-up of existing studies reporting outcomes for systemic chemotherapy use during pregnancy Development of prospective registries for pregnancy cases that necessitate systemic chemotherapy
What is the safety of tumor-treating fields during pregnancy?	Preclinical animal models and eventual clinical trials querying the safety of tumor-treating fields on fetal development
What characteristics of a brain tumor necessitate neurosurgical intervention, in comparison to observation?	Large prospective registries with histopathologic and clinical data as well as sufficient sample size to analyze pregnancy-related factors predictive of successful observation until term delivery
What is the ideal stage of pregnancy for neurosurgical intervention?	Meta-analyses of existing case reports on tumor resection during pregnancy Large prospective registries comparing perioperative outcomes for brain tumor resection at different stages of pregnancy (e.g. second vs. third trimester) Comparison of short-term and long-term fetal outcomes based on gestational age at delivery
What is the safety of ventriculoperitoneal shunt placement in pregnancy?	What are rates of uterine trauma and preterm labor following ventriculoperitoneal shunt placement? What is the safety profile and efficacy of alternative shunt placement techniques, such as laparoscopic-assisted placement of the peritoneal catheter?
What patients are appropriate candidates for vaginal delivery?	Meta-analyses of existing case reports on outcomes based on mode of delivery Large prospective registries with sufficient sample size to analyze maternal and tumor-related factors predictive of vaginal delivery without maternal or fetal morbidity

Summary of existing areas of controversy in the management of brain tumors during pregnancy as well as solutions and studies that may resolve these areas of uncertainty

Conclusion

Brain tumors during pregnancy are a challenging clinical entity associated with poorer maternal and fetal outcomes. Across tumor subtypes, several physiologic changes during pregnancy promote the growth and progression of intracranial neoplasms, which may remit with delivery and recur in subsequent pregnancies. Medical, neurosurgical, and obstetric management are all important components of treatment that may be utilized in tandem for especially complicated neoplasms with life-threatening sequelae.

References

1. Ostrom QT, Gittleman H, Liao P, et al. CBTRUS statistical report: primary brain and other central nervous system tumors diagnosed in the United States in 2010-2014. Neuro-Oncology. 2017;19(suppl_5):v1–v88.
2. Group USCSW. U.S. Cancer statistics data visualizations tool. U.S. Department of Health and Human

Services, Centers for Disease Control and Prevention and National Cancer Institute. https://www.cdc.gov/cancer/dataviz. Published 2021. Access.

3. Stevenson CB, Thompson RC. The clinical management of intracranial neoplasms in pregnancy. Clin Obstet Gynecol. 2005;48(1):24–37.

4. Isla A, Alvarez F, Gonzalez A, Garcia-Grande A, Perez-Alvarez M, Garcia-Blazquez M. Brain tumor and pregnancy. Obstet Gynecol. 1997;89(1):19–23.

5. Tewari KS, Cappuccini F, Asrat T, et al. Obstetric emergencies precipitated by malignant brain tumors. Am J Obstet Gynecol. 2000;182(5):1215–21.

6. Haas JF, Janisch W, Staneczek W. Newly diagnosed primary intracranial neoplasms in pregnant women: a population-based assessment. J Neurol Neurosurg Psychiatry. 1986;49(8):874–80.

7. Terry AR, Barker FG 2nd, Leffert L, Bateman BT, Souter I, Plotkin SR. Outcomes of hospitalization in pregnant women with CNS neoplasms: a population-based study. Neuro-Oncology. 2012;14(6):768–76.

8. Yust-Katz S, de Groot JF, Liu D, et al. Pregnancy and glial brain tumors. Neuro-Oncology. 2014;16(9):1289–94.

9. van Westrhenen A, Senders JT, Martin E, DiRisio AC, Broekman MLD. Clinical challenges of glioma and pregnancy: a systematic review. J Neuro-Oncol. 2018;139(1):1–11.

10. Roelvink NC, Kamphorst W, van Alphen HA, Rao BR. Pregnancy-related primary brain and spinal tumors. Arch Neurol. 1987;44(2):209–15.

11. Bonfield CM, Engh JA. Pregnancy and brain tumors. Neurol Clin. 2012;30(3):937–46.

12. Cohen-Gadol AA, Friedman JA, Friedman JD, Tubbs RS, Munis JR, Meyer FB. Neurosurgical management of intracranial lesions in the pregnant patient: a 36-year institutional experience and review of the literature. J Neurosurg. 2009;111(6):1150–7.

13. Frishberg BM. Neuroimaging in presumed primary headache disorders. Semin Neurol. 1997;17(4):373–82.

14. Eckenstein M, Thomas AA. Benign and malignant tumors of the central nervous system and pregnancy. Handb Clin Neurol. 2020;172:241–58.

15. Dias MS, Sekhar LN. Intracranial hemorrhage from aneurysms and arteriovenous malformations during pregnancy and the puerperium. Neurosurgery. 1990;27(6):855–65; discussion 865–856.

16. Committee Opinion No. 723: guidelines for diagnostic imaging during pregnancy and lactation. Obstet Gynecol. 2017;130(4):e210–6.

17. Simon RH. Brain tumors in pregnancy. Semin Neurol. 1988;8(3):214–21.

18. Webb JA, Thomsen HS, Morcos SK, Members of contrast media safety Committee of European Society of urogenital Radiology. The use of iodinated and gadolinium contrast media during pregnancy and lactation. Eur Radiol. 2005;15(6):1234–40.

19. Edelman RR, Warach S. Magnetic resonance imaging (1). N Engl J Med. 1993;328(10):708–16.

20. Sundgren PC, Leander P. Is administration of gadolinium-based contrast media to pregnant women and small children justified? J Magn Reson Imaging. 2011;34(4):750–7.

21. Marcos HB, Semelka RC, Worawattanakul S. Normal placenta: gadolinium-enhanced dynamic MR imaging. Radiology. 1997;205(2):493–6.

22. Schock H, Zeleniuch-Jacquotte A, Lundin E, et al. Hormone concentrations throughout uncomplicated pregnancies: a longitudinal study. BMC Pregnancy Childbirth. 2016;16(1):146.

23. Pritchard JA. Changes in the blood volume during pregnancy and delivery. Anesthesiology. 1965;26:393–9.

24. Evans P, Wheeler T, Anthony F, Osmond C. Maternal serum vascular endothelial growth factor during early pregnancy. Clin Sci (Lond). 1997;92(6):567–71.

25. Rodrigues AJ, Waldrop AR, Suharwardy S, et al. Management of brain tumors presenting in pregnancy: a case series and systematic review. Am J Obstet Gynecol MFM. 2021;3(1):100256.

26. Kareva I. Immune suppression in pregnancy and cancer: parallels and insights. Transl Oncol. 2020;13(7):100759.

27. Gonzalez-Aguero G, Gutierrez AA, Gonzalez-Espinosa D, et al. Progesterone effects on cell growth of U373 and D54 human astrocytoma cell lines. Endocrine. 2007;32(2):129–35.

28. Pallud J, Mandonnet E, Deroulers C, et al. Pregnancy increases the growth rates of World Health Organization grade II gliomas. Ann Neurol. 2010;67(3):398–404.

29. Pallud J, Duffau H, Razak RA, et al. Influence of pregnancy in the behavior of diffuse gliomas: clinical cases of a French glioma study group. J Neurol. 2009;256(12):2014–20.

30. Daras M, Cone C, Peters KB. Tumor progression and transformation of low-grade glial tumors associated with pregnancy. J Neuro-Oncol. 2014;116(1):113–7.

31. Peeters S, Pages M, Gauchotte G, et al. Interactions between glioma and pregnancy: insight from a 52-case multicenter series. J Neurosurg. 2018;128(1):3–13.

32. DeAngelis LM. Central nervous system neoplasms in pregnancy. Adv Neurol. 1994;64:139–52.

33. Cushing H, Eisenhardt L. Meningiomas arising from the tuberculum sellae. Arch Ophthalmol. 1929;1:168–205.

34. Stedman KE, Moore GE, Morgan RT. Estrogen receptor proteins in diverse human tumors. Arch Surg. 1980;115(3):244–8.

35. Blaauw G, Blankenstein MA, Lamberts SW. Sex steroid receptors in human meningiomas. Acta Neurochir. 1986;79(1):42–7.

36. Schoenberg BS, Christine BW, Whisnant JP. Nervous system neoplasms and primary malignancies of other sites. The unique association between meningiomas and breast cancer. Neurology. 1975;25(8):705–12.

37. Jaaskelainen J, Laasonen E, Karkkainen J, Haltia M, Troupp H. Hormone treatment of meningiomas:

lack of response to medroxyprogesterone acetate (MPA). A pilot study of five cases. Acta Neurochir. 1986;80(1–2):35–41.

38. Allen J, Eldridge R, Koerber T. Acoustic neuroma in the last months of pregnancy. Am J Obstet Gynecol. 1974;119(4):516–20.

39. Iuliano S, Laws ER Jr. Management of pituitary tumors in pregnancy. Semin Neurol. 2011;31(4):423–8.

40. Jan M, Destrieux C. Pituitary disorders in pregnancy. Neurochirurgie. 2000;46(2):88–94.

41. Molitch ME. Pituitary tumors and pregnancy. Growth Horm IGF Res. 2003;13(Suppl A):S38–44.

42. Bronstein MD, Paraiba DB, Jallad RS. Management of pituitary tumors in pregnancy. Nat Rev Endocrinol. 2011;7(5):301–10.

43. Gemzell C, Wang CF. Outcome of pregnancy in women with pituitary adenoma. Fertil Steril. 1979;31(4):363–72.

44. Hayes AR, O'Sullivan AJ, Davies MA. A case of pituitary apoplexy in pregnancy. Endocrinol Diabetes Metab Case Rep. 2014;2014:140043.

45. Domingue ME, Devuyst F, Alexopoulou O, Corvilain B, Maiter D. Outcome of prolactinoma after pregnancy and lactation: a study on 73 patients. Clin Endocrinol. 2014;80(5):642–8.

46. Nayak N, Kumar A. Cerebellar hemangioblastoma during pregnancy: management options and review of literature. Surg Neurol Int. 2020;11:123.

47. Frantzen C, Kruizinga RC, van Asselt SJ, et al. Pregnancy-related hemangioblastoma progression and complications in von Hippel-Lindau disease. Neurology. 2012;79(8):793–6.

48. Binderup ML, Budtz-Jorgensen E, Bisgaard ML. New von Hippel-Lindau manifestations develop at the same or decreased rates in pregnancy. Neurology. 2015;85(17):1500–3.

49. Burnette MS, Mann TS, Berman DJ, Nguyen TT. Brain tumor, pheochromocytoma, and pregnancy: a case report of a cesarean delivery in a patient with Von Hippel-Lindau disease. A A Pract. 2019;13(8):289–91.

50. Magge SN, Brunt M, Scott RM. Craniopharyngioma presenting during pregnancy 4 years after a normal magnetic resonance imaging scan: case report. Neurosurgery. 2001;49(4):1014–6; conclusion 1016–1017.

51. Ravindra VM, Braca JA 3rd, Jensen RL, Duckworth EA. Management of intracranial pathology during pregnancy: case example and review of management strategies. Surg Neurol Int. 2015;6:43.

52. Razak AR, Nasser Q, Morris P, Alcutt D, Grogan L. Medulloblastoma in two successive pregnancies. J Neuro-Oncol. 2005;73(1):89–90.

53. Wing LA, Conaglen JV, Meyer-Rochow GY, Elston MS. Paraganglioma in pregnancy: a case series and review of the literature. J Clin Endocrinol Metab. 2015;100(8):3202–9.

54. Muntcr MW, Wengenroth M, Fehrenbacher G, et al. Heavy ion radiotherapy during pregnancy. Fertil Steril. 2010;94(6):2329.e2325–7.

55. Eibye S, Kjaer SK, Mellemkjaer L. Incidence of pregnancy-associated cancer in Denmark, 1977-2006. Obstet Gynecol. 2013;122(3):608–17.

56. Vogelbaum MA, Suh JH. Resectable brain metastases. J Clin Oncol. 2006;24(8):1289–94.

57. Chen KY, Wang HC, Shih JY, Yang PC. Lung cancer in pregnancy: report of two cases. J Formos Med Assoc. 1998;97(8):573–6.

58. Sharma A, Nguyen HS, Lozen A, Sharma A, Mueller W. Brain metastases from breast cancer during pregnancy. Surg Neurol Int. 2016;7(Suppl 23):S603–6.

59. Goutham C, Kumar JP, Anil P, Peter SN, Ravi R, Chakravorthy VM. Malignant course of a metastatic melanoma during pregnancy: a case report. World J Oncol. 2011;2(2):79–82.

60. Mehta MP, Rodrigus P, Terhaard CH, et al. Survival and neurologic outcomes in a randomized trial of motexafin gadolinium and whole-brain radiation therapy in brain metastases. J Clin Oncol. 2003;21(13):2529–36.

61. Yuzhalin AE, Yu D. Brain metastasis organotropism. Cold Spring Harb Perspect Med. 2020;10(5):a037242.

62. Mamelak AN, Withers GJ, Wang X. Choriocarcinoma brain metastasis in a patient with viable intrauterine pregnancy. Case report. J Neurosurg. 2002;97(2):477–81.

63. Schechter NR, Mychalczak B, Jones W, Spriggs D. Prognosis of patients treated with whole-brain radiation therapy for metastatic gestational trophoblastic disease. Gynecol Oncol. 1998;68(2):183–92.

64. American College of O, Gynecology. ACOG Committee Opinion No. 390, December 2007. Ethical decision making in obstetrics and gynecology. Obstet Gynecol. 2007;110(6):1479–87.

65. Dietrich J, Rao K, Pastorino S, Kesari S. Corticosteroids in brain cancer patients: benefits and pitfalls. Expert Rev Clin Pharmacol. 2011;4(2):233–42.

66. Tomson T, Battino D, Perucca E. Teratogenicity of antiepileptic drugs. Curr Opin Neurol. 2019;32(2):246–52.

67. Patterson RM. Seizure disorders in pregnancy. Med Clin North Am. 1989;73(3):661–5.

68. Tomson T, Landmark CJ, Battino D. Antiepileptic drug treatment in pregnancy: changes in drug disposition and their clinical implications. Epilepsia. 2013;54(3):405–14.

69. Veroniki AA, Cogo E, Rios P, et al. Comparative safety of anti-epileptic drugs during pregnancy: a systematic review and network meta-analysis of congenital malformations and prenatal outcomes. BMC Med. 2017;15(1):95.

70. Hill DS, Wlodarczyk BJ, Palacios AM, Finnell RH. Teratogenic effects of antiepileptic drugs. Expert Rev Neurother. 2010;10(6):943–59.

71. Stupp R, Taillibert S, Kanner A, et al. Effect of tumor-treating fields plus maintenance Temozolomide vs maintenance Temozolomide alone on survival in

patients with glioblastoma: a randomized clinical trial. JAMA. 2017;318(23):2306–16.

72. Magne N, Marcie S, Pignol JP, Casagrande F, Lagrange JL. Radiotherapy for a solitary brain metastasis during pregnancy: a method for reducing fetal dose. Br J Radiol. 2001;74(883):638–41.

73. Mazonakis M, Damilakis J, Theoharopoulos N, Varveris H, Gourtsoyiannis N. Brain radiotherapy during pregnancy: an analysis of conceptus dose using anthropomorphic phantoms. Br J Radiol. 1999;72(855):274–8.

74. Nolan B, Balakrishna M, George M. Exposure to Temozolomide in the first trimester of pregnancy in a young woman with glioblastoma multiforme. World J Oncol. 2012;3(6):286–7.

75. Imran SA, Ur E, Clarke DB. Managing prolactin-secreting adenomas during pregnancy. Can Fam Physician. 2007;53(4):653–8.

76. Glezer A, Bronstein MD. Prolactinomas in pregnancy: considerations before conception and during pregnancy. Pituitary. 2020;23(1):65–9.

77. Maiter D. Prolactinoma and pregnancy: from the wish of conception to lactation. Ann Endocrinol (Paris). 2016;77(2):128–34.

78. O'Sullivan SM, Farrant MT, Ogilvie CM, Gunn AJ, Milsom SR. An observational study of pregnancy and post-partum outcomes in women with prolactinoma treated with dopamine agonists. Aust N Z J Obstet Gynaecol. 2020;60(3):405–11.

79. ACOG Committee Opinion No. 775: nonobstetric surgery during pregnancy. Obstet Gynecol. 2019;133(4):e285–6.

80. Lynch JC, Gouvea F, Emmerich JC, et al. Management strategy for brain tumour diagnosed during pregnancy. Br J Neurosurg. 2011;25(2):225–30.

81. Jayasekera BA, Bacon AD, Whitfield PC. Management of glioblastoma multiforme in pregnancy. J Neurosurg. 2012;116(6):1187–94.

82. Mazze RI, Kallen B. Reproductive outcome after anesthesia and operation during pregnancy: a registry study of 5405 cases. Am J Obstet Gynecol. 1989;161(5):1178–85.

83. Wang LP, Paech MJ. Neuroanesthesia for the pregnant woman. Anesth Analg. 2008;107(1):193–200.

84. Delaney AG. Anesthesia in the pregnant woman. Clin Obstet Gynecol. 1983;26(4):795–800.

85. Meng L, Han SJ, Rollins MD, Gelb AW, Chang EF. Awake brain tumor resection during pregnancy: decision making and technical nuances. J Clin Neurosci. 2016;24:160–2.

86. Al Mashani AM, Ali A, Chatterjee N, Suri N, Das S. Awake craniotomy during pregnancy. J Neurosurg Anesthesiol. 2018;30(4):372–3.

87. Wisoff JH, Kratzert KJ, Handwerker SM, Young BK, Epstein F. Pregnancy in patients with cerebrospinal fluid shunts: report of a series and review of the literature. Neurosurgery. 1991;29(6):827–31.

88. Naftel RP, Argo JL, Shannon CN, et al. Laparoscopic versus open insertion of the peritoneal catheter in ventriculoperitoneal shunt placement: review of 810 consecutive cases. J Neurosurg. 2011;115(1):151–8.

89. Marx GF, Zemaitis MT, Orkin LR. Cerebrospinal fluid pressures during labor and obstetrical anesthesia. Anesthesiology. 1961;22:348–54.

90. Verheecke M, Halaska MJ, Lok CA, et al. Primary brain tumours, meningiomas and brain metastases in pregnancy: report on 27 cases and review of literature. Eur J Cancer. 2014;50(8):1462–71.

91. Loren AW, Mangu PB, Beck LN, et al. Fertility preservation for patients with cancer: American Society of Clinical Oncology clinical practice guideline update. J Clin Oncol. 2013;31(19):2500–10.

92. Stone JB, Kelvin JF, DeAngelis LM. Fertility preservation in primary brain tumor patients. Neurooncol Pract. 2017;4(1):40–5.

93. Zwinkels H, Dorr J, Kloet F, Taphoorn MJ, Vecht CJ. Pregnancy in women with gliomas: a case-series and review of the literature. J Neuro-Oncol. 2013;115(2):293–301.

Pituitary Region Tumors in Pregnancy: Overview and Management Paradigms

John S. Herendeen, Elizabeth E. Ginalis, Rima Rana, Nitesh V. Patel, and Simon Hanft

Overview

The pituitary gland is a sensitive neuroendocrine structure in regard to both its anatomy and physiology. It receives neural and hormonal input through a number of biochemical pathways, each of which influences both the function and growth of its constituent cells. In turn, it exerts hormonal control over a number of organ systems, a feedback system that is critical to maintaining homeostasis and responding to external stimuli. The pituitary is dependent on a regular physiologic internal environment to function appropriately and is exquisitely susceptible to aberrant conditions. As a result, disruptions of normal gland activity can have profound implications.

Pregnancy presents a unique hormonal environment for the pituitary gland. Over the course of gestation, the pituitary undergoes a series of expected changes. Most notably, placental estro-gen stimulates lactotroph hyperplasia, resulting in an increase in pituitary volume of 40% during the second trimester and up to 70% during the third trimester [1, 2]. Somatotrophs progressively decline in number, due to negative feedback from placental secretion of a growth hormone variant which increases release of insulin-like growth factor 1 (IGF-1) [3]. Corticotrophs are stimulated by placental release of corticotropin-releasing hormone (CRH), whose serum levels rise several 100-fold during the course of pregnancy [4]. This represents a basic overview of the complex transformation undergone by the gland during pregnancy.

A variety of tumors within the sella turcica have been defined. These include functioning and nonfunctioning adenomas of the pituitary gland as well as tumors from adjacent structures, such as tuberculum sellae meningiomas. Each tumor uniquely responds to chemical signals and consequently imposes different influences on various body systems. Given the delicate nature of pituitary anatomy and physiology, these tumors may present a serious risk when they compress healthy pituitary tissue, and this risk may be magnified in the setting of pregnancy. Ideally, all sellar tumors should be met with a definitive management plan prior to conception. Depending on the unique clinical situation, pituitary region tumors in pregnancy may be monitored, treated medically, or even surgically removed. Generally, transsphenoidal surgery is considered during pregnancy in

J. S. Herendeen · E. E. Ginalis · N. V. Patel
Department of Neurosurgery, New Jersey Medical School, Rutgers University,
New Brunswick, NJ, USA

R. Rana
Department of Obstetrics and Gynecology, New Jersey Medical School, Rutgers University,
New Brunswick, NJ, USA

S. Hanft (✉)
Department of Neurosurgery, Westchester Medical Center, New York Medical College,
Valhalla, NY, USA
e-mail: simon.hanft@wmchealth.org

G. Gupta et al. (eds.), *Neurological Disorders in Pregnancy*,
https://doi.org/10.1007/978-3-031-36490-7_33

cases of severe symptoms unresponsive to medical therapy, symptomatic tumor enlargement, or pituitary apoplexy. Pituitary apoplexy is a feared complication of any pituitary tumor. The changes of pregnancy can cause a pituitary tumor to outgrow or compress the blood supply to the gland [5], compromising the function of the entire gland and leading to dreaded consequences including acute adrenal insufficiency and acute visual loss. The possibility of apoplexy during pregnancy remains low but is likely elevated compared to normal physiologic states [6].

Functioning Tumors

Prolactinoma

A prolactinoma is a functioning pituitary tumor comprised of lactotrophs and represents the most common primary pituitary tumor. Prolactinomas can be further classified as either microadenoma (<10 mm diameter) or macroadenoma (>10 mm diameter). This classification guides management of prolactinomas when they are recognized in pregnancy [7]. Just as the high estrogen environment of pregnancy stimulates normal pituitary lactotrophs, it also indiscriminately stimulates their neoplastic derivatives [8]. Consequently, increased estrogen levels may result in further growth of prolactinomas during pregnancy. Microprolactinomas carry a low risk of progression during pregnancy, with studies showing asymptomatic enlargement in 4.5% of cases and symptomatic enlargement in only 1.5–2.5% [8, 9]. Macroprolactinomas are associated with a higher risk of progression during pregnancy, with studies citing a range of 15.5–35.7% for symptomatic enlargement in tumors that were previously untreated [2, 8]. The risk of symptomatic enlargement in macroprolactinomas treated with surgery or radiation therapy prior to pregnancy is 3–7.1% [2, 7–9].

Many prolactinomas are actually discovered in young women attempting to become pregnant as the presence of a prolactinoma can interfere with fertility and normal menstruation. Thus women who are having difficulty conceiving often undergo a basic hormone panel including a prolactin level. If elevated, this leads to an MRI which nearly always detects the prolactinoma. These patients are then started on a dopamine agonist in order to restore fertility. Dopamine agonists include bromocriptine and cabergoline, both of which have well established efficacy in treating prolactinomas. In addition to cabergoline being better tolerated than bromocriptine in terms of side effects, cabergoline has also demonstrated a higher success rate in inducing pregnancy in infertile women [10]. Once pregnancy is confirmed, the dopamine agonist is typically withheld due to the lack of information with regard to its fetal safety profile [11]. For microprolactinomas, cabergoline can be confidently stopped by the treating endocrinologist without significant fear of optic chiasm compression from interval tumor growth. However, for macroprolactinomas, especially those already contacting the optic apparatus, this can be a much more difficult decision. Indeed, the general recommendation in such cases is to defer pregnancy until the tumor has demonstrated a radiographic response to medical therapy with a concomitant lowering of the prolactin level [12–14]. In rare medically refractory cases, transsphenoidal surgery to achieve at least a significant debulking is recommended prior to pursuing pregnancy [15]. The likelihood of discovering a symptomatic macroprolactinoma during pregnancy is extremely low due to the difficulty of conceiving with such a hyperactive tumor in place. In such an unusual circumstance the similar paradigm of medical therapy followed by surgery in the rare event of failure would be applied.

Once the dopamine agonist is withheld after pregnancy is confirmed, the prolactinoma can now grow unchecked and so patients are closely monitored for the development or worsening of visual symptoms [5, 7]. In patients with microprolactinomas, visual field examinations have been recommended every 3 months [16], though the likelihood of optic chiasmatic compression is so low that we would advocate for exams only in the setting of new onset visual complaints. For patients harboring macroadenomas, closer surveillance is recommended with visual field checks every 2–3 months along with clinical evaluation every 1–2 months [7]. If the patient develops symptoms in the interim, urgent evaluation must proceed. This includes a brain MRI though contrast agents (typically gadolinium) are held due to risk of fetal exposure [17]. Contrast can be considered in very specific circumstances, but in all likelihood a noncontrast MRI should be able to delineate a larger mass and its relationship to the chiasm. Routine surveillance brain MRIs during pregnancy are not recommended.

When medical treatment of prolactinoma during pregnancy is warranted, such as in symptomatic tumor enlargement, dopamine agonists remain the appropriate medical therapy [8]. Bromocriptine has not been associated with adverse pregnancy outcomes such as spontaneous abortions, multiple pregnancies, ectopic pregnancies, and congenital malformations. However, it has been suggested that it can precipitate apoplexy, which is why it is not used during pregnancy for asymptomatic tumors [6]. The dose can be rapidly titrated as tolerated to control symptoms [8]. Exposure to cabergoline, a newer age and more widely prescribed dopamine agonist, during pregnancy does not appear to increase incidence of adverse effects [2]. However, there is more information on the safety of bromocriptine during pregnancy as opposed to cabergoline [18] given the relative recency of cabergoline's use (approved for use in 1993 vs. bromocriptine in 1975). Bromocriptine, therefore, is most commonly prescribed during the first and second trimesters in the event of symptomatic tumor enlargement, although there has been an uptick in cabergoline usage based on some recent studies [19]. Ideally the medication will shrink the tumor and improve visual symptoms so that surgery can be avoided. Following delivery, remission of the elevated prolactin and tumor is often observed. Domingue et al. reported 41% remission of hyperprolactinemia following delivery and lactation in a median time of 22 months, while Auriemma et al. reported 68% remission after a maximum of 60 months [20, 21]. Of note, prolactin will rise during pregnancy (levels can rise above 200 ng/mL) and therefore cannot be used as an accurate indicator of whether the prolacti-

noma is growing or responding to medical therapy [22].

Surgical management of prolactinoma during pregnancy is rarely required but is appropriate in the instance of a worsening clinical picture that does not respond to dopamine agonist therapy, especially in the setting of worsening vision [2]. In these cases, transsphenoidal surgery during the second trimester is recommended [23]. Later in the pregnancy, delivery is an acceptable alternative to surgery [23]. Regardless of treatment strategy, close follow-up, including prolactin levels, is recommended for 2 months following delivery to monitor symptom progression [7]. Lactation can be attempted with the patient still off medication, as dopamine agonists can impair lactation, but if symptoms arise the obvious recommendation is to restart the medication and cease breastfeeding [24]. Figure 33.1 shows a summary of the management of prolactinomas in pregnancy.

ACTH-Secreting Adenoma and Cushing's Disease

Though far less common than prolactinomas, adrenocorticotropic hormone (ACTH)-secreting adenomas are another type of functioning pituitary tumor. Similar to prolactinomas, women with ACTH-secreting adenomas are very unlikely to conceive as hypercortisolism leads to infertility [25, 26]. This makes the incidence of Cushing's disease in pregnancy very rare. If an ACTH-secreting adenoma is encountered prior to pregnancy, the clear recommendation is to defer conception until surgical removal and subsequent remission of the cortisol level occurs.

Cushing's syndrome during pregnancy is also rare, with the syndrome caused by Cushing's disease only 40% of the time [16]. In contrast, ACTH-secreting tumors are responsible for closer to 70% of cases of Cushing's syndrome in the general population [27]. Furthermore, the signs and symptoms of Cushing's disease are challenging to differentiate from the standard sequelae of pregnancy, which may include weight gain, hypertension, fatigue, hyperglycemia, and emo-

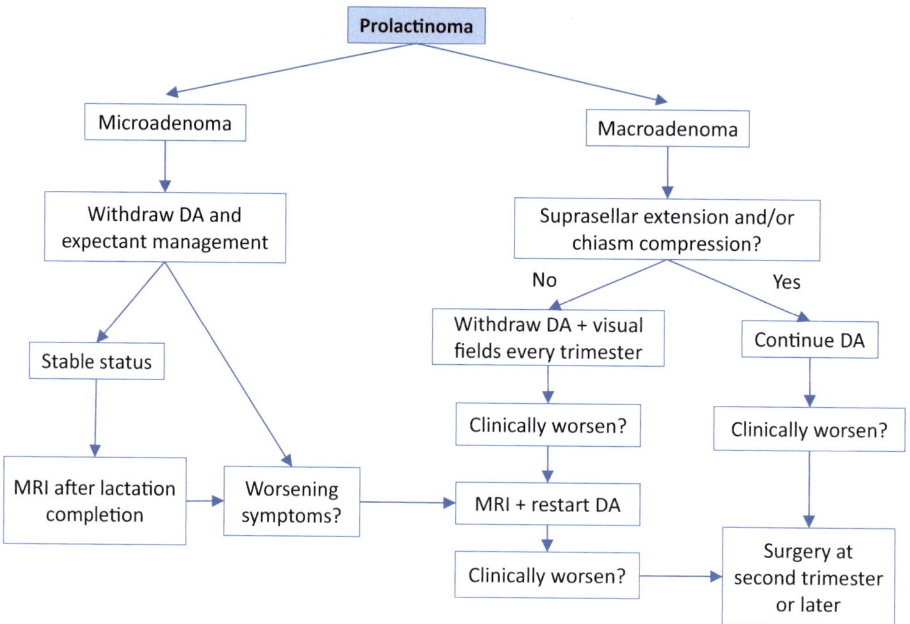

Fig. 33.1 Prolactinoma management paradigm during pregnancy. *DA* dopamine agonist

tional changes [3]. The physical exam findings of purple striae, hirsutism, acne, muscle weakness, and pathologic fractures should lead to increased suspicion for Cushing's syndrome. Traditional diagnostic testing, such as dexamethasone suppression tests, are less reliable during pregnancy, so clinical acumen is critical to establishing the diagnosis [16]. Inferior petrosal sinus sampling can be pursued judiciously especially if the clinical suspicion for an ACTH-secreting tumor is high and the MRI is negative for a microadenoma or shows a tumor <6 mm in size [28].

Cushing's syndrome during pregnancy is associated with increased maternal morbidity in 70% of cases [29] as well as inferior outcomes for the fetus [16]. Maternal complications include hypertension, diabetes, cardiomyopathy, and impaired wound healing in pregnancies requiring C-section. Premature labor is common, though reported incidence varies, ranging from 48 to 72% in untreated patients [8, 25, 30]. Studies by Bevan et al. and Buescher et al. reported that the incidence of premature labor was reduced to 20% and 47%, respectively, if the mother received treatment during pregnancy. Cushing's syndrome in the mother suppresses the developing fetal

adrenal glands [8], and fetal mortality rates have been reported at 9–24% [25, 30].

In contrast with the more common prolactinoma, ACTH-secreting pituitary adenomas are indications for prompt intervention due to the frequency of these aforesaid serious complications. Second trimester transsphenoidal surgical resection is the preferred first line treatment (Fig. 33.2) [3, 16]. For patients who cannot undergo surgery, medical therapy is available albeit with limited effectiveness [8]. Metyrapone is a widely used medication during the second and third trimesters for hypercortisolism, though it may worsen hypertension. Other medications include ketoconazole [28] and cabergoline [3, 31]. In patients with mild disease, vigilant monitoring may be considered with adequate control of comorbidities during pregnancy, and treatment can be pursued following delivery [9].

Growth-Hormone Secreting Adenoma and Acromegaly

Acromegaly is the syndrome resulting from excess growth hormone (GH) most often caused

Fig. 33.2 Cushing's disease management paradigm during pregnancy

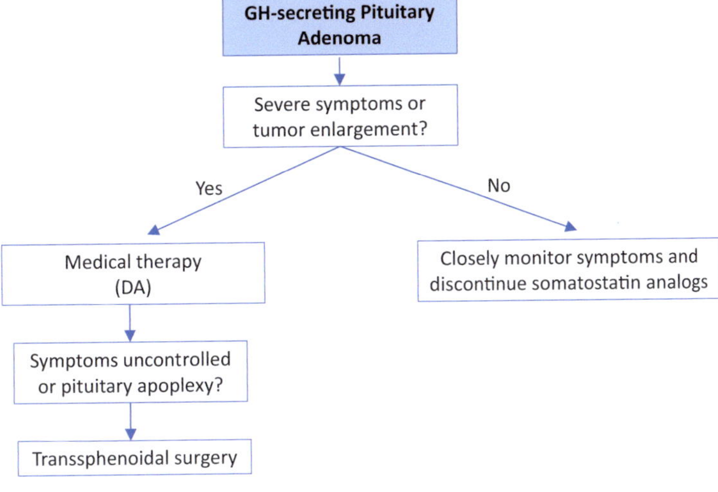

Fig. 33.3 GH-secreting pituitary adenoma management paradigm during pregnancy

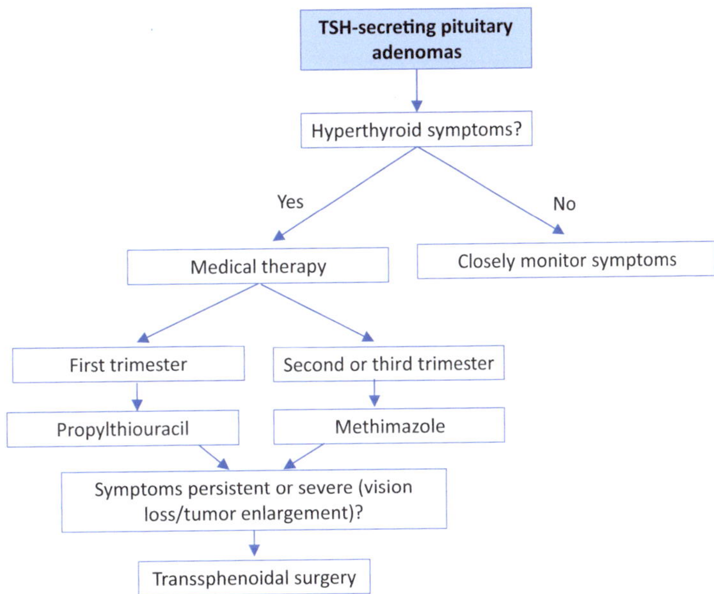

by GH-secreting pituitary adenomas and has unique clinical implications for pregnant patients. GH-secreting pituitary adenomas are derived from somatotropic cells and are another uncommon type of functioning pituitary tumor, with less than 100 cases reported during pregnancy [8]. In most instances, there are no complications in women with acromegaly and their fetuses. Most cases result in healthy infants at full birth weight [3]. In fact, many patients with existing symptomatic GH-secreting adenoma often report improvement in signs and symptoms during pregnancy [3]. There are only two

known instances of GH-secreting adenoma enlargement during pregnancy [8, 32, 33]. If discovered before pregnancy, the recommendation is to surgically remove the GH-adenoma prior to attempting conception, both to improve fertility and to lower the risks of acromegaly-related sequelae to the patient and fetus during gestation [34].

However, in few patients, pregnancy may exacerbate symptoms of acromegaly. Complications associated with acromegaly during pregnancy include gestational diabetes mellitus, hyperglycemia, hypertension, headache,

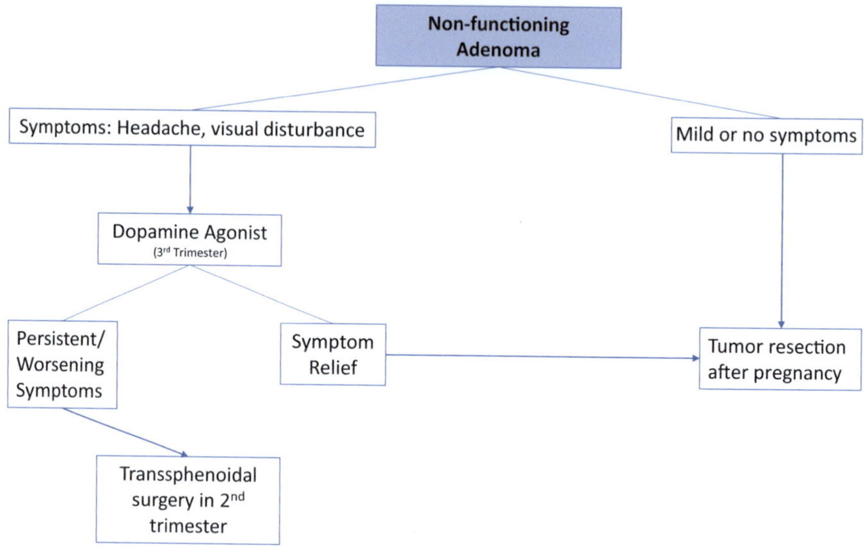

Fig. 33.4 TSH-secreting pituitary adenoma management paradigm during pregnancy

visual disturbances, and cardiac disease [8]. Few instances have resulted in low birth weight, but this has been related to gestational use of a somatostatin analog (i.e. octreotide) for treatment of acromegaly [3].

It is recommended that patients with acromegaly discontinue use of somatostatin analogs during pregnancy with close monitoring of symptoms (Fig. 33.3) [8]. Somatostatin analogs cross the placenta and may affect fetal growth. Thus, treatment with somatostatin analogs during pregnancy is reserved for severe symptoms attributed to acromegaly or tumor enlargement, including headaches or vision changes. Medical management with dopamine agonists may also be considered in these cases. Transsphenoidal surgery is indicated in cases of severe disease not controlled by medications, acute severe symptoms such as vision loss, and pituitary apoplexy. In these settings, transsphenoidal surgery is indicated preferentially during the second trimester and has yielded desirable outcomes.

cases have been reported during pregnancy [3, 36–40]. Clinical concerns center largely around symptoms from hyperthyroidism, which need to be monitored and, if necessary, controlled with standard antithyroid drugs [8], including propylthiouracil (preferred during the first trimester) and methimazole (during the second and third trimesters), or with octreotide.

No consensus has been reached regarding treatment of these tumors during pregnancy given their rarity. Case reports on this topic have managed pregnant patients with either close observation, medical therapy with propylthiouracil or octreotide, or transsphenoidal surgery [36–40]. In all cases, there were no reported maternal or fetal complications following therapy. Generally, management of TSH-secreting adenomas is individualized to each patient. In cases of severe symptoms such as vision loss or tumor enlargement, medical or surgical treatment can be considered without maternal-fetal adverse effects (Fig. 33.4).

TSH-Secreting Adenoma

Thyroid stimulating hormone (TSH)-secreting pituitary adenomas account for only 0.5–3% of all pituitary adenomas [35]. To date, only five

Nonfunctioning Tumors

Nonfunctioning Adenomas

Nonfunctioning adenomas make up approximately 30% of primary pituitary tumors [9]. They

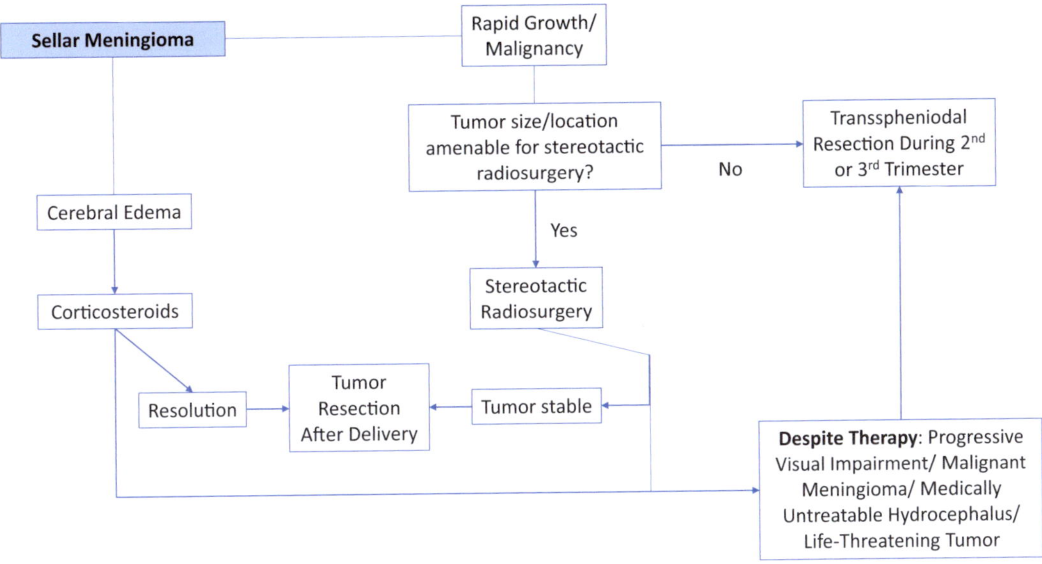

Fig. 33.5 Nonfunctioning pituitary adenoma management paradigm during pregnancy

can have considerable impact on pituitary gland function due to compression of neighboring healthy pituitary tissue in this confined space and may also lead to mass effect on nearby structures. These issues may be amplified in pregnancy. Though the size of most nonfunctioning adenomas does not change during pregnancy [7, 8], previously described physiologic lactotroph hyperplasia can exacerbate the mass effect of any tumor in the sella turcica [8]. In this setting, a previously undiscovered nonfunctioning adenoma may cause symptoms from increased mass effect, including visual disturbances and headache. Though not targeting the tumor directly, dopamine agonists can be used to relieve these symptoms by reducing hyperplasia [16]. Often, symptoms can be controlled through pregnancy, and the tumor can be resected after delivery [5]. If symptoms cannot be controlled medically during pregnancy, surgery may be performed during the second trimester (Fig. 33.5) [16].

The question of how to deal with a nonfunctioning adenoma before pregnancy is more complicated. Ultimately it is a judgment call shared by the endocrinologist and neurosurgeon. The question really only applies to macroadenomas, and even then the tumors that warrant consideration of upfront surgical removal would likely have to be at least in the 1.5–2.0 cm range and/or

within 2 mm of the optic chiasm. These are the tumors that have the potential to lead to optic chiasm compression with visual loss during pregnancy if they are displaced by lactotroph hyperplasia, but this is a rare phenomenon with only one case described in the literature [41]. As such, there is a role for upfront transsphenoidal removal of these tumors in patients who intend to become pregnant. But this operation should be endeavored upon very judiciously, as the surgery itself may lead to pituitary damage that in turn makes conception more challenging. There is no specific paradigm on how to proceed in these complicated cases. We would generally recommend avoiding surgery unless there are preoperative visual symptoms (very obvious indication for a pre-pregnancy operation) or clear optic chiasm compression without visual loss. In this latter circumstance, upfront surgery should be considered, and if pursued, we would recommend a conservative debulking so as to minimize the chance of pituitary gland injury [16, 22].

Meningioma

Not all sellar tumors are derived from the cells of the pituitary gland. Meningiomas are the most common primary benign intracranial neo-

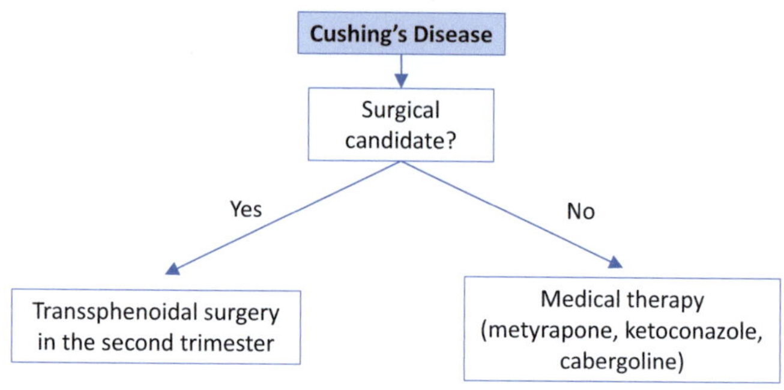

Fig. 33.6 Tuberculum sellae meningioma management paradigm during pregnancy

plasm in adults, representing one-third of primary intracranial tumors [42]. The skull base is a common location [43], and meningiomas account for 15% of nonadenomatous sellar masses [44]. They have an incidence of 5.6 per 100,000 pregnancies [45]. Specifically, tuberculum sellae meningiomas can compress the optic, abducens and oculomotor nerves, resulting in visual disturbance, or the pituitary stalk, leading to endocrine impairment [46].

It has been demonstrated that meningiomas are sensitive to a variety of hormones, including those that see major fluctuations during pregnancy. Meningioma growth is enhanced during the luteal phase of the menstrual cycle [42]. Approximately 80% of meningiomas in female patients have been found to have progesterone receptors [47]. Plasma progesterone levels rise during the second and third trimesters of pregnancy, which may contribute to meningioma growth during this period [42]. Follicle stimulating hormone and luteinizing hormone have been shown to have an inhibitory effect on tumor growth in vitro [48], so the suppression of these during pregnancy disinhibits proliferation. Curiously, human chorionic gonadotropin (hCG), which is elevated during pregnancy, has been shown to inhibit tumor growth as well [48]. The presence of prolactin receptors has been associated with meningioma growth rate [49, 50]. Human placental lactogen (hPL) has also been shown to stimulate tumor growth [42]. Prolactin and hPL are both elevated later in the course of pregnancy, which may explain associated meningioma growth during the second and third trimester [42].

Though representing only 1% of sellar masses [46], tuberculum sellae meningiomas in pregnancy are an important situation to consider. This is due to the substantial effect that the hormonal milieu of pregnancy has on tumor growth and the danger associated with rapid tumor progression. Despite the risks associated with the tumor in pregnancy, the preferred course of action is observation until delivery (Fig. 33.6) [42]. If encountered before surgery, in general we would recommend holding off on surgery in the absence of visual symptoms. Perhaps in the case of clear optic chiasm compression, even without symptoms, an upfront operation can be entertained, but these are challenging tumors to resect and the morbidity (including permanent damage to the pituitary stalk) should preclude upfront surgery in all but the most select circumstances.

If the tumor is leading to visual decline during pregnancy, corticosteroids can be considered to slow or improve symptom progression, though edema is less likely the issue as opposed to direct mass effect on the chiasm and prechiasmatic optic nerves. MRI of the pituitary region (or orbits) even without contrast can delineate the relationship of a tuberculum sella meningioma to the optic nerves. The T2 sequences can prove especially useful in the absence of contrast. In this rare circumstance of true progressive visual loss and a growing tumor on MRI, surgical intervention during pregnancy is warranted and is generally considered safe during the second and third trimesters [42].

Problems of Perfusion: Pituitary Vascular Disorders

Though not necessarily a direct consequence of sellar tumors themselves, pregnancy also increases the risk of vascular insult to the pituitary. Sheehan syndrome demonstrates the gland's heightened sensitivity as a result of changing physiologic demands. The increased metabolic activity requires increased metabolic resource utilization. A failure to adequately recruit these resources from the blood can be the result of compromised vascular supply, systemic shock, or simply overwhelming demand. In Sheehan syndrome, even a transient episode of hypoperfusion can lead to severe and lasting pituitary injury. By both threatening the vascular supply of the sella and further increasing the compartment's metabolic demands, a tumor of any kind increases the risk of such an episode.

Similarly, pituitary apoplexy can be a singular event with devastating and enduring consequences. As pregnancy increases local blood flow, the risk increases. In the setting of even a benign tumor, fragility of the vasculature increases the risk as well. Even if suspicion is low, any concern for apoplexy warrants further workup with clinical examination and possibly MRI given the potential consequences. If confirmed, it is a strong indication for immediate surgical intervention during pregnancy [51].

Conclusions

The limited volume within the sella turcica presents a uniquely perilous environment for tumor growth. Pregnancy is associated with a number of well-defined hormoal changes, which can have a profound impact on the precarious condition of pre-existing pituitary region tumors. In turn, these tumors can represent a significant threat to the pregnant mother and her fetus. Identification and appropriate management are critical to avoid complications during pregnancy. Determining the type of tumor will inform the approach to care. The management is overwhelmingly conservative, even in those tumors discovered in advance of pregnancy. Therefore, the emphasis is on increased surveillance for symptom development and medical management. Often, the goal is simply to suppress symptoms and defer more aggressive definitive treatment until after delivery. However, some cases cannot be controlled

conservatively or present a more acute hazard to the patient, especially in the setting of pituitary apoplexy. In these rare cases, surgical resection may be recommended.

Disclosures None.

References

1. Dinc H, Esen F, Demirci A, Sari A, Resit GH. Pituitary dimensions and volume measurements in pregnancy and post partum. MR assessment. Acta Radiol. 1998;39(1):64–9.
2. Frohman LA. Pituitary tumors in pregnancy. Endocrinologist. 2001;11(5):399–406.
3. Araujo PB, Vieira Neto L, Gadelha MR. Pituitary tumor management in pregnancy. Endocrinol Metab Clin N Am. 2015;44(1):181–97.
4. Stalla GK, Bost H, Stalla J, et al. Human corticotropin-releasing hormone during pregnancy. Gynecol Endocrinol. 1989;3(1):1–10.
5. Iuliano S, Laws ER Jr. Management of pituitary tumors in pregnancy. Semin Neurol. 2011;31(4):423–8.
6. Semple PL, Jane JA Jr, Laws ER Jr. Clinical relevance of precipitating factors in pituitary apoplexy. Neurosurgery. 2007;61(5):956–61; discussion 961–952.
7. Bronstein MD, Paraiba DB, Jallad RS. Management of pituitary tumors in pregnancy. Nat Rev Endocrinol. 2011;7(5):301–10.
8. Molitch ME. Pituitary tumors and pregnancy. Growth Horm IGF Res. 2003;13(Suppl A):S38–44.
9. Huang W, Molitch ME. Pituitary tumors in pregnancy. Endocrinol Metab Clin N Am. 2019;48(3):569–81.
10. Ono M, Miki N, Amano K, et al. Individualized high-dose cabergoline therapy for hyperprolactinemic infertility in women with micro- and macroprolactinomas. J Clin Endocrinol Metab. 2010;95(6):2672–9.
11. Melmed S, Casanueva FF, Hoffman AR, et al. Diagnosis and treatment of hyperprolactinemia: an Endocrine Society clinical practice guideline. J Clin Endocrinol Metab. 2011;96(2):273–88.
12. Ahmed M, Al-Dossary E, Woodhouse NJ. Macroprolactinomas with suprasellar extension: effect of bromocriptine withdrawal during one or more pregnancies. Fertil Steril. 1992;58(3):492–7.
13. Gemzell C, Wang CF. Outcome of pregnancy in women with pituitary adenoma. Fertil Steril. 1979;31(4):363–72.
14. Snyder PJ. Management of lactotroph adenoma (prolactinoma) during pregnancy. Waltham: UpToDate; 2019.
15. Molitch ME. Endocrinology in pregnancy: management of the pregnant patient with a prolactinoma. Eur J Endocrinol. 2015;172(5):R205–13.
16. Karaca Z, Tanriverdi F, Unluhizarci K, Kelestimur F. Pregnancy and pituitary disorders. Eur J Endocrinol. 2010;162(3):453–75.

17. Obstetricians ACo, Gynecologists. Guidelines for diagnostic imaging during pregnancy and lactation: committee opinion no. 723. Obstet Gynecol. 2017;130:e210–6.

18. Almalki MH, Alzahrani S, Alshahrani F, et al. Managing prolactinomas during pregnancy. Front Endocrinol. 2015;6:85.

19. Lebbe M, Hubinont C, Bernard P, Maiter D. Outcome of 100 pregnancies initiated under treatment with cabergoline in hyperprolactinaemic women. Clin Endocrinol. 2010;73(2):236–42.

20. Domingue ME, Devuyst F, Alexopoulou O, Corvilain B, Maiter D. Outcome of prolactinoma after pregnancy and lactation: a study on 73 patients. Clin Endocrinol. 2014;80(5):642–8.

21. Auriemma RS, Perone Y, Di Sarno A, et al. Results of a single-center observational 10-year survey study on recurrence of hyperprolactinemia after pregnancy and lactation. J Clin Endocrinol Metab. 2013;98(1):372–9.

22. Bronstein MD, Salgado LR, de Castro Musolino NR. Medical management of pituitary adenomas: the special case of management of the pregnant woman. Pituitary. 2002;5(2):99–107.

23. Molitch ME. Pregnancy and the hyperprolactinemic woman. N Engl J Med. 1985;312(21):1364–70.

24. Laway BA, Mir SA. Pregnancy and pituitary disorders: challenges in diagnosis and management. Indian J Endocrinol Metab. 2013;17(6):996–1004.

25. Buescher MA, McClamrock HD, Adashi EY. Cushing syndrome in pregnancy. Obstet Gynecol. 1992;79(1):130–7.

26. Nieman LK. Diagnosis and management of Cushing's syndrome during pregnancy. Waltham: UpToDate; 2020.

27. Newell-Price J, Bertagna X, Grossman AB, Nieman LK. Cushing's syndrome. Lancet. 2006;367(9522):1605–17.

28. Lindsay JR, Jonklaas J, Oldfield EH, Nieman LK. Cushing's syndrome during pregnancy: personal experience and review of the literature. J Clin Endocrinol Metab. 2005;90(5):3077–83.

29. Lindsay JR, Nieman LK. The hypothalamic-pituitary-adrenal axis in pregnancy: challenges in disease detection and treatment. Endocr Rev. 2005;26(6):775–99.

30. Bevan JS, Gough MH, Gillmer MD, Burke CW. Cushing's syndrome in pregnancy: the timing of definitive treatment. Clin Endocrinol. 1987;27(2):225–33.

31. Woo I, Ehsanipoor RM. Cabergoline therapy for Cushing disease throughout pregnancy. Obstet Gynecol. 2013;122(2 Pt 2):485–7.

32. Kupersmith MJ, Rosenberg C, Kleinberg D. Visual loss in pregnant women with pituitary adenomas. Ann Intern Med. 1994;121(7):473–7.

33. Okada Y, Morimoto I, Ejima K, et al. A case of active acromegalic woman with a marked increase in serum insulin-like growth factor-1 levels after delivery. Endocr J. 1997;44(1):117–20.

34. Caron P, Broussaud S, Bertherat J, et al. Acromegaly and pregnancy: a retrospective multicenter study of 59 pregnancies in 46 women. J Clin Endocrinol Metab. 2010;95(10):4680–7.

35. Beck-Peccoz P, Lania A, Beckers A, Chatterjee K, Wemeau JL. 2013 European thyroid association guidelines for the diagnosis and treatment of thyrotropin-secreting pituitary tumors. Eur Thyroid J. 2013;2(2):76–82.

36. Perdomo CM, Arabe JA, Idoate MA, Galofre JC. Management of a pregnant woman with thyrotropinoma: a case report and review of the literature. Gynecol Endocrinol. 2017;33(3):188–92.

37. Bolz M, Korber S, Schober HC. TSH secreting adenoma of pituitary gland (TSHom)—rare cause of hyperthyroidism in pregnancy. Dtsch Med Wochenschr. 2013;138(8):362–6.

38. Caron P, Gerbeau C, Pradayrol L, Simonetta C, Bayard F. Successful pregnancy in an infertile woman with a thyrotropin-secreting macroadenoma treated with somatostatin analog (octreotide). J Clin Endocrinol Metab. 1996;81(3):1164–8.

39. Blackhurst G, Strachan MW, Collie D, Gregor A, Statham PF, Seckl JE. The treatment of a thyrotropin-secreting pituitary macroadenoma with octreotide in twin pregnancy. Clin Endocrinol. 2002;57(3):401–4.

40. Chaiamnuay S, Moster M, Katz MR, Kim YN. Successful management of a pregnant woman with a TSH secreting pituitary adenoma with surgical and medical therapy. Pituitary. 2003;6(2):109–13.

41. Masding M, Lees P, Gawne-Cain M, Sandeman D. Visual field compression by a non-secreting pituitary tumour during pregnancy. J R Soc Med. 2003;96:27–8.

42. Hortobagyi T, Bencze J, Murnyak B, Kouhsari MC, Bognar L, Marko-Varga G. Pathophysiology of meningioma growth in pregnancy. Open Med. 2017;12:195–200.

43. Kanaan I, Jallu A, Kanaan H. Management strategy for meningioma in pregnancy: a clinical study. Skull Base. 2003;13(4):197–203.

44. Famini P, Maya MM, Melmed S. Pituitary magnetic resonance imaging for sellar and parasellar masses: ten-year experience in 2598 patients. J Clin Endocrinol Metab. 2011;96(6):1633–41.

45. Dumitrescu BC, Tataranu LG, Gorgan MR. Pregnant woman with an intracranial meningioma-case report and review of the literature. Rom Neurosurg. 2014;21(4):489.

46. Kwancharoen R, Blitz AM, Tavares F, Caturegli P, Gallia GL, Salvatori R. Clinical features of sellar and suprasellar meningiomas. Pituitary. 2014;17(4):342–8.

47. Carroll RS, Glowacka D, Dashner K, Black PM. Progesterone receptor expression in meningiomas. Cancer Res. 1993;53(6):1312–6.

48. Boyle-Walsh E, Shenkin A, White MC, Fraser WD. Effect of glycoprotein and protein hormones on human meningioma cell proliferation in vitro. J Endocrinol. 1995;145(1):155–61.

49. Carroll RS, Schrell UM, Zhang J, et al. Dopamine D1, dopamine D2, and prolactin receptor messenger ribonucleic acid expression by the polymerase chain reaction in human meningiomas. Neurosurgery. 1996;38(2):367–75.

50. Jimenez-Hakim E, el-Azouzi M, Black PM. The effect of prolactin and bombesin on the growth of meningioma-derived cells in monolayer culture. J Neuro-Oncol. 1993;16(3):185–90.

51. Luger A, Broersen LHA, Biermasz NR, et al. ESE clinical practice guideline on functioning and non-functioning pituitary adenomas in pregnancy. Eur J Endocrinol. 2021;185(3):G1–G33.

Chiari Malformation and Pregnancy

Katherine G. Holste and Karin M. Muraszko

Introduction

Chiari malformation type 1 (CM) is defined as cerebellar tonsillar herniation of 5 mm or more through the foramen magnum. The prevalence is about 0.8–3.7% in children and 0.24–0.9% in adults [1]. As more and more MRIs are being completed for various reasons, CM is increasingly identified, although only a fraction is symptomatic [1, 2]. Syringomyelia may occur in 25–50% of patients with CM and may be an indication that there is aberrant cerebrospinal fluid (CSF) flow dynamics due to crowding at the foramen magnum [3, 4]. There is an increasing incidence of CM decompression surgery (CMD) in both the pediatric and adult populations [1]. As more patients with CM are identified, some incidentally, and more patients are undergoing CMD, neurosurgeons are increasingly asked about the safety of pregnancy and labor in these patients. Unfortunately, most of the evidence in the literature is based on two large database reviews [1, 5], a few retrospective reviews [3, 6, 7], case series/reports [8, 9], and expert opinion [10]. The lack of prospective analyses is an impediment to critical appraisal and informed counseling. In this

chapter we will discuss the peripartum management of patients with CM with and without syringomyelia Fig. 34.1.

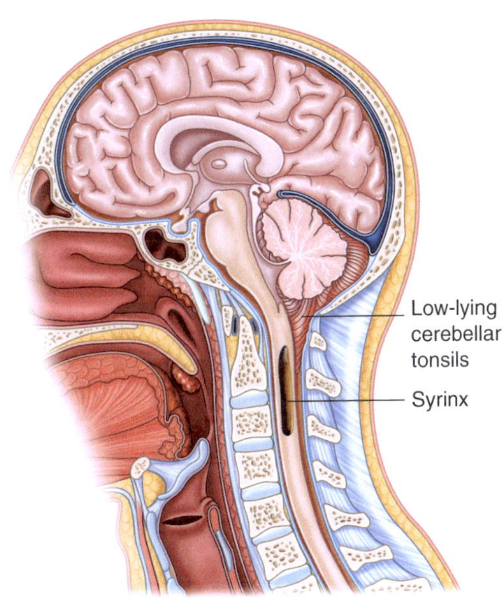

Fig. 34.1 Chiari malformation is defined as at least 5 mm of cerebellar tonsillar ectopia below the level of the foramen magnum and may be associated with a syrinx, a fluid filled cavity in the spinal cord

K. G. Holste (✉) · K. M. Muraszko
Department of Neurosurgery, University of Michigan, Ann Arbor, MI, USA
e-mail: karinm@med.umich.edu

Preconception Counseling

One of the more common questions from parents with CM is whether they will pass this along to their child. Most cases of CM are thought to be sporadic. There is some evidence, using twin-twin studies, that demonstrate a higher concordance of CM in monozygotic twins compared to dizygotic twins, but were discordant for other factors such as presence of a syrinx or severity of tonsillar herniation or symptoms [11–13]. There are also reports of familial aggregation or clustering of CM. In 31 families in which 2 or more had CM, 21% of asymptomatic first degree relatives also had CM [14]. In another study of 500 pediatric patients undergoing CMD, 3% had a positive family history of CM [15], suggesting a higher prevalence of CM in those families than that of the general population, about 1 in 1280 or 0.078% [11]. Conversely, familial history of CM may lead to more MRIs obtained in even relatively asymptomatic patients. Inheritance of CM is likely polygenic, complex, and affected by environmental factors and therefore making predictions is challenging.

Patients with CM are also more likely to have other bony or connective tissue developmental problems. Examples include Ehlers Danlos syndrome, Klippel-Feil anomaly, tethered cord, and achondroplasia to name a few [10]. This is because CM is thought to be a disorder of bony and connective tissue during fetal development leading to the tonsillar herniation seen on imaging. In a prospective study of patients with CM, 5% had a hereditary disorder of connective tissue as well [16]. Patients with severe kyphosis due to connective tissue disorders may require pulmonary function evaluation before proceeding with general anesthesia [4]. General principles of preconception counseling are discussed in Chap. 1.

Pregnancy Management

Most women with CM do not experience any change in their symptoms during pregnancy. In one study of 51 deliveries, 21 women had chronic

Table 34.1 Development of symptoms during labor is rare in women with CM, but appears to be more common in women who have an associated syrinx

Patient characteristics	Symptoms during labor
With CMD	Rare
Without CMD	Uncommon, but usually worse tussive headache
With syrinx	Uncommon, but includes headache, numbness, weakness

headaches prior to pregnancy and there was no report of worsening headaches during pregnancy, delivery, or postpartum [6]. Conversely, there was actually improvement of chronic headaches during pregnancy in some women. In one case series, 4 out of 7 women endorsed improvement in their chronic headaches during the second and third trimesters [17]. Worsening of neurologic symptoms during labor is reported rarely in the literature. In untreated women, those who had not undergone CMD, the most common symptom was worsened tussive headache [6]. Women with CM and a syrinx more commonly reported new or worsened neurologic symptoms during labor, including headache, numbness, and weakness, but even this appears to be uncommon (Table 34.1) [3].

Method of Delivery

A trial of natural childbirth is not contraindicated in women with treated or untreated CM. There have been many reports of women successfully delivering vaginally [6, 7, 9, 17–19]. In women who are asymptomatic or incidentally diagnosed, some experts propose that vaginal delivery is the method of choice unless there are obstetric concerns [20]. The main concern raised about vaginal delivery in the setting of CM is the potential for increasing ICPs during labor in patients with already elevated ICPs. Rarely, CM can be associated with increased ICP and it is unclear whether ICP is the cause of the CM or a result of the CM.

Valsalva maneuver can increase spinal fluid pressures. In a study of CSF pressure during delivery-related Valsalva, CSF pressures increased by 20–51 mmHg, from a basal pressure of around 13 mmHg. During the second and third stages of labor, when most of the bearing down occurred, there was an overall increase of 8 mmHg in CSF pressures [4]. For women who have elevated basal ICPs from CM, that small increase in CSF pressure during the second stage of labor could theoretically be the tipping point for further herniation and a devastating neurologic outcome. Some argue that the elevation in ICP is temporary and the risks mentioned above are only theoretical, as few patients in the literature are symptomatic from high ICPs during delivery [6]. In one multicenter retrospective review of 185 deliveries in 148 patients, 43% underwent vaginal delivery without any catastrophic neurologic complication [7]. To mitigate that theoretical risk, similar to patients with shunted hydrocephalus, some obstetricians recommend against prolonged second stage of labor and for instrument assisted delivery [9, 21]. Unfortunately for obstetricians, neurosurgeons, and anesthesiologists, there is a lack of evidence-based guidelines and no uniform recommendations.

There have been a few retrospective reviews and large database studies examining the outcomes of vaginal delivery in patients with CM. The safety of delivery in women who had undergone prior CMD has been documented in case reports and case series [4, 17, 22]. One could argue that patients who have had their CM treated have restored normal CSF flow by removing the crowding of the posterior fossa and eliminating the theoretic risk of neurologic complications. Safety of vaginal delivery in the untreated CM population is supported in the larger studies. In a cohort of patients who delivered before their diagnosis of CM, 14 vaginal deliveries were performed without complication or symptoms of worsening ICPs [18]. In a cohort of 63 women who had not undergone CMD, none of the patients who delivered vaginally had evidence of elevated ICPs or new or worsened neurologic deficits. The size of cerebellar tonsillar herniation in patients who delivered vaginally varied up to 19 mm [6]. Finally, in another retrospective study of 21 women and 23 pregnancies, 65% had a vaginal delivery, without neurological complications [19].

Patients who had prior CMD had similar outcomes to those who were untreated. Wilkinson et al. examined US medical records for 1048 deliveries in 866 women with CM. Of the 103 deliveries in women who had a CMD at any time point, 66 deliveries occurred prior to surgery and 37 after surgery. Interestingly, only 4 (7%) of those patients that went on to have CMD after their delivery even had a diagnosis of CM before delivery. The patients that were symptomatic enough to require surgical intervention had successful deliveries prior to their diagnosis. There were no cases or serious maternal morbidity or mortality in any of the 103 deliveries [2]. This finding is supported in other primary literature as well [19]. Vaginal delivery is possible in women with CM, especially so in patients with a prior CMD, without report of catastrophic neurologic decline, symptoms of elevated ICPs or new or worsening neurologic symptoms during delivery.

Most, but not all, experts agree that a successful vaginal delivery is possible, but in untreated women or symptomatic patients, obstetricians argue for a low threshold for performing a cesarean (C)-section if vaginal delivery is expected to be difficult, prolonged, or complicated [10, 19, 20]. Worsening ICPs or new neurologic symptoms are rare in the literature and appear to be more common in women with an associated syrinx [3, 19]. The most common reason for C-section in one cohort of CM patients was prior C-section or other obstetrical reason, followed by neurosurgical or neurologic recommendation in 21% of cases [7]. Physician recommendation for C-Section was based on the size of tonsillar herniation, presence of a syrinx and at times presence of CM alone [6]. This conflicts with the findings of the Waters study, in which there was no difference in size of tonsillar herniation or patient characteristics in women who were recommended to have a C-section and those who underwent vaginal delivery [6]. This conflict is indicative of the variability of physician comfort in treating women with CM and lack of guidelines.

Two nationwide studies on inpatient samples for women with CM admitted for delivery demonstrated they were more likely to deliver by C-section than women without CM [2, 5]. The Wilkinson study included 400 deliveries after diagnosis of CM and 648 before diagnosis of CM. In patients with a known history of CM, the rate of C-section was higher than those who had not yet been diagnosed (42.3 compared to 36.2%) [2]. The higher rate of C-section among mothers with CM was also demonstrated in 1280 deliveries examined in another nationwide inpatient sample [5]. The diagnosis of CM appears to bias clinicians in favor of recommending or performing a C-section.

Anesthesia

The safety of performing neuraxial anesthesia in women with CM has been debated in the literature. Much of the fear of herniation or worsening symptoms of increased ICPs are based on three early cases (Table 34.2). One patient who underwent spinal anesthesia prior to their diagnosis of CM developed recurrent headaches with vision changes not responsive to an epidural blood patch. On further workup she was found to have a CM and her headache resolved after 6 weeks of prednisone. Continuous spinal anesthesia was used in another woman leading to worsening headache that resolved after an epidural blood patch. Finally, one woman with CM developed

headaches and gait instability 1 year after accidental dural puncture during an epidural [4, 18]. These cases lead to the idea that neuraxial anesthesia may be contraindicated in CM patients, as any egress of CSF would lead to changes in the cranial and spinal compartment pressures and cause further cerebellar herniation. Since then there have been numerous reports of safe use of both spinal and epidural anesthesia [6, 18, 19] in patients before or after diagnosis of CM [18]. Outside of case reports, two larger studies support this claim. In one single center study of women with untreated CM, neuraxial anesthesia was used in 62 deliveries, 38 epidurals, and 24 spinals without signs of increased ICPs or neurologic complications [6]. In another multicenter retrospective review of 185 deliveries, 73% underwent neuraxial anesthesia without report of any catastrophic neurologic complications, although 3 did have a positional headache afterward [7].

The choice between epidural and spinal anesthesia appears to be clinician dependent. Epidural anesthesia has been used successfully in the literature, even in women with syrinxes, without a change in symptoms [9, 10, 17, 18, 21, 23]. There are two main considerations in the use of epidural anesthesia: accidental dural puncture and elevation of ICPs caused by epidural bolus of anesthetic. Epidural anesthesia should be performed with caution to avoid dural puncture given the larger size of the needle. If patients become symptomatic with positional headaches, then epidural blood patch should be performed immediately so as not to obscure any CM related symptoms surrounding labor and delivery [10]. Epidural boluses of anesthesia can increase ICPs, ranging from 6 to 39 mmHg, thought to be due to the rapid deformation of the thecal sac after a bolus. This abrupt rise in ICP can be minimized when the bolus volume is halved, which increases ICP by 5 mmHg instead, and can be further mitigated with a slower rate of administration [4, 9]. In the case of spinal anesthesia, although one purposefully enters into the intrathecal space, it is performed with a smaller needle and the space is usually only accessed once so the amount of CSF that leaves the space is very small [8]. The use of

Table 34.2 Three historical cases in the literature which were thought to indicate that neuraxial anesthesia was contraindicated in CM. Subsequently there have been numerous cases of safe use of neuraxial anesthesia

Patient characteristics	Type of anesthesia	Outcome
Undiagnosed CM	Spinal	Recurrent headaches and vision changes refractory to epidural blood patch. Later diagnosed with CM
Undiagnosed CM	Spinal	Headache, resolved after epidural blood patch
Diagnosed CM	Epidural with accidental dural puncture	Headaches and gait instability for 1 year after epidural

spinal anesthesia is less common than epidural in women with CM; 50% underwent epidurals compared to 39% spinal in one study [7]. In women who have not had CMD, single access spinal anesthesia has been used successfully [3, 18, 19, 23]. If there is a spinal fluid leak, then epidural blood patch should be performed immediately for the same reasons detailed above [10].

General anesthesia is preferred when patients are showing symptoms of elevated ICPs, although this is rare in laboring patients with CM [3, 19]. General anesthesia can avoid the risk of dural puncture in symptomatic patients with the added benefit of controlling the airway and blood pressure if patients do decompensate. Conversely, laryngeal manipulation and endotracheal intubation can lead to abrupt increases in ICPs; therefore, some authors prefer awake fiberoptic intubation or rapid sequence intubation [4, 22]. When performing general anesthesia, extreme and prolonged neck extension should be avoided as patients with CM can have comorbidities such as Ehlers Danlos syndrome and cranio-cervical instability [10]. Overall, use of general anesthesia for increased ICPs is rare in the literature in this population with the exception in few cases of patients with CM and syringomyelia which will be discussed below.

Syringomyelia

Patients with CM can have concomitant syringomyelia in up to 25–50% of cases [21]. The presence of a syrinx is likely due to impaired spinal fluid dynamics from obstruction of the foramen magnum which can either force fluid through the obex into the central canal or through the perivascular spaces into a syrinx [3]. The presence of a syrinx in patients with CM indicates that the crowding of the foramen magnum is significant, and the syrinx is usually resolved with CMD [24]. Symptoms of syringomyelia include weakness, burning pain in the neck, back, or extremities, paresthesias, or referred chest pain. In patients with CM and a large syrinx, Bolognese et al. recommend repeat MRI of the spine around the 25th week to see if the syrinx has increased in size. If it has enlarged or if the patient has new or worsening symptoms of syringomyelia, then they recommend early delivery and CMD based on their expert experience at two multidisciplinary centers [10]. Conversely, no other authors recommend repeat imaging of the spine during pregnancy [3, 4, 17, 21] unless the patient is symptomatic.

Most of the outcome data on women with CM and syringomyelia were limited to case reports and case series with little conclusions drawn until a recent systematic review [3]. Their cohort consisted of 39 patients with syringomyelia, 21 of which were due to CM. Of the 43 total deliveries, 30 were delivered by C-section and the most common reason sited was to avoid Valsalva and aggravation of the syrinx. Six of the 13 vaginal deliveries were instrumented to prevent prolonged second stage of labor. General anesthesia was most commonly used in 21 of the 30 C-sections as neuraxial anesthesia was thought to possibly cause neurologic worsening. There were 5 patients who had worsening of neurologic symptoms prior to delivery thought to be due to worsening ICPs [3]. Of the cases of worsened neurologic symptoms during delivery, headaches, paresthesias, numbness, and weakness were most commonly cited. In most cases, the symptoms resolved within 24 h of delivery via C-section [3, 4, 19, 21]. Cases of worsening neurologic symptoms are rare in the CM literature but appear to be more common when there is a concomitant syrinx.

Data on vaginal delivery for women with CM and syringomyelia is limited. In the above systematic review, the cohort of women with CM associated syringomyelia was too small to draw meaningful conclusions [3]. In the few cases reported in the literature vaginal delivery appeared to be successful with epidural anesthesia. [6, 17, 21, 23] In one case, passive second stage of labor was performed without complication [21]. One woman with a large syrinx had worsening upper extremity numbness tingling, muscle jerks, and tinnitus during the third trimester which resolved after vaginal delivery [17]. The reason for this limited amount of data is likely related to the preference for clinicians to recommend or perform C-section when someone with CM has a syrinx [6, 19]. Therefore, it is difficult to assess how safe vaginal delivery is in this population.

Postpartum Care

Data on postpartum outcomes in women with CM is extremely limited. Most of the data focuses instead on delivery method and use of anesthetic. In the Orth database study, women with CM were 2.2 times more likely to develop severe medical complications including respiratory distress syndrome, stroke, CVA, sepsis, or seizures. They were also more likely to present with preeclampsia or eclampsia. The reasoning behind this is unknown [5]. This directly conflicts with the Wilkinson study which reported a severe morbidity rate of 0.9% in CM patients; no different than patients without CM [2]. Neonatal outcomes were reported as good, without complications, in a few case reports as well as the systematic review of patients with syringomyelia [3, 17, 21]. Ultimately, the postpartum outcomes of women with CM remain poorly understood. Neonatal outcomes appear to be good, from the limited data available, although no real conclusions can be drawn.

Conclusion

The incidence of CM diagnosis has been increasing over time with the use of MRI along with an increasing rate of CMD. As such, more women with CM are becoming pregnant and delivering. There are no evidence-based guidelines for obstetricians, anesthesiologists, and neurosurgeons to rely on which further complicates the care of women with CM. Overall, it is rare in the literature for women with CM to have worsening symptoms of elevated ICPs during labor but appears to be more common when a syrinx is present. Vaginal delivery is not contraindicated and is preferred if there are no obstetric complications and no symptoms of elevated ICPs. Neuraxial anesthesia can also be used, at the discretion of the anesthesiologist, with very few reports of neurologic complications.

References

1. Wilkinson DA, Johnson K, Garton HJ, Muraszko KM, Maher CO. Trends in surgical treatment of Chiari malformation type I in the United States. J Neurosurg Pediatr. 2017;19(2):208–16.
2. Wilkinson DA, Johnson K, Castaneda PR, et al. Obstetric management and maternal outcomes of childbirth among patients with Chiari malformation type I. Neurosurgery. 2019;87:45.
3. Garvey GP, Wasade VS, Murphy KE, Balki M. Anesthetic and obstetric Management of syringomyelia during Labor and delivery: a case series and systematic review. Anesth Analg. 2017;125(3):913–24.
4. Ghaly RF, Tverdohleb T, Candido KD, Knezevic NN. Management of parturients in active labor with Arnold Chiari malformation, tonsillar herniation, and syringomyelia. Surg Neurol Int. 2017;8:10.
5. Orth T, Gerkovich M, Babbar S, Porter B, Lu G. 716: maternal and pregnancy complications among women with Arnold Chiari malformation: a national database review. Am J Obstet Gynecol. 2015;212(1):S349.
6. Waters JFR, O'Neal MA, Pilato M, Waters S, Larkin JC, Waters JH. Management of Anesthesia and Delivery in women with Chiari I malformations. Obstet Gynecol. 2018;132(5):1180–4.
7. Gruffi TR, Peralta FM, Thakkar MS, et al. Anesthetic management of parturients with Arnold Chiari malformation-I: a multicenter retrospective study. Int J Obstet Anesth. 2019;37:52–6.
8. Landau R, Giraud R, Delrue V, Kern C. Spinal anesthesia for cesarean delivery in a woman with a surgically corrected type I Arnold Chiari malformation. Anesth Analg. 2003;97(1):253–5. table of contents.
9. Semple DA, McClure JH. Arnold-Chiari malformation in pregnancy. Anaesthesia. 1996;51(6):580–2.
10. Bolognese PA, Kula RW, Onesti ST. Chiari I malformation and delivery. Surg Neurol Int. 2017;8:12.
11. Capra V, Iacomino M, Accogli A, et al. Chiari malformation type I: what information from the genetics? Childs Nerv Syst. 2019;35(10):1665–71.
12. Stovner LJ, Cappelen J, Nilsen G, Sjaastad O. The Chiari type I malformation in two monozygotic twins and first-degree relatives. Ann Neurol. 1992;31(2):220–2.
13. Turgut M. Chiari type I malformation in two monozygotic twins. Br J Neurosurg. 2001;15(3):279–80.
14. Speer MC, George TM, Enterline DS, Franklin A, Wolpert CM, Milhorat TH. A genetic hypothesis for Chiari I malformation with or without syringomyelia. Neurosurg Focus. 2000;8(3):E12.

15. Small JA, Sheridan PH. Research priorities for syringomyelia: a National Institute of Neurological Disorders and Stroke workshop summary. Neurology. 1996;46(2):577–82.
16. Thomas HM, Paolo AB, Misao N, Nazli BM, Clair AF. Syndrome of occipitoatlantoaxial hypermobility, cranial settling, and Chiari malformation type I in patients with hereditary disorders of connective tissue. J Neurosurg. 2007;7(6):601–9.
17. Mueller DM, Oro J. Chiari I malformation with or without syringomyelia and pregnancy: case studies and review of the literature. Am J Perinatol. 2005;22(2):67–70.
18. Chantigian RC, Koehn MA, Ramin KD, Warner MA. Chiari I malformation in parturients. J Clin Anesth. 2002;14(3):201–5.
19. Roper JC, Al Wattar BH, Silva AHD, Samarasekera S, Flint G, Pirie AM. Management and birth outcomes of pregnant women with Chiari malformations: a 14 years retrospective case series. Eur J Obstet Gynecol Reprod Biol. 2018;230:1–5.
20. Agrawal A, Moscote-Salazar LR, Gomez-Rhenals E, Garcia-Ballestas E. Letter: obstetric management and maternal outcomes of childbirth among patients with Chiari malformation type I. Neurosurgery. 2020;86(5):E473.
21. Parker JD, Broberg JC, Napolitano PG. Maternal Arnold-Chiari type I malformation and syringomyelia: a labor management dilemma. Am J Perinatol. 2002;19(8):445–50.
22. Sicuranza GB, Steinberg P, Figueroa R. Arnold-Chiari malformation in a pregnant woman. Obstet Gynecol. 2003;102(5 Pt 2):1191–4.
23. Choi CK, Tyagaraj K. Combined spinal-epidural analgesia for laboring parturient with Arnold-Chiari type I malformation: a case report and a review of the literature. Case Rep Anesthesiol. 2013;2013:512915.
24. Chotai S, Chan EW, Ladner TR, et al. Timing of syrinx reduction and stabilization after posterior fossa decompression for pediatric Chiari malformation type I. J Neurosurg Pediatrics. 2020;26:1–7.

Katherine G. Holste and Karin M. Muraszko

Introduction

Neural tube defects (NTD)s are one of the most common birth defects and occur in 1 in 1000 live births worldwide [1]. Spina bifida, a large portion of NTDs, can be further divided into spina bifida occulta (SBO), failure of fusion of the vertebral arch without exposure of the neural elements, and spina bifida cystica, a midline defect in which the neural elements are exposed. Myelomeningocele (MMC) makes up a majority of spina bifida cystica cases. As the treatment of MMC has advanced over time, women are more frequently living to childbearing age [2]. In fact, live births in women with MMC have been increasing dramatically within the last 15 years [2]. Unfortunately, since the first published case report in 1973, the data on women with SBO and MMC is limited to case series and a couple of national database reviews [2–4]. The recommendations for management are therefore based on the limited data and expert opinion. Having SBO or MMC is not a contraindication for pregnancy. In fact, many women with MMC have had successful pregnancies and deliveries, but there are unique considerations of which clinicians and patients should be aware

[4, 5]. In this chapter we will discuss the peripartum management of women with spina bifida, focusing primarily on MMC.

Preconception Counseling

Patients with MMC have a variety of neurologic and non-neurologic comorbidities as a result of their open NTD during fetal development. Based on the level of their defect, patients will have differing function in their lower extremities, bladder, and bowels. They may also have Chiari II malformations and shunt dependent hydrocephalus [6]. As such, preconception counseling needs to be tailored to the individual with considerations of these factors (Table 35.1). Currently, there is no compelling evidence to suggest patients with MMC have an increased risk of miscarriage. One study of mothers with shunted hydrocephalus reported that 12 of their 32 reported miscarriages were in three mothers with MMC, but this is too small of a cohort to draw any generalizable conclusions [7]. Unfortunately, most of the large cohort studies are based on patients with MMC admitted to hospitals for delivery, which excludes miscarriages and spontaneous abortions [2, 8].

Part of preconception counseling in MMC is the recurrence rate of NTDs in the fetus. The recurrence rate according to the literature is about 1–5% if one parent is affected and up to 15% if

K. G. Holste · K. M. Muraszko (✉)
Department of Neurosurgery, University of Michigan, Ann Arbor, MI, USA
e-mail: karinm@med.umich.edu

© The Author(s), under exclusive license to Springer Nature Switzerland AG 2023
G. Gupta et al. (eds.), *Neurological Disorders in Pregnancy*,
https://doi.org/10.1007/978-3-031-36490-7_35

Table 35.1 Preconception and prepartum risks in patients with MMC as well as potential management strategies. Patient specific considerations should be taken into account

Risk	Management strategies
Increased risk of NTDs	High dose daily folic acid preconception and until 12th week of pregnancy
Use of AEDs	Discussion with neurologist to ideally be on the lowest effective dose of a non-teratogenic agent
Maternal obesity	Encourage to lose weight before conception
Increased risk of UTIs and renal damage	Involvement from urology may need screening renal function testing and treatment of asymptomatic bacteriuria
Kyphoscoliosis	May obtain pulmonary function tests and echocardiogram to assess pulmonary impact during pregnancy
Hypertension	Medical management of hypertension similar to women without MMC
Shunted hydrocephalus	Higher index of suspicion for shunt malfunction or failure

both parents are affected. The inheritance of MMC is controversial and it is thought to be multifactorial in origin with influence of environmental and multiple genetic factors. There is not a single gene attributed to MMC, but the most common genes are those related to folate homocysteine metabolism and are thought to be inherited in an autosomal dominant manner with reduced penetrance [1, 9]. In order to reduce the risk of a NTD in the offspring, 5 mg of folic acid daily taken prior to pregnancy is recommended for mothers with a personal history of NTD or who have had a baby with a NTD [9]. Previous randomized control trials have demonstrated the effectiveness of folic acid supplementation in this population with one study demonstrating 72% reduction in NTD cases in women with a previously affected fetus given 4 mg of folic acid daily [10]. This supplementation should be started 3 months before conception and should be continued until the 12th week of pregnancy [9]. This is especially important if the patient is on certain antiepileptic drugs (AEDs; discussed in detail in Chap. 28).

Another aspect of caring for these patients involves further mitigating their risk of adverse maternal and fetal outcomes. About 12% of patients with MMC have epilepsy and as such they will be on AEDs [11]. Ideally, they should be on the lowest effective dose of a single, non-teratogenic agent. Patients with diabetes, regardless of a NTD, are at increased risk of fetal malformations of the central nervous system. Diabetic control should be optimized preconception to help reduce this risk [9]. Finally, maternal obesity alone increases the risk of fetal NTD by 1.9–3.5 times [12]. Patients with MMC are 50% more likely to be obese than the general population, likely in part due to reduced mobility [13]. Antenatal and intrapartum complications are increased two to three fold by maternal obesity [9]. Patients should be encouraged to lose weight, if possible, before conception to reduce their maternal and fetal risks.

Pregnancy Management

Managing Comorbidities

Patients with MMC can have many comorbidities outside of neurologic deficits such as bladder/bowel dysfunction, kyphoscoliosis, and other orthopedic complications. Neurogenic bladder is a very common chronic problem in patients with MMC [6]. Their risk of urinary tract infections (UTIs) and renal damage from hydronephrosis is well documented in the literature. This risk is particularly elevated during pregnancy. The reason for this is multifactorial: prostaglandins and hormones during pregnancy decrease ureter peristalsis causing urine stasis and the gravid uterus causes mechanical obstruction [8, 9]. Recurrent UTIs are associated with low birth weight and preterm delivery [14]. Some authors recommend obtaining baseline renal function and then screening regularly throughout pregnancy as well as performing regular urinalysis [5]. This is clinically supported by data demonstrating that treatment of asymptomatic bacteriuria in pregnant patients was beneficial and reduced the risk of symptomatic UTI, low birth weight, and preterm delivery in a meta-analysis [14]. Some patients with MMC require frequent intermittent straight catheterization which does have an increased risk of UTIs associated with it as well. Other patients will have urinary diversion procedures or bladder augmentation complicating their intraabdominal anatomy [5].

Kyphoscoliosis in MMC ranges in its severity and its effect on pregnancy is multifactorial. Historically, kyphoscoliosis had been a contraindication for pregnancy due to risk of cardiopulmonary compromise, but continued evidence refutes this claim and shows that women with kyphoscoliosis can have safe pregnancies and deliveries [15]. In the more severe cases, mechanical restriction of the ribcage causes reduced lung volumes, diminished forced vital capacity, right heart strain, and remodeling [15]. Adding in the gravid uterus diminishes the pulmonary function further. In this case, the clinician may opt to obtain pulmonary function tests and an echocardiogram during pregnancy to assess the impact. Patients may need positive pressure ventilation to improve oxygen saturations, especially overnight [9]. From a biomechanics standpoint, kyphoscoliosis reduces the volume of the abdominal and pelvic cavity causing fetal growth restriction [5]. Some authors recommend obtaining more frequent growth ultrasounds due to potential compression of the fetus. It can also reduce the pelvic outlet, making vaginal delivery more difficult, if not impossible [5].

Patients with MMC are also more likely to have hypertension at a younger age. They have a 6% increase in risk of hypertension, especially in the fourth decade of life. This may be due to longstanding renal disease or obesity [16]. Medical management of hypertension is similar to that in other pregnant women. There is also a theoretical increase in risk of deep vein thrombosis, especially in pregnant patients who are immobile. There is no consensus on upfront prophylaxis, but the general recommendations are screening with deep vein ultrasound and prophylactic anticoagulation if the patient is immobile and has multiple risk factors [9, 17]. A significant portion of the MMC population

have shunted hydrocephalus. Women with shunts are more likely to experience shunt malfunction or failure requiring revision during the peripartum period [7]. For more information on that subject, see the chapter on hydrocephalus and pregnancy (Chap. 36).

Mode of Delivery

Having MMC is not a contraindication for vaginal delivery. There have been a number of reported successful vaginal deliveries in mothers with MMC and SBO [4, 18, 19]. Two of the largest studies on a nationwide database examining delivery outcomes in women with MMC were performed by Shepard et al. [2, 8]. They examined the United States Healthcare Cost and Utilization's National Inpatient Sample comparing 10,147 deliveries from women with MMC and SBO to 42 million deliveries among women without a NTD. About 1/3 of their cohort had SBO and 18% had MMC with shunted hydrocephalus. They found only 43.8% of women with MMC or SBO had normal vaginal deliveries compared to 62.4% in women without NTD [2]. When separating the two populations, patients with SBO were more likely to have a normal vaginal delivery, whereas those with MMC and those with hydrocephalus in particular, had higher rates of cesarean (C)-section (64.3% had C-section compared to the national average of 31.9%). In another large Canadian study by Auger et al. examining 397 women with MMC and 720 births, women with MMC were twice as likely to have a C-section [3]. Having paraplegia does not immediately subject a woman to a C-section. Robertson et al. reported successful vaginal delivery in 26 women with paraplegia due to a mix of trauma and congenital causes with lesions above the tenth thoracic level [20]. Of the 39 deliveries in this series, 21 were delivered normally, 15 required instrument assistance, and 3 required C-section for obstetric reasons. The group argued that though the innervation of the uterus was disrupted, it still had polarizing contractions [20]. In women with paraplegia, there may be a reduced ability to bear down resulting in need for instrument assistance to achieve safe, efficient vaginal delivery [3, 5, 9].

In the obstetric literature, vaginal delivery is preferred over C-section for women with MMC [2, 19]. C-section may be required for typical obstetrical complications such as fetal distress or failure of progression of labor. Malposition and obstruction of labor were common indications for C-section in the MMC and spinal cord injury population [17, 20]. Uniquely in the MMC population, vaginal delivery may not be indicated for women with small pelvic inlets due to kyphoscoliosis, severe contractures in the lower extremities or shunt complications including existing elevated intracranial pressure [2, 5]. C-section can put a ventriculoperitoneal shunt at risk of infection or damage [18]. Also, women with MMC may have had multiple intraabdominal procedures such as ileal or bladder augmentation which can make a C-section complicated by adhesions or complex anatomy [4, 5, 18]. In a few of the reported cases, damage to patients' ileal conduits or bladder reconstructions were reported during C-section [5, 19]. For this reason, if a woman has known complicated urologic history, some obstetricians recommend having a urologist nearby during the operation [2, 5].

Anesthetic

The choice of regional anesthetic for delivery in the setting of NTD is quite controversial in the literature. There is agreement that the high prevalence of tethered cord in MMC confers higher risk of spinal cord injury during spinal anesthesia. Patients with SBO can also have tethered cord and require assessment of the level at which the conus medullaris terminates. In the case of tethered cord, the conus medullaris may terminate at a lower lumbar level, complicating the use of normal anatomic landmarks for lumbar puncture/spinal anesthesia. Therefore, MRI of the spine is recommended to evaluate where the conus ends before performing spinal anesthesia. Patients with SBO and no tethered cord tend to tolerate spinal and epidural anesthesia well without increased risk of complication [9, 21].

In MMC, spinal anesthesia becomes more complicated owing to the tethered cord as well as the unique anatomy resulting from fetal and possible subsequent surgeries. Some authors recommend against spinal anesthesia in patients with MMC, while others report spinal anesthesia being used without complication in a few cases [9, 18]. Epidural anesthesia is possible and can be successful, but anatomic issues may make placement of the epidural catheter difficult resulting in patients experiencing patchy anesthesia. There may be extreme scarring of the epidural space due to previous spinal surgeries. Importantly, the epidural space in patients with MMC is obliterated at the level of the defect but can be significantly scarred in a broader area. Patients with MMC will lack spinous processes at the level of their lesion and will have undergone at least one surgery, if not more in the case of tethered cord. Tidmarsh et al. recommend placement of the epidural catheter above the level of their lesion where the anatomy is more normal [21]. Some patients, however, may have insufficient perineal anesthesia due to poor caudal spread of the anesthetic. In this case, either a second epidural catheter can be placed to obtain adequate perineal anesthesia or a pudendal nerve block can be attempted [9, 18, 21]. The choice of anesthetic is generally determined by the comfort level of the anesthesiologist and a discussion with the obstetrician and patient.

Postpartum Outcomes and Management

In the Auger study, women with MMC had a higher prevalence of maternal and fetal adverse outcomes (Fig. 35.1). Mothers with MMC were 9.5 times more likely to have a respiratory morbidity such as pulmonary embolism, amniotic fluid embolism, acute pulmonary edema, respiratory distress, etc. and they were 23 times more likely to be intubated. They had longer lengths of stay, ICU admission, and increased risk of maternal death or near miss events as compared to the general population [3]. This was echoed in the Shepard study: women with MMC were more

Fig. 35.1 Increased risk of adverse maternal and infant morbidity in women with MMC

- Increased risk of Respiratory Morbidity
  - Pulmonary embolism
  - Acute pulmonary edema
  - Respiratory distress
  - Need forintubation
- Longer length of hospital stay and ICU admission
- Increased risk of maternal death
- Increased risk of preterm delivery
- Increased risk of UTI
- Infants had a higher rate of preterm birth, low birth weight, intracranial hemorrhage, respiratory distres, birth hypoxia, and need for intubation.
- Increased risk of shunt failure up to 1 year postpartum

likely to have preterm delivery (<37 weeks), 6 times more likely to have UTIs and overall were more likely to have adverse neurologic (seizures, shunt malfunctions), pulmonary (pneumonia, respiratory distress), renal (kidney injury, UTI), and cardiac complications than the general population [8]. The exact reasoning for the increased risk of adverse events postpartum is unclear, but could be due to the multiple medical comorbidities often found in women with MMC such as obesity, hypertension, diabetes, and baseline urologic dysfunction.

In the Auger study, infants born to women with MMC had a higher rate of preterm birth (<37 weeks), low birth weight, intracranial hemorrhage, respiratory distress, birth hypoxia, need for intubation, and length of stay >14 days [3]. There was no significant increased risk of death, preterm birth (<32 weeks), or very low birth weight (<1500 g). There was a significantly increased risk of oral clefts and abdominal wall diaphragmatic defects, but no significant increased rate of NTD [3]. Preterm labor and low birth weight in babies of mothers with MMC have been demonstrated in the literature before this 2019 study [5, 18, 19]. Preterm birth and low birth weight are not just restricted to women with MMC; women with spinal cord injury due to trauma were also more likely to have preterm delivery and low birth weight as well as increased risk of UTIs and pyelonephritis [17]. Some authors postulate that most of the adverse neonatal outcomes are a result of preterm delivery. Recurrent UTI is also known to cause preterm labor, and in this population where recurrent UTI and kidney injury are already a problem, it likely

contributes [8, 14, 17, 19]. Additionally, midline schisis abnormalities such as cleft lip, omphalocele, and diaphragmatic hernias tend to cluster in individuals and families along with NTDs [3]. Interestingly, there does not appear to be an increased risk of NTDs in this population.

The data on postpartum care for women with MMC is extraordinarily sparse, especially outside of the immediate postpartum window. It appears that UTIs and hypertension persist during the postpartum period. Hypertension in some cases worsened in the postpartum period [9, 19]. Perhaps the most striking complication in the postpartum period is the risk of shunt malfunction and failure, which can linger up to 1 year after delivery [7, 22]. Shunt infection and resultant shunt malfunction may occur in a delayed fashion after C-section and must always be considered particularly for indolent organisms such a P. acnes which may present months after surgical manipulation. CSF obtained in sick patients to rule out infection should be cultured for at least 2 weeks to assess for low grade pathogens such as P. acnes. Breastfeeding may be difficult in women with kyphoscoliosis from a mechanical/positioning standpoint. Eliciting support from breastfeeding specialists can be helpful if the mother desires to breastfeed [9].

Conclusion

In conclusion, pregnancy is not contraindicated in women with MMC and SBO. Preconception counseling includes the increased risk of NTDs in their offspring, recommended initiating folic acid supplementation prior to pregnancy, shunt care, and urologic care as these women are at increased risk of shunt malfunction or failure, UTIs, and renal complications. Vaginal delivery is not contraindicated and is even preferred, as long as there are no obstetric issues, no evidence of elevated intracranial pressure, appropriate pelvic parameters, and no contractures. C-section can be complicated as these patients may have had multiple prior surgeries and unique anatomy. Use of regional anesthesia, spinal or epidural, depends on the comfort level of the anesthetist, but the patients' complicated anatomy after MMC repair or presence of tethered spinal cord increases risk of incomplete anesthesia and spinal cord injury, respectively. Women with MMC are at increased risk of adverse outcomes and are more likely to deliver preterm with a low weight infant. Infants of mothers with MMC are also more likely to have adverse outcomes, likely related to prematurity. A healthy pregnancy and delivery are possible in women with MMC and SBO with the careful observation of their multidisciplinary clinical team.

References

1. Deak KL, Siegel DG, George TM, Gregory S, Ashley-Koch A, Speer MC. Further evidence for a maternal genetic effect and a sex-influenced effect contributing to risk for human neural tube defects. Birth Defects Res A Clin Mol Teratol. 2008;82(10):662–9.
2. Shepard CL, Yan PL, Hollingsworth JM, Kraft KH. Pregnancy among mothers with spina bifida. J Pediatr Urol. 2018;14(1):11.e11–6.
3. Auger N, Arbour L, Schnitzer ME, Healy-Profitos J, Nadeau G, Fraser WD. Pregnancy outcomes of women with spina bifida. Disabil Rehabil. 2019;41(12):1403–9.
4. Powell B, Garvey M. Complications of maternal spina bifida. Ir J Med Sci. 1984;153(1):20–1.
5. Richmond D, Zaharievski I, Bond A. Management of pregnancy in mothers with spina bifida. Eur J Obstet Gynecol Reprod Biol. 1987;25(4):341–5.
6. Cavalheiro S, da Costa MDS, Moron AF, Leonard J. Comparison of prenatal and postnatal Management of Patients with myelomeningocele. Neurosurg Clin N Am. 2017;28(3):439–48.
7. Liakos AM, Bradley NK, Magram G, Muszynski C. Hydrocephalus and the reproductive health of women: the medical implications of maternal shunt dependency in 70 women and 138 pregnancies. Neurol Res. 2000;22(1):69–88.
8. Shepard CL, Yan PL, Kielb SJ, et al. Complications of delivery among mothers with spina bifida. Urology. 2019;123:280–6.
9. Sivarajah K, Relph S, Sabaratnam R, Bakalis S. Spina bifida in pregnancy: a review of the evidence for pre-conception, antenatal, intrapartum and postpartum care. Obstet Med. 2019;12(1):14–21.
10. Anon. Prevention of neural tube defects: results of the Medical Research Council vitamin study. MRC vitamin study research group. Lancet. 1991;338(8760):131–7.
11. Werhagen L, Gabrielsson H, Westgren N, Borg K. Medical complication in adults with spina bifida. Clin Neurol Neurosurg. 2013;115(8):1226–9.
12. Watkins ML, Rasmussen SA, Honein MA, Botto LD, Moore CA. Maternal obesity and risk for birth defects. Pediatrics. 2003;111(5 Pt 2):1152–8.
13. Dosa NP, Foley JT, Eckrich M, Woodall-Ruff D, Liptak GS. Obesity across the lifespan among persons with spina bifida. Disabil Rehabil. 2009;31(11):914–20.
14. Koves B, Cai T, Veeratterapillay R, et al. Benefits and harms of treatment of asymptomatic bacteriuria: a systematic review and meta-analysis by the European Association of Urology urological infection guidelines panel. Eur Urol. 2017;72(6):865–8.
15. Bhardwaj A, Nagandla K. Musculoskeletal symptoms and orthopaedic complications in pregnancy: pathophysiology, diagnostic approaches and modern management. Postgrad Med J. 2014;90(1066):450–60.
16. Imamura M, Hayashi C, Kim WJ, Yamazaki Y. Renal scarring on DMSA scan is associated with hypertension and decreased estimated glomerular filtration rate in spina bifida patients in the age of transition to adulthood. J Pediatr Urol. 2018;14(4):317.e311–5.
17. Crane DA, Doody DR, Schiff MA, Mueller BA. Pregnancy outcomes in women with spinal cord injuries: a population-based study. PM R. 2019;11(8):795–806.
18. Rietberg CC, Lindhout D. Adult patients with spina bifida cystica: genetic counselling, pregnancy and delivery. Eur J Obstet Gynecol Reprod Biol. 1993;52(1):63–70.
19. Arata M, Grover S, Dunne K, Bryan D. Pregnancy outcome and complications in women with spina bifida. J Reprod Med. 2000;45(9):743–8.
20. Robertson DN. Pregnancy and labour in the paraplegic. Paraplegia. 1972;10(3):209–12.
21. Tidmarsh MD, May AE. Epidural anaesthesia and neural tube defects. Int J Obstet Anesth. 1998;7(2):111–4.
22. Wisoff JH, Kratzert KJ, Handwerker SM, Young BK, Epstein F. Pregnancy in patients with cerebrospinal fluid shunts: report of a series and review of the literature. Neurosurgery. 1991;29(6):827–31.

Hydrocephalus and Pregnancy

36

Katherine G. Holste and Karin M. Muraszko

Introduction

As surgical and medical management have advanced over time, hydrocephalus patients have experienced improved length and quality of life. Importantly, women with hydrocephalus are more commonly surviving to childbearing age, and as such neurosurgeons, neurologists, obstetricians, and anesthesiologists are faced with the management of peripartum patients with shunts. Case reports of pregnancy and childbirth in patients with shunted hydrocephalus were first published in 1979 [1] with only 26 publications by the year 2000 in the neurosurgical, obstetric, and anesthesiology literature [2]. Since then, there have been a handful of additional studies [3–8]. Most reports on management of pregnant patients with hydrocephalus are case reports or case series, with a few notable exceptions which we will discuss later in this chapter [2, 9, 10]. The recommendations on management of these patients remain dependent on a limited sample of literature including case series, one prospective survey, a few larger retrospective chart reviews, and expert opinion. In this chapter, we will summarize the current evidence, including that derived from case reports, and highlight areas where more research is needed. The multiple modalities of cerebrospinal fluid (CSF) shunts, including ventriculoperitoneal (VP), ventriculoatrial (VA), and ventriculopleural (VPl), will be grouped together with unique considerations discussed as needed (Fig. 36.1).

K. G. Holste · K. M. Muraszko (✉)
Department of Neurosurgery, University of Michigan,
Ann Arbor, MI, USA
e-mail: karinm@med.umich.edu

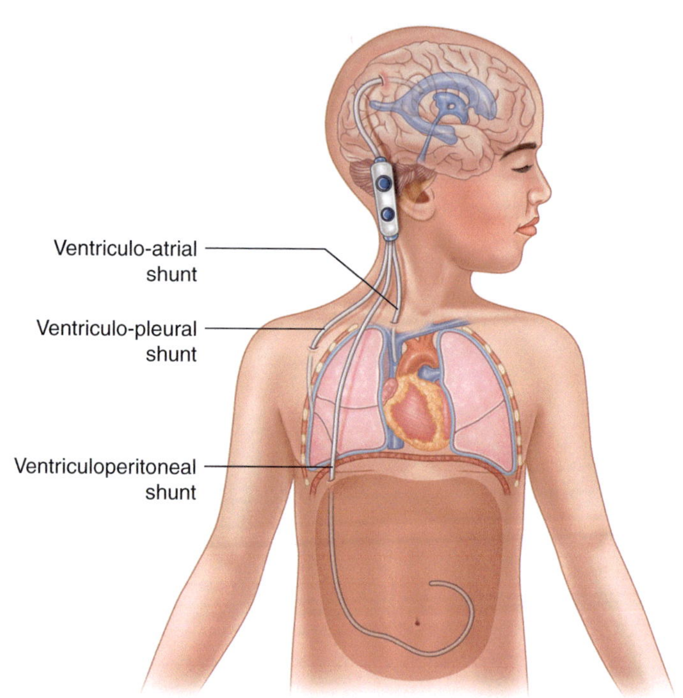

Fig. 36.1 A single diagram representing three of the most common shunt terminuses used. The proximal shunt catheter is connected to a valve which is connected to a single distal catheter which can terminate in the peritoneum, pleura or atrium of the heart. Less common shunt terminuses are not represented in this diagram

Preconception Management

One of the most important points of consensus regarding hydrocephalus and pregnancy is that shunted hydrocephalus is not a contraindication for pregnancy. However, patients with shunts are at increased risk of shunt malfunction during and after pregnancy and therefore require close monitoring from a multidisciplinary team including their obstetrician, neurosurgeon, neurologist, and other care providers. The prevalence of symptoms indicative of elevated intracranial pressures (ICPs) including headache, nausea, vomiting, altered sensorium, cranial neuropathies, or other new neurologic deficits has been reported to be as high as 59–76% of women with shunted hydrocephalus during pregnancy [2, 10]. Moreover, 25–50% of patients experience shunt failure requiring surgical revision [10]. To identify patients at risk of these complications, it is absolutely critical to obtain baseline imaging prior to conception, either in the form of head CT or, preferably, brain MRI. For patients who have had multiple shunt revisions in their lifetime, they may already have optimized baseline imaging

that demonstrates ventricular size while the patient is not being evaluated for shunt failure. Other patients without readily accessible baseline imaging including those without prior shunt revisions, those who have not followed up with a surgeon in many years, or those who are new to a healthcare system should undergo intracranial MRI. It is valuable to establish baseline ventricular size and CSF space appearance prior to pregnancy.

Generally speaking, other areas of preconception counseling should follow obstetrical guidelines. Of note, patients with shunted hydrocephalus may be on anti-epileptic drugs (AEDs) which can exhibit teratogenicity. These medications should be thoroughly reviewed and an appropriate regimen can be determined by the neurology team can. For AEDs with unfavorable fetal safety profiles, it may be necessary to discontinue or substitute the agent. In all patients, changing the dose should be considered to account for changes in metabolism and body volume changes during pregnancy. Any changes should be made under supervision of the treating neurologist or neurosurgeon [10]. Considerations for AED management during pregnancy are discussed in detail in Chap. 28. Patients with shunts must also be counseled on the elevated risk of miscarriage or abortion owing to the underlying hydrocephalus [2, 11].

Pregnancy Management

Symptoms During Pregnancy

As discussed above, more than half of patients with shunted hydrocephalus reported new or worsened symptoms of elevated ICPs during pregnancy. The quoted prevalence of 59% is derived from the combined publications of Liakos [2] and Bradley [12] et al., the former an update to the latter, which represents one of the largest studies on pregnancy in women with shunted hydrocephalus. These results reported by the same group were obtained by prospective survey of 70 women with shunted hydrocephalus, a combination of VP, VA, and VPl shunts, about their collective 138 pregnancies. The cause of hydrocephalus in these women was varied and consisted of a combination of congenital and acquired cases. This cohort included 54 patients with VP, 10 with VA, and 1 with VPl shunts; 5 patients had multiple shunt configurations. The cohort was followed throughout pregnancy and 6 months post-partum. Shunt malfunction and shunt failure were examined separately; shunt malfunction was defined as any symptoms of elevated ICP which required medical attention but did not require surgical intervention, while shunt failures were those cases that required surgical revision. Over the course of 138 pregnancies, there were 19 malfunctions and 7 revisions, of which 5 revisions occurred in 2 patients. Of the patients who did not require surgery during pregnancy, many of them experienced resolution of their symptoms after delivery.

Increased incidence of headaches and other symptoms of possibly elevated ICP clustered around the second and third trimester of pregnancy. In one of the other larger studies of pregnant women with shunted hydrocephalus, a retrospective examination of 18 patients and 21

pregnancies published by Wisoff et al. in 1991, it was demonstrated that 6% of patients had severe headaches without any other symptoms of elevated ICP or imaging evidence of ventriculomegaly during pregnancy [10]. Interestingly, four patients with acquired hydrocephalus in this series required index shunt placement following the development of symptoms of elevated ICPs during the second and third trimesters; their symptoms resolved after shunt placement. Similarly, Olatunbosun et al. reported on three cases of index shunting during pregnancy at 1, 12, and 24 weeks without neurosurgical or obstetric complication [13].

There are a few hypotheses as to why headaches and other symptoms of elevated ICP may increase during pregnancy. The first is that the gravid uterus causes increased abdominal pressure which then exerts pressure onto the distal shunt tubing in the case of VP shunts and causes a functional rather than mechanical obstruction. In the case of the other shunt configurations, the increased intra-abdominal pressure may cause venous congestion leading to elevated ICPs [2]. Conversely, Finfer et al. argued that there are other aspects of pregnancy that contribute to elevated ICPs including increased salt and water retention causing cerebral edema, venous distention, increased blood volume, and increased cardiac output during pregnancy [14]. Notably, these changes reach peaks during the second and third trimesters (see Chap. 7 for details). In the case of acquired hydrocephalus due to tumors, hormones circulating during pregnancy may contribute to tumor growth or even hemorrhage in certain types of mass lesions (see Chaps. 32 and 33) [15]. Further complicating matters, these symptoms are very similar to symptoms of pre-eclampsia and may go unrecognized [7].

Conservative measures reported in these analyses for the treatment of headaches and symptoms of elevated ICP without imaging evidence of shunt failure included elevating the head of the bed, bed rest, fluid restrictions, and at times diuretics [10]. Fluid restriction and diuretic use was under careful monitoring and direction of obstetricians to prevent fetal-placental hypoperfusion. In a few cases, shunt pumping was utilized during the third trimester by the patients' neurosurgeons; notably, this procedure was no longer needed after delivery [8, 16]. Because the shunt was thought to be functionally obstructed by reduced pressure differential incited by the gravid uterus rather than a true mechanical obstruction, temporizing measures were felt to be safe and prevented subjecting the patient to the risks of a shunt revision operation.

While shunt-related complications may occur, they are relatively uncommon and difficult to predict. In the Liakos and Bradley studies, there were 77 pregnancies without shunt malfunction or failure [2, 11, 13]. Moreover, in the Wisoff study, the clinical course of one pregnancy did not predict the clinical course of the subsequent pregnancies. In 3 patients who each had 2 pregnancies, one was asymptomatic in both pregnancies, one was symptomatic in both pregnancies not needing revision and one was asymptomatic in one pregnancy and in the subsequent pregnancy required revision [10]. One group recommended the use of ultrasound during routine checkups to examine the peritoneal catheter for kinking, deviation, or cyst formation. In their cohort of 3 patients with VP shunts, they also used the ultrasound to mark the course of the catheter on the skin at the end of pregnancy in case an emergent C-section was needed [4].

Other considerations during pregnancy include seizures, abdominal pain, and fetal testing. In patients with shunted hydrocephalus, 12% had an exacerbation of their seizure disorder during pregnancy, possibly due to alterations in medication metabolism [10]. Adjustment of dosing should be considered as discussed above and in Chap. 28. About 22% of patients with VP shunts reported sharp stabbing abdominal pain during the first trimester of pregnancy, which resolved in the second trimester and did not require any shunt revisions [2]. In regard to fetal testing, amniocentesis has been performed in a limited number of reported patients (18 in one study) with VP shunts without report of neurosurgical complications such as infection or damage to the shunt tubing [2].

Method of Revision

In cases requiring revision, the type of shunt to implant during pregnancy is controversial. Generally, there was no relationship in the literature between the type of shunt and number of revisions [2, 10]. Okagaki et al. suggested that if revision is required, then VP shunts should be converted to VA shunts to avoid the elevated intra-abdominal pressures in the second and third trimester; notably, this assertion was based on a single case report [17]. VA shunts come with their own set of risks and complications including a few cases of mitral valve prolapse and distal catheter migration in these cohorts [2, 10], as well as infection, pulmonary hypertension, endocarditis, renal damage, and even end-stage renal disease in the setting of VA shunt infection [18]. Furthermore, inserting a VA shunt does not circumvent the increased venous pressure of pregnancy, although one could argue that the movement of the right atrium functions as a siphon, making it less likely to have a distal obstruction, even during pregnancy [19]. Others have suggested that VPl may be a good alternative as it circumvents the potential complications of both VP and VA shunts. However, this assertion is based primarily in theory due to scarce reports of VPl shunts during pregnancy in the literature; therefore, generalization should be taken with caution [12]. When placing a VP shunt during pregnancy, Wisoff et al. argued that placement in the normal fashion was safe during the first trimester, but the tunneling trocar should not be used during the third trimester to avoid damage to the gravid uterus or induction of preterm labor and recommended placement of VA or VPl shunts in the third trimester [10].

ETV

Endoscopic third ventriculostomy (ETV) has been used for the treatment of obstructive hydrocephalus and works by creating a stoma between the third ventricle and subarachnoid spaces to bypass an area of CSF flow obstruction, usually at the cerebral aqueduct. Recently, there was a small cohort of pregnant patients with obstructive hydrocephalus who underwent successful ETVs. Riffaud et al. reported a cohort of 5 patients, two of which were not shunt dependent prior to pregnancy who were successfully treated. These two patients had acquired triventriculomegaly due to compressive midbrain and tectal lesions and became symptomatic during pregnancy due to lesion expansion and hemorrhage, respectively. It might be argued that the underlying cause of their hydrocephalus was affected by pregnancy rather than the shunt being affected by pregnancy. The other three patients had prior VP shunts for cerebral aqueductal stenosis and developed shunt failure with triventriculomegaly during pregnancy. All 5 patients underwent ETV, with VP shunt removal in the latter 3, and had symptom resolution without need for implantation/reimplantation at 1 year follow-up [15]. Though limited in sample size, these data showed that for patients with worsening acquired obstructive hydrocephalus or shunt failure during pregnancy, ETV is a good alternative to shunt revision that mitigates concerns of implanting foreign materials and obtaining intra-abdominal access. It is important to note that ETV is indicated for obstructive, not communicating, hydrocephalus and does still carry risk of infection, hemorrhage, and closure of the stoma resulting in continued hydrocephalus.

Hydrocephalus associated with increased venous pressures will not be improved without shunting, improvement in venous outflow, and/or correction of the etiology of idiopathic intracranial hypertension (IIH). Such causes of IIH include venous thrombosis, jugular foraminal stenosis, obesity, and a wide variety of medications. Addressing the cause of the IIH and resulting hydrocephalus are the ideal solution.

Delivery Management

Mode of Delivery

The presence of shunted hydrocephalus itself is not a contraindication for vaginal delivery. Many **asymptomatic** patients have undergone successful vaginal delivery of their infants and when obstetrically feasible vaginal delivery is preferred in this population [1, 3, 4, 9, 13, 16]. Cesarean (C)-section is felt to pose a greater threat to a VP shunt as the tubing could be exposed and infected or damaged during surgery and adhesions could form around the end of the catheter [2, 16]. A few authors recommend that the second stage of labor be shortened in all patients with shunted hydrocephalus to reduce the duration of intracranial hypertension that occurs with such a significant Valsalva maneuver [5, 11]. The second stage of labor can be shortened by the use of episiotomy and/or delivery augmentation with vacuum or forceps. Conversely, some argue that pushing is not contraindicated in asymptomatic shunt patients as the one-way valve prevents reverse flow and the ICP elevation is temporary [16]. In patients undergoing C-section, as with any intra-abdominal procedure, there is risk of delayed shunt infection with more indolent bacterial species such as P. acnes; infection should, therefore, be considered as a possible cause of shunt malfunction after C-section.

In the setting of shunted hydrocephalus, C-section is generally performed for obstetric reasons, such as fetal complications or failure of progression of labor [16]. Of 13 patients in one study for whom C-section was performed due to their shunt, 4 were performed for symptoms of elevated ICPs and 9 because the treating obstetricians thought it was protective of shunt function. Two other patients who were previously asymptomatic developed symptoms of elevated ICP during delivery but had relief of their symptoms after delivery and did not require shunt revision [2].

Anesthesia

The use of various modes of anesthesia during delivery in patients with shunted hydrocephalus has been hotly contested. The majority feel that spinal and epidural anesthesia are not contraindicated in these patients [11, 16]. In the Liakos study, epidural anesthesia was used in about 39% of vaginal deliveries and 43% of C-sections, while spinal anesthesia was used only in 1 patient undergoing vaginal delivery and in 6 undergoing C-section (13.6%) [2]. Prophylactic antibiotics before epidural or spinal anesthesia to mitigate risk of CSF infection has been discussed, although the literature remains inconclusive [20].

A theoretical risk of draining CSF during spinal anesthesia in patients with hydrocephalus is that it may change in the differential pressure between the intracranial and spinal CSF compartments [20]. When using a small gauge needle, most commonly 27G, for spinal anesthesia, only about 11 mL of CSF escapes over 5 h from the small hole in the dura. Considering that 20 mL of CSF is produced per hour, this is a negligible amount and should not be significant enough to meaningfully alter the shunt mechanics [20]. One important consideration is that post-procedural headaches after spinal anesthesia could be confused with shunt malfunction and lead to misdiagnosis; however, this can be avoided with a detailed clinical exam and history. Most notably, post-procedural spinal headaches should improve with lying flat and worsen when the head is raised, whereas those related to high ICP should worsen in the supine position and improve when the head is raised owing to the effect of gravity on CSF drainage. While conservative management of post-procedural spinal headaches involves lying flat for 24 h, patients with already elevated ICPs related to hydrocephalus/shunt malfunction may experience worsened headaches in the supine position and, according to one report, this can lead to need for shunt revision [2, 4]. A few groups recommend early treatment of post-procedural headaches with epidural blood patch so these patients do not need to lay flat for an extended period of time [2, 20]. Aside from altered CSF dynamics and ICP, there has been report that patients with lumboperitoneal shunts may exhibit shorter duration of regional anesthetic, thought to be due to migration of the drug from the CSF to peritoneal space [21].

General anesthesia can be used for asymptomatic or symptomatic patients with elevated ICPs to help with ICP control [7]. General anesthesia is preferred for patients with high ICP or those who are exhibiting neurological deterioration [2,

7]. In one report, anesthesia providers opted to use general anesthesia for asymptomatic patients to mitigate the risk of elevating their ICP. This was done successfully without neurosurgical or obstetric complication in 17 C-sections [2]. Due to the ambiguity in selection of anesthesia for these patients in the literature, the decision for any individual patient should be based on their clinical appearance, symptomatology, risk of intracranial hypertension, and the comfort and experience of the treating obstetrician and anesthesiologist.

Antibiotics

The use of antibiotics during delivery is controversial for patients undergoing vaginal delivery. Some feel that antibiotics should be used in all cases, similar to use in endocarditis, to avoid infection of the shunt due to the risk of bacteremia with delivery [13]. In this case, the antibiotic of choice should cover for reproductive tract pathogens including group B streptococcus, enterococcus, and gram negative organisms. Typical treatment includes a penicillin like ampicillin, or vancomycin for penicillin allergic, as well as an aminoglycoside [1]. Patients with VA shunts would be particularly vulnerable to seeding of their shunt in the case of bacteremia. Therefore, some experts contend that antibiotics should only be given to patients with VA shunts as the risk of seeding a VP shunt with bacteremia is much lower during vaginal delivery [16]. In the literature, there has been just one patient whose VP shunt was contaminated by group B streptococcus after vaginal delivery resulting in delayed meningitis 6 months post-partum [22]. In another retrospective review of 8 patients with 25 pregnancies, none of the 11 vaginal deliveries received prophylactic antibiotics and there were no cases of shunt infection [4, 11].

Patients undergoing C-section may receive prophylactic antibiotics per the institutions normal surgical guidelines [11]. There was a recent case report of Corynebacterium infection of a shunt after C-section [5]. In this case, the patient with a previously placed VP shunt developed fever, confusion, vomiting, and abdominal pain 10 days after C-section. Ventriculomegaly was discovered on head CT which prompted VP shunt removal and EVD placement. Although her CSF cultures were negative for any organisms, culturing the distal tip produced gram-positive bacilli identified as *Corynebacterium xerosis*. In a separate report, a patient developed late onset meningitis from group B streptococcus infection of her VP shunt following C-section. This infection was hypothesized to have resulted from contamination of the shunt's distal tip during surgery [6]. Accordingly, these authors recommended prophylactic antibiotics in patients with VP shunts and known group B streptococcus colonization undergoing C-section.

Post-Partum Management

Concern for shunt malfunction and failure should not be limited to the pregnancy period. There have been a number of cases of post-partum shunt malfunction and failure requiring shunt revision up to 6 months and 1 year from delivery. Wisoff et al. reported 4 of 17 shunts requiring revision within 1 year post-partum [10]. Liakos reported 13 patients who developed shunt malfunction with transient symptoms and 23 shunt failures within 7 months post-partum; 15 of which clustered in 5 patients [2]. The reasoning for this is not clear but could be due to continued salt and water retention, cerebral edema, or disordered cerebral autoregulation that can persist after pregnancy [23]. Regardless of the mechanism, clinicians should have an elevated index of suspicion for shunt malfunction or failure in patients who are recently post-partum presenting with symptoms of possibly elevated ICP.

Conclusion

In conclusion, pregnancy is not contraindicated in women with shunted hydrocephalus. The use of multidisciplinary teams with obstetricians, neurosurgeons, neurologists, anesthesiologists, and other care providers is beneficial for patient outcome in pregnant women with shunted hydro-

cephalus [4]. More than half of these patients will experience headaches and symptoms of elevated ICPs and about 25–50% required shunt revision during pregnancy. To assess the need for revision, it is crucial to have baseline imaging for comparison. It remains unclear as to why there is an increased risk of shunt malfunction and failure during pregnancy and which type of shunt to use when revision is necessary during pregnancy. Vaginal delivery is preferred in asymptomatic patients, especially those with VP shunt to avoid damage, infection, or adhesions around the distal catheter secondary to C-section. The use of antibiotics and type of anesthesia are also controversial and depend on patient factors as well as the comfort of the treating physicians. These patients continue to be at increased risk of shunt failure in the post-partum period, up to 1 year from delivery, so close monitoring and increased index of suspicion are necessary when caring for a post-partum mother with a shunt.

References

1. Gast MJ, Grubb RL Jr, Strickler RC. Maternal hydrocephalus and pregnancy. Obstet Gynecol. 1983;62(3 Suppl):29s–31s.
2. Liakos AM, Bradley NK, Magram G, Muszynski C. Hydrocephalus and the reproductive health of women: the medical implications of maternal shunt dependency in 70 women and 138 pregnancies. Neurol Res. 2000;22(1):69–88.
3. Cohen-Gadol AA, Friedman JA, Friedman JD, Tubbs RS, Munis JR, Meyer FB. Neurosurgical management of intracranial lesions in the pregnant patient: a 36-year institutional experience and review of the literature. J Neurosurg. 2009;111(6):1150–7.
4. Häussler B, Laimer E, Hager J, Putz G, Marth C, Haeussler R. Pregnancy, delivery and postpartum care of women with ventriculo-peritoneal shunted hydrocephalus: a case series. Int J Gynecol Obstet. 2010;12:12.
5. Hocaoglu M, Turgut A, Eminoglu EM, Yilmaz Karadag F, Karateke A. Maternal ventriculoperitoneal shunt infection due to Corynebacterium xerosis following caesarean section. J Obstet Gynaecol. 2019;39(3):400–2.
6. Kane JM, Jackson K, Conway JH. Maternal postpartum group B beta-hemolytic streptococcus ventriculoperitoneal shunt infection. Arch Gynecol Obstet. 2004;269(2):139–41.
7. Schiza S, Stamatakis E, Panagopoulou A, Valsamidis D. Management of pregnancy and delivery of a patient

with malfunctioning ventriculoperitoneal shunt. J Obstet Gynaecol. 2012;32(1):6–9.

8. Sasagawa Y, Sasaki T, Fuji T, Akai T, Iizuka H. Ventriculoperitoneal shunt malfunction due to pregnancy. No Shinkei Geka. 2006;34(2):181–7.

9. Brkic M, Dermit K, Galic T, Orlovic M, Krznaric Lovosevic AM, Plesa I, Blagaic V. Managing pregnancy in women with ventriculoperitoneal shunt: a review of the literature. Biomed Surg. 2017;1(3):141–3.

10. Wisoff JH, Kratzert KJ, Handwerker SM, Young BK, Epstein F. Pregnancy in patients with cerebrospinal fluid shunts: report of a series and review of the literature. Neurosurgery. 1991;29(6):827–31.

11. Landwehr JB Jr, Isada NB, Pryde PG, Johnson MP, Evans MI, Canady AI. Maternal neurosurgical shunts and pregnancy outcome. Obstet Gynecol. 1994;83(1):134–7.

12. Bradley NK, Liakos AM, McAllister JP 2nd, Magram G, Kinsman S, Bradley MK. Maternal shunt dependency: implications for obstetric care, neurosurgical management, and pregnancy outcomes and a review of selected literature. Neurosurgery. 1998;43(3):448–60; discussion 460–441.

13. Olatunbosun OA, Akande EO, Adeoye CO. Ventriculoperitoneal shunt and pregnancy. Int J Gynaecol Obstet. 1992;37(4):271–4.

14. Finfer SR. Management of labour and delivery in patients with intracranial neoplasms. Br J Anaesth. 1991;67(6):784–7.

15. Riffaud L, Ferre JC, Carsin-Nicol B, Morandi X. Endoscopic third ventriculostomy for the treatment of obstructive hydrocephalus during pregnancy. Obstet Gynecol. 2006;108(3 Pt 2):801–4.

16. Cusimano MD, Meffe FM, Gentili F, Sermer M. Management of pregnant women with cerebrospinal fluid shunts. Pediatr Neurosurg. 1991;17(1):10–3.

17. Okagaki A, Kanzaki H, Moritake K, Mori T. Case report: pregnant woman with a ventriculoperitoneal shunt to treat hydrocephalus. Asia Oceania J Obstet Gynaecol. 1990;16(2):111–3.

18. Hung AL, Vivas-Buitrago T, Adam A, et al. Ventriculoatrial versus ventriculoperitoneal shunt complications in idiopathic normal pressure hydrocephalus. Clin Neurol Neurosurg. 2017;157:1–6.

19. Rymarczuk GN, Keating RF, Coughlin DJ, et al. A comparison of Ventriculoperitoneal and Ventriculoatrial shunts in a population of 544 consecutive pediatric patients. Neurosurgery. 2019;87:80.

20. Littleford JA, Brockhurst NJ, Bernstein EP, Georgoussis SE. Obstetrical anesthesia for a parturient with a ventriculoperitoneal shunt and third ventriculostomy. Can J Anaesth. 1999;46(11):1057–63.

21. Kaul B, Vallejo MC, Ramanathan S, Mandell GL, Krohner RG. Accidental spinal analgesia in the presence of a lumboperitoneal shunt in an obese parturient receiving enoxaparin therapy. Anesth Analg. 2002;95(2):441–3; table of contents.

22. Fox BC. Delayed-onset postpartum meningitis due to group B streptococcus. Clin Infect Dis. 1994;19(2):350.

23. Janzarik WG, Jacob J, Katagis E, et al. Preeclampsia postpartum: impairment of cerebral autoregulation and reversible cerebral hyperperfusion. Pregnancy Hypertens. 2019;17:121–6.

Management of Pseudotumor Cerebri in Pregnancy

Stephen A. Johnson

Introduction

Pseudotumor cerebri, also known as idiopathic intracranial hypertension (IIH) is a disease characterized by increased intracranial pressure (ICP) with unknown etiology. Symptoms often mimic a mass lesion, or tumor, which led to the term *pseudotumor*. IIH has a female to male predominance of 8:1 [1]. Obese women carry a 20x greater risk of the disease than the general population [1, 2]. IIH occurs primarily in women of childbearing age and is subsequently of particular importance from an obstetric perspective. Weight gain and exogenous estrogen in pregnancy are thought to worsen IIH symptoms [1, 2], with one study noting worsening symptoms in 9 of 11 IIH pregnancies [3]. However, IIH occurs in pregnancy at the same rate as the general population; the perceived association of pregnancy with IIH is a reflection that IIH affects women of childbearing age [4].

Presentation

Headache is the most common presenting symptom in IIH. Headaches are usually diffuse or retro-orbital. Pulsatile tinnitus and emesis are also common. Subjective and transient blurry vision, objective visual field defects, papilledema, decreased visual acuity, and even blindness may occur with advanced disease. Diplopia may occur secondary to abducens nerve palsy. Aside from vision and diplopia, there should be no other neurological deficits.

Radiology

Magnetic resonance imaging (MRI) and computed tomography (CT) of the brain are negative for mass lesion, sinus thrombosis, or ischemia. Ventricular size is normal.

Diagnosis

IIH is a diagnosis of exclusion, delineated by the modified Dandy criteria:

1. Signs and symptoms of increased ICP.
2. No other focal neurological deficits with the exception of vision loss or abducens nerve palsy.
3. Cerebral spinal fluid (CSF) opening pressure > 25 cm H_2O with normal composition.
4. No evidence of hydrocephalus, mass lesion, or sinus thrombosis on imaging.
5. No other identifiable cause of increased ICP.

S. A. Johnson (✉)
Department of Neurosurgery, Rutgers Robert Wood Johnson Medical School, New Brunswick, NJ, USA
e-mail: stephen.a.johnson@rutgers.edu

© The Author(s), under exclusive license to Springer Nature Switzerland AG 2023
G. Gupta et al. (eds.), *Neurological Disorders in Pregnancy*,
https://doi.org/10.1007/978-3-031-36490-7_37

Papilledema, while not a part of the Dandy criteria, is also present in the vast majority of IIH patients [4].

Evaluation and Surveillance

Pregnant women with known IIH should be counseled to report any subjective visual changes and should be formally monitored for papilledema, changes in visual acuity and visual fields in each trimester. Since the majority of IIH patients already have documented papilledema, it is important to note changes from baseline. Weight gain during pregnancy should be limited to what is healthy and expected for pregnancy in coordination with an obstetrician, as it has been suggested that excessive weight gain may lead to poor symptomatic control during pregnancy [1, 5]. Patients taking any medications for IIH that are higher risk than category A, such as acetazolamide, should consider a trial off the medication while planning for pregnancy. This will help both patient and physician to anticipate the evolution and subsequent management of their symptoms in advance.

Imaging strategies are the principal difference in the evaluation of pregnant versus non-pregnant IIH patients. In pregnant patients, MRI/MRV should be obtained to rule out mass lesion, venous sinus thrombosis, and hydrocephalus. Contrast dye and CT head should be avoided in the pregnant patient.

Pregnant patients with existing shunts and suspected shunt failure may be tapped and interrogated safely. Increased opening pressure suggests distal shunt malfunction, while failure of spontaneous CSF flow is concerning for ventricular catheter obstruction. Shunt series X-rays and shuntogram with radiotracer should be avoided.

Management

The primary treatment goal is vision preservation and palliation of symptoms, chiefly headache. Expectant management is appropriate in patients with controlled symptoms and stable vision. However, several options are available for patients with intractable headaches and/or visual changes.

Acetazolamide

Acetazolamide, trade name Diamox, is the mainstay of medical management for IIH. Acetazolamide is a carbonic anhydrase inhibitor; it is a clinical diuretic that reduces blood volume, decreases CSF production, and subsequently reduces edema and ICP. It is an FDA category C agent; teratogenicity (limb defects) has been noted in animal studies with 10x normal human doses [6]. There is no clinical evidence to substantiate this in humans. However, acetazolamide is avoided when possible, especially in the first trimester. Occasionally, the benefit of acetazolamide may outweigh the risks of withholding it, especially in the case of severe, intractable headaches and vision loss after the first trimester. Of note, one report of 12 women with refractory IIH symptoms treated with acetazolamide showed no adverse outcomes or congenital malformations [2]. A second, larger study followed 50 women who required acetazolamide for IIH before 13 weeks gestation; they reported similar spontaneous abortion risk to the control group with no major obstetric complications [6]. The authors concluded that while liberal use of acetazolamide should be avoided in pregnancy, the medication should remain a treatment option when clinically indicated.

Corticosteroids

Corticosteroids are not routine treatment for IIH in pregnant or non-pregnant patients. They are typically reserved for emergent treatment as a temporizing measure with acute, progressive vision loss. They are FDA category B due to reports of low birth weight and cleft palate [4]. However, they may be considered in the urgent setting of progressive vision loss.

Lumbar Puncture

Lumbar puncture without fluoroscopic guidance is a safe procedure in the pregnant patient. It may be both diagnostic (opening pressure) and therapeutic (CSF drainage). This is the preferred method to temporize symptoms in the first trimester in lieu of category C medications.

Surgery

Surgery is indicated in the setting of progressive vision loss despite medical management and temporizing lumbar punctures. The two primary options are shunting procedures or optic nerve sheath fenestrations. Both have demonstrated safety and efficacy in pregnant patients; normal delivery can be expected post-operatively [7]. Neurosurgical coordination with a dedicated abdominal surgeon for distal catheter placement of ventriculoperitoneal shunts in pregnant patients is recommended. Shunting procedures may address both vision loss and refractory headaches, whereas optic nerve sheath fenestration will only preserve vision.

Transverse sinus stenting to reduce ICP via increasing venous outflow is an emerging and controversial new treatment for IIH. This should be avoided in pregnant patients due to the radiation exposure with fluoroscopy.

Labor Planning

IIH is not a contraindication to vaginal delivery [1, 2, 4]. The uterine contractions, prolonged Valsalva maneuvers, and fluid shifts of vaginal delivery have not been shown to complicate obstetric or visual outcomes in IIH patients [2]. However, peripartum anesthetic management remains controversial. A literature review by Karmaniolou et al. noted the safety and efficacy of both spinal and epidural anesthesia in peripartum IIH patients with no reports of uncal herniation [8]. Others prefer epidural anesthesia to minimize any potential effect on CSF dynamics and pressure [2]. For cesarean deliveries, regional anesthesia (spinal or epidural) has been encouraged over general anesthesia, which can be associated with transient spikes in intracranial pressure [2].

Summary

The general consensus is that IIH does not constitute a high-risk pregnancy and is not a contraindication to vaginal delivery [1, 4, 5]. There is no increase in birth defects or complications when compared to the general population [2, 4, 9, 10]. Additionally, there is no increase in visual defects in pregnant versus non-pregnant IIH patients [2, 4, 9, 11]; reports of severe vision loss in pregnant IIH patients are exceedingly rare [12]. Katz et al. did note an increase in headache symptoms in 9 of 11 IIH pregnancies; however, there were no obstetric complications [3]. Patients with newly diagnosed IIH during pregnancy will often experience symptomatic relief after delivery [2]. In summary, IIHC can be safely managed in pregnancy with excellent outcomes provided there is vigilant observation, communication, and management between patient and physician.

References

1. Evans R, Lee AG. Idiopathic intracranial hypertension in pregnancy. Headache. 2010;50:1513–5.
2. Bagga R, Jain V, Gupta KR, et al. Choice of therapy and mode of delivery in idiopathic intracranial hypertension during pregnancy. MedGenMed. 2005;4:42.
3. Katz VL, Peterson R, Cefalo RC. Pseudotumor cerebri and pregnancy. Am J Perinatol. 1989;6:442–5.
4. Kesler A, Kupferminc M. Idiopathic intracranial hypertension and pregnancy. Clin Obstr Gyn. 2013;56:389–96.
5. Evans R, Friedman D. The management of pseudotumor cerebri during pregnancy. Headache. 2000;40:495–7.
6. Falardeau J, Lobb BM, Golden S, et al. The use of acetazolamide during pregnancy in intracranial hypertension patients. J Neuroophthalmol. 2013;33:9–12.
7. Shapiro S, Yee R, Brown H. Surgical management of pseudotumor cerebri in pregnancy: case report. Neurosurgery. 1995;37:829–31.
8. Karmaniolou I, Petropoulos G, Theodoraki K. Management of idiopathic intracranial hyperten-

sion in parturients: anesthetic considerations. Can J Anaesth. 2011;58:7.

9. Tang R. Management of idiopathic intracranial hypertension in pregnancy. MedGenMed. 2005;7:40.

10. Bashiri A, Mazor M, Maymon E, et al. Pseudotumor Cerebri during pregnancy. Harefuah. 1996;131:397–402.

11. Peterson CM, Kelly JV. Pseudotumor cerebri in pregnancy: case reports and review of literature. Obstet Gynecol Surv. 1985;40:323–9.

12. Zamecki KJ, Frohman LP, Turbin RE. Severe visual loss associated with idiopathic intracranial hypertension in pregnancy. Clin Ophthalmol. 2007;1:99–103.

Index